Anesthesia for Aortic Surgery

Anesthesia for Aortic Surgery

Joseph I. Simpson, M.D.

Associate Professor of Anesthesiology, Albert Einstein College of Medicine, Bronx, New York; Director of Quality Management, Education, and Research, Department of Anesthesiology, Long Island Jewish Medical Center, New Hyde Park, New York

Butterworth–Heinemann

Boston   Oxford   Johannesburg   Melbourne   New Delhi   Singapore

Library of Congress Cataloging-in-Publication Data

Anesthesia for aortic surgery / [edited by] Joseph I. Simpson.
        p.   cm.
      Includes bibliographical references and index.
      ISBN 0-7506-9578-1
      1. Aorta--Surgery.   2. Anesthesia in cardiology.   I. Simpson,
Joseph I.
      [DNLM: 1. Aorta--surgery. 2. Aortic Diseases--surgery.
3. Anesthesia.   WG 410 A579 1997]
      RD598.6.A53   1997
      617.9'67413--dc21
      DNLM/DLC
      for Library of Congress   96-50468
                                                                                                        CIP

British Library Cataloguing-in-Publication Data
A catalogue record for this book is available from the British Library.

The publisher offers special discounts on bulk orders of this book.
For information, please contact:

Manager of Special Sales
Butterworth–Heinemann
313 Washington Street
Newton, MA 02158–1626
Tel: 617-928-2500
Fax: 617-928-2620

For information on all medical publications available, contact our World Wide Web home page at:
http://www.bh.com/med

10 9 8 7 6 5 4 3 2 1

Printed in the United States of America

To my wife Judy and my children Shoshana, Tova, Tzvi, and Ariella
for their constant love and encouragement

Contents

Contributing Authors

Mark Badach, M.D.
Assistant Professor of Anesthesiology, Seton Hall University, South Orange, New Jersey; Attending Physician, Department of Anesthesia, St. Joseph's Hospital and Medical Center, Paterson, New Jersey

Pierre A. Casthely, M.D.
Professor of Anesthesiology, Seton Hall University, South Orange, New Jersey; Attending Physician, Department of Cardiac Anesthesia, St. Joseph's Hospital and Medical Center, Paterson, New Jersey

Meir Chernofsky, M.D.
Attending Anesthesiologist, Elias Sourasky-Tel Aviv Medical Center, Sackler Faculty of Medicine, Tel Aviv University, Israel

John Francis Clagnaz, M.D.
Attending Anesthesiologist, Division of Cardiothoracic Anesthesia, Department of Anesthesia, Long Island Jewish Medical Center, New Hyde Park, New York

Jacob Cynamon, M.D.
Associate Professor of Radiology, Albert Einstein College of Medicine; Associate Chief of Vascular and Interventional Radiology, Department of Radiology, Montefiore Medical Center, Bronx, New York

Thomas R. Eide, M.D.
Director of Resident Education, Department of Anesthesiology, Long Island Jewish Medical Center, New Hyde Park, New York

Nabil Ghabrial, M.D.
Resident in Anesthesiology, Department of Anesthesiology, Maimonides Medical Center, Brooklyn, New York

L. Michael Graver, M.D.
Assistant Professor of Surgery, Albert Einstein College of Medicine, Bronx, New York; Chief, Division of Cardiothoracic Surgery, Department of Surgery, Long Island Jewish Medical Center, New Hyde Park, New York

Michael Hanania, M.D.
Assistant Professor of Anesthesiology, Albert Einstein College of Medicine, Bronx, New York; Director of Pain Management, Department of Anesthesiology, Long Island Jewish Medical Center, New Hyde Park, New York

Ronald S. Levy, M.D.
Resident in Anesthesiology, Department of Anesthesiology, Long Island Jewish Medical Center, New Hyde Park, New York

Sarojini Rao, M.D.
Associate Attending Anesthesiologist, Department of Anesthesiology, Maimonides Medical Center, Brooklyn, New York

Gerald A. Schiff, M.D.
Assistant Professor of Anesthesiology, Albert Einstein College of Medicine, Bronx, New York; Attending Anesthesiologist, Department of Anesthesiology, Long Island Jewish Medical Center, New Hyde Park, New York

Steven B. Schulman, M.D.
Attending Anesthesiologist, St. Francis Medical Center, Roslyn, New York

Ketan Shevde, M.D.
Chairman, Department of Anesthesiology, Maimonides Medical Center, Brooklyn, New York

Michael B. Simon, M.D.
Resident in Anesthesiology, Department of Anesthesiology, Columbia-Presbyterian Medical Center, New York, New York

Joseph I. Simpson, M.D.
Associate Professor of Anesthesiology, Albert Einstein College of Medicine, Bronx, New York; Director of Quality Management, Education, and Research, Department of Anesthesiology, Long Island Jewish Medical Center, New Hyde Park, New York

Ruth S. Spector, M.D.
Clinical Instructor of Anesthesiology, Albert Einstein College of Medicine, Bronx, New York; Attending Physician, Department of Anesthesiology, Long Island Jewish Medical Center, New Hyde Park, New York

Samuel I. Wahl, M.D.
Instructor of Radiology, Albert Einstein College of Medicine; Assistant Attending Physician, Division of Vascular and Interventional Radiology, Department of Radiology, Montefiore Medical Center, Bronx, New York

David S. Weiss, Ph.D., C.N.I.M.
Department of Rehabilitation Medicine, Long Island Jewish Medical Center, New Hyde Park, New York; Department of Surgery, Northshore University Hospital, Manhasset, New York

Kevin Whitrock, M.D.
Attending Anesthesiologist, Department of Anesthesiology, Long Island Jewish Medical Center, New Hyde Park, New York

Jonathan Zelen, M.D.
Assistant Professor of Cardiothoracic Surgery and Attending Surgeon, Department of Cardiothoracic Surgery, State University of New York at Stony Brook

Preface

As the practice of medicine in general and the practice of anesthesiology in particular become more technologically advanced and complex, we find ourselves taking care of older and sicker patients—taking on challenges we never before dreamed possible. The use of transesophageal echocardiography, retrograde cerebral perfusion, and selective spinal cord cooling are but a few examples of how these changes have affected the practice of anesthesia for aortic surgery.

Traditionally, anesthesia for surgery on the aorta has been covered in part in various types of textbooks. Anesthesia for surgery on the ascending aorta and, to a lesser degree, anesthesia for surgery on the aortic arch are usually covered in textbooks on cardiac anesthesia. Anesthesia for surgery on the descending thoracic aorta is usually covered in textbooks on thoracic anesthesia and, in the case of coarctation surgery, in textbooks of pediatric anesthesia or pediatric cardiac anesthesia. Anesthesia for surgery on the abdominal and peripheral aorta is usually covered in textbooks on vascular anesthesia. There are, however, many similar underlying themes that apply equally to the anesthetic management of all these procedures.

Over the past few years the practice of anesthesia in many institutions has become highly subspecialized. In addition to the well-recognized areas of cardiac anesthesia, pediatric anesthesia, obstetric anesthesia, thoracic anesthesia, pain management, and anesthesia in intensive care, vascular anesthesia has emerged as yet another area of specialization at some of the larger academic institutions. However, anesthesia for aortic surgery does not fit neatly into any of these categories and crosses into the domains of all of them (with the possible exception of obstetric anesthesia). In this book, I have attempted to include all the relevant information for the practice of anesthesia for all types of aortic surgery—thoracic, abdominal, and pediatric. In addition, I have attempted to take the reader through the anesthetic management of the entire perioperative period, including the preoperative evaluation, the intraoperative management, and the postoperative intensive care unit and pain management of these patients. This book is not meant to function as an introductory anesthesia textbook, and a basic level of general anesthesia knowledge is assumed.

Conceptually, this book is divided into three parts. The first five chapters are introductory and cover the general areas that apply to all types of aortic surgery. The topics of these chapters include anatomy, preoperative risk assessment, radiologic evaluation, monitoring (including a large section on monitoring of the brain and spinal cord), and, finally, bleeding and coagulation. In addition to providing the background knowledge necessary for the anesthetic management of aortic surgery patients, this section introduces the reader to the various ways these patients present for treatment and their proper preoperative evaluation.

The second part of the book (Chapters 6–10) discusses the anesthetic management of the specific aortic surgical procedures. These chapters are divided by anatomic location. Topics include the ascending aorta, the aortic arch, the descending thoracic aorta, and the abdominal aorta. In addition, one chapter is devoted to the anesthetic management of the pediatric patient presenting for aortic coarctation surgery. These topics are covered in separate chapters because each presents unique challenges and anesthetic considerations.

The last three chapters of the book are devoted to the postoperative care of the aortic surgery patient. Chapters 11 and 12 discuss the postanesthesia recovery and intensive care management of these patients. Chapter 13 discusses the issues involved in postoperative pain management of the aortic surgery patient.

This book is not meant to function as a manual. Rather, I have tried to focus on the pathophysiology of specific disease processes and its interaction with anesthetic and surgical techniques. Nevertheless, where appropriate, specific recommendations are made. Although this book is multi-authored, I have tried to maintain consistency in style and to eliminate as much overlap as possible.

I would like to thank all of the authors who have contributed to this book. I also thank Susan F. Pioli for her continued faith in me and her never-ending patience and Marianne Graff for all her help. Finally, I would like to thank my wife Judy and my children Shoshana, Tova, Tzvi, and Ariella for their continued support, understanding, and patience.

J.I.S.

Chapter 1

Anatomy and Pathology of the Aorta

L. Michael Graver and Jonathan Zelen

I profess both to learn and to teach anatomy, not from books but from dissections; not from positions of philosophers but from the fabric of nature.

William Harvey, 1628[1]

The great English physician and father of modern medicine, William Harvey, knew that understanding of the treatment of disease must begin with a first-hand understanding of anatomy and pathology. The cardiovascular anesthesiologist and surgeon are uniquely situated to observe anatomy and pathology of the aorta in the living human being. Successful management of pathologic conditions affecting the aorta is the result of careful observation and understanding gained in the operating room. This didactic review of anatomy and pathology of the aorta should serve as a framework on which to base continuing observation in patients. Ultimately, first-hand experience is the best instructor.

The Aorta and Its Branches

The aorta is the central conduit for the arterial vascular system. It arises from the left ventricle just above the aortic valve and ascends anteriorly, superiorly, and to the right before arching backward and to the left, superior to the pulmonary hilum. It descends posteriorly from the level of the fourth thoracic vertebral border, coursing caudad through the diaphragm (aortic hiatus) at the level of the twelfth thoracic vertebra and into the abdomen. Continuing its descent along the vertebral column, the aorta bi-

furcates at the level of the fourth lumbar vertebra giving rise to the left and right common iliac arteries.

The aorta is divided into four anatomically continuous segments termed ascending, transverse, descending, and abdominal. (1) The ascending aorta is that portion from the aortic annulus to the innominate artery. The ascending aorta can be conceptually subdivided into three segments: annular, sinus, and suprasinus. (2) The transverse aorta begins at the innominate artery and continues to the ligamentum arteriosum opposite and just distal to the left subclavian artery. (3) The descending aorta begins at the left subclavian artery and becomes the abdominal aorta at the diaphragm. (4) The abdominal aorta is that portion from the diaphragm to the bifurcation of the iliac vessels (Figure 1-1).

The right and left coronary arteries, which arise within the aortic sinuses, are the two main branches of the ascending aorta. They most commonly arise from separate ostia midway between the aortic valve commissures. The aortic sinuses are commonly named right, left, and noncoronary sinuses (Figure 1-2). A single coronary ostium giving rise to both coronary arteries as well as dual coronary ostia arising from the same sinus are possible (Figure 1-3).[2]

The right coronary artery emerges anteriorly from the right coronary sinus between the aorta and pulmonary artery. Coursing rightward and inferiorly it enters the right atrioventricular sulcus giving off three small branches (conal, marginal, and atrioventricular nodal). As it continues along a straight path to the acute margin of the right heart it bifurcates to form the posterior lateral and poste-

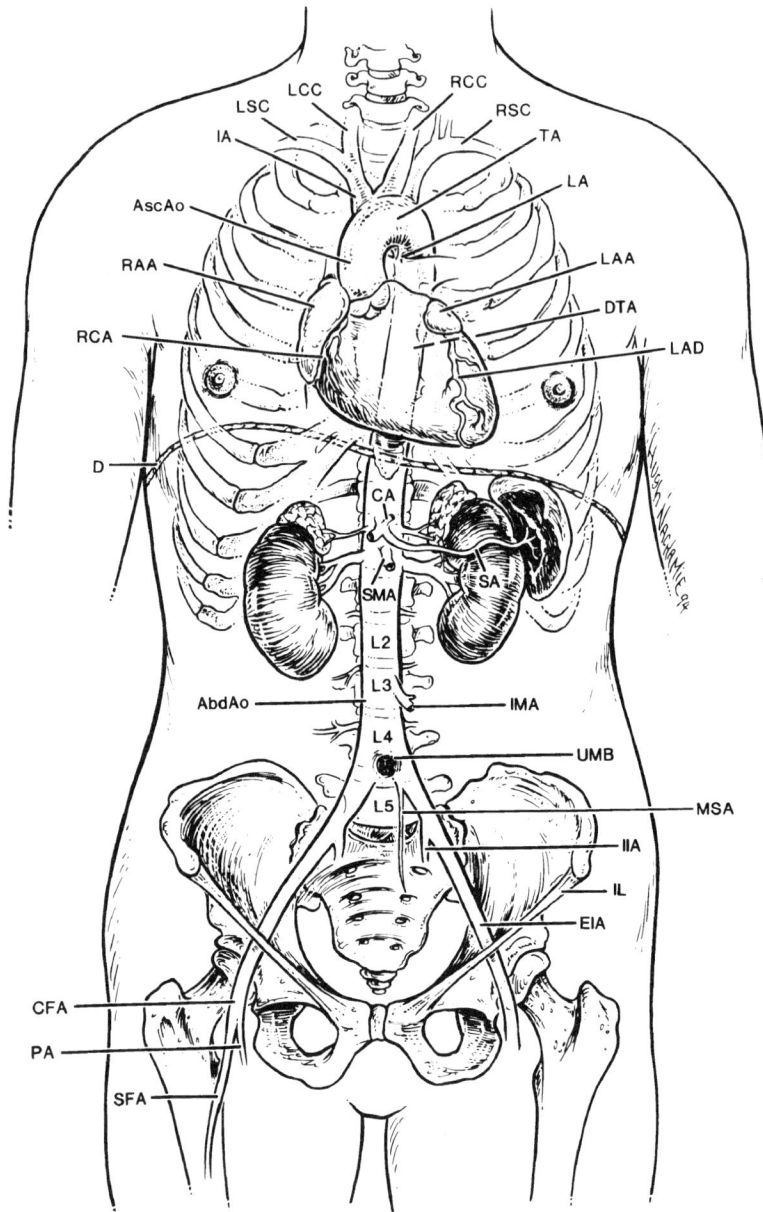

Figure 1-1. Surface landmarks and major branches of the ascending, transverse, descending, and abdominal aorta. (LCC = left common carotid artery; LSC = left subclavian artery; IA = innominate artery; AscAo = ascending aorta; RAA = right atrial appendage; RCA = right coronary artery; CA = celiac axis; SMA = superior mesenteric artery; AbdAo = abdominal aorta; IL = inguinal ligament; CFA = common femoral artery; SFA = superficial femoral artery; RCC = right common carotid artery; RSC = right subclavian artery; TA = transverse aorta [aortic arch]; LA = ligamentum arteriosum; LAA = left atrial appendage; DTA = descending thoracic aorta; LAD= left anterior descending coronary artery; D = diaphragm; SA = splenic artery; IMA = inferior mesenteric artery; UMB = umbilicus; MSA = middle sacral artery; EIA = external iliac artery; IIA = internal iliac artery; PA = profunda femoris artery.) (Courtesy of Hugh Nachamie, 1994.)

rior descending (PD) arteries. The posterior lateral artery supplies marginal branches to the inferior surface of the left ventricle while the PD artery contributes to the interventricular septum. Coronary dominance is defined by the origin of the vessel supplying the inferior intraventricular septum. In 90% of hearts the right coronary artery supplies the PD artery (right dominance). In 10% of hearts the PD artery is a terminal branch of the circumflex (left dominance). Infrequently, there are two PD arterial branches arising from both the right and left coronaries (codominance).

The left coronary artery begins in the posterior aortic sinus and courses between the pulmonary artery and left atrial appendage for a variable distance. Here, the artery is large and has no major branches. As it continues to curve left, it enters the left atrioventricular sulcus where it either bifurcates into the left anterior descending (LAD) and circumflex (CFX) arteries or trifurcates into the LAD

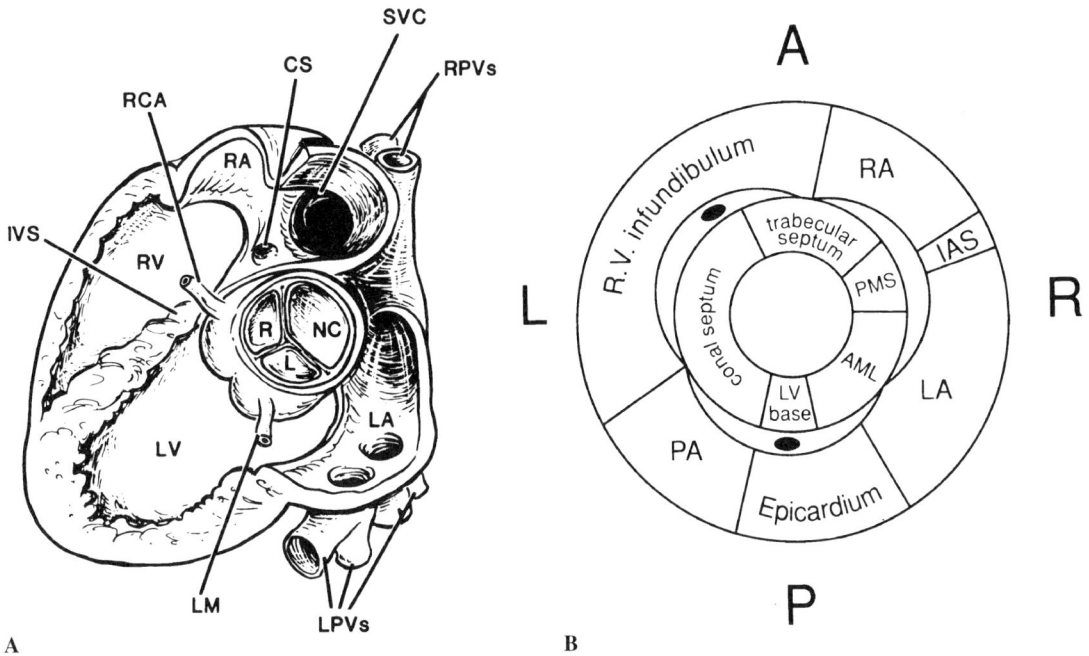

Figure 1-2. Anatomy of the aortic root and its related structures. A. Aortic root viewed from above with the pulmonary outflow tract removed to allow visualization of the aortic valve. The right-left commissure points to the normal position of the pulmonary trunk. B. Anatomic relationships of the structures inferior to the valve (inner circle) and superior to the valve (outer circle). The atrioventricular (AV) node lies beneath the noncoronary cusp and the common branching portion of the AV bundle lies beneath the perimembranous septum. (A = anterior; R = right; L = left; P = posterior; IVS = interventricular septum; RV = right ventricle; RCA = right coronary artery; CS = coronary sinus; SVC = superior vena cava; RPVs = right pulmonary veins; LPVs = left pulmonary veins; LM = left main coronary artery; LV = left ventricle; RA = right atrium; IAS = intra-atrial septum; LA = left atrium; PA = pulmonary artery; AML = anterior mitral leaflet; PMS = perimembranous septum.)

artery, ramus marginalis, and CFX artery. The LAD artery gives off a major diagonal branch and together they supply the anterior and anterolateral surfaces and anterior interventricular septum of the left ventricle. The CFX artery curves around the obtuse margin of the heart in the atrioventricular sulcus and gives off at least three large and multiple small marginal arteries supplying the lateral wall, apex, and inferior wall of the left ventricle (LV). When present, the ramus marginalis supplies the obtuse margin of the LV and can be an important tributary. Blood supply to the conduction system of the heart is variable (Table 1-1).

The transverse aorta most commonly (approximately 65%) has three branches: the brachiocephalic (innominate artery), left common carotid artery, and the left subclavian artery. In 27% of patients, the left common carotid originates from the innominate artery.[2] Other variations in transverse arch anatomy

such as four branches (2.5%), a single common trunk (<1%), or aberrant right subclavian forming a vascular ring with compression of the trachea and esophagus have been described (Figure 1-4).

The blood supply to the brain is constant, even if the origins of the great vessels are not (Table 1-2). The common carotid artery divides to form the internal and external carotid arteries on both the right and left sides. The external carotid artery supplies the soft tissues of the face and neck and the internal carotid artery continues cephalad without branching to provide blood supply to the brain. The internal carotid arteries provide approximately 90% of total brain blood flow and the vertebral system provides the remainder. The internal carotid artery first branches to form the ophthalmic artery and then ends by branching into the anterior cerebral, middle cerebral, and posterior communicating arteries. The middle cerebral artery is a large colinear

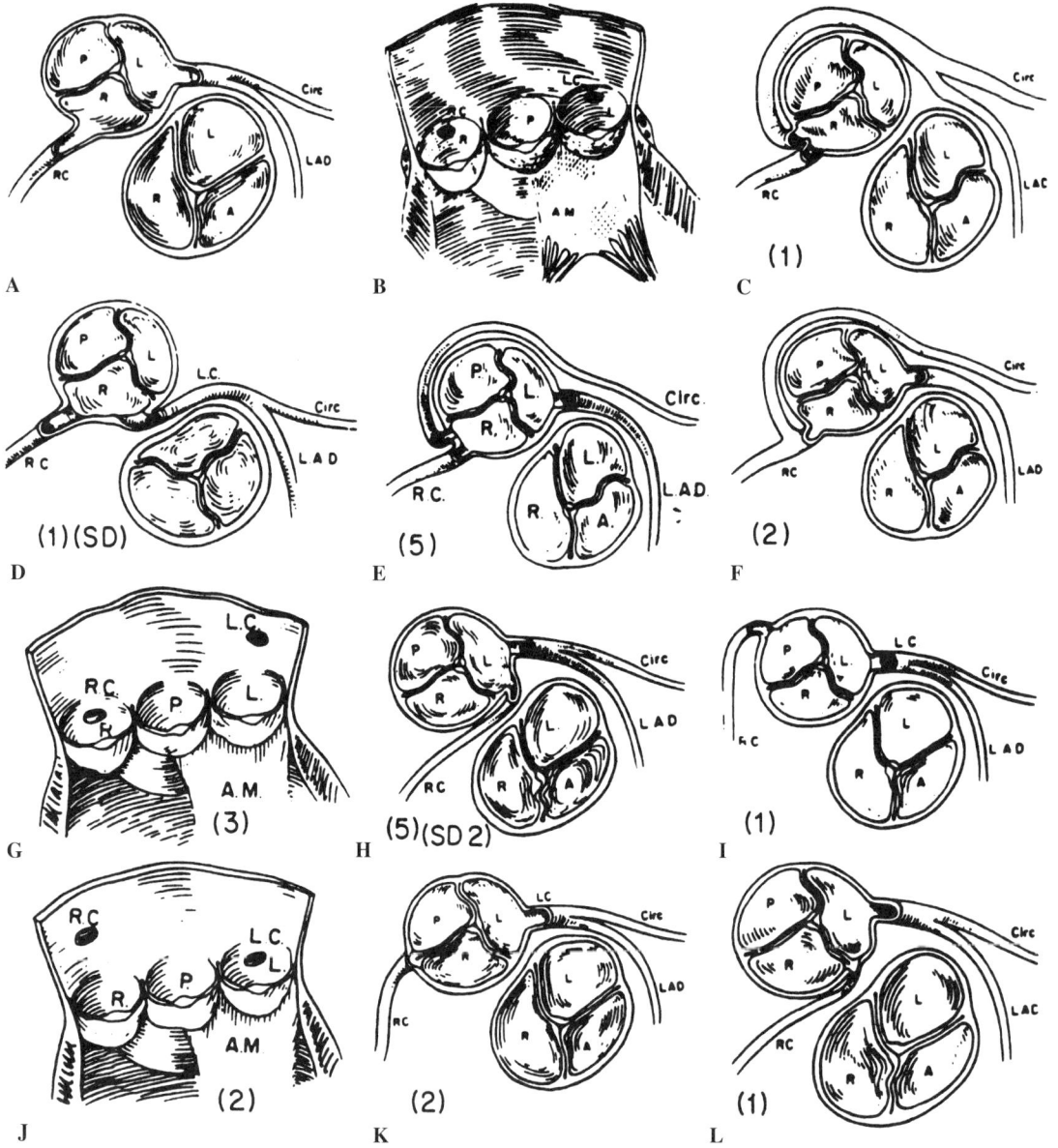

Figure 1-3. Patterns of the coronary ostia and coronary arteries. A, B. Normal. C. Left coronary from right aortic sinus; posterior course. D. Left coronary artery from right aortic sinus; anterior course. E. Circumflex coronary artery from right aortic sinus. F. Circumflex coronary artery from right coronary artery. G. Left coronary artery from above left aortic sinus. H. Right coronary artery from left aortic sinus. I. Right coronary artery from posterior aortic sinus. J. Right coronary artery from above right aortic sinus. K. Right coronary artery from above right-posterior commissure. L. Right coronary artery from above right-left commissure. Numbers in parentheses represent number of cases out of 23 total. (P = posterior aortic sinus; L = left aortic sinus; R = right aortic sinus; RC = right coronary; AM = anterior mitral leaflet; Circ = circumflex coronary artery; A = anterior; LC = left coronary; LAD = left anterior descending coronary artery; SD = sudden death.) (Reprinted with permission from JM Mahowald, LC Blieden, JI Coe, JE Edwards. Ectopic origin of a coronary artery from the aorta. Chest 1986;89:668.)

Table 1-1. Frequency of Origin of Blood Supply to the Sinoatrial and Atrioventricular Nodes

Origin	Sinoatrial Node (Percentage)	Atrioventricular Node (Percentage)
Right coronary	60	90
Circumflex coronary	40	10

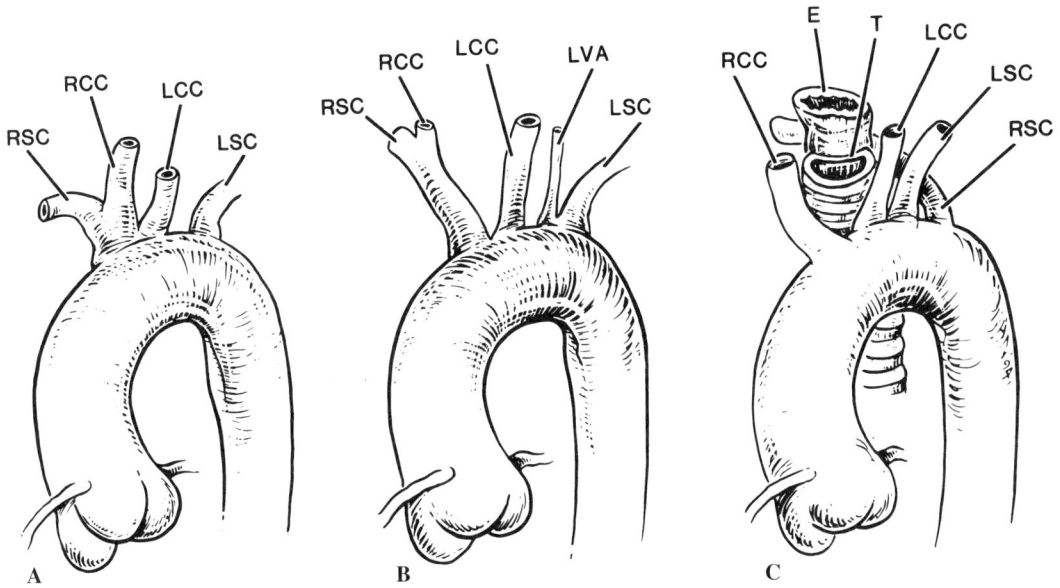

Figure 1-4. Variations in the anatomy of the aortic arch. A. Innominate artery gives right subclavian and right common carotid arteries and left common carotid artery in 26% of patients. B. Left common carotid, left vertebral, and left subclavian arteries arise from separate origins in 2.5% of patients. C. Right subclavian artery arises distal and posterior to left subclavian artery, causing potential tracheal and esophageal constriction (rare). (RSC = right subclavian artery; RCC = right common carotid artery; LCC = left common carotid artery; LVA = left vertebral artery; LSC = left subclavian artery; T = trachea; E = esophagus.) (Courtesy of Hugh Nachamie, 1994.)

Table 1-2. Blood Supply of the Brain and Spinal Cord

Origin	Main Branch	Major Terminal Artery Branch	Distribution
Common carotid	Internal carotid	Anterior cerebral	Medial and superior frontal lobes
Common carotid	Internal carotid	Middle cerebral	Lateral temporal lobes
Vertebral	Basilar	Posterior cerebral	Inferior and occipital lobes
Vertebral	Basilar	Anterior inferior cerebellar	Anterior cerebellar
Vertebral	Basilar	Posterior inferior cerebellar	Posterior cerebellar
Vertebral	None	Anterior spinal	Anterior spinal cord*

*The blood supply to the anterior spinal cord is not continuous. Segments of the anterior spinal cord are supplied via local communicating arteries from the intercostals.

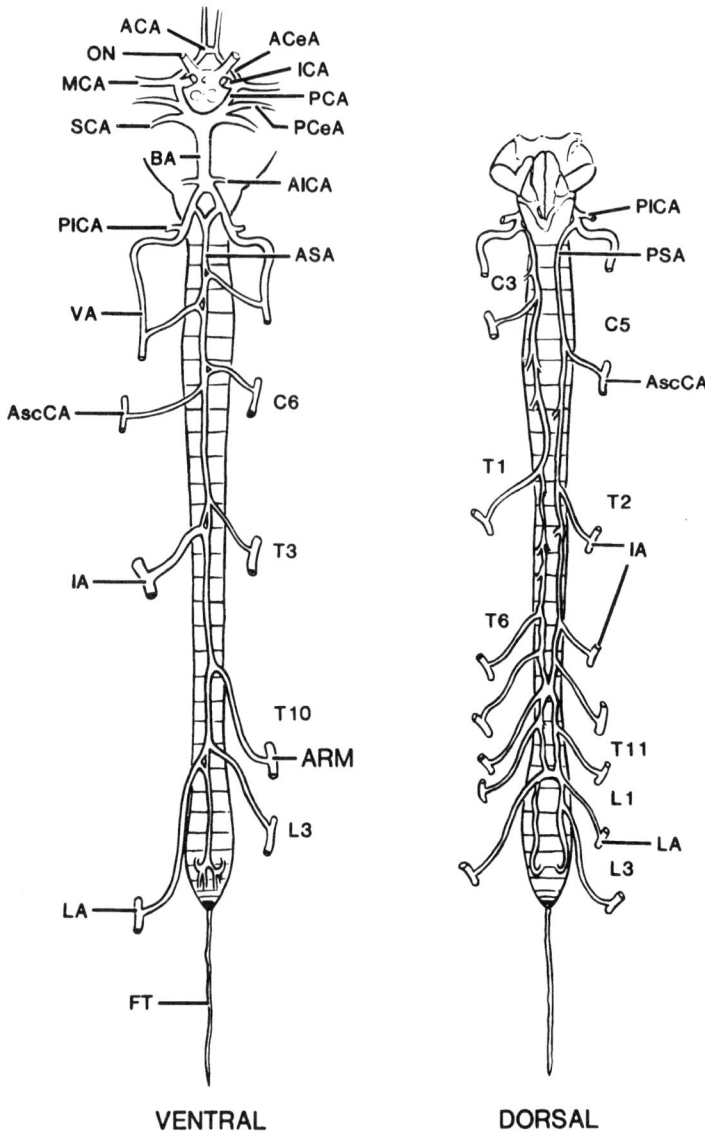

Figure 1-5. Ventral and dorsal blood supply of the brain and spinal cord. Note that the large ventral intercostal around T10 (ARM) provides variable collateralization through the anterior spinal artery collaterals in the cervical spinal cord. (ACA = anterior communicating artery; ON = optic nerve; MCA = middle cerebral artery; SCA = superior cerebellar artery; BA = basilar artery; PICA = posterior inferior cerebellar artery; VA = vertebral artery; AscCA = ascending cervical artery; IA = intercostal artery; LA = lumbar artery; FT = filum terminale; PSA = posterior spinal artery; ACeA = anterior cerebral artery; ICA = internal carotid artery; PCA = posterior communicating artery; PCeA = posterior cerebral artery; AICA = anterior inferior cerebellar artery; ASA = anterior spinal artery; ARM = arteria radicularis magna [artery of Adamkiewicz].)

continuation of the internal carotid artery. This explains the propensity of arterial emboli entering the carotid circulation to lodge in the middle cerebral distribution. The right and left anterior cerebral arteries are connected via the anterior communicating artery. The posterior communicating arteries from the right and left form connections with the posterior cerebral artery, a branch of the basilar artery that originates from the fusion of the right and left vertebral arteries. This circular communication of arterial supply to the brain is termed the "circle of Willis" (Figure 1-5). The full collateralization provided by the circle of Willis is present in only 25–40% of patients. Frequently, one or more of the posterior communicating arteries is absent.

The descending thoracic aorta begins at the left subclavian at the level of the fourth thoracic vertebra. It continues to the level of the diaphragm at the twelfth thoracic vertebra. Multiple paired and unpaired posterior vessels originate from this portion of the aorta. These branches supply the chest wall and spinal cord. Anteriorly, small unpaired segmen-

Table 1-3. The Abdominal Aortic Branches and Their Distribution

Branch	Derivative Branches	Organs Supplied
Inferior phrenic	Anterior and posterior branches	Adrenals, cavae, pericardium, chest wall
Celiac	Left gastric, splenic, hepatic	Stomach, spleen, liver, duodenum, pancreas, omentum, gall bladder, common duct
Middle suprarenal	—	Adrenal
First lumbar	—	Vertebrae, psoas, quadratus lumborum, oblique muscles, spinal cord
Superior mesenteric	Inferior pancreaticoduodenal, intestinal, middle colic, right colic, ileocolic	Duodenum, jejunum, ileum, colon, appendix
Renal	—	Kidney, adrenal
Spermatic, ovarian	Ureteral, cremasteric, epi-didymal, testicular	Testes, scrotum, ovary, fallopian tube
Second lumbar	—	Vertebrae, psoas, quadratus lumborum, oblique muscles, spinal cord
Inferior mesenteric	Left colic, sigmoid, superior hemorrhoidal	Sigmoid colon, rectum
Third lumbar	—	Vertebrae, psoas, quadratus lumborum, oblique muscles, spinal cord
Fourth lumbar	—	Vertebrae, psoas, quadratus lumborum, oblique muscles, spinal cord
Common iliac	Internal iliac, external iliac	Rectum, bladder, uterus, perineum
Middle sacral	Lowest lumbar, lateral sacral, rectal	Sacral canal, rectum

tal arteries supply the pericardium, pleura, diaphragm, lungs, bronchi, and esophagus. A large radicular artery called the arteria radicularis magna or artery of Adamkiewicz arises from the aorta at a variable level (T5–T12) to supply the lower two-thirds of the spinal cord. The artery is said to arise between the fifth and eight thoracic vertebral levels in 15% of patients and between the ninth and twelfth thoracic vertebral levels in approximately 60% of patients. In 25% of individuals it is located at the first lumbar vertebra. Occasionally this large dominant vessel can be visualized by the radiologist or surgeon.[3] Because the natural collaterals between the circle of Willis and the thoracic cord arterial supply may be incomplete, interruption of the artery of Adamkiewicz can result in watershed ischemia or infarct of the spinal cord (see Figure 1-5). Surgical procedures on the descending thoracic aorta allow for antegrade perfusion of the cerebral, vertebral, and coronary vessels. However, the blood supply to the lower thoracic spinal cord via the anterior and posterior spinal arteries may be adequate only to the level of the midcervical spinal cord. The importance of reimplantation of the large intercostal vessels during aortic resection is a widely debated issue (see Chapter 8).

The abdominal aorta is that portion of the aorta from the diaphragm to its bifurcation at the level of the fourth lumbar vertebra. The major branches of the abdominal aorta are celiac, superior mesenteric, right and left renal, gonadal, inferior mesenteric, and right and left common iliac arteries (see Figure 1-1). There are multiple minor branches that may vary greatly in number, origin, and distribution including the inferior phrenic, adrenal, lumbar, and median sacral arteries. The blood supply to the abdominal viscera is listed in Table 1-3.

Histology

Histologically the aorta is divided into three layers: intima, media, and adventitia. The intima is composed of an innermost continuous layer of vasoactive polygonal endothelial cells held together by intracellular junctions. These tight junctions prevent extravasation of intraluminal contents but contribute little to the overall structural integrity of the aortic wall. Below the endothelium there is a fine layer of collagen and elastin fibers with a few fibroblasts. Deeper in the intima there are smooth muscle cells and an internal elastic membrane composed of two or more lamellae of elastin fibers.

Beyond the intima, the media is composed of highly organized lamellae of smooth muscle, collagen, elastin, and proteoglycans. The media gives strength and elasticity to the aortic wall. Elastin rings together with smooth muscle and collagen are organized with structural proteins to form lamellar units. In mammalian species the density of lamellar units is proportional to the wall tension. Interestingly, the human abdominal aorta has fewer lamellar units than would be anticipated based on its diameter and wall tension. Wolinsky and colleagues have suggested that the lower number of lamellar units with corresponding greater thickness may be related to the observed increased propensity of the abdominal aorta to atherosclerotic and aneurysmal diseases.[4]

The adventitia is the outermost layer of the aortic wall. It contains the nutritive vasa vasorum and is composed of a dense network of fibrous tissue. Vasa vasorum are epiarterial vessels that provide most of the nutritive supply to the arterial wall. Large arteries have a relatively constant avascular inner zone that derives its nutrition directly from intraluminal circulating blood elements. Loss of the vasa vasorum in disease states does not cause fullthickness necrosis of the aorta but leads to necrosis of a significant portion of the outer media.[5] The adventitia provides an important part of the structural integrity of the aorta, which accounts for the ability of large arterial vessels (including the aorta) to sustain arterial pressure after endarterectomy without developing aneurysmal dilatation.[6] Collagen and elastin are important structural proteins in the media and adventia. Loss of these proteins has been implicated in aneurysm formation.[7]

Embryology

The formation of the aorta and its major branches occurs during the fourth and fifth weeks of gestation. The embryo develops a single ventral aorta as an anterior prolongation of the heart tube. Posteriorly, two dorsal aortae develop along the endodermal gut. These primitive vessels are connected

sequentially in a craniocaudal sequence by six pairs of aortic arches (Figure 1-6). The dorsal aortae fuse to a single unpaired vessel in the trunk. As each successive arch forms and involutes, a portion or all of the vessel remains as an adult structure. Table 1-4 lists the adult derivatives of the six aortic arches of the embryo. The right dorsal aorta involutes completely, leaving the left dorsal aorta to form the adult descending aorta. The ascending aorta is formed from the ventral aorta. The fifth arch normally fails to develop significantly and has no adult remnant. The third, fourth, and sixth branchial arches give rise to the transverse aorta and components of its branches. Defects in the involution of the branchial arches, right dorsal aorta, or intersegmental artery (unpaired seventh arch) may lead to congenital malformations of the aorta or its major branches.[8] A summary of these abnormalities is listed in Table 1-5 (see also Chapter 9).

Pathology of the Aorta

Arteriosclerosis

Loss of elasticity with concomitant thickening of the arterial wall is generally referred to as arteriosclerosis. The patterns of arteriosclerosis have been classified as atherosclerosis, Mönckeberg's medial calcific sclerosis, and arteriolosclerosis.

Atherosclerosis of the aorta is by far the most prevalent form of arteriosclerosis involving the aorta. Atherosclerosis accounts for over 90% of the arteriosclerotic lesions of the aorta seen clinically in Western society. It is characterized early in the disease by raised, fibrofatty intimal plaques harboring liquid lipid-rich centers mixed with fibroblasts and smooth muscle cells. As the atherosclerotic plaques project into the lumen of the artery they cause progressive luminal narrowing and flow disturbance. With time the plaques enlarge, deepen, and disturb the underlying media, leading to fragmentation of the organized lamellae. Damage to the media results in ulceration, thrombosis, intraplaque hemorrhage, and ultimately calcification of the damaged areas. Eventually, fibrosis of the media and adventitia lead to a generalized loss of elasticity and weakening of the aortic wall. The result is a ragged, narrowed lumen with greatly increased potential for thrombosis, embolization, dissection, and

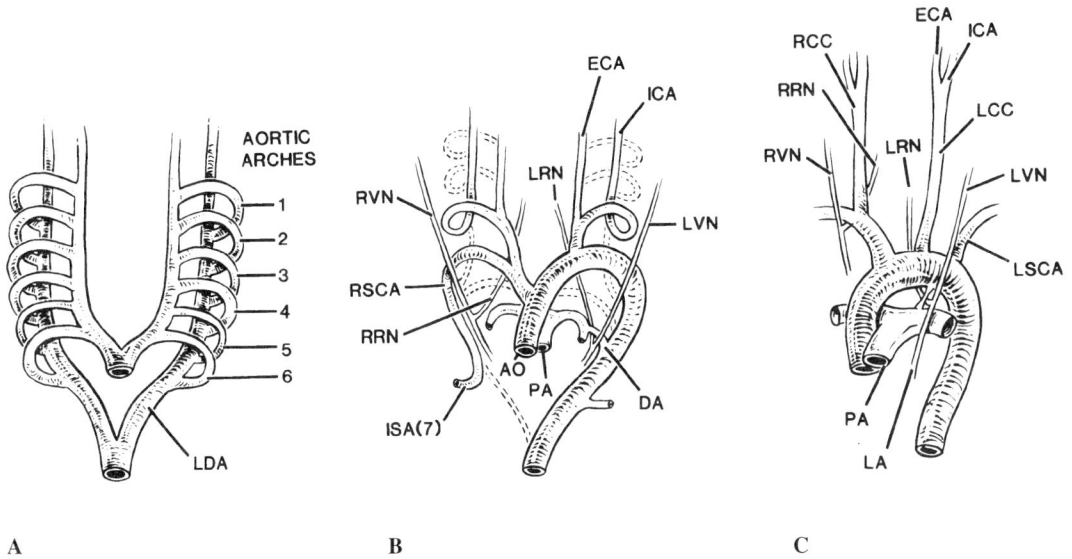

Figure 1-6. Embryology of the aorta and pulmonary artery. A. Diagrammatic development of the aortic arches and dorsal aortas before transformation into the definitive vascular pattern. B. Diagram of the aortic arches and dorsal aortas after the transformation. The broken lines indicate obliterated structures. C. The aortic arch and great arteries in the adult. Note the position of the recurrent laryngeal nerve on the left and right relative to the ductus arteriosus and right subclavian artery, respectively. (LDA = left dorsal aorta; RVN = right vagus nerve; RSCA = right subclavian artery; RRN = right recurrent nerve; ISA(7) = seventh unpaired intersegmental artery; AO = ascending aorta; PA = main pulmonary artery; LA = ligamentum arteriosum; LRN = left recurrent nerve; ECA = external carotid artery; ICA = internal carotid artery; LCC = left common carotid; LVN = left vagus nerve; DA = ductus arteriosus; RCC = right common carotid artery; LSCA = left subclavian artery.) (Reprinted with permission from Cardiovascular System. In J Langman [ed], Medical Embryology [4th ed]. Baltimore: Williams & Wilkins, 1981;186.)

aneurysm formation. Early atherosclerotic lesions can be seen in childhood but generally do not become clinically manifest until the fifth and sixth decades of life. Certain risk factors for development of the disease have become well established by epidemiologic studies. Hyperlipidemia, hypertension, cigarette smoking, male sex, and diabetes mellitus all emerge as independent risk factors in large groups of individuals observed prospectively for development of the disease. Age and genetic predisposition play an important role as well.[9]

Mönckeberg's medial calcific sclerosis is a nonatherosclerotic form of arteriosclerosis. This medial degenerative disease is characterized by calcification of the media by irregular plaques or rings. These calcifications create a loss of elasticity within the wall of the aorta, which spares the intima and does not encroach on the lumen. As the disease progresses, the plaques may coalesce and ossify to form a continuous band of calcium between the intima and adventitia. Surgically and ra-

diographically this is described as a "porcelain aorta."[10] This disease can and often does coexist with intimal atherosclerosis.

Arteriolosclerosis is a disorder involving small blood vessels and is not itself a disease of the aorta. Arteriolosclerosis can, however, affect the vasa vasorum, the nutritive supply of the aortic wall, and lead indirectly to fibrosis and loss of elasticity within the aortic wall. Thus, the aortic wall becomes weakened and predisposed to dissection and aneurysm formation.

Medial Degeneration

Cystic medial degeneration is an idiopathic disorder characterized by focal loss of both connective tissue (elastin and collagen) and muscular (smooth muscle) tissue within the media of the aortic wall. The term medionecrosis or cystic medial necrosis is probably not appropriate because the cystic areas noted histo-

Table 1-4. Embryology of the Aorta: Derivatives of the Branchial Arches

Arch	Normal Arterial Component
First	Maxillary artery
Second	Hyoid and stapedial arteries
Third	Common carotid artery
Fourth	Right: forms part of the right subclavian
	Left: forms part of the transverse aortic arch
Fifth	No remnant
Sixth	Right: forms part of the right pulmonary artery
	Left: forms the ductus arteriosus

logically are probably the result of "dropout of degenerated elastin fibers and smooth muscle cells" rather than purely cellular necrosis.[11] The intima, adventitia, and vasa vasorum all remain histologically normal. The weakened aortic wall becomes predisposed to longitudinal dissection and aneurysm formation. The defect in cystic medial degeneration involves the connective tissue lamellae, which are composed of collagen, elastin, and smooth muscle tissue. It is not clear whether the process is an acquired progressive degenerative disease or a normal consequence of aging of the arterial wall.

Cystic medial degeneration has been described with inherited disorders of collagen synthesis, the most prevalent of which are Marfan's syndrome and Ehlers-Danlos syndrome. Other, less common inherited disorders of collagen, elastin, and mu-

copolysaccharides have also been associated. These are neurofibromatosis, mucopolysaccharidosis, Hunter's syndrome, Hurler's disease, Sanfilippo's syndrome, and Morquio's disease.[12]

Marfan's syndrome is characterized by lax ligaments, lens dislocation, tall stature with reduced muscle mass, chest wall deformities, arachnodactyly, scoliosis, mitral valve prolapse, and dilatation and dissections of the aorta. The association of cystic medial degeneration with Marfan's syndrome has been linked to a structural defect in synthesis of elastin fibrillogenesis.[13]

Ehlers-Danlos syndrome is characterized by velvety, hyperextensible skin, hypermobile joints, fragile tissue, and a bleeding diathesis. Of the ten subtypes of Ehlers-Danlos syndrome that have been described and characterized, types I, III, and IV are associated with vascular complications. Type IV, called Sack-Barabas type, is the best known of these and has been demonstrated to be caused by a defect in the synthesis of type III collagen. Patients with type IV Ehlers-Danlos syndrome are more prone to aortic rupture secondary to the thinness of the aortic wall and also have an increased propensity for aortic dissection.[14]

Infectious Aortitis

Infectious aortitis most commonly results from hematogenous bacterial invasion of the aortic intima. A generalized arteritis involving the full thickness of the aortic wall ensues, which results in a weaken-

Table 1-5. Common Abnormalities During Formation of the Aorta and Great Vessels

Abnormality	Involved Structures
Patent ductus arteriosus	Persistent sixth branchial arch (when present without other congenital heart defect)
Coarctation of the aorta	Abnormality in the aortic media in association with intimal hyperplasia
Anomalous origin of the right subclavian	Fourth arch inappropriately involutes and the right subclavian forms as an extension of the right dorsal aorta
	The subclavian crosses behind the esophagus, which may lead to a vascular ring
Double aortic arch	Persistence of the right dorsal aorta and right fourth branchial arch
Right aortic arch	Obliteration of left fourth branchial arch and dorsal aorta with persistence of the right fourth arch and dorsal aorta
Interrupted aortic arch	Abnormal obliteration of the left fourth arch with or without an abnormal origin of the right subclavian artery

Table 1-6. Clinical Criteria for Diagnosis of Takayasu's Disease

Age of onset ≤40 years
Claudication of an extremity
Decreased brachial artery pulse
Greater than 10 mm Hg difference in systolic blood pressure between arms
Bruit of the subclavian arteries or aorta
Arteriographic evidence of narrowing or occlusion of the entire aorta, its primary branches, or large arteries in the proximal upper or lower extremities

ing of the wall and usually subsequent aneurysm formation. Contiguous perivascular inflammation and infection can also result in infectious aortitis such as is seen with primary aortoduodenal fistula and aortoesophageal fistula.[15] Aneurysms that result from embolic bacterial infections are generally referred to as mycotic aneurysms although the term *mycotic* as used by Osler et al. generally referred to fungal vegetations on the heart valves.[16] The most common organisms responsible for mycotic infection are salmonellae, staphylococci, and streptococci. An aneurysm with or without thrombus may precede development of bacterial aortitis, but it is possible for certain organisms (especially salmonellae) to hematogenously infect the normal aorta. The true incidence of mycotic aortitis is not known because a significant percentage of aortic infections do not progress to aneurysm formation and may be healed with antimicrobial therapy. Although endarterial infection is rarely etiologic in abdominal aortic aneurysm, Schwartz and colleagues noted a 10% incidence of aortic thrombus colonization in patients undergoing abdominal aortic aneurysm resection.[17]

Syphilitic aortitis is primarily a disease of historical interest in developed countries. This form of aortitis occurs during the tertiary stages of syphilitic infection, which may occur 15–20 years after the primary infection. Pathologically, the spirochete infects the vasa vasorum of the aorta typically near the aortic sinuses, but any portion of the aorta (and infrequently great vessels) can be affected. The infection produces swelling and hyperplasia of the endothelium. Medial necrosis results from occlusion of the vasa vasorum. Eventually, a transmural inflammatory lesion develops that causes "tree barking" of the intima and can result in aneurysm formation. When the proximal root is involved, aortic insufficiency (from annular dilation) and coronary obstruction (from intimal hyperplasia) can result.[18,19] Rupture is less frequently a

cause of death from syphilitic aortitis than is aortic regurgitation and congestive heart failure. The diagnosis can be confusing even at surgery or postmortem examination because the organism is not always observed in the tissues and the "tree bark" appearance of the intima can occur with other immune-mediated aortitis entities.[20]

Immunomediated Arteritis

Distant systemic infections and autoimmune disorders, which do not directly infect the wall of the aorta and other autoimmune processes, can produce inflammatory changes in the aorta. It is believed that the reticuloendothelial system can become temporarily overwhelmed with antigen-antibody complexes, resulting in the deposition of these immune complexes in the intima of blood vessels. The reaction of the immune system to these deposited complexes is that of a localized inflammatory reaction with invasion by polymorphonucleocytes. Inflammatory cells secrete proteolytic enzymes that disrupt the ultrastructure of the vascular wall and cause transmural inflammation. Ultimately, when this process affects the aortic wall, the result is a damaged wall with a propensity for fibrosis, thrombosis, and late aneurysm formation.[12,21] Immunomediated arteritides that can affect the aorta are Takayasu's disease, Kawasaki's disease, giant cell arteritis, polyarteritis nodosa, Cogan's syndrome, and Behçet's disease. The most common of these, Takayasu's disease, or pulseless disease, occurs principally in young women and is diagnosed clinically by the presence of three or more of the signs and symptoms listed in Table 1-6. Treatment is directed at the immune mechanism, and only occasionally is surgical therapy initiated to palliate the ischemic symptoms after reducing the inflammation of affected vessels.[22]

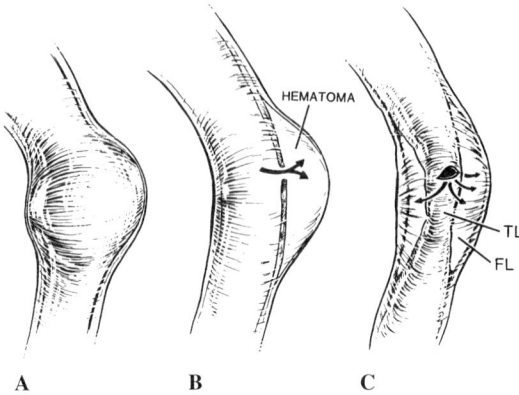

Figure 1-7. Pathophysiology of aneurysmal dilatation. A. True aneurysm. All layers of the aorta are involved in the dilatation. The aortic wall is generally thinned and stretched. Wall tension is increased locally and the lumen may contain laminated thrombus. Formation of an aneurysm may predispose to subsequent dissection. B. Pseudoaneurysm. A disruption of the intima and media leads to formation of a subadventitial or extra-adventitial hematoma. This may thrombose or may remain liquefied and in continuity with arterial flow and pressure. The aneurysm is generally contained by contiguous tissues. C. Dissecting aneurysm. An intimal disruption allows entry of blood under pressure into the plane of the media. The separation of medial layers propagates antegrade and retrograde and narrows the true lumen (TL) of the vessel, creating a false lumen (FL). The false lumen may persist and may reenter the true lumen at a distant site. The aneurysm results from stretching and dilatation of the weakened wall of the false lumen. Both obstruction and rupture can result. (Courtesy of Hugh Nachamie, 1994.)

Aneurysms of the Aorta

Aneurysms of the aorta can be classified as either true or false aneurysms. A true aneurysm is a dilatation of all layers of the aortic wall (intima, media, and adventitia). Progressive mural thinning and expansion of the aortic diameter accompany an increase in wall tension. Aneurysms can be saccular or fusiform. Saccular aneurysms tend to result from a localized infectious or traumatic process. Fusiform or cylindrical aneurysms result from a more generalized disease process in the aorta. Characteristically, ascending and proximal descending aortic dilatation eventually results in dissection. Aneurysms of the abdominal aorta and thoracoab-

dominal segment have a greater propensity to rupture rather than dissect.

A false aneurysm does not involve all layers of the aortic wall and generally occurs following a breach in the integrity of the intima (Figure 1-7). Blood under pressure disrupts the media, but the adventitia remains intact. The adventitia then expands while the central lumen of the aorta remains the same or is compressed by the expanding subadventitial or extra adventitial hematoma. Dissection is the result of a breach of the intima and development of a cleavage plane in the media. The process tends to propagate longitudinally and is limited only by the presence of atherosclerotic plaques and surgical suture lines. This explains the tendency of young Marfan's syndrome patients to sustain total aortic dissection, whereas older patients with atheromatous diseases have more limited dissections. Aneurysmal disease of the aorta can predispose to aortic dissection resulting in a so-called dissecting aortic aneurysm. Indeed many localized aneurysms of the descending aorta are found to contain a localized area of dissection. It is possible, however, to develop a dissection in a normal caliber aorta.[23]

Aneurysms of the aorta virtually always increase in size over time. The rate of expansion of the aneurysm is not particularly related to sex or age, but may be related to absolute size.[24] Rupture of a descending aneurysm is rare if the absolute size of the aneurysm is less than or equal to the size of the body of the third lumbar vertebra.[25] Repair of all aneurysms of any site in the aorta in emergency circumstances carries a higher risk than elective repair. Further, population-based studies suggest that the life expectancy of a patient is markedly diminished by the presence of aneurysmal disease in the thoracic aorta (Figure 1-8). Because of these facts, aggressive surgical management of aneurysmal disease of the aorta is warranted unless the patient has a significant other life-limiting pathology.

Ascending Aortic Aneurysms

Until shortly after World War II, treatment for aortic aneurysms consisted of wrapping the aortic wall with materials intended to prevent expansion. Results of these palliative operations were poor.[26] With the advent of cardiopulmonary bypass and the pioneering techniques of Cooley and DeBakey, the first proximal aortic repair was accomplished in 1956.[27]

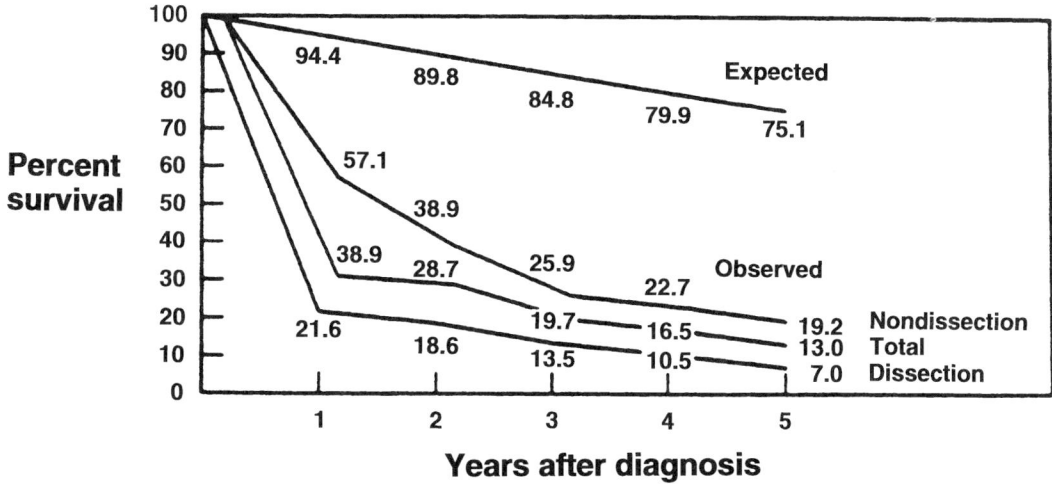

Figure 1-8. Estimated survival of 72 Rochester, Minnesota, residents with thoracic aortic aneurysm (total, dissecting, and nondissecting) initially diagnosed in the period from 1951–1980. (Reprinted with permission from LK Bickerstaff, PC Pairolero, LH Hollier, et al. Thoracic aortic aneurysms: a population-based study. Surgery 1982;92:1103.)

Since that time, improved surgical technique, extra-corporeal perfusion, advances in prosthetics, and preoperative and intraoperative management have made ascending aortic surgery routine, with relatively low mortality (10–16%) and a good long-term survival rate (80–90% at 5 years).[28–30]

Pathophysiology.   The overall incidence of thoracic aneurysms is 6 in 100,000 person-years, with a slight male predilection. Degenerative medial disease resulting from atherosclerosis and connective tissue disorders are the most common causes of aneurysm formation in the ascending aorta. Table 1-7 and Figure 1-9 discuss the causes of ascending aortic aneurysm.

When marked dilation of the ascending aorta is associated with cystic medial degeneration, frequently annuloaortic ectasia occurs as well. Annular dilatation with thinning of the aortic sinuses results in valvar insufficiency. Although the aortic valve may appear anatomically normal, its leaflets are frequently thinned and diaphanous and central valvar incompetence develops as a result of commissural widening. An operative procedure to spare the valve and resuspend the commissures from a normal caliber prosthetic conduit has been proposed by David.[31] Others have taken the position that the aortic leaflets have intrinsic connective tissue disease and should be replaced by a prosthetic valve or homograft. If left untreated, a severely dilated proxi-

mal aortic root will eventually progress to an aortic dissection or frank rupture through the sinuses into the pericardium. Although studies of the natural history of ascending aortic aneurysm are scarce, some conclusions can be made from existing literature. Generally, a patient who is otherwise fit should be offered surgery if the ascending aorta reaches 6 cm or if the diameter increases more than 0.5 cm in 6 months.[32] In young patients undergoing aortic valve replacement with incidental ascending aortic dilatation, the surgeon should evaluate the diameter and thinness of the aortic wall. Ascending aortic replacement is performed prophylactically if the aortic diameter is greater than 4.5–5.0 cm, or if the aortic media is thinned.

Diagnosis.   Patients with ascending aneurysm are generally asymptomatic. Some aneurysms are discovered as a result of an abnormal shadow on the chest radiograph. Pain from adventitial stretching and direct contact and erosion into the chest wall is possible. Symptoms from compression of local structures can occur, causing superior vena cava syndrome or tracheal compression. Pulmonary artery compression and erosion with development of aortopulmonary fistula have also been reported. When aortic valvular incompetence occurs, classical findings of congestive heart failure and "water-hammer pulses" are present. Acute dissection can cause sudden aortic insufficiency, which presents

Table 1-7. Predisposing Etiologies
for Aneurysms of the Aorta

Cystic medial degeneration
   Marfan's syndrome
   Ehlers-Danlos syndrome
Atherosclerosis
Aortitis
   Takayasu's disease
   Giant cell arteritis
Infectious
   Syphilis
   Bacterial
      Salmonellae
      Staphylococci
      Streptococci
      Escherichia coli
Hemodynamic
   Poststenotic dilatation
   Aortic valve stenosis
   Aortic coarctation
Trauma (pseudoaneurysm)
   Deceleration injury
   Prior surgery

with massive congestive heart failure (see the section on aortic dissection). It is important for the anesthesiologist to know the status of the aortic valve and coronary arteries as well as the extent of dilatation of the aortic arch. Usually, transesophageal echocardiography and cardiac catheterization are sufficient to evaluate the ascending aorta. A computed tomography scan or magnetic resonance angiography may also demonstrate the anatomy, but are not required. In patients with a history of transient ischemic attacks or in whom cervical bruits are detected, aortography is indicated to evaluate the great vessels.

Aortic Arch Aneurysms

Isolated aortic arch aneurysm is unusual, but presents a particularly challenging problem to the surgeon. Etiologic factors in the development of aortic arch aneurysms are the same as those for ascending aneurysms. Chronic dissection propagated from the proximal descending thoracic aorta is a common cause as well. The clinical presentation of arch dilatation is diverse and usually related to compression of adjacent structures. In addition to venous and airway compression, these aneurysms can cause dysphagia by direct compression of the esophagus and typically cause stretching and neuropraxia of the left recurrent nerve as it passes adjacent to the arch around the ligamentum arteriosum. Occasionally cerebrovascular manifestations can announce the presence of atheroembolic material within the lumen. Erosion into the pulmonary vessels or lung parenchyma may be heralded by development of arteriovenous fistula or hemoptysis.

Arch aneurysms are uncommon, and therefore natural history studies are not available. It is not, however, unreasonable to use operability criteria similar to those used for ascending aortic aneurysm. There is a natural tendency on the part of the surgeon to be more cautious in the selection of patients for arch resection because of the greater inherent risks of surgery (see Chapter 7). Like aneurysms of the ascending aorta, dissection and subsequent free rupture are common endpoints. Contained ruptures, like those occurring in the abdominal aorta, are not common.

Diagnostic modalities too are similar to those used for ascending aortic aneurysm. Transesophageal echocardiography may be somewhat more limited than other modalities in evaluation of proximal transverse aortic dilatation. Conventional or magnetic resonance angiography is useful preoperatively to evaluate the aortic arch anatomy and is performed in essentially all elective patients (see Chapter 3).

*Descending Thoracic and Thoracoabdominal
Aneurysms*

The presentation of descending thoracic aneurysms is frequently back pain or a symptom of compression of an adjacent organ such as the esophagus. Erosion into the vertebrae, chest wall, lung, and esophagus have all been reported. Frank rupture of descending and thoracoabdominal aneurysms is associated with a higher mortality than that which occurs with abdominal rupture. Further, the complexity of surgical approach and repair makes it more difficult for the surgical and anesthetic teams to intervene in the setting of an acute rupture. Patients with asymptomatic descending dilatation should be treated aggressively because operative therapy can alter the very poor natural history of thoracic aneurysm.[33]

An aortogram is helpful if not essential in defining the visceral arterial anatomy for the surgeon.

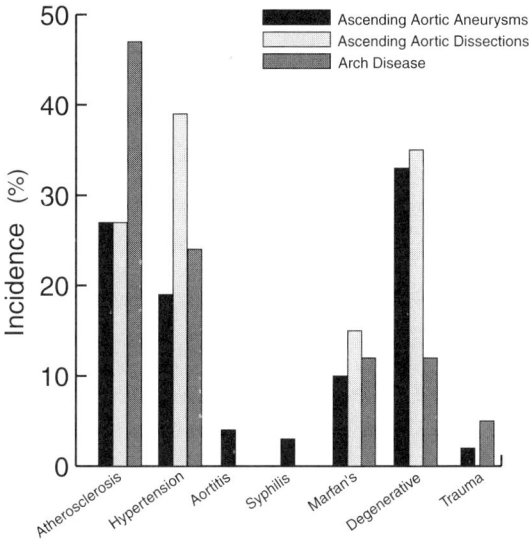

Figure 1-9. Relative frequency of various etiologies of ascending and transverse aortic aneurysm in 95 patients treated surgically. Degenerative changes and atherosclerosis were the main causes of ascending aneurysms. Hypertension and atherosclerosis were predominant causes of ascending dissections and arch disease. (Reprinted with permission from JS Ikonomidis, RD Weisel, MS Mouradian, et al. Thoracic aortic surgery. Circulation 1991;84[Suppl 3]:1.)

Aortography, however, should not be the sole diagnostic modality because a laminated intraluminal clot can give the false impression of mild ectasia where significant dilatation exists. Computed tomography can also have significant inaccuracy when used to measure the diameter of an aneurysm because the transverse measurement of a tortuous aorta may yield an elliptical diameter that overestimates the true luminal size of the aorta (see Chapter 3).[25]

In a study of thoracic aortic aneurysms presenting for medical care in Rochester, Minnesota, between 1951 and 1980, Bickerstaff and colleagues found that 27 of 72 patients had aneurysms located in the descending aorta that were etiologically diverse in comparison with abdominal aneurysms.[34] Atherosclerosis, medial degeneration, and dissection are the most commonly cited causes; however, inflammatory diseases of the aorta, postsurgical aneurysms, and posttraumatic aneurysms are also sporadically reported. Several observers have noted as much as a 25% coincidence of abdominal aortic aneurysm with descending thoracic aneurysm.[35]

The term *thoracoabdominal aneurysm* is used to denote a dilatation that would require replacement of portions of the aorta in the chest and abdomen. This should be distinguished from the separately occurring but coincidental thoracic and abdominal aortic aneurysms that can be resected separately. The anatomy of the blood supply to the spinal cord and viscera makes thoracic and thoracoabdominal aneurysms especially challenging to the surgeon and anesthesiologist and presents substantial risk of morbidity to the patient. The most significant predictors related to paraplegia after resection are length and location of the excluded aortic segment (see Chapter 8).

Classification of Thoracoabdominal Aneurysm. Crawford and colleagues proposed a system of anatomic classification of four types that is widely accepted.[36] Type I involves the entire descending thoracic aorta and the abdominal aorta up to the celiac trunk. Type II involves most of the descending thoracic aorta and the abdominal aorta up to the bifurcation. Type III involves the distal half of the descending thoracic aorta and the abdominal aorta down past the renal arteries. Type IV involves only the distal portion of the descending thoracic aorta and the abdominal aorta to its bifurcation. All four types occur with an approximate frequency of 25%.

Abdominal Aortic Aneurysms

Presentation and Diagnosis. Abdominal aortic aneurysms have a reported incidence of approximately 22 of 100,000 person-years.[37] The retroperitoneal location of the abdominal aorta alters significantly the presentation and the likelihood of death when these aneurysms rupture. Rather than an exsanguinating hemorrhage, many patients have a premonitory leak into the retroperitoneal tissues. This event provokes symptoms that allow time for surgical intervention. Abdominal aneurysms that rupture freely within the peritoneum usually result in death.[38] Other presentations of abdominal aneurysm disease include aortocaval fistula with sudden heart failure, repetitive cholesterol embolization, spontaneous aortoenteric fistula, infection, and thrombosis.

Most abdominal aneurysms are asymptomatic and are discovered during the course of a routine examination by a radiologist or internist. The diagnosis is relatively easily confirmed with abdominal ultrasonography, which gives an accurate estimate of the diameter of the aneurysm. Computed tomography is useful for evaluation of the character and extent of the lesion and is frequently used as a screening tool to exclude retroperitoneal hemorrhage. Patients with a known history of aneurysm presenting with abdominal pain (with or without anemia) and hypotension are presumed to have contained ruptures. Delay in therapy to obtain a certain diagnosis is not indicated and can be fatal.

Pathology and Classification.   Most abdominal aneurysms begin below the renal arteries and extend to the aortic bifurcation. Approximately 10% are said to be suprarenal and perhaps as many as 3–5% are supraceliac but confined to the abdomen. The distinctions are important to recognize because of the potential visceral and renal ischemia during repair. The risk of surgical repair is increased in extensive abdominal aneurysm disease.

Most abdominal aneurysms are atherosclerotic in origin, with involvement of all layers of the aorta. The pathogenesis of abdominal aortic aneurysmal disease is beyond the scope of this discussion, but investigators have identified proteolysis and deficiencies in the structural proteins that make up the aortic wall as important etiologic factors.[39]

Natural History.   The risk of rupture of an abdominal aneurysm is related to size, rate of growth, and perhaps to the recent postsurgical status of the patient.[40] The risk of rupture is proportional to the diameter of the aneurysm, with the chance of rupture of a 5-, 6-, or 7-cm aneurysm at 5 years being 25%, 35%, and 95%, respectively. It has been argued that smaller aneurysms can be safely watched because they have a slower rate of growth.[24,41] The surgeon's evaluation of risk of operation compared with the risk of rupture should be the primary determinant of timing of elective operative repair.

Aortic Dissection

Aortic dissection is the most common catastrophic pathology involving the aorta. It can be one of the most perplexing problems diagnostically and therapeutically that a cardiologist, cardiac surgeon, and cardiovascular anesthesiologist can face. In addition

to the mechanical disruption of the aortic wall, patients who sustain aortic dissection seem to have a systemic disease of excessive catecholamines. It is important to treat this problem aggressively during the initial management and long-term follow-up of these patients (see Chapters 6 and 7).

Diagnosis

Ninety percent of acute aortic dissections present with pain. The classical tearing or ripping pain is usually greatest at onset and subsides with control of anxiety and blood pressure. Frequently, there is migration of the pain, providing evidence as to whether the dissection is propagating antegrade or retrograde. Approximately 30% of patients present also with arterial occlusion and symptomatic ischemia of the lower extremities, viscera, central nervous system, or myocardium. Because symptoms can be remote from the origin of the dissection, erroneous initial diagnoses are common. The diagnosis should come immediately to mind in a patient with markedly elevated blood pressure, abdominal, back, or chest pain, and differential pulses in the extremities.

Table 1-8 lists common etiologies known to predispose the aorta to dissection. Medial degenerative disease, formerly thought to be present in virtually all aortic dissection, is histologically identifiable in only 31% of patients. Hypertension is present in 75–90% of patients presenting with acute dissection and frequently continues to be a problem for these patients after treatment.[42] Iatrogenic causes such as aortic cannulation for cardiopulmonary bypass, proximal aortotomy for aortic valve replacement, clamp injury during coronary bypass, aortography, and intra-aortic balloon pump counterpulsation have been occasionally reported. The incidence of aortic dissection in coronary bypass is less than 1%, but carries a significant mortality when it occurs.[43]

Classification of Aortic Dissection

The classification schemes depicted in Figure 1-10 are widely used.[44,45] The important clinical contributions of Daily and colleagues and later of Wheat have made it logical to divide aortic dissections into two groups: (1) those that involve the ascending aorta (type A), and (2) those that do not (type B).[46,47] Dissections older than 2 weeks are considered chronic

Table 1-8. Predisposing Factors and Etiologies to Acute Aortic Dissection

Hereditary diseases
   Marfan's syndrome
   Ehlers-Danlos syndrome (type IV)
   Turner's syndrome
   Noonan's syndrome
   Familial aortic dissection
Hypertension
Pregnancy
Cystic medial degeneration
Bicuspid aortic valve
Atherosclerosis
Aortitis
Iatrogenic
   Cardiopulmonary bypass
   Aortotomy
   Arteriography
   Intra-aortic balloon pump

echocardiography as well as magnetic resonance imaging and computed tomography (Table 1-9).[48] In these studies, they found that transthoracic echocardiography cannot be relied on to evaluate dissections of the arch and descending aorta. Magnetic resonance imaging proved the most accurate in diagnosis of all thoracic dissections. There may, however, be practical limitations in obtaining an emergency magnetic resonance imaging study in an acutely ill patient in some institutions. Computed tomography and transesophageal echocardiography used together can provide highly specific and reliable diagnostic information in the emergency situation. The incidence of coronary disease in association with ascending dissection is very low and therefore coronary angiography is not essential unless there is an ischemic history that warrants investigation preoperatively.

and may have different management from those identified acutely.

The precise diagnosis of aortic dissection can be enigmatic. In the past aortography was considered essential to define the entry point and extent of dissection. Recently, Nienaber and coworkers studied the accuracy of transthoracic and transesophageal

Natural History and Treatment of Aortic Dissection

The important contributions of Daily and coworkers and Wheat have defined the roles for medical and surgical therapy in acute aortic dissection.[46,47] Table 1-10 lists the mortality of patients with type A

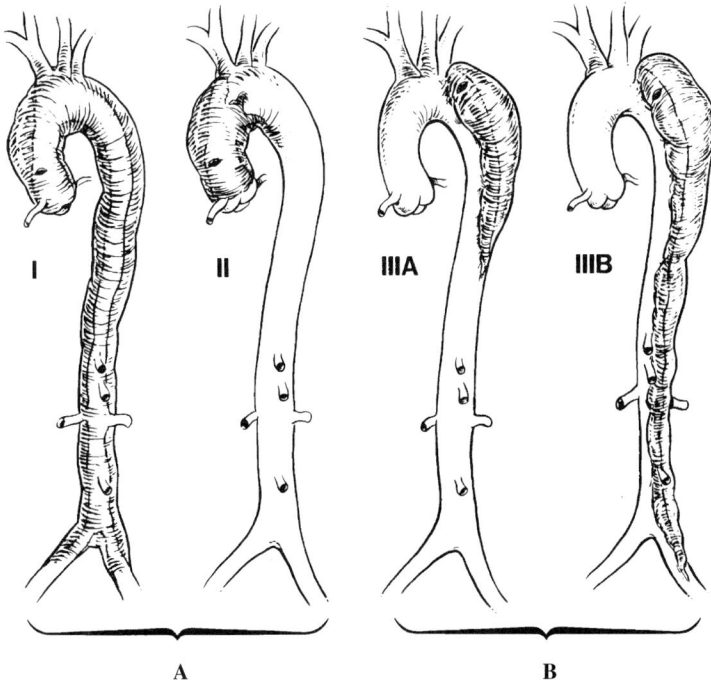

I   **II**   **IIIA**   **IIIB**

A   **B**

Figure 1-10. Classification of aortic dissection. The DeBakey scheme (types I, II, IIIA, and IIIB) describes the site of intimal tear and extent of dissection. The Stanford classification (type A and type B) is based on the presence or absence of ascending dissection. (Modified with permission from ME DeBakey, CH McCollum, ES Crawford, et al. Dissection and dissecting aneurysms of the aorta: twenty-year follow-up of five hundred twenty-seven patients treated surgically. Surgery 1982;92:1118; and DC Miller, EB Stinson, PE Oyer, et al. Operative treatment of aortic dissections. J Thorac Cardiovasc Surg 1979;78:365.)

Table 1-9. Identification of Thoracic Aortic Dissection According to Imaging Procedure

Imaging Procedure	Sensitivity (Percentage)	Specificity (Percentage)	Positive Predictive Value (Percentage)	Negative Predictive Value (Percentage)
Ascending dissection				
TTE	78.1	86.7	71.4	90.3
TEE	96.4	85.7	81.8	97.3
CT	82.6	100.0	100.0	93.3
MRI	100.0	98.7	96.8	100.0
Arch dissection				
TTE	35.7	97.4	83.3	80.4
TEE	95.0	93.6	86.4	97.8
CT	89.5	96.7	89.5	96.7
MRI	96.1	100.0	100.0	98.7
Descending dissection				
TTE	31.3	100.0	100.0	59.8
TEE	97.1	94.4	94.3	97.1
CT	90.2	86.8	88.1	89.2
MRI	98.0	100.0	100.0	98.1

TTE = transthoracic echocardiography; TEE = transesophageal echocardiography; CT = computed tomography; MRI = magnetic resonance imaging.
Source: Modified from CA Nienaber, Y von Kodolitsch, V Nicolas, et al. The diagnosis of thoracic aortic dissection by noninvasive imaging procedures. N Engl J Med 1993;328:1.

and type B dissections managed medically and surgically. In general, descending dissection is managed medically unless a complication arises. Loss of a pulse, visceral ischemia, rupture, aneurysm formation, and uncontrolled pain or hypertension are all complications that may indicate early surgical repair. Glower et al. have suggested that there may be an even greater role for operative therapy in descending dissection in patients with low operative risk and no complicating features.[49] Chronic aortic dissection is managed surgically when the complications of aortic dilatation, branch occlusion, and aortic insufficiency develop.

Table 1-10. Medical and Surgical Therapies of Thoracic Aortic Dissection: Mortality by Site and Therapy

Site	Medical Therapy (Percentage)	Surgical Therapy (Percentage)
Ascending	83	38
Descending	22	36

Source: Modified from MW Wheat. Acute dissecting aneurysms of the aorta: diagnosis and treatment—1979. Am Heart J 1980;99:373.

Aortic Occlusive Disease

Ninety percent of the occlusive disease of the aorta itself and of its major branches is caused by atherosclerosis. Aortitis, aortic dissection, neoplastic obstruction, and trauma account for the remaining 10%. Leriche's syndrome refers to the characteristic symptoms caused by chronic obstruction of the aortic bifurcation and iliac arteries. Typically there is claudication in the low back, buttocks, and thighs. Men also frequently report impotence. Because collateral circulation around the aortic bifurcation is abundant and the obstruction develops gradually, distal gangrene is unusual unless there is coexistent distal arterial disease. Treatment is directed at restoration of distal pressure and flow with anatomic and extra-anatomic bypass techniques.

Acute obstruction of the aorta is generally the result of embolism or proximal dissection. Emboli of sufficient size to obstruct the distal aorta usually arise from the chambers of the heart or occasionally from the atherosclerotic wall of the proximal aorta. Acute aortic obstruction is a surgical emergency that requires embolectomy and occasionally a reconstructive procedure.

Aortic Embolic Disease

Distal embolization from atherosclerotic debris from the aortic wall can occur spontaneously or can be the result of surgical manipulation of the aorta. Repetitive cholesterol embolization from the wall of the abdominal or thoracic aneurysm can cause localized distal gangrene. Anticoagulation does not generally provide protection from this type of embolization and resection is required to prevent recurrent distal vascular occlusion and gangrene.

Surgical manipulation of the ascending aorta during cardiac surgery is a major cause of cerebrovascular and other embolic injuries. There is currently no definitive technique to recognize and prevent inadvertent embolization from the atherosclerotic ascending aorta. Mills and Everson have characterized the patterns of ascending atherosclerosis and suggested techniques for intraoperative management (Figure 1-11).[50] Mills' type II and type III ascending atherosclerosis may be missed if they are not carefully sought. Careful review of the cardiac catheteri-

zation and chest radiography may give clues to the presence of calcium in the aorta. Surgical palpation and intraoperative transesophageal echocardiography should also be used routinely. Barzilai and colleagues have advocated routine epiarterial and epicardial echocardiography to increase the sensitivity of the examination.[51] Modification of the technique of operation when aortic atherosclerotic disease is identified during coronary bypass can reduce the incidence of intraoperative systemic embolization.

Aortic Trauma

Transection of the aorta can result from closed chest injuries that cause sudden deceleration of the chest wall and expose the intrathoracic contents to torsion and shearing stresses at points of relative fixation.[52] Eighty percent of patients sustaining an aortic deceleration injury die from exsanguination within an hour of the injury. Of the remaining patients, only 1% survive more than 2 weeks and go on to develop

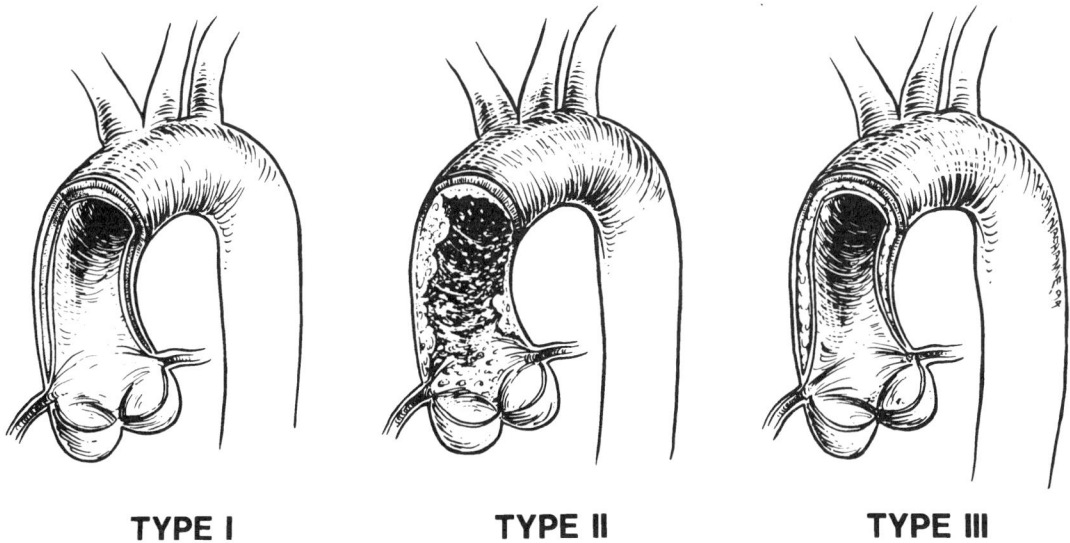

TYPE I   **TYPE II**   **TYPE III**

Figure 1-11. Mills' classification of aortic atherosclerosis. Type I: Porcelain aorta. Calcified media that is generally visible on fluoroscopy or plain radiography. This type is palpable and may be associated with little intimal disease. The surgeon risks cracking the vessel during clamp application. Type II: Irregular raised, ragged and friable atheromatous debris replacing the intima. This type may be discovered on transesophageal or epiarterial echo. Clamping results in massive, multiple emboli. Type III: Smooth, but thickened, liquefied intima. This type is the most elusive of the three and may be suggested by thickening of the wall of the aorta and a pale appearance of the adventia. Clamping results in liberation of liquid debris. (Modified with permission from NL Mills, CT Everson. Atherosclerosis of the ascending aorta and coronary artery bypass. J Thorac Cardiovasc Surg 1991;102:546.)

a chronic pseudoaneurysm. For those who make it to the hospital alive, survival is dependent on prompt recognition and treatment.

The aortic isthmus (that portion between the left subclavian artery and the ligamentum arteriosum) is characteristically the site of disruption. The deceleration injury has a predilection for this area because it is a natural site of shearing and torsional aortic wall stress between the mobile transverse aorta and the fixed descending segment. The hematoma may be initially contained by the mediastinal pleura and will rupture freely with the slightest provocation. In a small percentage of patients, the tear is just above the aortic valve or just proximal to the innominate artery. Disruption in the distal aorta at the diaphragm or in the abdomen is much less common.

References

1. The Concise Columbia Encyclopedia (Microsoft Bookshelf). New York: Columbia University Press, 1991.

2. Williams PL, Warwick R, Dyson M, Bonnister LH. Angiology. In PL Williams, R Warwick (eds), Gray's Anatomy (36th ed). Philadelphia: Saunders, 1980.

3. Wadouh F, Lindemann EM, Arndt CF, et al. The arteria radicularis magna anterior as a decisive factor influencing spinal cord damage during aortic occlusion. J Thorac Cardiovasc Surg 1984;88(Suppl 1):1.

4. Wolinsky H, Glagov S. Comparison of abdominal and thoracic aortic medial structure in mammals. Circ Res 1969;25:677.

5. Mahowald JM, Blieden LC, Coe JI, Edwards JE. Ectopic origin of a coronary artery from the aorta: sudden death in 3 of 23 Patients. Chest 1986;89:668.

6. White JV, Hass K, Phillips S, Comerota AJ. Adventitial elastolysis is a primary event in aneurysm formation. J Vasc Surg 1993;17(Suppl 2):371.

7. Rizzo RJ, McCarthy WJ, Dixit SN, et al. Collagen types and matrix protein content in human abdominal aortic aneurysms. J Vasc Surg 1989;10:365.

8. Cardiovascular System. In J Langman (ed), Medical Embryology (4th ed). Baltimore: Williams & Wilkins, 1981;157.

9. Ross R. Factors Influencing Atherogenesis. In JW Hurst, RC Schlant, CE Rackley, et al (eds), The Heart Arteries and Veins (7th ed). New York: McGraw-Hill, 1990;877.

10. Coselli JS, Crawford ES. Aortic valve replacement in the patient with extensive calcification of the ascending aorta (the porcelain aorta). J Thorac Cardiovasc Surg 1986;91:184.

11. Lindsay J, Beall AC, DeBakey ME. Diseases of the Aorta. In JW Hurst, RC Schlant, CE Rackley, et al (eds), The Heart Arteries and Veins (7th ed). New York: McGraw-Hill, 1990;1408.

12. Porter JM, Taylor LM, Harris EJ. Nonarteriosclerotic Arterial Disease. In LJ Greefield, MW Mulholland, KT Oldham, GB Zelenock (eds), Surgery: Scientific Principles and Practice. Philadelphia: Lippincott, 1993;1458.

13. Perejda AJ, Abraham PA, Carnes W, et al. Marfan's syndrome: structural, biochemical and mechanical studies of aortic media. J Lab Clin Med 1985;106:376.

14. Hunter GC, Malone JM, Moore WS, et al. Vascular manifestations in patients with Ehlers-Danlos syndrome. Arch Surg 1982;117:495.

15. Gable DS, Stoddard LD. Acute bacterial aortitis resulting in an aortoesophageal fistula. A fatal complication of untreated esophageal carcinoma. Pathol Res Pract 1989;184:318.

16. Osler MC, Brener BJ, Buda JA. A ten-year experience with bacterial aortitis. J Vasc Surg 1989;10:439.

17. Schwartz JA, Powell TW, Burnham SJ, Johnson G Jr. Culture of abdominal aortic aneurysm contents. An additional series. Arch Surg 1987;122:177.

18. Nakashima H, Takahara A, Yoshioka M, et al. A case of left coronary ostial obstruction due to syphilitic aortitis. Kokyu To Junkan 1991;39:831.

19. Gore I. Blood and Lymphatic Vessels. In WA Anderson (ed), Pathology (6th ed). St. Louis: Mosby 1971;728.

20. MacLeon DB, Johnson D, Frable WJ. "Tree-barking" of the ascending aorta. Syphilis or systemic lupus erythematosus? Am J Clin Pathol 1992;97:58.

21. Lie JT. The classification and diagnosis of vasculitis in large- and medium-sized blood vessels. Pathol Annu 1987;22:125.

22. Arend WP, Michel BA, Block DA, et al. The American College of Rheumatology 1990: criteria for the classification of Takayasu arteritis. Arthritis Rheum 1990;33:1129.

23. DeSanctis RW, Doroghazi RM, Austen WG, Buckley MJ. Aortic dissection. N Engl J Med 1987;317:1060.

24. Brown PM, Pattenden R, Gutelius JR. The selective management of small abdominal aortic aneurysms: The Kingston Study. J Vasc Surg 1992;15:21.

25. Ouriel K, Green RM, Donayre C, et al. An evaluation of new methods of expressing aortic aneurysm size: relationship to rupture. J Vasc Surg 1992;15:12.

26. Cohen JR, Graver LM. The ruptured abdominal aortic aneurysm of Albert Einstein. Surg Gynecol Obstet 1990;170:455.

27. Cooley DA, DeBakey ME. Resection of the entire ascending aorta in fusiform aneurysm using cardiac bypass. JAMA 1956;162:1158.

28. Ikonomidis JS, Weisel RD, Mouradian MS, et al. Thoracic aortic surgery. Circulation 1991;84(Suppl 3):1.

29. Ottino G, Biratta L, Del Ponte S, et al. Ascending aortic aneurysms: composite conduit replacement. Texas Heart Institute Journal 1984;11:338.

30. Kidd JN, Reul GJ, Cooley DA, et al. Surgical treatment of aneurysms of the ascending aorta. Circulation 1976;54(Suppl 3):18.

31. David TE. Aortic valve repair in patients with Marfan's syndrome and ascending aneurysms due to degenerative disease. J Card Surg 1994;9(Suppl 2):182.

32. McNamara JJ, Pressler BM. Natural history of arteriosclerotic thoracic aortic aneurysms. Ann Thorac Surg 1978;26:468.

33. Crawford ES, Hess KR, Cohen ES, et al. Ruptured aneurysm of the descending thoracic and thoracoabdominal aorta. Analysis according to size and treatment. Ann Surg 1991;213:417.

34. Bickerstaff LK, Pairolero PC, Hollier LH, et al. Thoracic aortic aneurysms: a population-based study. Surgery 1982;92:1103.

35. McNamara JJ, Pressler V. Natural history of arteriosclerotic thoracic aneurysms. Ann Thorac Surg 1978;26:468.

36. Crawford ES, Crawford JL, Safi HJ, et al. Thoracoabdominal aortic aneurysms: preoperative and intraoperative factors determining immediate and long-term results of operations in 605 patients. J Vasc Surg 1986;3:389.

37. Bickerstaff LK, Hoolier LH, Van Peenen HJ, et al. Abdominal aortic anerysms: the changing natural history. J Vasc Surg 1984;1:6.

38. Martin P. On abdominal aortic aneurysms. J Cardiovasc Surg (Torino) 1978;19:597.

39. Cohen JR, Mandell C, Wise L. Characterization of human aortic elastase found in patients with abdominal aortic aneurysms. Surg Gynecol Obstet 1987;165:301.

40. Durham SJ, Steed DL, Moosa HH, et al. Probablility of rupture of an abdominal aortic aneurysm after an unrelated operative procedure: a prospective study. J Vasc Surg 1991;13:248.

41. Limet R. Determination du taux d'expansion et de l'incidence de rupture des aneurysmes de l'aorte abdominale. Bull Mem Acad R Med Belg 1992;147:253.

42. Svensson LG, Crawford S. Aortic dissection and aortic aneurysm surgery: clinical observations, experimental investigations, and statistical analyses part II. Curr Probl Surg 1992;29:923.

43. Murphy DA, Craver JM, Jones EL, et al. Recognition and management of ascending aortic dissection complicating cardiac surgical operations. J Thorac Cardiovasc Surg 1983;85:247.

44. DeBakey ME, McCollum CH, Crawford ES, et al. Dissection and dissecting aneurysms of the aorta: twenty-year follow-up of five hundred twenty-seven patients treated surgically. Surgery 1982;92:1118.

45. Miller DC, Stinson EB, Oyer PE, et al. Operative treatment of aortic dissections: experience with 125 patients over a sixteen-year period. J Thorac Cardiovasc Surg 1979;78:365.

46. Daily PO, Trueblood HW, Stinson EB, et al. Management of acute aortic dissection. Ann Surg 1970;10:237.

47. Wheat MW. Acute dissecting aneurysms of the aorta: diagnosis and treatment—1979. Am Heart J 1980;99:373.

48. Nienaber CA, von Kodolitsch Y, Nicolas V, et al. The diagnosis of thoracic aortic dissection by noninvasive imaging procedures. N Engl J Med 1993;328:1.

49. Glower DD, Fann JI, Speir RH, et al. Comparison of medical and surgical therapy for uncomplicated descending aortic dissection. Circulation 1990;82(Suppl 4):39.

50. Mills NL, Everson CT. Atherosclerosis of the ascending aorta and coronary artery bypass. J Thorac Cardiovasc Surg 1991;102:546.

51. Barzilai B, Marshall WB Jr, Saffitz JE, Kouchoukos N. Avoidance of embolic complications by ultrasonic characterization of the ascending aorta. Circulation 1989;80:275.

52. Parmley LF, Mattingly TW, Manion WC, et al. Nonpenetrating traumatic injury of the aorta. Circulation 1958;17:1086.

Chapter 2

Preoperative Evaluation of the Patient with Aortic Disease

Thomas R. Eide and Michael B. Simon

Perioperative Risk Assessment

Risk is the exposure to a harm or loss. In a surgical patient this is the possible morbidity or mortality the patient is exposed to as a result of receiving an anesthetic and undergoing a surgical procedure. Studies that attempt to define and quantitate morbidity and mortality based on patient characteristics form the basis for understanding risk. These studies are extremely valuable in that they clarify which of the many conditions or disease states are important predictors of outcome. This "risk stratification" allows clinicians and researchers to specifically address certain patient characteristics in order to improve outcome.

Perioperative risk assessment is important in aortic surgical patients due to the large incidence of coronary disease in this patient population and to the urgency and inherent mortality of untreated aneurysmal disease. It should also be appreciated that most of the literature on risk assessment, coronary artery disease, and patient outcome tends to address vascular surgical patients as a group and only occasionally singles out patients with abdominal aortic disease. Furthermore, it is unusual for studies to include patients with diseases of the thoracic aorta or to distinguish between patients with atherosclerotic disease and aneurysmal disease of the abdominal aorta. Most of the comments about aortic surgical patients should be clearly understood to be derived from studies from vascular surgical patients as a group unless specifically stated to be about aortic surgical patients.

Coronary Artery Disease in the Aortic Surgical Patient

Coronary artery disease continues to represent the largest and most clinically significant factor contributing to perioperative morbidity and anesthetic management decisions in the aortic surgical patient. There is a highly significant relationship between the presence of coronary artery disease and patients evaluated for and undergoing major vascular surgical procedures. In a series[1] of 1,000 vascular surgical patients beginning in 1978 at the Cleveland Clinic, 25% were found to have severe, correctable coronary disease. Within this group, only 34% of patients were suspected by history and clinical findings of having coronary disease. Severe correctable coronary disease was found in 31% of patients whose primary vascular diagnosis was abdominal aortic aneurysm, in 26% of patients with cerebral vascular disease, and in 21% of patients with lower extremity disease.[2] There is no doubt that coronary artery disease in aortic surgical patients continues to be the most profound factor affecting intraoperative management and postoperative outcome.

Myocardial Ischemia

Myocardial ischemia occurs in a large percentage of aortic surgical patients. In a prospective study by Baron and coworkers[3] of 457 patients undergoing abdominal aortic surgery, 19% developed postoperative cardiac complications that included prolonged myocardial ischemia, congestive failure, ventricular arrhythmias, and myocardial infarction (MI). Eisenberg and colleagues[4] monitored for intraoperative myocardial ischemia using the 12-lead electrocardiogram (ECG) and transesophageal echocardiography in 332 noncardiac surgical patients who were considered at high risk for coronary artery disease by such inclusion criteria as the need for vascular surgery, hypertension, diabetes, a Q wave on the ECG, or a history of angina. They found that 39% of patients developed an episode of myocardial ischemia. The study of Raby and coworkers[5] of elective vascular surgical patients who had ECG monitors before, during, and after surgery showed that 18% of patients developed intraoperative myocardial ischemia and that 30% developed myocardial ischemia during the postoperative period.

Many studies now indicate that the majority of perioperative cardiac ischemic episodes occurs postoperatively and that patients with perioperative ischemic episodes are at risk for postoperative cardiac events and have poorer outcomes. Mangano and colleagues[6] prospectively studied 474 men with coronary artery disease undergoing elective noncardiac surgery and found that 41% had ECG findings of myocardial ischemia during the postoperative period as compared with 20% before surgery and 25% during surgery. In another study, Mangano and colleagues[7] also found that postoperative myocardial ischemia within 48 hours after surgery conferred a ninefold increase in the risk of cardiac death, a nonfatal MI, or unstable angina. Long-term follow-up of this group found that the occurrence of a postoperative ischemic episode and a postoperative adverse cardiac event greatly increased the risk for a subsequent cardiac complication over a 2-year period.

Myocardial Infarction

The risk of perioperative MI has a major impact on the management of aortic surgical patients. The rate of perioperative MI in studies of vascular surgical patients that included peripheral, carotid, and aortic disease and emergency procedures,[8,9] has been found to range from 0.7% to 3.9%, with an overall rate of 2–3% found most consistently.

It has been shown that MI has a significant impact on overall outcome in postsurgical follow-up studies.

In a group of 273 patients who underwent lower extremity revascularization, fatal MI occurred in 3.3% of patients and accounted for 52% of the deaths that occurred within 30 days of surgery.[10] In 335 patients undergoing carotid endarterectomy, fatal MI accounted for 60% of early postoperative deaths and occurred postoperatively in 1.8% of patients.[11] In 343 patients who underwent repair of an abdominal aortic aneurysm, fatal MI accounted for 37% of all postoperative deaths and occurred in 6% of patients.[12]

These studies consistently show that the rate of perioperative MI is significant in all vascular surgical patients and represents a major cause of perioperative and long-term morbidity and mortality.

Risk Stratification

In a risk stratification strategy proposed by Eagle and coworkers,[13] patients with no clinical indicators for coronary disease would probably not benefit from additional laboratory tests. In patients whose clinical symptoms already indicate that they have unstable coronary disease, therapy, not additional risk stratification, is needed. In patients with one or two clinical indicators of coronary disease, however, additional noninvasive testing can identify which patients are truly at high risk (e.g., patients with large areas of myocardium susceptible to infarction). In this intermediate group of patients overall risk may be decreased by coronary angiography and either coronary angioplasty or coronary bypass surgery prior to elective aortic surgery. This strategy, however, remains controversial as few studies have rigorously looked at the merits of coronary bypass or angioplasty before elective aortic surgery.

Clinical Factors for Identifying Risk of Poor Outcome

Performing coronary arteriography on all aortic surgical patients is currently not recommended as an initial means to evaluate cardiac status due to intrinsic procedural risks and increased cost. Identifying patients at risk for perioperative cardiac events by means other than coronary arteriography and understanding the nature of perioperative myocardial ischemia are important in assessing risk and taking steps to minimize perioperative morbidity.

Many clinical characteristics common in vascular surgical patients have been studied as predictors of perioperative myocardial ischemia and poor outcome. The presence of left ventricular hypertrophy on ECG, hypertension, diabetes mellitus, the known presence of coronary artery disease (i.e., angina, heart failure, previous MI) and the use of digoxin have been identified as significant predictors of perioperative cardiac morbidity.[14] These risk factors are also common in the aortic surgical patient population.

Goldman et al.,[15] Detsky et al.,[16] Eagle et al.,[13] and others have constructed weighted clinical risk scales that attempt to predict risk for perioperative cardiac complications (Table 2-1). Recurring risk indicators in the many studies that have attempted to use clinical factors as predictors of postoperative outcome are prior MI, cardiac failure, preoperative ventricular arrhythmias, and preoperative hypertension.

Clinical Risk Factors and Preoperative Recommendations

Prior Myocardial Infarction

Patients with a history of a prior MI have a higher rate of perioperative reinfarction when compared with patients without a prior MI (5–7% compared with 0.1–0.5% for general surgical patients). Rao and colleagues[17] studied two groups of patients who had a previous MI and were undergoing noncardiac surgery. Their first group was a retrospective review of 364 patients from 1973–1976. This group had a reinfarction rate of 7.7%. A second group of 733 patients followed prospectively from 1977–1982 had a reinfarction rate of 1.9%. This second group of patients was managed with arterial lines, pulmonary artery catheters, a 3- to 4-day stay in a postoperative intensive care unit, and aggressive intraoperative control of blood pressure (BP) and heart rate. This study implies that optimization of cardiovascular status, invasive monitoring, and aggressive intervention and control of intraoperative hemodynamic parameters served to dramatically reduce the rate of reinfarction in these patients.

The study by Rao and colleagues[17] also addressed the length of delay of elective surgery that would be prudent after a recent MI. In their prospectively followed group, the rate of reinfarction after surgery was 5.7% in patients with an infarct less than 3 months before surgery and 2.3% in patients with an infarction of 4–6 months. Steen and colleagues[18] found reinfarction rates of 27% for an MI occurring less than 3 months before surgery and 11% for an MI occurring 4–6 months before surgery. These percentages are much less in comparison with many other studies that address the rate of reinfarction relative to the length of time between an MI and elective surgery. Despite the large differences in rates found in this study as compared with other studies, nearly all studies have found that waiting 3 months after an MI before proceeding with elective surgery significantly reduces the risk of reinfarction. Waiting 6 months further decreases the risk of reinfarction, but to a lesser degree.

Cardiac Failure

The presence of impaired cardiac function, which can be determined clinically by evidence of pulmonary congestion, an S_3, or jugular venous distension, or measured as an ejection fraction by an imaging technique, is widely recognized as a significant factor associated with perioperative morbidity. The multifactorial index of Goldman and colleagues[15] that measures cardiac risk in noncardiac surgery ascribes the highest number of risk points to the presence of jugular venous distension or an S_3. In the study by Mangano and colleagues[7] of long-term cardiac events following noncardiac surgery, the presence of preexisting congestive failure was found to correlate with adverse cardiac events for the in-hospital period and for up to 2 years after discharge. In a large study[19] of preoperative predictors of perioperative adverse outcomes in 17,201 patients, a history of congestive heart failure carried a 7.3% risk of a severe outcome event (e.g., myocardial ischemia, MI, cardiac failure, respiratory failure, or bronchospasm).

Cardiac failure in a surgical patient should be treated aggressively and well in advance of the surgical procedure with every reasonable effort made to optimize cardiac performance.

Ventricular Arrhythmias

In a patient population considered at risk for coronary artery disease, the presence of asymptomatic ventricular arrhythmias (frequent premature ventric-

Table 2-1. Clinical Risk Factors for a Perioperative Cardiac Event for Noncardiac Surgery

Goldman Index	Detsky Index	Eagle Risk Factors
S_3 or jugular venous distension	Prior myocardial infarction	Congestive heart failure
Myocardial infarction <6 months	Emergency surgery	Angina
Premature ventricular contractions >5/minute	Angina (Canadian Cardiovascular Society Class 3 or 4)	Prior myocardial infarction
Nonsinus rhythm	Unstable angina—last 3 months	Diabetes
Age >70 years	Pulmonary edema	Q wave on electrocardiogram
Intra-abdominal, intrathoracic, or aortic surgery	Critical aortic stenosis	
Emergency surgery	Nonsinus rhythm or atrial premature contractions	
Significant aortic stenosis	Premature ventricular contractions >5/minute	
Poor general medical condition	Age >70 years	

Source: Modified from L Goldman, DL Caldera, SR Nussbaum, et al. Multifactorial index of cardiac risk in noncardiac surgical procedures. N Engl J Med 1977;297:845; AS Detsky, HB Abrams, N Forbath, et al. Cardiac assessment for patients undergoing noncardiac surgery: a multifactorial clinical risk index. Arch Intern Med 1986;146:2131; and KA Eagle, DE Singer, DC Brewster, et al. Dipyridamole-thallium scanning in patients undergoing vascular surgery. JAMA 1987;257:2185.

ular contractions or ventricular tachycardia) is regarded as a manifestation of underlying cardiac pathology. The aortic surgical patient population, however, is already presumed to be at a significantly increased risk for cardiac disease, and the presence of perioperative ventricular arrhythmias may not, by itself, be an independent marker for further increased risk of an adverse cardiac outcome. Shah and colleagues[20] prospectively studied 688 patients with coronary artery disease undergoing noncardiac surgery and found no correlation between arrhythmias and perioperative MI. This study, as with most previous studies addressing the significance of arrhythmias, did not continuously record the ECG on patients throughout surgery. In a more recent study using continuous Holter monitoring beginning 24 hours preoperatively, O'Kelly and colleagues[21] prospectively followed 230 major noncardiac surgical patients with known or presumed cardiac disease. They found that ventricular arrhythmias were common, occurring in 44% of patients, and that there was no relationship between ventricular arrhythmias and perioperative MI or in-hospital cardiac death. Increased intraoperative arrhythmias were associated with preoperative arrhythmias and preoperative congestive failure and were found during new episodes of myocardial ischemia.

There is a need to make reasonable recommendations for patients with asymptomatic ventricular arrhythmias and patients receiving chronic antiarrhythmic therapy. Asymptomatic patients found to have ventricular arrhythmias not thought secondary to ongoing ischemia are not considered to be at increased risk for an adverse cardiac outcome.

The physiologic changes (e.g., alterations in blood pCO_2, pH, electrolytes, temperature, and sympathetic activity) that are intrinsic to the induction of general anesthesia and the perioperative period can increase arrhythmia activity and may require intraoperative treatment with an antiarrhythmic agent. Patients with these changes should have their ECG monitored continuously for a least 24 hours postoperatively to demonstrate a return to baseline arrhythmia activity, but they need not be committed to chronic antiarrhythmic therapy.

Patients currently on chronic antiarrhythmic therapy should continue their medications up to surgery and may require intravenous supplementation of their medications during the procedure (depending on the length of surgery and the half-life of the agents) to maintain therapeutic blood levels.

Hypertension

Hypertension is commonly found in patients presenting for aortic surgery and especially in those presenting for emergency aortic surgery, such as the patient presenting with a dissecting aortic aneurysm.

Interpreting outcome studies of hypertensive disease is inherently difficult. The definition of a controlled BP varies from study to study and includes subsets of patients whose medications have multiple effects (e.g., antihypertensive, anti-ischemic, and antiarrhythmic) in addition to medications with only antihypertensive effects. These agents variably affect cardiac output, systemic vascular resistance, intravascular volume status, and sympathetic tone.

The degree of control of chronic hypertensive disease as a necessary preoperative step to minimize anesthetic risk and improve postoperative outcome remains controversial and unresolved. A history of hypertension was found to be an independent predictor of in-hospital mortality among patients undergoing noncardiac surgery by Browner and colleagues[22] and was found to be a predictor of postoperative myocardial ischemia by Hollenberg and colleagues.[14] However, it was not found to be a predictor of intraoperative or postoperative myocardial ischemia in vascular surgical patients by Raby and colleagues.[5] Prys-Roberts and coworkers[23] found that hypertension was associated with intraoperative lability of BP. However, in a large prospective study of both treated and untreated hypertensive patients, Goldman and Caldera[24] found that the patients did not develop more perioperative cardiac complications or postoperative renal failure, nor did they require more intraoperative fluid challenges or adrenergic agents to control BP decreases than normotensive patients.

The preoperative withdrawal of beta-antagonists and clonidine has been studied and found to result in intraoperative BP lability and to exacerbate anginal symptoms.[25,26] This is the basis for the general recommendation that antihypertensive medications should be continued and given on the morning of surgery.

When weighing the many conflicting results of studies of perioperative complications in patients with a history of hypertension, it cannot be determined whether the presence of hypertension, adequately treated or not, exposes the patient to more risk.

Nevertheless, common sense recommendations would seem to dictate that (1) patients on chronic antihypertensive medications should continue their medication up to and including the morning of surgery, (2) patients with inadequately treated BP (diastolic pressure >115 mm Hg) scheduled for elective surgery should have surgery postponed until their hypertension is controlled, (3) patients with a history of hypertension may have a more labile intraoperative course and require intraoperative antihypertensive medications, and (4) patients presenting for urgent or emergent aortic surgery for repair of dissecting aneurysms should have vigorous control of their BP together with reduction of cardiac output whenever possible prior to surgery as these may contribute to extension of the dissection or rupture of the aorta before the patient can present to the operating room.

It is clear that some cardiovascular conditions are more strongly associated with poor outcomes than others (e.g., congestive heart failure and ischemic heart disease as compared with chronic hypertension or arrhythmias). The optimization of a patient's cardiac and hemodynamic status before surgery remains important, however, and includes the establishment of appropriate and stable drug regimens for control of cardiac failure, ischemic heart disease, arrhythmias, and hypertension.

Laboratory Tests for Identifying Risk of Perioperative Myocardial Ischemia

The large incidence of coronary artery disease and the role it plays in perioperative morbidity in aortic surgical patients is well established. Patients with areas of myocardium at risk for ischemia or infarction can be identified with noninvasive laboratory testing. These tests are also associated with their own morbidity and economic costs, and therefore, many studies have sought to determine which test will most reliably identify those patients at risk for developing perioperative cardiac complications.

Table 2-2 presents the sensitivity and specificity of some commonly performed tests for detecting cardiac ischemia in a nonsurgical setting.[27–31] These different tests have been correlated to coronary pathology in an attempt to discern which test would be the most clinically useful and reliable. Sensitivities and specificities are expressed as ranges because the study populations differ. For example, when nuclear medicine tests (thallium) are judged against angiographic findings, the sensitivities and specificities are different for single vessel coronary disease than for multivessel coronary disease. The accuracy of these tests also depends on selection of the study group. Did the study population include

Table 2-2. Laboratory Tests for Identifying Patients with Coronary Artery Disease

Test	Sensitivity (Percentage)	Specificity (Percentage)
Exercise electrocardiography[27,28]	60–78	43–65
Dipyridamole-thallium scintigraphy[29,30]	72–100	80–88
Dobutamine-stress echocardiography[27,31]	79–96	66–91
Exercise thallium scintigraphy[28]	100	93
Exercise echocardiography[28]	93	96

or exclude patients with known coronary disease or major risk factors for coronary disease?

Specific Tests

Exercise Stress Testing

The use of exercise stress testing as a tool for identifying patients with significant coronary artery disease requires relatively inexpensive equipment and is simple to perform. This test places ECG-monitored patients on a treadmill and requires the attainment of a high percentage of a predicted maximal heart rate, usually 75–85%. Exercise testing requires a certain amount of physical endurance to achieve a targeted heart rate and patients with significant vascular disease are often not able to complete the test. In two studies by Cutler and coworkers[32] and McPhail and coworkers,[33] only 30–35% of patients were able to complete the stress test. Depending on the criteria used, the results of these studies also show a relatively low value, ranging from 11% to 24%, for predicting perioperative cardiac events, compared with other methods of laboratory investigation. Another study by McPhail and colleagues[34] compared exercise stress testing and dipyridamole-thallium imaging in 60 patients undergoing aortic surgery and found that exercise stress testing was a comparatively insensitive predictor for perioperative cardiac events.

Holter Monitor

Raby and colleagues[35] monitored 176 elective vascular surgical patients, who were not preselected on the basis of risk factors for coronary disease, through their operative course using Holter moni-

toring beginning 24 hours before surgery. They found that 18% of these patients had preoperative ischemic events, nearly all of which were asymptomatic. Of patients who had preoperative ischemic events, 38% had postoperative cardiac events (fatal and nonfatal MI and unstable angina) as compared with less than 1% of patients without preoperative ischemic events. In a similar study of 115 patients, Raby and colleagues[5] were able to show that preoperative Holter screening for ischemic events could identify a group of patients particularly at risk for postoperative cardiac events. In this study, 18% of patients had preoperative ischemia and 30% had postoperative ischemia. Preoperative ischemia was present in 57% of patients with postoperative ischemia as compared with only 4% without postoperative ischemia.

The use of Holter monitoring as a simple, risk-free, and cost-effective means of identifying patients at risk for perioperative cardiac events is promising. However, more investigation is required before the routine use of preoperative Holter monitoring can be recommended for this group of patients.

Dipyridamole-Thallium Scintigraphy

Dipyridamole-thallium scintigraphy (DTS) consists of an intravenous injection of dipyridamole, an agent that maximally dilates the coronary circulation, which diverts flow to nonstenosed coronary circulation at the expense of stenosed coronary circulation. (This can also be accomplished by the use of intravenous adenosine.) This "coronary steal phenomenon" is identified by injecting thallium 201, which distributes to regions of the myocardium in proportion to blood flow. The initial defects seen can represent old scarring or infarcts. These defects are reexamined 4 hours later (after the dipyridamole effect is gone) for evidence of increased thallium uptake. If uptake has occurred in these areas, they are considered to represent regions of viable myocardium placed at risk due to the presence of coronary arterial stenosis. It is this redistribution phenomenon that indicates the presence of a significant coronary lesion.

Findings of studies on the usefulness of DTS in predicting adverse perioperative cardiac events have ranged from DTS being a highly sensitive and specific predictor of perioperative myocardial ischemia[36] to DTS having no predictive value.[37] However, most of the studies consistently point to the usefulness of DTS in its high negative predictive accuracy. That is, if no redistribution is found, the chances for an uneventful operative course are very high. In a study of 61 consecutive vascular surgical patients, Eagle and colleagues[13] found that perioperative cardiac events occurred in 8 of 18 patients who had redistribution on their DTS, as compared with no events in 43 patients with no redistribution on their DTS. Lette and coworkers,[38] in a study of 125 vascular surgical patients (89 of whom were aortic surgical patients), found that 13 of 62 patients with redistribution abnormalities had postoperative cardiac complications, whereas none of the 63 patients with no redistribution defect had postoperative cardiac complications. The value of DTS for risk stratification or as a routine screening test in aortic surgical patients without clinical risk factors of coronary disease, however, remains unproven as studies continually question its worth. For example, in their study of 457 consecutive aortic surgical patients Baron and colleagues[3] found that the only factors correlated with adverse cardiac outcome were age greater than 65 years and definite clinical evidence of coronary disease (i.e., angina, MI by history or ECG), and not DTS.

Ejection Fraction

The left ventricular ejection fraction can be measured by echocardiography or by a nuclear medicine test that is called *gated blood pool scanning*. The nuclear medicine test is done by injecting in vitro radiolabeled red blood cells and analyzing the radioactive counts from the end-systolic and end-diastolic points of the cardiac cycle.

It is a commonly held view that patients with impaired cardiac function (e.g., reduced left ventricular ejection fraction) are at an increased risk for developing postoperative cardiac complications, and studies have compared the value of using the preoperative ejection fraction to predict postoperative cardiac complications.

McPhail and coworkers[39] compared the use of dipyridamole-thallium imaging to ejection fraction to predict postoperative cardiac complications and found that thallium imaging had a higher sensitivity (91% as compared with 27%) but a similar specificity (79% as compared with 85%) when compared with reduced ejection fraction.

Other studies have not found measuring ejection fraction to be a worthwhile preoperative test for identifying patients at high risk of postoperative cardiac complications. An outcome study in aortic surgical patients by Baron and colleagues[3] comparing clinical indicators, dipyridamole-thallium imaging, and left ventricular ejection fraction obtained from gated blood pool imaging showed that a decreased preoperative left ventricular ejection fraction (<35%) was related only to postoperative cardiac failure and not to other major postoperative cardiac complications such as ischemia, infarction, or severe ventricular arrhythmias. Similarly, Franco and coworkers[40] found no relationship between preoperative ejection fraction and perioperative MI in peripheral vascular surgical patients.

Dobutamine-Stress Echocardiography

The earliest sign of new myocardial ischemia is considered to be the appearance of a new wall motion abnormality seen with echocardiography. Therefore, provoking an echocardiographic wall motion abnormality with the use of a chronotropic and inotropic agent such as dobutamine may reveal a group of patients at risk for the development of a perioperative ischemic event. Dobutamine is infused intravenously into patients (1–40 µg/kg/minute) to an end point of 85% maximal heart rate for a given age, or ischemic changes seen on ECG. The usefulness of this new test has been studied by Poldermans and colleagues.[41] In their study, patients with a negative dobutamine-stress echo (DSE) test result had no perioperative ischemic events (indicating a high negative predictive value);

however, only 19% of patients with a positive test result developed a perioperative ischemic event (indicating a low positive predictive value). Another study by Eichelberger and coworkers[42] demonstrated only a 45% positive predictive value.

From these results, it appears that this test may be useful only to exclude patients from the need for further risk assessment tests. A positive DSE result would still require further evaluation in order to reliably predict a perioperative ischemic event. Also, the DSE exposes the patient to some risk because these patients may develop angina or ventricular arrhythmias. This test is relatively new and needs considerably more study to assess its value for risk assessment.

Coronary Artery Bypass or Coronary Angioplasty Prior to Elective Aortic Surgery

A goal of identifying patients at high risk for perioperative cardiac complication is to intervene and optimize cardiac status. A definitive way to accomplish this is to perform coronary angiography and either percutaneous coronary angioplasty (PTCA) or bypass surgery, if anatomically possible, before elective aortic surgery. This should, in theory, improve perioperative outcome because there would be few, if any, areas of myocardium subject to the risk of perioperative ischemia or infarction.

In a study by Foster and colleagues[43] of 1,600 patients undergoing noncardiac surgery, operative mortality for patients without coronary artery disease was 0.5%, for those with coronary artery disease and no prior coronary bypass surgery the operative mortality was 2.4%, and for patients with coronary artery disease who underwent coronary artery bypass before the noncardiac surgery the operative mortality was 0.9%. In the study by Hertzer and colleagues[2] of coronary artery disease in peripheral vascular surgical patients, 130 patients who had a coronary artery bypass prior to vascular surgery had a surgical mortality of 0.8% as compared with a mortality of 2.0% in 796 patients who did not have coronary bypass surgery. In a study by Elmore and coworkers[44] of a total of 2,452 patients who underwent abdominal aortic aneurysm repair at the Mayo Clinic, perioperative MI occurred in 5.8% of 86 patients who had

prior coronary bypass and 0% of 14 patients with prior PTCA.

However, in reviewing the studies addressing prior coronary bypass or prior PTCA before aortic surgery, the following factors make overall conclusions difficult to draw:

1. The definitions of a bad outcome vary from study to study, making comparisons difficult (e.g., perioperative ischemic event—pulmonary edema, ventricular arrhythmia, angina, prolonged ischemia; perioperative ischemia seen on intraoperative ECG, Holter monitor, transesophageal ECG; MI; surgical mortality; cardiac mortality).
2. The larger studies were retrospective, spanning many years and beginning as early as the 1970s.
3. Overall surgical mortality has improved independently for aortic surgery as well as for coronary bypass surgery requiring larger numbers of study patients in order to draw meaningful conclusions.
4. PTCA has been performed extensively only since the late 1980s.
5. The patients selected to receive a coronary bypass before aortic surgery were selected because they had more severe cardiac symptoms and hence more severe coronary disease than those undergoing PTCA or those patients allowed to proceed with elective aortic surgery.

Coronary bypass grafting or percutaneous transluminal coronary angioplasty prior to aortic surgery for those patients with severe, correctable coronary artery disease is most probably beneficial. However, the benefit remains controversial because no large, randomized, prospective controlled studies have addressed the risks of elective aortic surgery with or without prior coronary artery bypass graft or PTCA.

Preoperative Pulmonary Dysfunction

Preoperative pulmonary dysfunction greatly affects the intraoperative course and postoperative pulmonary status of the patient. A history of smoking, sputum production, or obstructive or restrictive lung disease greatly contributes to perioperative pulmonary dysfunction. Reversible pulmonary conditions should be identified and corrected prior to elective aortic surgery.

Aortic surgery involves the administration of considerable amounts of intravenous fluid, often resulting in decreases in body temperature, and requires an extensive incision, which can result in postoperative pulmonary dysfunction. Computed tomography studies on patients with normal lungs have shown that patients administered general anesthesia with muscle relaxation and mechanical ventilation will develop atelectasis in dependent areas of the lungs in both the supine and lateral decubitus positions.[45] Further studies on patients with normal lungs have found that general anesthesia with muscle relaxation and mechanical ventilation causes a decrease in functional residual capacity,[46] cephalad displacement of the diaphragm, and a reduction of total thoracic volume.[47] This causes a mismatching of ventilation and perfusion that results in an increased shunt fraction and an impairment of arterial oxygenation.[48]

Preoperative pulmonary dysfunction and unresolved pulmonary diseases increase the likelihood of developing greater amounts of pulmonary and bronchial secretions, atelectasis, bronchospasm, and pneumonia. These conditions contribute negatively to the fundamental changes in pulmonary physiology that occur with the administration of a general anesthetic. In particular, any unresolved pulmonary condition will be a crucial factor in surgery for repair of a descending thoracic aortic aneurysm, because there is a surgical requirement for exposure of the descending thoracic aorta by deflation of the left lung with the use of a double-lumen endotracheal tube. One-lung ventilation with no gas exchange and continued blood flow through the nondependent lung will produce a large shunt fraction that may not be tolerated with an ongoing disease process in the dependent lung.

A preoperative respiratory history, pulmonary function testing such as a forced expiratory spirogram, and an arterial blood gas when impaired gas exchange is suspected will help identify patients at risk for postoperative complications. A forced vital capacity of less than 20 ml/kg, a forced expiratory volume in 1 second to forced vital capacity ratio of less than 50%, and signs and symptoms of pneumonia, bronchitis, or asthma place a patient at high risk for pulmonary dysfunction. Therapeutic interventions such as bronchodilators, cessation of smoking, preoperative chest physical therapy for the mobilization and clearance of bronchial secretions,

and antibiotic therapy for any suspected underlying bronchial or pulmonary infection will result in an improvement of vital capacity and reduce the possibility of developing intraoperative and postoperative pulmonary dysfunction.

Preoperative Renal Dysfunction

The incidence of renal failure as a complication of aortic surgery has not changed appreciably throughout the years.[49] Crawford and coworkers[50] identified preoperative renal insufficiency as the only independent significant determinant of postoperative renal failure. Hence, the evaluation of preoperative renal function is of prime importance for intraoperative management as well as for patient outcome.

Renal dysfunction has been shown to be present in 2–5% of all adult patients admitted to general medical and surgical services of major medical centers, while the development of new renal insufficiency in any hospitalized patient has been shown to be associated with a high mortality. Shusterman et al.[51] reported a 35% mortality for hospital-acquired renal failure. Other studies have reported mortalities in the range of 25–64%.[52–56] In addition, aortic surgery, in and of itself, predisposes the patient with normal preoperative renal function to renal failure as dramatic changes of blood flow to the kidneys occur with the application of a cross clamp to the aorta. Although no studies have specified any factor as being responsible for postoperative renal failure, decreased cardiac output, the location of the aortic cross clamp, cross-clamp time, and emboli of atheromatous plaque are probably all contributory.

Perioperative Outcome

Patients with preoperative renal dysfunction are at risk for the development of further postoperative renal impairment, potentially to the point of requiring dialysis. In a retrospective analysis of 26 patients undergoing abdominal aortic aneurysm repair, Cohen and coworkers[57] examined the effects of preoperative renal failure. They divided patients into three groups based on preoperative serum creatinine (Table 2-3). The data indicate that patients with moderate-to-severe preoperative renal dysfunction who have not yet come to require dialysis fare

Table 2-3. Postoperative Outcome in Patients with Renal Disease Undergoing
Abdominal Aortic Aneurysm Repair

Study Group	Preoperative Creatinine	Number of Patients in Each Group	Patients Requiring Postoperative Dialysis	30-Day Mortality (Number of Patients in Each Group)	One-Year Survival (Percentage of Each Preoperative Group)
I	2–4 mg/dl	16	0	0	100
II	>4 mg/dl and no dialysis	6	4	1	33
III	>4 with chronic dialysis	4	4	1	75

Source: Modified from JR Cohen, JA Mannick, NP Couch, Whittemore AD. Abdominal aortic aneurysm repair in patients with preoperative renal failure. J Vasc Surg 1986;3:867.

worse than either patients with known renal failure who receive chronic hemodialysis prior to surgery or those with mild renal dysfunction.

Patients who develop acute renal failure following aortic surgery have a significantly higher mortality than those who do not. The increased mortality accompanying renal failure has been reiterated by many studies, beginning with Crawford and coworkers[50] who reported that in a series of 39 patients undergoing repair of thoracoabdominal aortic aneurysms, 67% of those patients (26 of 39) died secondary to acute renal failure. Other studies have shown that patients who develop acute renal failure following aortic surgery have a significantly higher mortality than those who do not (Table 2-4).[58–62] Therefore, every attempt should be made to identify patients with compromised renal function to improve function when possible and to more accurately predict a patient's true perioperative risk.

Laboratory Abnormalities of Renal Insufficiency

The kidneys are responsible for the body's electrolyte and extracellular fluid homeostasis and possess intrinsic endocrine function. Under normal circumstances, the kidneys maintain a balance between solute and water intake and excretion as well as elimination of metabolic end products.

Electrolyte abnormalities can be seen to varying degrees in both acute and chronic renal dysfunction and in the setting of chronic dialysis. Table 2-5 lists some of the biochemical and electrolyte disturbances most often encountered with chronic renal failure.

Blood Urea Nitrogen and Serum Creatinine. Blood urea nitrogen (BUN) and serum creatinine are indicators of renal function but have limitations. BUN results from protein metabolism, but may become elevated in the face of dehydration, increased protein intake, gastrointestinal bleeding, accelerated tissue catabolism, and recent trauma or surgery. Another factor that makes BUN a poor indicator of renal function is its ability to be reabsorbed. This resorption is inversely proportional to urinary flow.

Serum creatinine results from the breakdown of skeletal muscle proteins, with a normal range of 0.5–1.2 mg/dl. Creatinine production varies with age, sex, and muscle mass, with a lower rate of production in the elderly and in women. In the range of 0.8–1.5, the serum creatinine is an insensitive marker of residual functional renal mass. However, an elevated creatinine (>1.5) is an indicator of the loss of significant renal function and not only should be investigated, but also conveys an increased risk for further deterioration of renal function during surgery on the aorta.

The collection of urine creatinine and the calculation of a creatinine clearance as an approximation of glomerular filtration rate allows for an accurate determination of renal function. A 2-hour urine sample has been deemed as accurate as a traditional 24-hour collection.[63] The following formula is applied: glomerular filtration rate = (U)(V)/P, where U = urinary concentration of creatinine (mg/dl); V = volume of urine (ml/minute); and P = plasma creatinine concentration (mg/dl).

Anemia. Anemia results from chronic renal failure and is present in the hemodialysis patient.

Table 2-4. Mortality for Aortic Aneurysm Surgery Complicated by Renal Dysfunction

	Total Number of Patients in the Study	Patients with Post-operative Renal Dysfunction	Perioperative Mortality (Percentage of Patients Who Developed Renal Dysfunction)
Crawford et al.[58]	717	44	25
Svensson et al.[59]	1,233	68	63
Olsen et al.[60]	656	81	58
Hesdorffer et al.[61]	61	6	67
Berisa et al.[62]	70	70	61

Anemia results from both a decrease in erythropoietin production[64] and a reduction in red blood cell survival time.[65] The patient with renal dysfunction may manifest a decreased hematocrit, yet tolerate this very well. Many physiologic changes occur as anemia progresses chronically. Blood viscosity decreases while organ perfusion increases. There is an accumulation of hydrogen ions and an increase in 2,3 diphosphoglycerate,[66] which causes a shift of the oxyhemoglobin dissociation curve to the right. These changes serve to maintain tissue oxygen delivery as the anemia progresses and eventually stabilizes.

The necessity to achieve a minimum hematocrit prior to surgery (i.e., 30%) has never been proven and remains controversial. Contributing to this unknown, the patient with chronic preoperative renal dysfunction has, to a large degree, adapted to a lower hematocrit. Efforts to enable presurgical patients to intrinsically increase their own hematocrit levels may prove beneficial. In two studies, Eschbach and colleagues[67,68] looked at the effects of recombinant human erythropoietin on the anemia resulting from progressive renal failure. They looked at patients who did not require hemodialysis, but had significantly impaired kidneys (serum creatinine > 4.0). Through their use of erythropoietin, they demonstrated an increase in the median hematocrit of ten percentage points. They also noted a "subjective improvement in well-being and appetite as [the patients'] hematocrits increased." Routine preoperative erythropoietin therapy to improve operative outcome has not been studied.

Platelet Dysfunction.   Renal insufficiency and failure results in the accumulation of bodily waste products that affect platelet function and often result in a prolongation of the bleeding time.[69]

Platelet activation involves the release of cytoplasmic granules whose contents include adenosine diphosphate (ADP), serotonin, catecholamines, and platelet factors.[70] Platelet factor III, factor VIII antigen, von Willebrand's factor, and ADP contribute to platelet aggregation and clot formation. In the face of renal dysfunction, platelets fail to release and respond to ADP.[71] Factor VIII and platelet factor III levels are decreased, further diminishing platelet function.

Factor VIII levels and platelet function can be increased through transfusion of either fresh frozen plasma or cryoprecipitate or with the use of arginine vasopressin. Janson and coworkers[72] examined the use of cryoprecipitate to correct prolonged bleeding times resulting from uremia. They found that cryoprecipitate infusion corrects bleeding times to normal within 24–36 hours, but fails to fully correct faulty platelet aggregation. Arginine vasopressin increases factor VIII and von Willebrand's factor and causes bleeding times to decrease in uremic patients.[73] Although dialysis may correct many of the biochemical abnormalities of uremia, platelet dysfunction does not always correct completely and

Table 2-5. Physiologic and Biochemical Disturbances of Renal Insufficiency

Elevated blood urea nitrogen and creatinine
Hypocalcemia
Hyperkalemia
Hypermagnesemia
Hyperphosphatemia
Hyperuricemia
Glucose intolerance
Anemia
Platelet dysfunction
Metabolic acidosis

bleeding times may remain prolonged.[74] This is an important issue to resolve preoperatively because the insertion of an epidural catheter has in recent years become increasingly popular for perioperative analgesia and early postoperative extubation.

Diabetes Mellitus

The kidney is to a great extent responsible for degrading and eliminating insulin, hence in chronic renal insufficiency, circulating insulin levels are increased. However, there is a peripheral insensitivity to the effects of insulin that results in a small but definable glucose intolerance.

A significant number of patients requiring aortic surgery are afflicted with diabetes, ranging from the mild, diet-controlled to the insulin-dependent. There is a significant interrelationship between diabetes, renal insufficiency, and atherosclerotic vascular disease. It is the pathology that develops in other organ systems in a patient with diabetes that contributes to increasing perioperative risk. The presence of diabetes and the management of glucose intolerance during surgery is an important aspect of both the intraoperative and postoperative care of the patient.

Diabetes is closely associated with hypertension, obesity, and abnormalities of lipid metabolism. Diabetes also encompasses additional concerns of poor wound healing and the increased incidence of wound complications.[75] These factors, in conjunction with the known association of coronary artery disease and diabetes, place the diabetic at a dramatically increased perioperative risk.

Preoperative Hemodynamic Optimization

There is a growing acceptance of the use of the intensive care unit preoperatively to optimize a patient's hemodynamic status prior to a major surgical procedure. This involves placing a pulmonary artery catheter and the use of inotropic and vasodilating agents such as dobutamine and sodium nitroprusside. The goal is to optimize systemic vascular resistance and cardiac output to achieve a total oxygen delivery of greater than 600 ml/min/m^2 (see Chapter 11).

The concept of preoperative hemodynamic optimization has been considered in the past. In 1968,

Thompson and colleagues[76] studied the value of preoperative volume loading. They found that by infusing balanced salt solution, both preoperatively and intraoperatively, they were able to significantly decrease the mortality resulting from renal failure. Bush and coworkers[77] advocated volume loading with pulmonary artery catheter monitoring as a preoperative intervention to minimize postoperative renal failure.

Shoemaker and coworkers[78] studied 98 patients undergoing "high-risk" surgical procedures and correlated organ system failure and mortality with an increased tissue oxygen consumption deficit. Berlauk and colleagues,[79] in a study of 89 patients undergoing limb-salvage arterial surgery, found that patients who had preoperative hemodynamic optimization had a lower mortality (3.4% as compared with 9.5%), and a lower rate of postoperative cardiac morbidity. Boyd and coworkers[80] divided a group of 107 high-risk surgical patients into two groups: (1) those who would have their oxygen delivery increased to 600 ml/min/m^2, and (2) a control group receiving standard perioperative care (without oxygen delivery and hemodynamic optimization). A lower mortality (5.7% as compared with 22.2%) with a lower rate of multiple organ system dysfunction was found in the study group. However, recently a study of 109 critically ill surgical and nonsurgical patients by Hayes and coworkers[81] contradicted these findings.

Preoperative Interview

Nonemergent Surgery

The preoperative evaluation of the surgical patient by the anesthesiologist is an important step in the preparation of the patient for surgery. It begins with an often overlooked, yet extremely important aspect—emotional and psychological preparation for surgery.

Most people are at the very least apprehensive when confronted with the acceptance of their own mortality, the loss of bodily control, possible permanent disability, and the thought of postsurgical pain. These are frightening unknowns. Hence, one of the primary purposes of the preoperative visit is to educate and reassure the patient. This is accomplished by demonstrating a competent and caring image and discussing in reasonable terms what the patient will experience on the day of surgery and in the intensive care unit during the postoperative period. Administering premedication agents cannot inform, educate, and reassure a patient. Premedication agents are not substitutes for the preoperative visit because there is no substitute for the personal interaction and reassurance the anesthesiologist can provide to the patient before the operation.

A major purpose of the preoperative evaluation is to gather information for assessing risk and formulating the anesthetic plan. The patient's medical and surgical history, physical examination, and laboratory data form the basis of the anesthetic plan and risk assessment.

A preoperative interview is conducted that seeks to identify medical and anesthetic issues that may contribute to perioperative morbidity. A thorough review of systems is performed, the past medical history, previous surgery including surgical and anesthetic complications, and current medications are noted. Objective laboratory results from the patient's chart (blood work, chest radiography, ECG, pulmonary studies) and informed consent for the anesthetic care to be provided are obtained. To provide informed consent, the anesthetic plan, along with possible complications, which are either common or severe, must be explained and discussed in language that the patient can understand.

Premedication prior to surgery is given for specific reasons such as to reduce gastric volume and acidity, provide amnesia and prophylaxis against nausea, relieve pain, and provide sedation to assist with relief of anxiety. Premedication can be accomplished with combinations of agents that have different pharmacologic properties and include H_2 antagonists, gastrokinetic agents (metoclopramide), anxiolytics (benzodiazepines), and analgesics (opioids). The agents prescribed depend not only on the patient's individual medical conditions, but significantly on the habits and traditions of individual practitioners and institutions.

Finally, a preoperative note is written in the patient's chart that briefly discusses the relevant medical and surgical histories, allergies, medications, and physical and laboratory findings. It is concluded with a statement of the informed consent, an assessment of physical status (ASA classification), and the invasive monitoring and type of anesthesia planned.

A safe, uneventful anesthetic and perioperative course together with the least possible perioperative morbidity is the desired goal.

Emergent Surgery

The patient brought to the operating room for emergent aortic aneurysmal surgery presents additional concern to the anesthesiologist. The key factor in this group of patients is how quickly they can be diagnosed with a life-threatening condition (dissecting or leaking aorta) and how quickly surgical control can be obtained. There may be little time for a standard preoperative history, review of systems, physical examination, or the gathering of laboratory data as anesthetic management is directed toward securing basic monitors (ECG, BP cuff, pulse oximeter) and intravenous lines to rapidly and safely anesthetize the patient for quick surgical intervention. However, during the stressful and challenging anesthesia of the emergency aortic surgical patient, a brief examination of the patient may provide additional important information that is unique to this group of patients.

An acute dissection of the aorta can involve any of the major arteries that arise from the thoracic and abdominal aorta. This can cause a decrease in perfusion to the brain (innominate and left carotid arteries), kidneys (renal arteries), spinal cord (intercostal arteries), or extremities. Dissection may progress back to the aortic valve to cause acute aortic regurgitation (with a new diastolic murmur) or cardiac tamponade from blood leaking into the pericardial sac. Depending on how much time is available, these conditions can be diagnosed prior to proceeding with anesthetic care and may have a great impact on a patient's anesthetic and surgical course.

Premedication issues in the patient requiring emergency aortic surgery must be tailored to the individual situation. These will usually be limited to treating the critical and immediate hemodynamic conditions directly related to a dissecting or leaking aorta and stabilizing hemodynamics as much as possible while an operating room is being made ready. The patient with an acute aortic dissection who is hemodynamically stable may require that hypertension and tachycardia be controlled to limit the extent of a dissection. This will be done in a critical care setting immediately prior to the operating room. There is usually little time to address the premedication issues of the emergent aortic surgical patient prior to surgery (amnesia, anxiety, gastric contents, analgesia), and these will have to be considered during the anesthetic and after surgical control has been obtained.

References

1. Hertzer NR. Clinical experience with preoperative coronary angiography. J Vasc Surg 1985;2:510.

2. Hertzer NR, Beven EG, Young JR, et al. Coronary artery disease in peripheral vascular patients. A classification of 1000 coronary angiograms and results of surgical management. Ann Surg 1984;199:223.

3. Baron JF, Mundler O, Bertrand M, et al. Dipyridamole-thallium scintigraphy and gated radionuclide angiography to assess cardiac risk before abdominal aortic surgery. N Engl J Med 1994;330:663.

4. Eisenberg MJ, London MJ, Leung JM, et al. Monitoring for myocardial ischemia during noncardiac surgery. JAMA 1992;268:210.

5. Raby KE, Barry J, Creager MA, et al. Detection and significance of intraoperative and postoperative myocardial ischemia in peripheral vascular surgery. JAMA 1992;268:222.

6. Mangano DT, Browner WS, Hollenberg M, et al. Association of perioperative myocardial ischemia with cardiac morbidity and mortality in men undergoing noncardiac surgery. N Engl J Med 1990,323:1781.

7. Mangano DT, Browner WS, Hollenberg M, et al. Long term cardiac prognosis following noncardiac surgery. JAMA 1992;268:233.

8. Bunt TJ. The role of a defined protocol for cardiac risk assessment in decreasing perioperative MI on vascular surgery. J Vasc Surg 1992;15:626.

9. Taylor LM, Yeager RA, Moneta GL, et al. The incidence of perioperative MI in general vascular surgery. J Vasc Surg 1992;15:52.

10. Hertzer NR. Fatal MI following lower extremity revascularization. Two-hundred seventy-three patients followed six to eleven postoperative years. Ann Surg 1981;193:492.

11. Hertzer NR. Fatal MI following abdominal aortic aneurysm resection. Three-hundred forty-three patients followed six to eleven years postoperatively. Ann Surg 1980;192:667.

12. Hertzer NR. Fatal MI following carotid endarterectomy. Three-hundred thirty-five patients followed six to eleven years after operation. Ann Surg 1981;194:212.

13. Eagle KA, Singer DE, Brewster DC, et al. Dipyridamole-thallium scanning in patients undergoing vascular surgery. JAMA 1987:257:2185.

14. Hollenberg M, Mangano DT, Browner WS, et al. Predictors of postoperative myocardial ischemia in patients undergoing noncardiac surgery. JAMA 1992;268:205.

15. Goldman L, Caldera DL, Nussbaum SR, et al. Multifactorial index of cardiac risk in noncardiac surgical procedures. N Engl J Med 1977;297:845.

16. Detsky AS, Abrams HB, Forbath N, et al. Cardiac assessment for patients undergoing noncardiac surgery: a multifactorial clinical risk index. Arch Intern Med 1986;146:2131.

17. Rao TL, Jacobs KH, El-Etr AA. Reinfarction following anesthesia in patients with MI. Anesthesiology 1983;59:499.

18. Steen PA, Tinker JH, Tarhan S. Myocardial reinfarction after anesthesia and surgery. JAMA 1978;239:2566.

19. Forrest JB, Rehder K, Cahalan MK, Goldsmith CH. Multicenter study of general anesthesia: III. Predictors of severe perioperative adverse outcomes. Anesthesiology 1992;76:3.

20. Shah KB, Kleinman BS, Rao TLK, et al. Angina and other risk factors in patients with cardiac diseases undergoing noncardiac operations. Anesth Analg 1990;70:240.

21. O'Kelly B, Browner WS, Massie B, et al. Ventricular arrhythmias in patients undergoing noncardiac surgery. JAMA 1992;268:217.

22. Browner WS, Li J, Mangano DT. In-hospital and long-term mortality in male veterans following noncardiac surgery. JAMA 1992;268:228.

23. Prys-Roberts C, Meloche R, Foex P. Studies of anaesthesia in relation to hypertension 1: cardiovascular responses of treated and untreated patients. Br J Anaesth 1971;43:122.

24. Goldman L, Caldera DL. Risks of general anesthesia and elective operation in the hypertensive patient. Anesthesiology 1979;50:285.

25. Miller RR, Olson HG, Amsterdam EA, Mason ST. Propranolol-withdrawal rebound phenomenon. Exacerbation of coronary events after abrupt cessation of anti-anginal therapy. N Engl J Med 1975;293:416.

26. Bruce DL, Croley TF, Lee JS. Preoperative clonidine withdrawal syndrome. Anesthesiology 1979;51:90.

27. Previtali M, Lanzarini L, Fetiveau R, et al. Comparison of dobutamine stress echocardiography, dipyridamole stress echocardiography and exercise stress testing for diagnosis of coronary artery disease. Am J Cardiol 1993;72:865.

28. Galanti G, Sciagra R, Comeglio M, et al. Diagnostic accuracy of peak exercise echocardiography in coronary artery disease: comparison with thallium 201 myocardial scintigraphy. Am Heart J 1991;122:1606.

29. Chikamori T, Doi Y, Yonezawa Y, et al. Coronary artery disease: noninvasive identification of significant narrowing of the left main coronary artery by dipyridamole thallium scintigraphy. Am J Cardiol 1991;68:472.

30. Jukema JW, van der Wall EE, van der Vis-Melsen MJ, et al. Dipyridamole thallium 201 scintigraphy for improved detection of left anterior descending coronary artery stenosis in patients with left bundle branch block. Eur Heart J 1993;14:53.
31. Marcovitz PA, Armstrong WF. Coronary artery disease: accuracy of dobutamine stress echocardiography in detecting coronary artery disease. Am J Cardiol 1992;69:1269.
32. Cutler BS, Wheeler HB, Paraskos JA, Cardullo PA. Applicability and interpretation of electrocardiographic stress testing in patients with peripheral vascular disease. Am J Surg 1979;137:484.
33. McPhail N, Calvin JE, Shariatmadar A, et al. The use of preoperative exercise testing to predict cardiac complications after arterial reconstruction. J Vasc Surg 1988;7:60.
34. McPhail N, Ruddy TD, Calvin JE, et al. A comparison of dipyridamole-thallium imaging and exercise stress testing in the prediction of postoperative cardiac complications in patients requiring arterial reconstruction. J Vasc Surg 1989;10:51.
35. Raby KE, Goldman L, Creager MA, et al. Correlation between preoperative ischemia and major cardiac events after peripheral vascular surgery. N Engl J Med 1989;321:1296.
36. Boucher CA, Brewster DC, Darling RC, et al. Determinations of cardiac risk by dipyridamole-thallium imaging before peripheral vascular surgery. N Engl J Med 1985;312:389.
37. Mangano DT, London J, Tubau F, et al. Dipyridamole thallium-201 scintigraphy as a preoperative screening test—a reexamination of its predictive potential. Circulation 1991;84:493.
38. Lette J, Waters D, Lassonde J, et al. Multivariate clinical models and quantitative dipyridamole-thallium imaging to predict cardiac morbidity and death after vascular reconstruction. J Vasc Surg 1991;14:160.
39. McPhail N, Ruddy TD, Calvin JE, et al. Comparison of left ventricular function and myocardial perfusion for evaluating perioperative cardiac risk of abdominal aortic surgery. Can J Surg 1990;33:224.
40. Franco CD, Goldsmith J, Veith FJ, et al. Resting gated pool ejection fraction: a poor predictor of perioperative MI in patients undergoing vascular surgery for infrainguinal bypass grafting. J Vasc Surg 1989;10:656.
41. Poldermans D, Fioretti PM, Forster T, et al. Dobutamine stress echocardiography for assessment of perioperative cardiac risk in patients undergoing major vascular surgery. Circulation 1993;87:1506.
42. Eichelberger JP, Schwarz KQ, Black EF, et al. Predictive value of dobutamine echocardiography just before noncardiac vascular surgery. Am J Cardiol 1993;72:602.
43. Foster ED, Davis KB, Carpenter JA, et al. Risk of noncardiac operation in patients with defined coronary disease: The Coronary Artery Surgery Study (CASS) registry experience. Ann Thorac Surg 1986;41:42.
44. Elmore JR, Hallett JW, Gibbons RJ, et al. Myocardial revascularization before abdominal aortic aneurysmorrhaphy: effect of coronary angioplasty. Mayo Clin Proc 1993;68:637.
45. Brismar B, Hedenstierna G, Lundquist H, et al. Pulmonary densities during anesthesia with muscular relaxation—a proposal of atelectasis. Anesthesiology 1985;62:422.
46. Hedenstierna G, Strandberg A, Brismar B, et al. What causes the lowered FRC during anesthesia? Clin Physiol 1985;5(Suppl 3):133.
47. Hedenstierna G, Strandberg A, Brismar B, et al. Functional residual capacity, thoracoabdominal dimensions, and central blood volume during general anesthesia with muscle paralysis and mechanical ventilation. Anesthesiology 1985;62:247.
48. Hedenstierna G, Tokics L, Strandberg A, et al. Correlation of gas exchange impairment to development of atelectasis during anaesthesia and muscle paralysis. Acta Anaesthesiol Scand 1986;30:183.
49. Abbott WM. Renal Failure Complicating Vascular Surgery. In VM Bernhard, JB Towne (eds), Complications in Vascular Surgery. New York: Grune & Stratton, 1980;3647.
50. Crawford ES, Crawford JL, Safi HJ, et al. Thoracoabdominal aortic aneurysms, preoperative and intraoperative factors determining immediate and long-term results of operations in 605 patients. J Vasc Surg 1986;3:389.
51. Shusterman N, Strom BL, Murray TG, et al. Risk factors and outcome of hospital acquired acute renal failure: clinical epidemiologic study. Am J Med 1987;83:65.
52. McMurry SD, Luft FE, Maxwell DR. Prevailing patterns and predictive variables in patients with acute tubular necrosis. Arch Intern Med 1978;138:950.
53. Butkus DE. Persistent high mortality in acute renal failure: are we asking the right questions? Arch Intern Med 1983;143:209.
54. Hou SH, Buchinsky DA, Wish JB, et al. Hospital acquired renal insufficiency: a prospective study. Am J Med 1983;74:243.
55. Rasmussen HH, Pitt EA, Ibels LSS, McNeil DR. Prediction of outcome in acute renal failure by discriminant analysis of clinical variables. Arch Intern Med 1985;145:2015.
56. Lien J, Chan V. Risk factors influencing survival in acute renal failure treated by hemodialysis. Arch Intern Med 1985;145:2067.
57. Cohen JR, Mannick JA, Couch NP, Whittemore AD. Abdominal aortic aneurysm repair in patients with preoperative renal failure. J Vasc Surg 1986;3:867.
58. Crawford ES, Coselli JS, Hess KR. Surgical treatment of aneurysm and/or dissection of the ascending aorta, transverse aortic arch, and ascending aorta and transverse aortic arch. J Thorac Cardiovasc Surg 1989;98:659.

59. Svensson LG, Coselli JS, Safi HJ, et al. Appraisal of adjuncts to prevent acute renal failure after surgery on the thoracic or thoracoabdominal aorta. J Vasc Surg 1989;10:230.

60. Olsen PS, Schroeder T, Agerskon K, et al. Surgery for abdominal aortic aneurysms. J Cardiovasc Surg (Torino) 1991;32:636.

61. Hesdorffer CS, Milne JF, Meyers AM, et al. The value of Swan-Ganz catheterization and volume loading in preventing renal failure in patients undergoing abdominal aneurysmectomy. Clin Nephrol 1987;28:272.

62. Berisa F, Berman M, Adu D, et al. Prognostic factors in acute renal failure following aortic aneurysm surgery. QJM 1990;279:689.

63. Sladon RN, Ondo E, Harrison T. Two-hour versus 22-hour creatinine clearance in critically ill patients. Anesthesiology 1987;67:1013.

64. Adamson JW, Eschbach JW, Finch CA. The kidney and erythropoiesis. Am J Med 1968;44:725.

65. Shaw AB. Haemolysis in chronic renal failure. BMJ 1967;2:213.

66. Lichtman MA, Murphy MS, Byer BJ, Freeman RB. Hemoglobin affinity for oxygen in chronic renal disease: the effect of hemodialysis. Blood 1974;43:417.

67. Eschbach JW, Kelly MR, Haley NR, et al. Treatment of the anemia of progressive renal failure with recombinant human erythropoietin. N Engl J Med 1989;321:158.

68. Eschbach JW, Egrie JC, Downing MR, et al. Correction of the anemia of end stage renal disease with recombinant human erythropoietin. N Engl J Med 1987;316:73.

69. Rabiner SF. Uremic bleeding. Prog Hemost Thromb 1972;1:233.

70. Ellison N. Hemostasis and Hemotherapy. In PG Barash, BF Cullen, RK Stoelting (eds), Clinical Anesthesia. Philadelphia: Lippincott, 1992;253.

71. Dodds A, Nicholls M. Haematological aspects of renal disease. Anaesth Intensive Care 1983;11:361.

72. Janson PA, Jubelirer SJ, Weinstein MJ, Deykin D. Treatment of the bleeding tendency in uremia with cryoprecipitate. N Engl J Med 1980;303:1318.

73. Kohler M, Hellstern P, Tarrach H, et al. Subcutaneous injection of desmopressin (DDAVP): evaluation of a new, more concentrated preparation. Haemostasis 1989;19:38.

74. Remuzzi G, Livio M, Marchiaro G, et al. Bleeding in renal failure: altered platelet function in chronic uremia only partially corrected by haemodialysis. Nephron 1978;22:347.

75. Gurri JA, Burnham SJ. Effect of diabetes mellitus on distal lower extremity bypass. Ann Surg 1982;48:75.

76. Thompson JE, Vollman RW, Austin DJ. Prevention of hypotensive and renal complications of aortic surgery using balanced salt solution. Ann Surg 1968;167:767.

77. Bush HL, Huse JB, Johnson WC, et al. Prevention of renal insufficiency after abdominal aortic aneurysm resection by optimal volume loading. Arch Surg 1981;116:1517.

78. Shoemaker WC, Appel PL, Kram HB. Tissue oxygen debt as a determinant of lethal and nonlethal postoperative organ failure. Crit Care Med 1988;16:1117.

79. Berlauk JF, Abrams JH, Gilmour IJ, et al. Preoperative optimization of cardiovascular hemodynamics improves outcome in peripheral vascular surgery. Ann Surg 1991;214:289.

80. Boyd O, Grounds MR, Bennett DE. A randomized clinical trial of the effect of deliberate perioperative increase of oxygen delivery on mortality in high risk surgical patients. JAMA 1993;270:2699.

81. Hayes MA, Timmins AC, Yau EHS, et al. Elevation of systemic oxygen delivery in the treatment of critically ill patients. N Engl J Med 1994;330:1717.

Chapter 3

Radiographic Evaluation of the Aorta

Jacob Cynamon and Samuel I. Wahl

Preoperative radiographic evaluation of aortic pathology may include a plain radiograph, computed tomography (CT) scan, ultrasound, or magnetic resonance imaging (MRI). The surgical urgency of a case or the availability of a particular modality in a given institution may influence what imaging studies are performed and available for preoperative review. The surgeon's preference and experience may also play a role. For example, some surgeons require ultrasound, CT, and angiography before operating on abdominal aortic aneurysms, whereas others operate based on an ultrasound alone. In this chapter, we review the radiographic appearance of the normal and pathologic thoracic and abdominal aorta using the various imaging modalities available. We also discuss a new minimally invasive approach to vascular repair of aortic pathology, the endoluminal stent graft.

Normal Aorta

A normal frontal and lateral chest radiograph is seen in Figure 3-1. The radiograph should be evaluated for abnormal calcifications, masses, widened mediastinum, rib fractures, or other evidence of trauma, pleural effusions, and so on. Representative slices of a normal chest CT (with contrast) are seen in Figure 3-2. Angiography of the thoracic aorta usually includes two views—a left anterior oblique (Figure 3-3) and either an anteroposterior (AP) or a right anterior oblique view. The right and left coronary arteries arise from the right and left aortic sinuses. The brachiocephalic artery, which bifurcates into the right

subclavian and right carotid arteries, is the first branch of the arch. Next, the left carotid artery and last, the left subclavian artery arise directly from the arch. Occasionally, the brachiocephalic and the left common carotid arteries arise together (Figure 3-4). There are also several other normal variants (Table 3-1) of aortic anatomy. (See Table 3-2 and Figure 3-5 for congenital abnormalities of the thoracic arch.)

The thoracic aorta is divided into four segments[1]: the ascending aorta, the aortic arch, the isthmus (between last great vessel and the attachment of the ductus arteriosus), and the descending aorta (see Chapter 1). Occasionally, there is a fusiform dilatation of the proximal descending aorta, a ductus diverticulum (Figure 3-6), that should not be confused with a traumatic injury. There are usually nine pairs of intercostal arteries, occurring between the third through the eleventh intercostal spaces. There are many variations to the intercostal anatomy. Most commonly, there are between two and four bronchial arteries, with multiple bronchial arteries being more common on the left. Bronchial arteries may arise directly from the aorta or have a common origin with an intercostal artery, thus forming an intercostal bronchial trunk.[2]

Thoracic Aortic Disease

Trauma

The thoracic aorta can be injured by rapid deceleration or by crushing injuries. If aortic disruption occurs, the victim is likely not to survive long enough

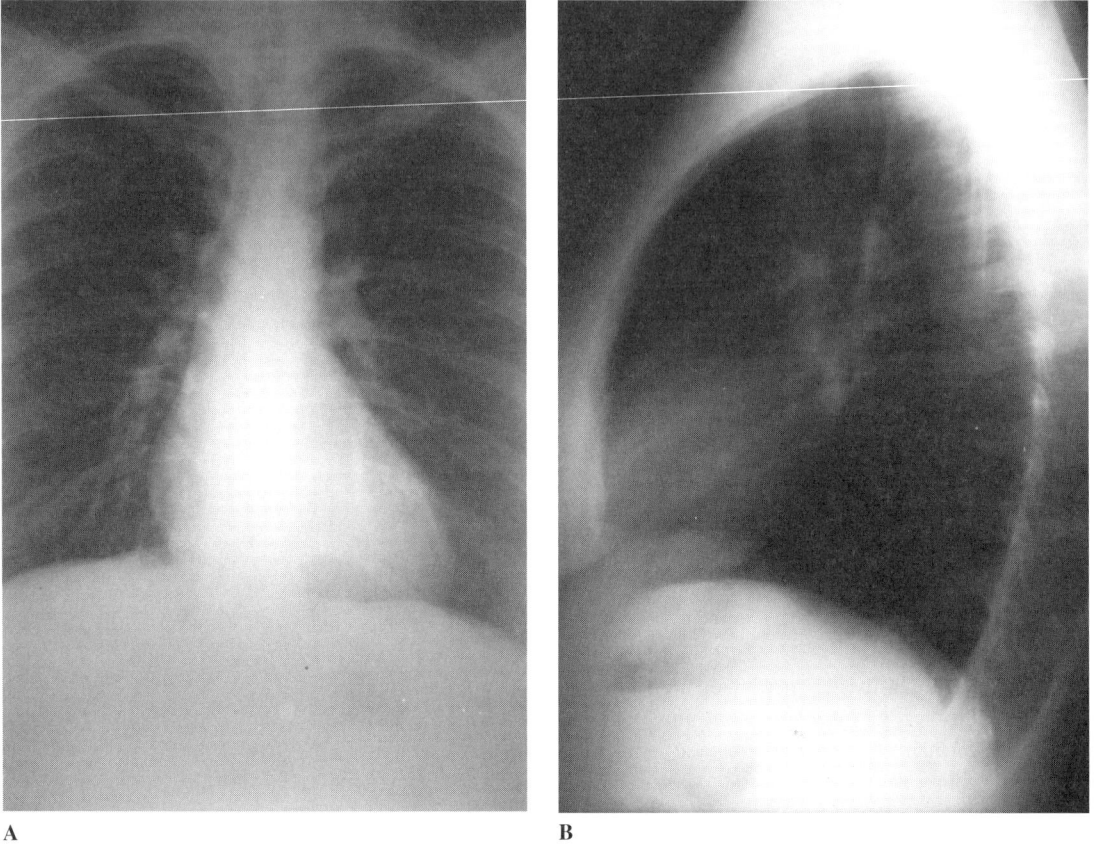

Figure 3-1. Normal frontal (A) and lateral (B) chest radiographs.

to receive medical attention.[3–5] If aortic injury is suspected by the nature of the injury or by plain film findings (Figure 3-7 and Table 3-3), an aortogram should be performed. The most common location of injury (80–86%) is the aortic isthmus.[4–5] The aorta at this site is relatively fixed by the ligamentum arteriosus, which joins the aorta and the pulmonary artery. The shear stresses that are produced here by the rapid deceleration cause the injury. Injury to the aortic root accounts for 9% of aortic injuries and a small number of tears occur at the diaphragm.[5] Injuries to the ascending aorta are more often fatal and these patients do not present for a workup. The findings in aortic injury (Figures 3-8 and 3-9) may range from minimal wall irregularity, which may represent focal intimal injury, to complete transection. Undiagnosed or untreated injury can develop into a chronic pseudoaneurysm with calcified walls and may continue to enlarge and eventually rupture.[6] If a

thoracic arteriogram is obtained, two views are necessary. The presence of one injury does not negate other injuries and therefore the entire thoracic aorta should be evaluated. One should not confuse a ductus bulge (see Figure 3-6), which typically has a smooth margin with no delay in washout of contrast, with injury to the aortic isthmus.

Thoracic Aortic Dissection

Aortic dissection or separation of the arterial wall layers occurs most commonly in patients with hypertension (see Chapter 1).[7] It may also occur in a number of patients who have Marfan's syndrome, coarctation of the aorta, or during pregnancy.[8–10] The separation of the aortic wall layers, which is most likely to occur in the outer third of the media, is usually secondary to one or more intimal tears.

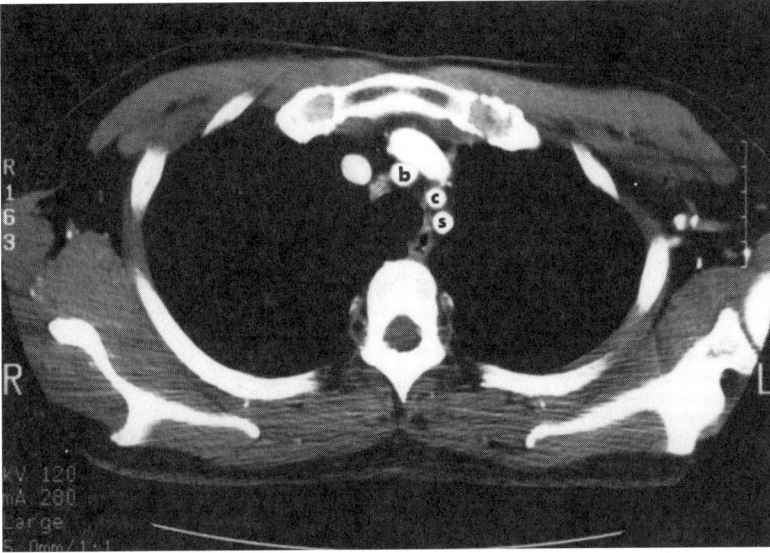

A

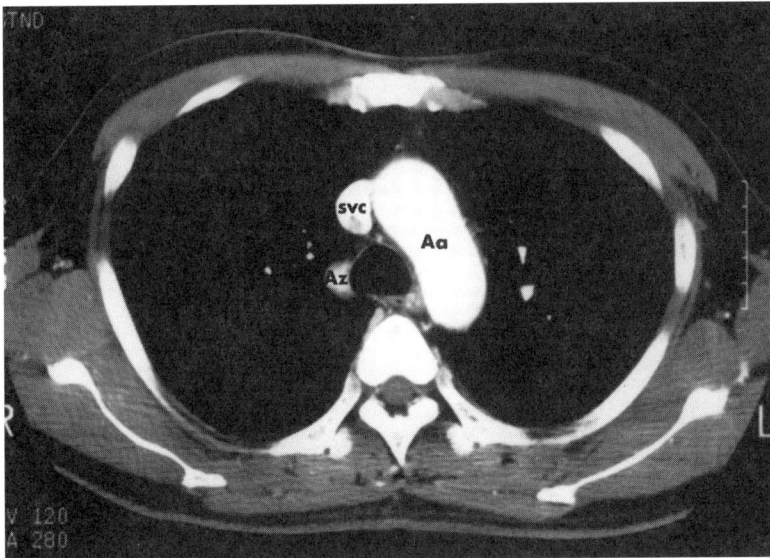

B

Figure 3-2. Axial images of a normal chest computed tomography scan. A. Normal great vessels. (s = left subclavian; c = left common carotid; b = brachiocephalic.) B. Axial image at the level of the aortic arch. (Aa = aortic arch; svc =superior vena cava; Az = azygous vein.)

In some cases, however, no tear is identified, and the dissection may be caused by bleeding from and into the vasa vasorum. These patients may present with severe chest, back, abdominal, or neck pain. If the dissection extends into the aortic root, these patients may have diastolic murmurs of aortic insufficiency.[11] Death from pericardial tamponade may occur in these patients. With extension of the dissection into the descending thoracic aorta, there can be unequal peripheral pulses re-

sulting in peripheral ischemia. Mesenteric or renal ischemia may also occur (see Chapter 1 for a more complete discussion).[12]

There are two classifications for aortic dissections—the DeBakey types I, II, and III[13] and the modification for this classification, Stanford types A and B, which was proposed by Daily et al.[14] in 1970 (Table 3-4). See Figures 3-10 and 3-11 for examples of aortograms and CT scans of aortic dissections. The location of the tear is irrelevant in the classifi-

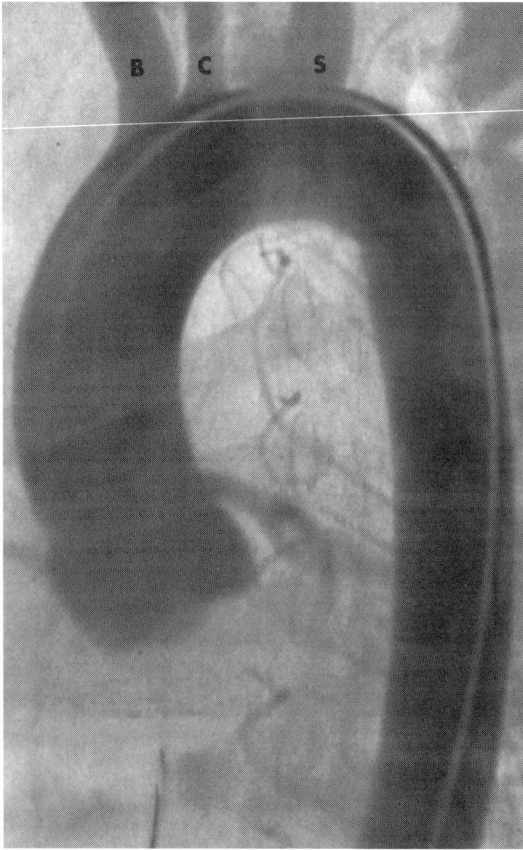

Figure 3-3. Normal left anterior oblique arch aortogram in a young individual. (B = brachiocephalic; C = left common carotid; S = left subclavian.)

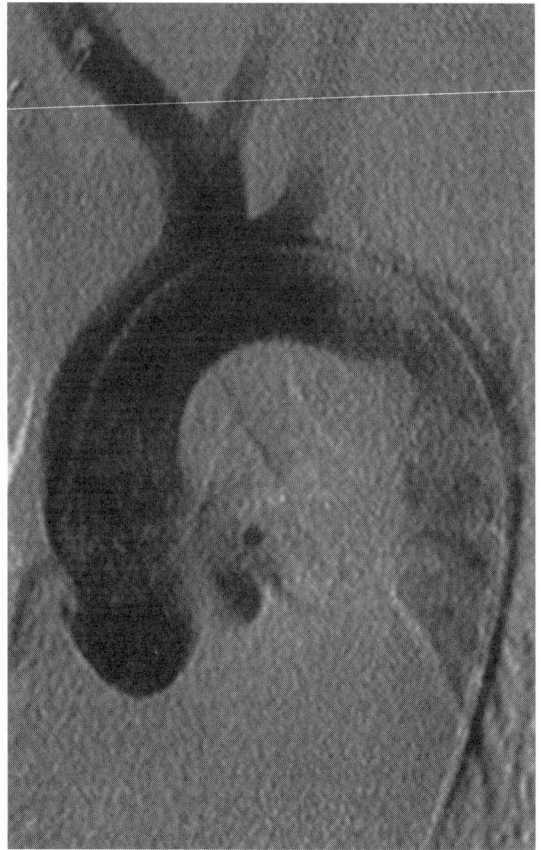

Figure 3-4. Left anterior oblique view of a left aortic arch demonstrating a common origin of the brachiocephalic and left common carotid arteries.

Table 3-1. Incidence of Normal Arch Anatomy and Its Variants

Anatomy	Incidence (Percentage)
Normal arch	70
Common origin of the brachiocephalic and left common carotid artery (see Figure 3-4)	22
Left vertebral artery directly off the aorta	4–6
Right and left common carotid artery with common origin	<1.0
Two brachiocephalic arteries	<1.0
All four great vessels with separate origins	0.1

Table 3-2. Congenital Variants for the Aortic Arch

Variant	Frequency
Left aortic arch with aberrant right subclavian artery (see Figure 3-5)[a]	1%
Right aortic arch 60% mirror image branching[b] 35% with aberrant right subclavian and left ductus or ligamentum arteriosus[c]	1–2%
Cervical aortic arch not associated with intracardiac anomalies	Rare
Coarctation, localized narrowing of the aorta[d]	—

[a]Associated with congenital heart disease (10–15%).
[b]Associated with cyanotic heart disease (98%).
[c]Associated with congenital heart disease (12%).
[d]Associated with congenital heart disease (50%).

cation of dissection, because the extent of the dissection determines prognosis. For instance, a tear in the descending aorta may retrograde dissect into the ascending aorta, affecting the great vessels and the aortic root, and therefore be classified as a type A dissection. The chest radiograph may be normal. See Table 3-5 for the possible abnormal radiographic finding in patients with aortic dissections.

Rapid-injection intravenous contrast CT scanning, with repeat scanning at the aortic root, mid ascending aorta, and aortic arch, or spiral CT (see Figure 3-10B) can be more accurate than angiography in the diagnosis of dissection.[15] However, if the patient is a surgical candidate due to ascending aorta involvement or visceral or extremity ischemia, an aortogram should be performed.[16,17] Aortography is usually performed via the femoral route. An attempt should be made to catheterize the true lumen and advance a pigtail catheter in the true lumen to the ascending aorta. The aortogram should be performed from just above the aortic valve to demonstrate any aortic regurgitation or coronary artery occlusion secondary to dissection. At least two views are necessary to exclude an aortic dissection. The diagnosis is definitively made when an intimal flap is noted separating a true and false lumen. The lumina may opacify simultaneously or sequentially. If the dissection is chronic or if there is no gross communication between the two lumen, the false lumen may not fill. If the true lumen is compressed or if the extraluminal border is widened, the diagnosis of aortic

dissection can be suggested; however, an aneurysm with mural thrombus can have a similar appearance. An abdominal aortogram should be obtained when a dissection is suspected. Dissections tend to follow the outer curve of the aorta; therefore, when the dissection extends into the abdominal aorta, the left renal artery often arises from the false lumen (see Figure 3-10C).

If the false lumen is entered during catheterization and the true lumen cannot be reentered, it is safe to perform the diagnostic arteriogram from the false lumen. The flow rates of the injection should be modified to match the observed flow in the false lumen. The sinuses of Valsalva will not opacify under these circumstances and aortic regurgitation cannot be determined. However, the proximal extent of the dissection can be diagnosed. It should be noted that there may be several entry and exit sites throughout the length of the dissection. It is not necessary to determine the location of all of these sites as it does not alter therapy in these cases.

Thoracic aortic dissections can also be well visualized with the use of transesophageal echocardiography (TEE). Because of the close proximity of the esophagus to the thoracic aorta, TEE is especially useful for the diagnosis of ascending (Figure 3-12) and descending (Figure 3-13) aortic aneurysms and dissections. This is especially true when a multiplane TEE probe is used. It is, however, less useful for the diagnosis of transverse aortic (arch) aneurysms and dissections because the trachea and

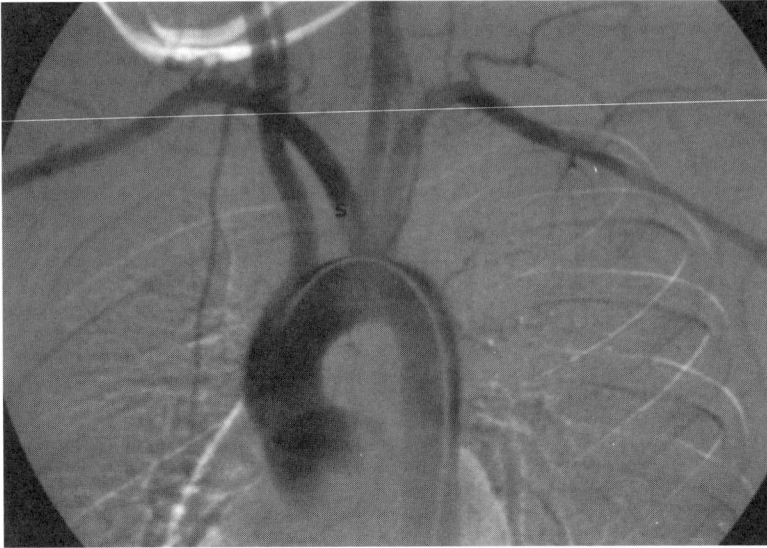

A

Figure 3-5. A. Digital subtraction left anterior oblique arch aortogram demonstrating an aberrant right subclavian artery arising as the last branch of the aortic arch (S). B. Axial computed tomographic image of the thorax through the upper aortic arch demonstrating the retroesophageal location of an aberrant right subclavian artery arising as the last branch of the arch (S).

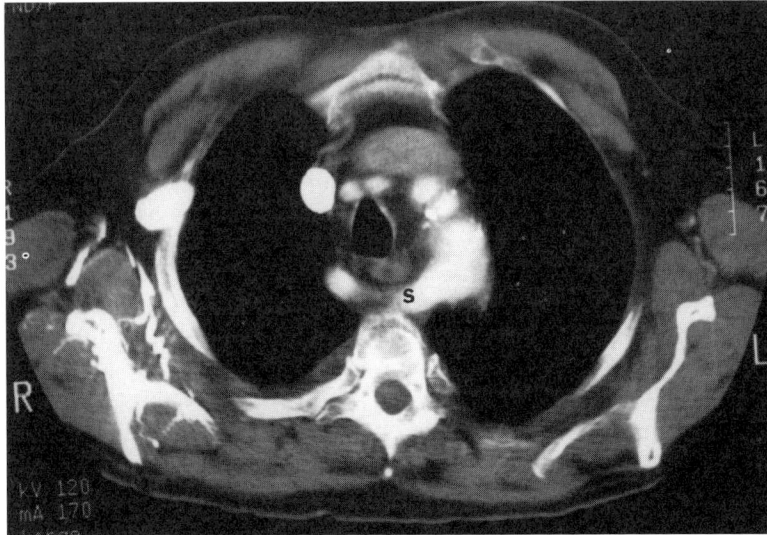

B

left main stem bronchus may lie between the esophagus and the aorta at this level (see Chapters 6 and 8). TEE may also be useful in distinguishing between true and false lumens in aortic dissection; this can be done by two-dimensional echocardiography, M-mode, or color-flow Doppler. TEE is also useful intraoperatively for determining the severity of aortic insufficiency, pericardial tamponade, or both, as well as the location of the intimal tear.

Thoracic Aortic Aneurysmal Disease

An aneurysm is an abnormally dilated vessel. In a true aneurysm, all three layers (i.e., intima, media, and adventitia) are intact. In a pseudoaneurysm, there is disruption of at least the intima with bulging of the remaining layers. All three layers of the arterial wall may be involved and this type of pseudoaneurysm can also be termed a *contained hematoma*.

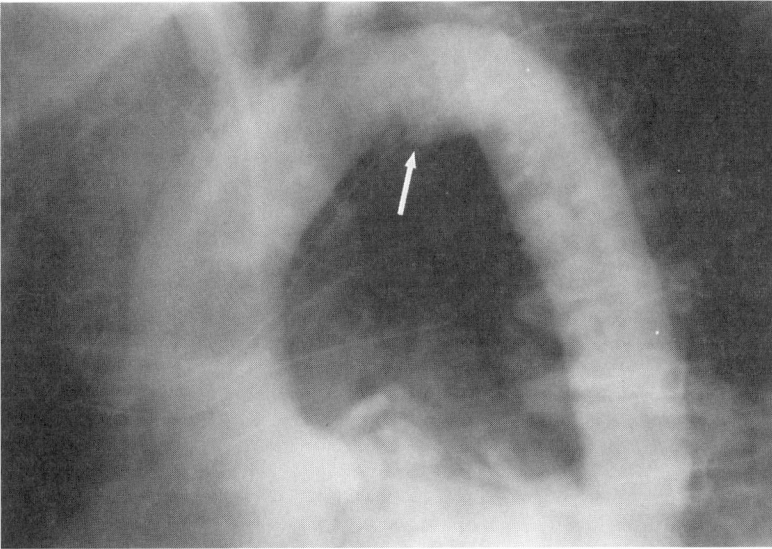

Figure 3-6. Left anterior oblique arch aortogram showing the arteriographic appearance of the ductus diverticulum (arrow).

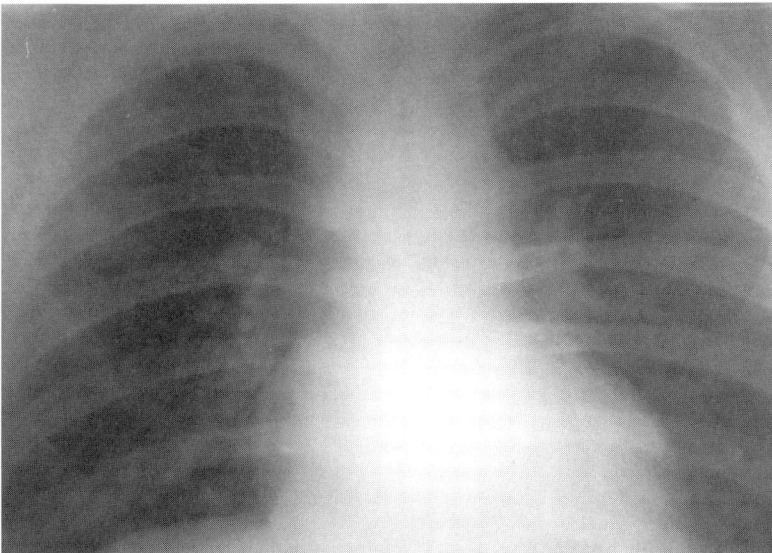

Figure 3-7. Anteroposterior plain film radiograph of the chest with mediastinal widening is the only suggestion of thoracic aortic injury in this 16-year-old patient who sustained steering wheel trauma to the chest from a motor vehicle accident.

Atherosclerotic aneurysms are the most common true aneurysms of the thoracic aorta.[18,19] They most often affect the descending thoracic aorta (Figure 3-14).

Abdominal Aorta

Atherosclerosis of the abdominal aorta may manifest as occlusive disease or aneurysms.[20] A normal plain film of the abdomen is depicted in Figure 3-15. Unsuspected aneurysms can be identified by the presence of curvilinear calcification in the midabdomen (Figure 3-16A and B). Ultrasound is a quick and efficient means of identifying the presence and size of an aneurysm (Figure 3-17). However, the relationship of the aneurysm to the renal arteries and the aortic bifurcation cannot always be determined by ultrasound.

Table 3-3. Plain Film Findings in Aortic Injury

Mediastinal widening (see Figure 3-7)
Shift of the nasogastric tube to the right
Depression of left bronchus
Tracheal deviation
Apical cap
Pneumothorax
Hemothorax
Pulmonary contusion
Rib or clavicular fracture

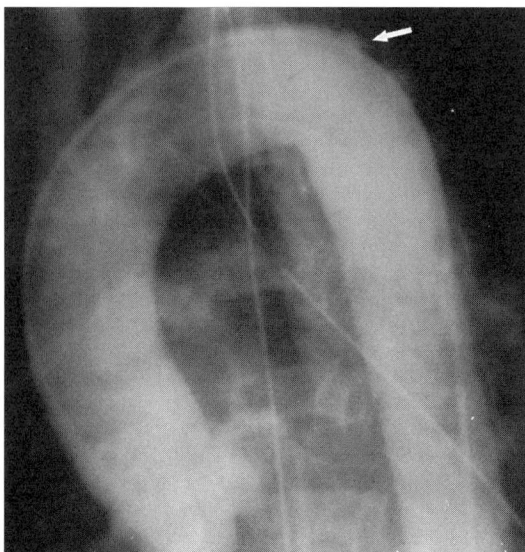

Figure 3-9. Deceleration injury. Anteroposterior thoracic aortogram shows a transmural injury involving the lateral proximal descending thoracic aorta (arrow).

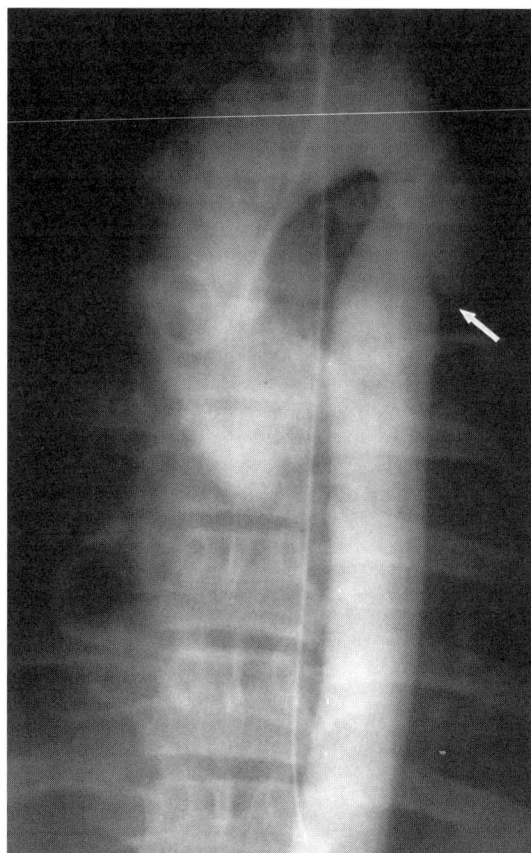

Figure 3-8. Aortic laceration due to deceleration injury. Left anterior oblique aortogram shows a focal intimal tear in the superior aspect of the aortic arch post–motor vehicle accident (arrow).

A normal CT scan of the abdominal aorta is seen in Figure 3-18. AP and lateral views of an abdominal aortic angiogram are depicted in Figure 3-19.

More than 90% of abdominal aortic aneurysms start below the renal arteries.[21] The distance between the renal arteries and the start of the aneurysms is known as the upper neck (Figure 3-20A). If the aneurysms end before the aortic bifurcation, the distance between the end of the aneurysm and the bifurcation is known as the lower neck (Figure 3-20B). If a proximal and distal neck are present, a tube graft can be used to repair the aneurysm. Often, the aneurysm extends into the common iliac arteries (Figure 3-21).[22] The external iliac arteries are rarely, if ever, involved. Aortoiliac aneurysms may also involve the hypogastric arteries (Figure 3-22).[23,24]

Many surgeons require aortography before aneurysm repair due to its ability to precisely define the proximal neck of the aneurysm and mesenteric perfusion (Figure 3-23).[21,25] In addition, the num-

Table 3-4. Classifications for Aortic Dissections

DeBakey	Daily
Type I: ascending arch and descending	Type A: ascending aorta
Type II: confined to ascending aorta and arch	Type B: all others
Type III: only descending or abdominal aorta	—

Table 3-5. Chest Radiographic Findings in Aortic Dissection

Mediastinal widening
Increased diameter of aortic knob
Pleural effusion
Cardiac enlargement
Separation of intimal calcification from
   the margin of the aortic knob by more than 4 mm

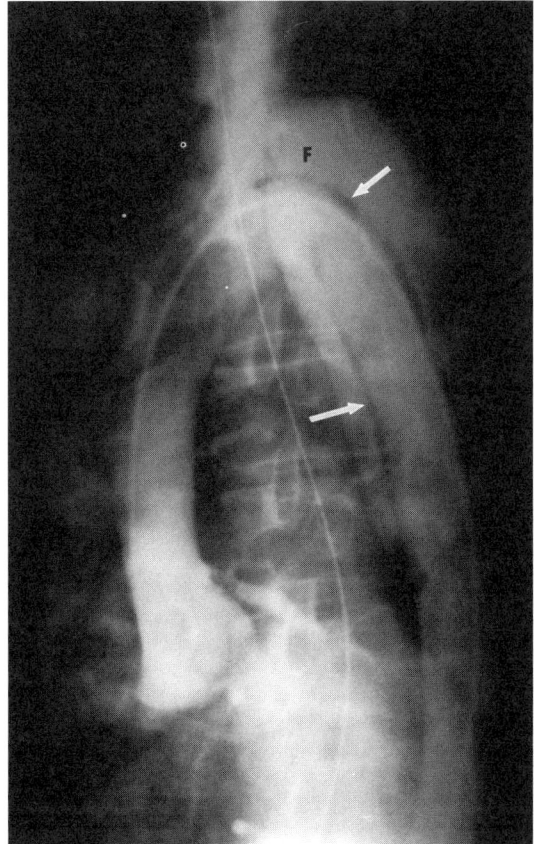

A

Figure 3-10. Aortic dissection. A. Left anterior oblique arch aortogram shows a type A or DeBakey's type I dissection. Multiple intimal flaps are visualized (arrows). Note the compression of the true lumen of the ascending and descending aorta by the false channel (F).

ber and size of the patent lumbar arteries can be determined preoperatively. Aortography for abdominal aortic aneurysm must include an AP and a lateral view. The lateral view is essential for demonstrating the proximal celiac axis and superior mesenteric artery. An additional injection with the catheter at the L3 level should be performed to determine if the inferior mesenteric artery is patent (Figure 3-23C). Since many aortic aneurysms are lined by mural clot, catheter manipulation within an aneurysm should be performed with extreme care to prevent embolization. This mural clot prevents accurate measurement of the size of an aneurysm on aortography. Ultrasound, CT scanning, or MRI are superior to aortography in this regard.

Patients with the triad of a known abdominal aortic aneurysm, pain, and syncope should be suspected of having a ruptured abdominal aortic aneurysm and should immediately be brought to the operating room for exploration and repair. In these circumstances, no additional imaging should be obtained because delay may increase the risk of death. Mortality associated with emergent surgery for rupture is on the order of 60%.[26,27] If this triad is not present, a CT scan may be performed. A CT scan of a ruptured aneurysm may be seen in the patient depicted in Figure 3-24, who presented with a known abdominal aortic aneurysm and new onset abdominal pain, but no syncope.

Inflammatory abdominal aortic aneurysms can be diagnosed by CT as a thickened aortic wall with retroperitoneal adhesions. The third portion of the duodenum may adhere to the anterior surface of the aneurysm, making surgical repair difficult (Figure 3-25).

Atherosclerotic occlusive disease of the abdominal aorta typically affects the infrarenal segment and is manifested as either focal stenoses, diffuse disease (Figure 3-26), or occlusions.[28,29] This pat-

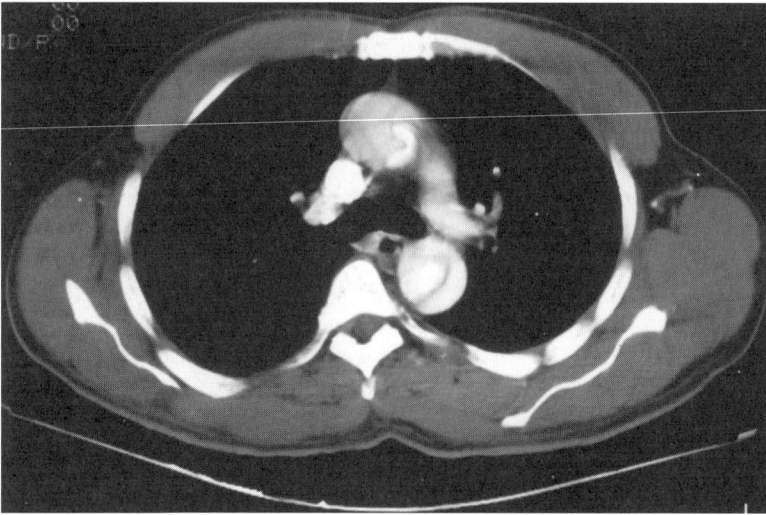

B

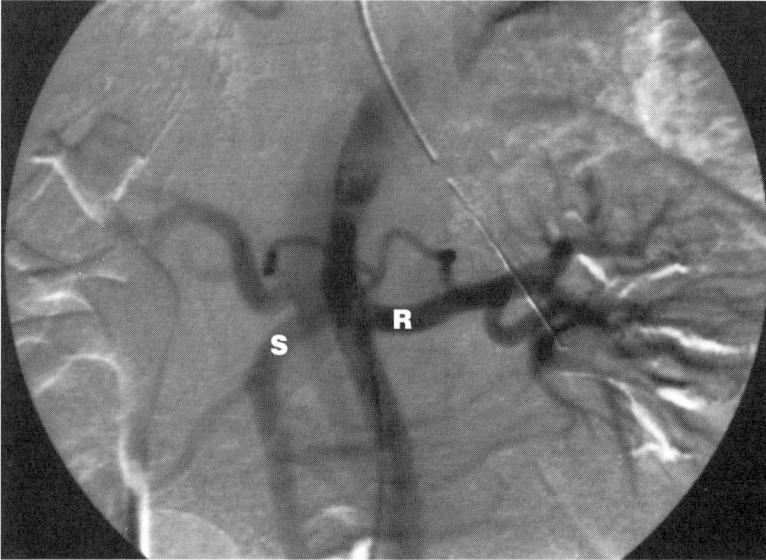

C

Figure 3-10. *(continued)*
B. Computed tomographic scan of the same patient at the level of the pulmonary artery shows the intimal flap involving both the ascending and descending aorta separating two aortic channels. Note the marked compression of the true lumen of the ascending aorta by the false channel. C. Anteroposterior abdominal aortogram of the same patient showing distal extension of the thoracic aortic dissection. Note the more densely opacified true lumen. The renal arteries (R) and superior mesenteric artery (S) arise from separate lumens.

tern of disease most often affects smokers. Men may present with the classic Leriche's syndrome consisting of thigh or buttock claudication and impotence. Women who smoke and have small aortoiliac vessels may have a similar pattern of disease and present with severe claudication.[30,31]

Aortoiliac reconstruction for occlusive disease can be undertaken surgically or percutaneously. Surgical reconstruction includes an anatomic bypass, such as an aortofemoral graft, or an extra-anatomic bypass, such as an axillary artery to femoral artery bypass, which alleviates the need for an aortic procedure, presumably reducing the risks of revascularization. If the aorta is occluded, and it is deemed a recent occlusion, then thrombolysis can be attempted.[32,33] Any underlying lesions can be treated with balloon angioplasty and stents if necessary (Figure 3-27). Some chronic occlusions of the distal aorta and iliac arteries can be primarily stented percutaneously (Figure 3-28), precluding the need for an aortic operation.[34]

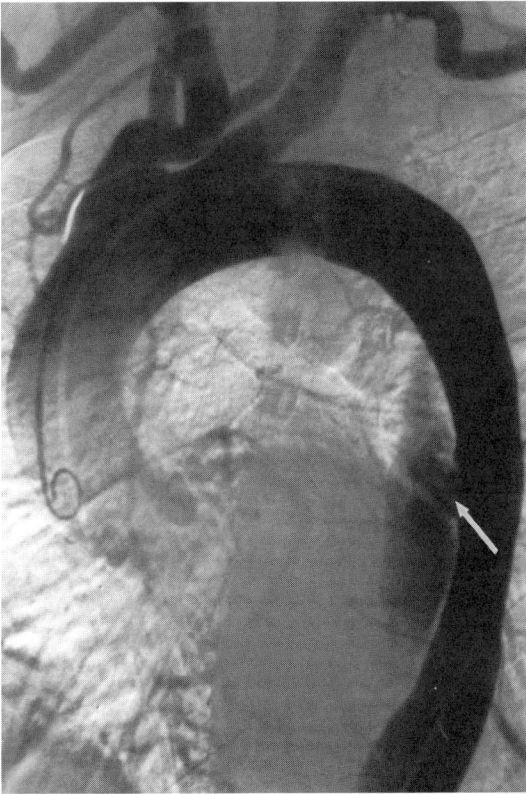

Figure 3-11. Left anterior oblique arch aortogram shows a type B or DeBakey's type III dissection. Normal ascending aorta and great vessels are seen. Note the communication of the false lumen with the true lumen at the midthoracic level (arrow). The true lumen is compressed and more densely opacified.

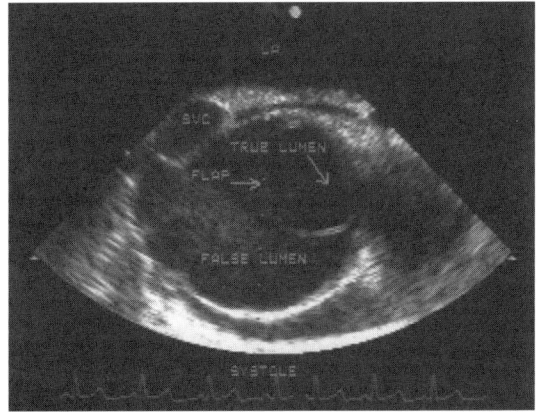

A

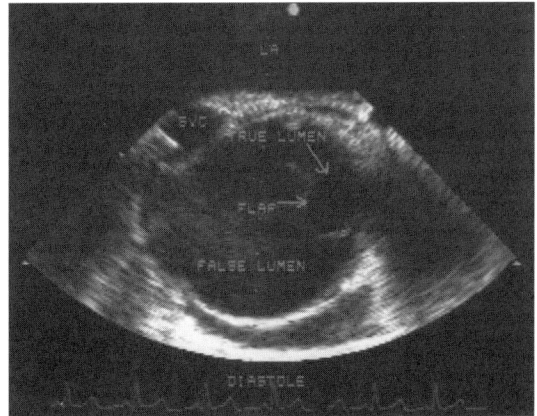

B

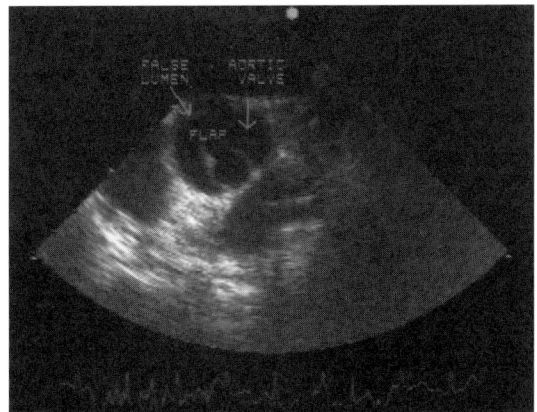

C

Figure 3-12. A. Transesophageal echocardiographic image of a patient with an ascending thoracic aortic dissection in systole. Note that the false lumen is much larger than the true lumen. Note also the round, convex appearance of the flap during systole. B. The same patient in diastole. Note the compressed true lumen, and the concave indentation of the flap during diastole. C. Transesophageal echocardiographic image of another patient whose ascending thoracic aortic dissection extends all the way down to the level of the aortic valve. (SVC = superior vena cava; LA = left atrium.)

Stent Grafts

An alternative approach to treating aneurysms and atherosclerotic occlusive disease of the aorta and peripheral vessels is the use of endoluminal stent grafts.[34–44] Endoluminal stent grafts are stents sutured to prosthetic material and delivered into position endoluminally usually via cutdown of the common femoral artery. The first clinical use of a stent graft was in 1990 by Parodi and colleagues,[35,38] who repaired an abdominal aortic aneurysm endoluminally via a common femoral artery approach. More recently, stent grafts have been used to treat traumatic injuries of large vessels, true and false aneurysms, and aortoiliac occlusive disease.

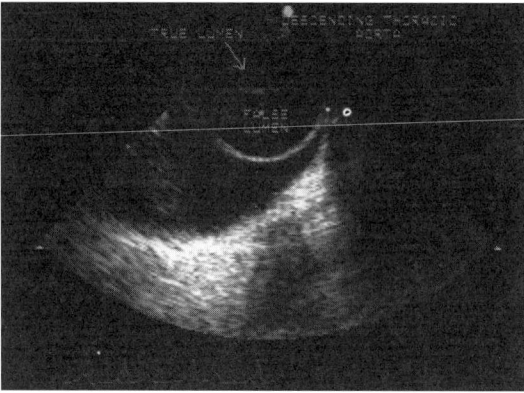
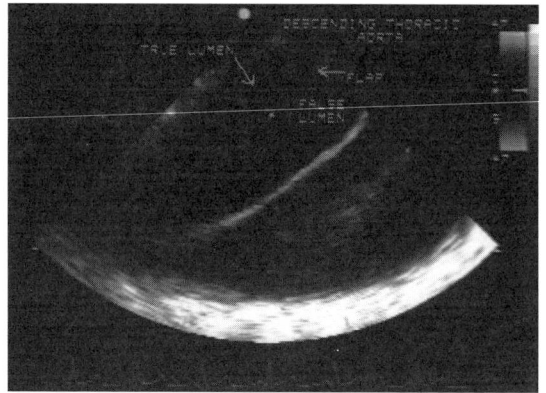

A   B

Figure 3-13. A. Short axis transesophageal echocardiographic image of a patient with a descending thoracic aortic dissection. B. The same patient with the descending thoracic aorta viewed at 90 degrees (longitudinal).

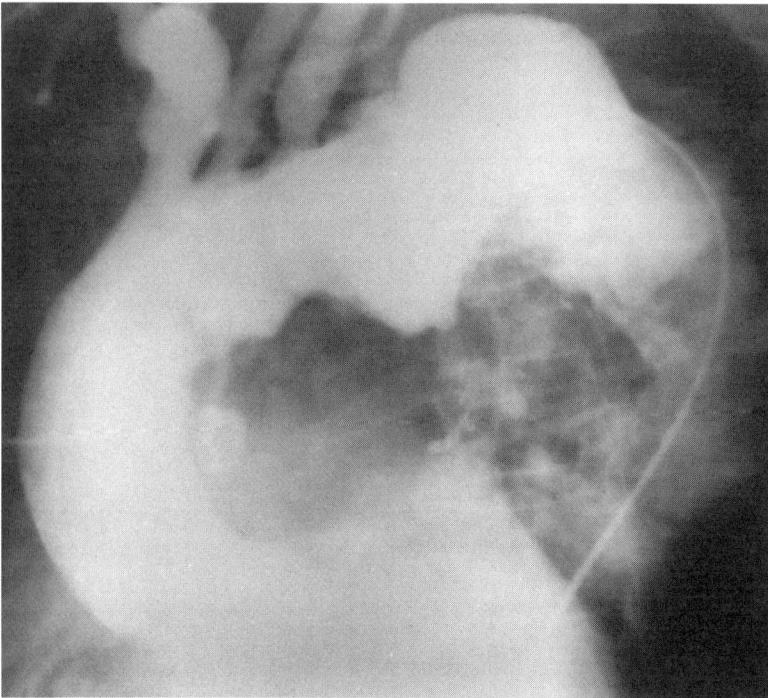

Figure 3-14. Atherosclerotic aneurysm. A. Left anterior oblique thoracic aortogram shows a markedly irregular descending thoracic aorta containing a saccular aneurysm arising distal to the left subclavian artery. B. Axial computed tomographic image of the same patient at the level of the aortic arch.

A

Figure 3-14. *(continued)*

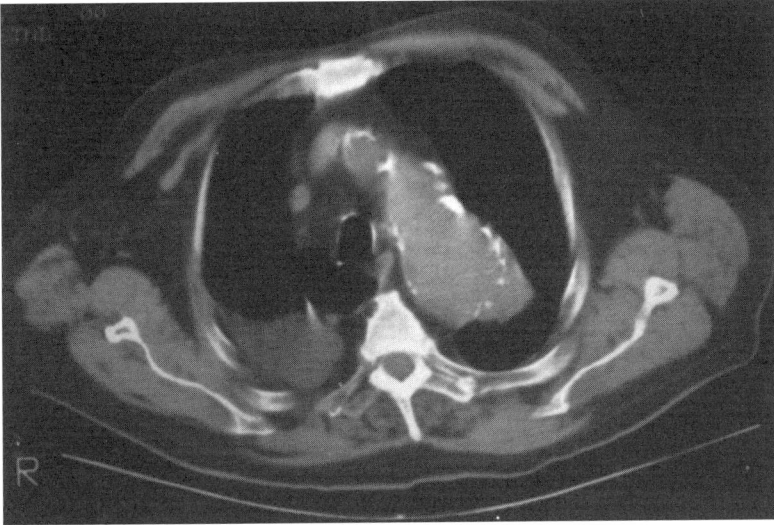

B

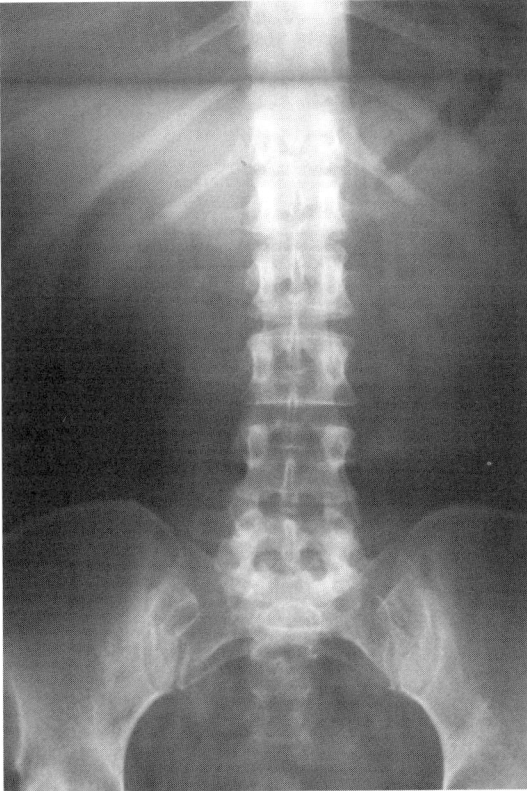

Figure 3-15. Frontal plain film radiograph of a normal abdomen.

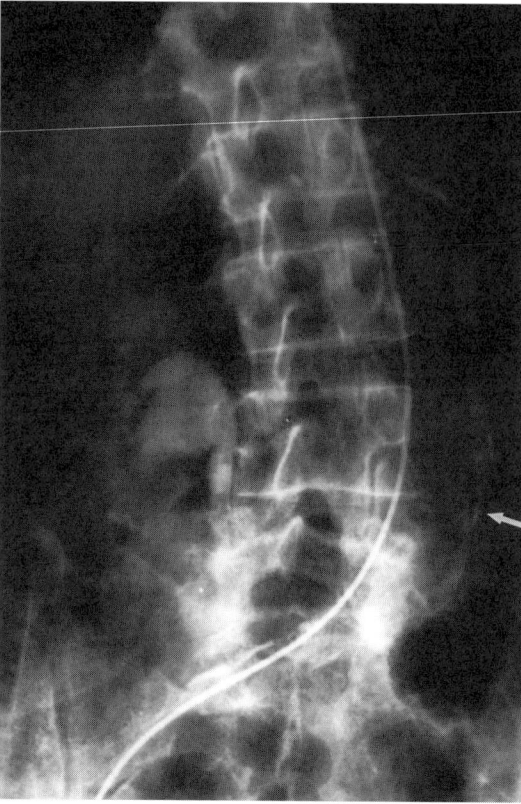 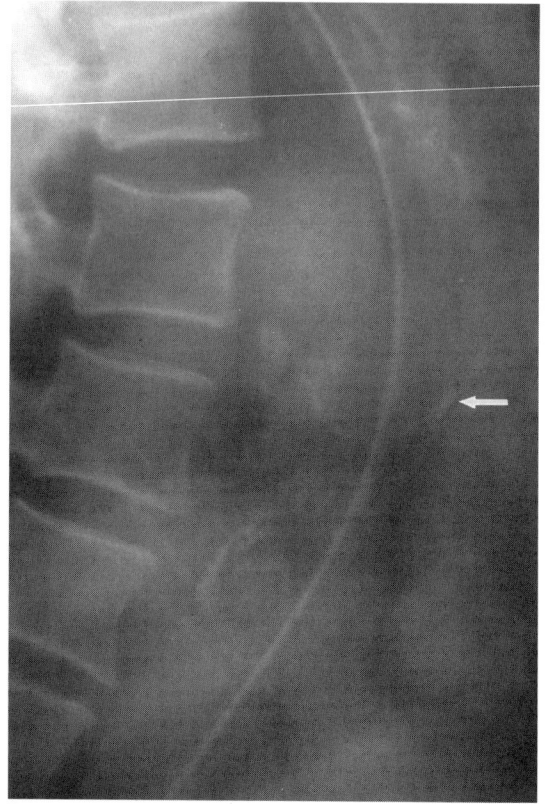

A B

Figure 3-16. Fusiform atherosclerotic infrarenal aortic aneurysm. A. Anteroposterior plain film of the abdomen. B. Lateral view of fusiform atherosclerotic aneurysm showing curvilinear calcification of the aneurysm (arrows).

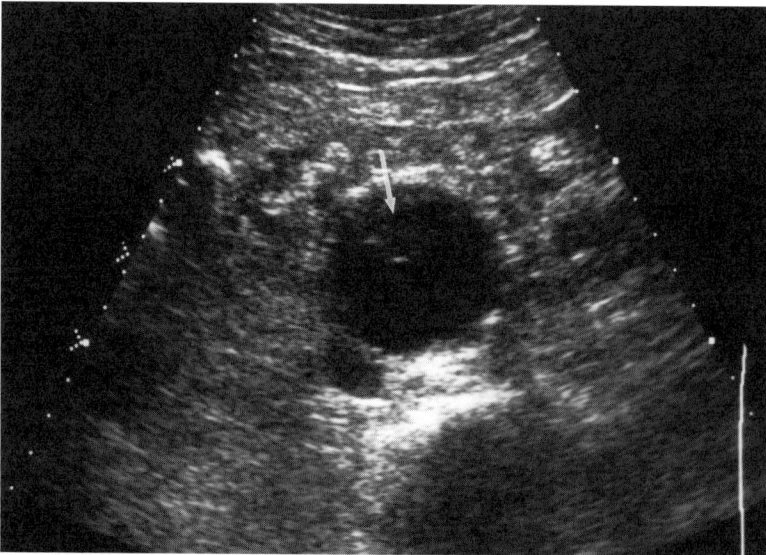

Figure 3-17. Transverse ultrasound of the abdominal aorta reveals an infrarenal aneurysm. There is a moderate amount of echogenic thrombus (arrow) anteriorly.

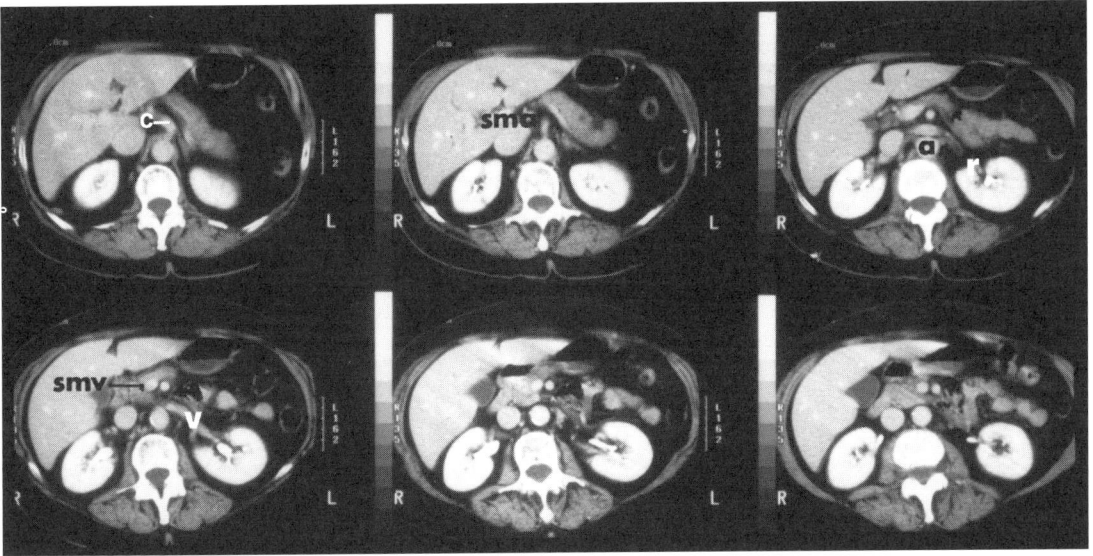

Figure 3-18. Sequential axial computed tomographic sections through the level of the kidneys demonstrating the normal abdominal aorta (a), superior mesenteric artery (sma), celiac artery (c), renal artery (r), left renal vein (v), and superior mesenteric vein (smv).

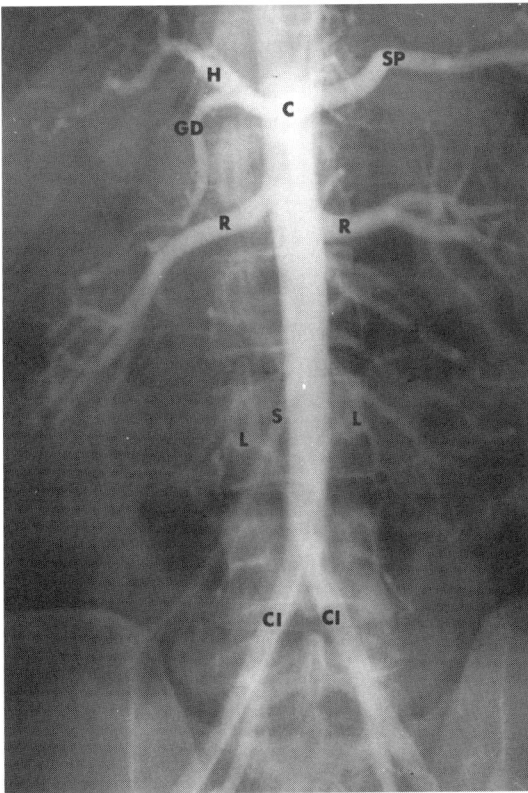

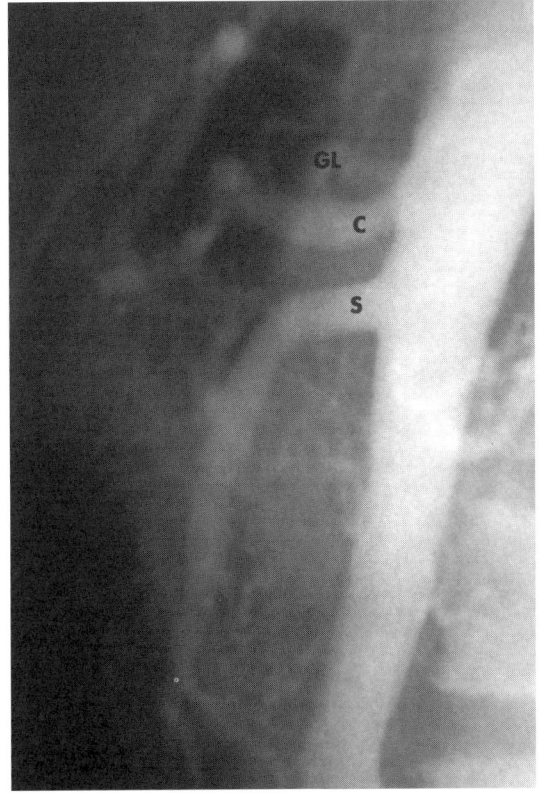

A

B

Figure 3-19. Normal anteroposterior (A) and lateral (B) abdominal aortogram. (C = celiac; CI = common iliac; GD = gastroduodenal; H = hepatic; R = renal; L = lumbar; GL = left gastric; S = superior mesenteric; SP = splenic.)

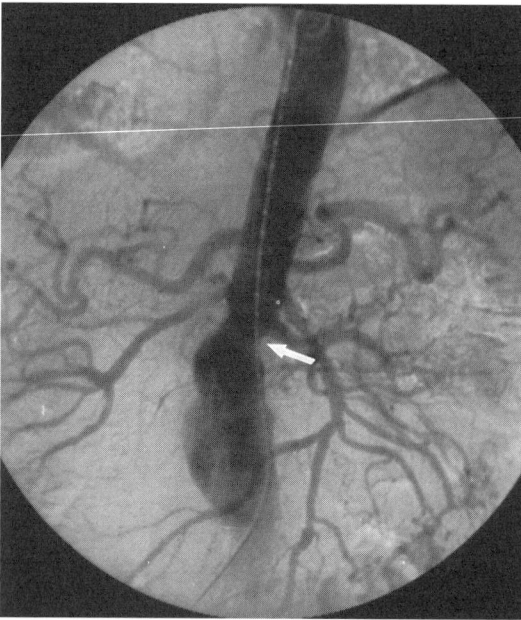

A

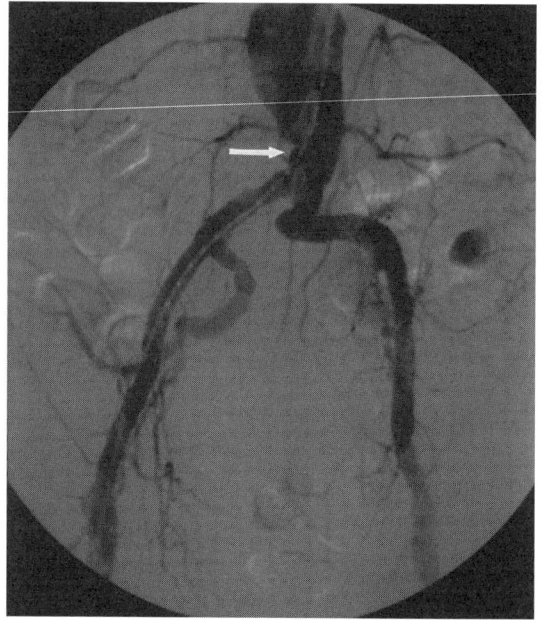

B

Figure 3-20. Abdominal aortic aneurysm. A. Digital subtraction arteriogram of an infrarenal abdominal aortic aneurysm showing the upper infrarenal neck (arrow). B. Same patient. Note the aneurysm ends prior to the aortic bifurcation. The distance between the end of the aneurysm and bifurcation is known as the lower neck (arrow).

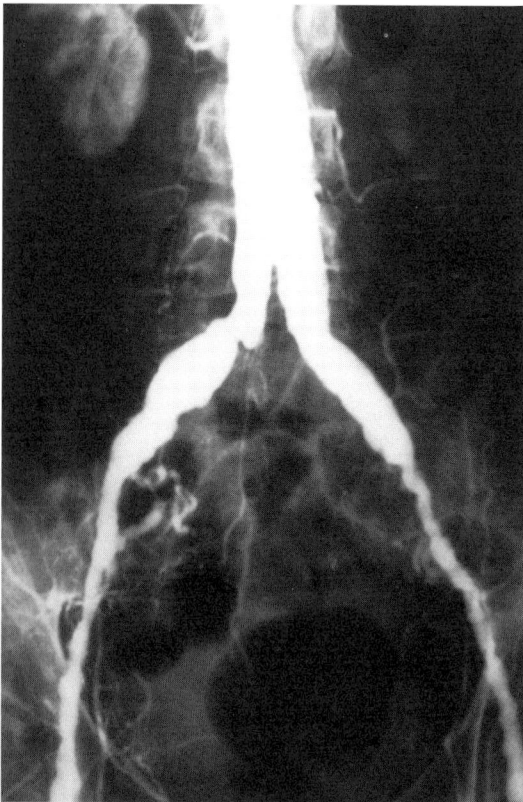

A

Figure 3-21. Infrarenal abdominal aortic aneurysm with extension into the common iliac arteries. A. Anteroposterior arteriogram of the abdominal aorta and iliac segments. Thrombus lining the aneurysm sac may give a relatively normal appearance to the aorta and the impression that no aneurysm exists. The iliac segments show fusiform dilatation with diffuse atherosclerotic changes. B. Computed axial tomography of the same patient through the lower abdomen demonstrates aneurysmal enlargement of the abdominal aorta. The aortic wall is calcified, and there is circumferential thrombus. The lumen of the aorta enhances with intravenous contrast (L). C. Scan below the aortic bifurcation demonstrates aneurysmal enlargement of the common iliac arteries, again showing circumferential thrombus and central luminal enhancement (L).

Figure 3-21. *(continued)*

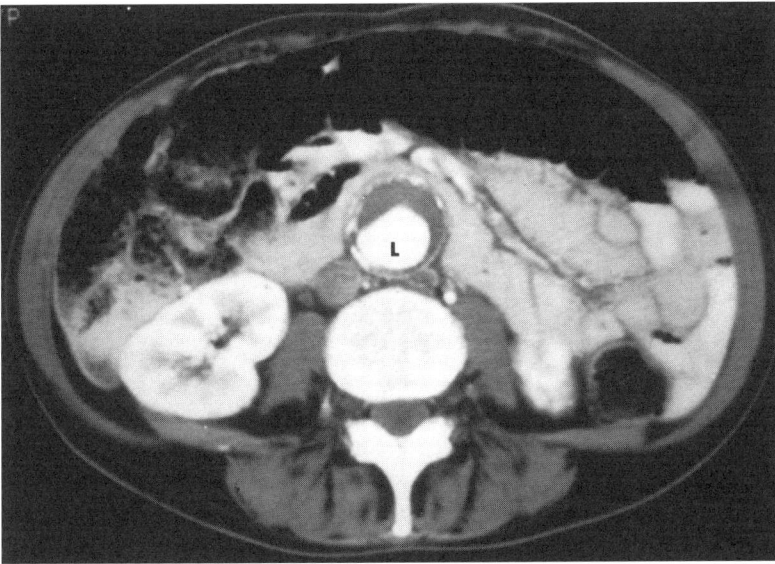

B

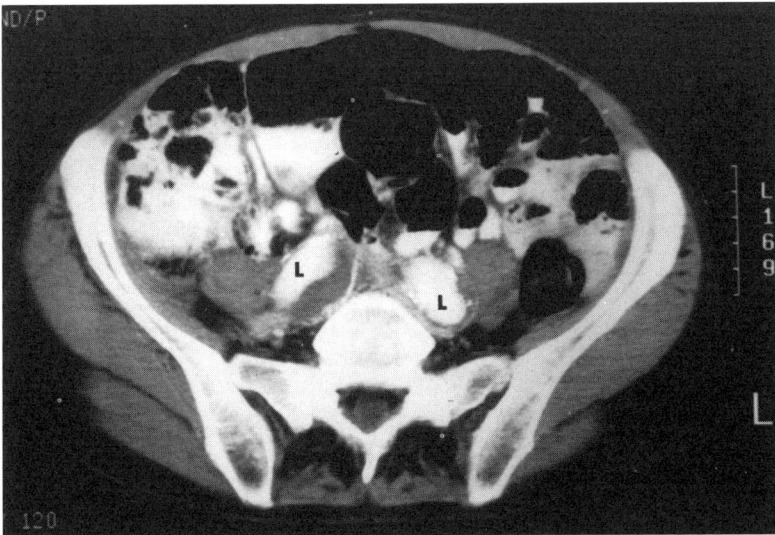

C

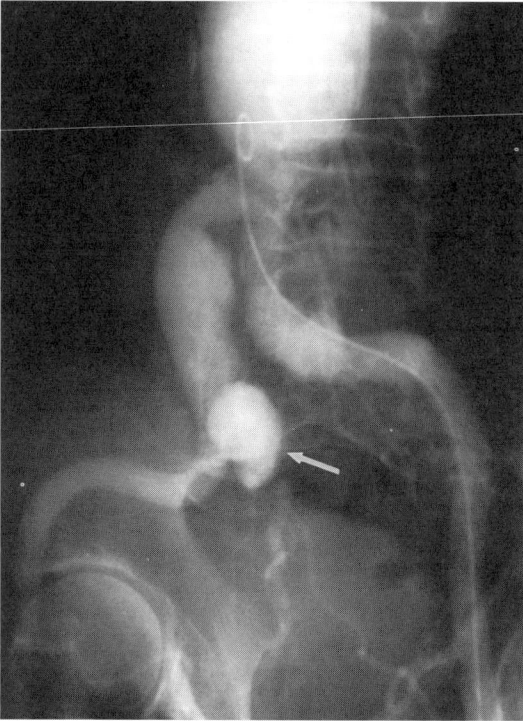

Figure 3-22. Anteroposterior view pelvic arteriogram showing a fusiform abdominal aortic aneurysm with an isolated aneurysm of the right common iliac artery. A saccular aneurysm of the right internal iliac (hypogastric) artery is also present (arrow).

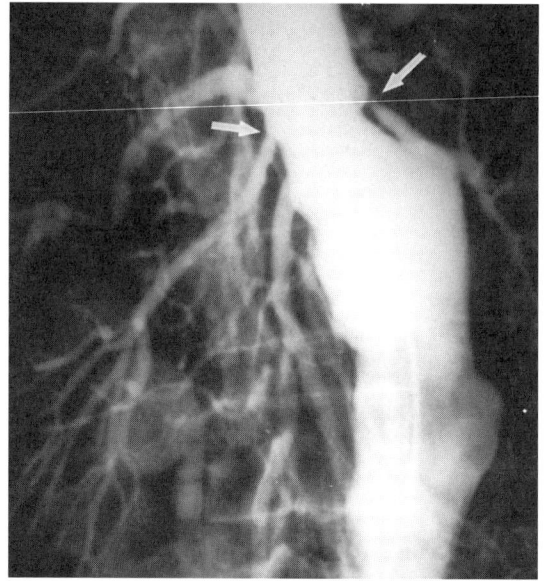

A

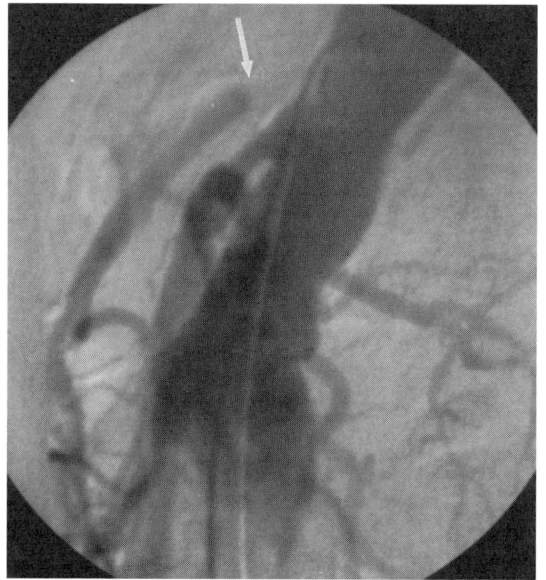

B

Figure 3-23. A. Anteroposterior view abdominal aortogram demonstrating an infrarenal abdominal aortic aneurysm and mesenteric perfusion. Bilateral renal artery stenosis is present (arrows). Note the paucity of normal lumbar arteries. B. Lateral view of the same patient. The celiac trunk is occluded (arrow) and was noted to fill retrograde via the gastroduodenal artery. C. Pelvic arteriography shows nonvisualization of the inferior mesenteric artery suggesting inferior mesentric artery occlusion.

Figure 3-23. *(continued)*

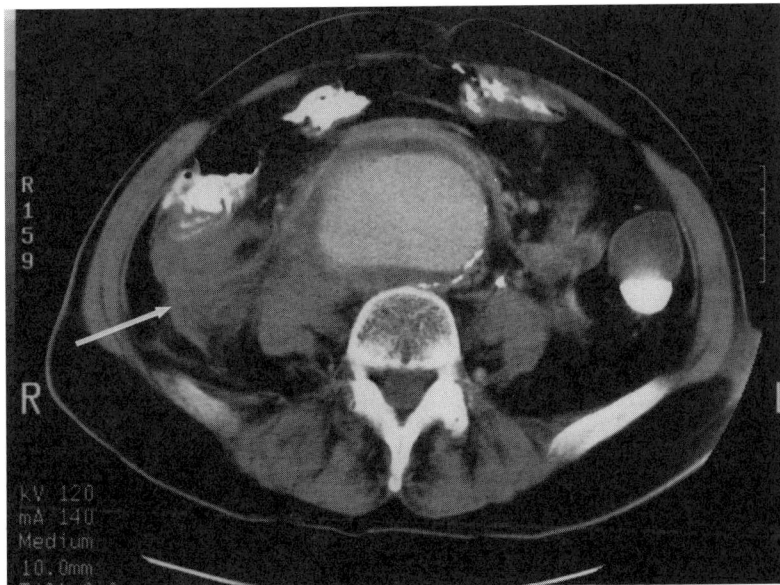

C

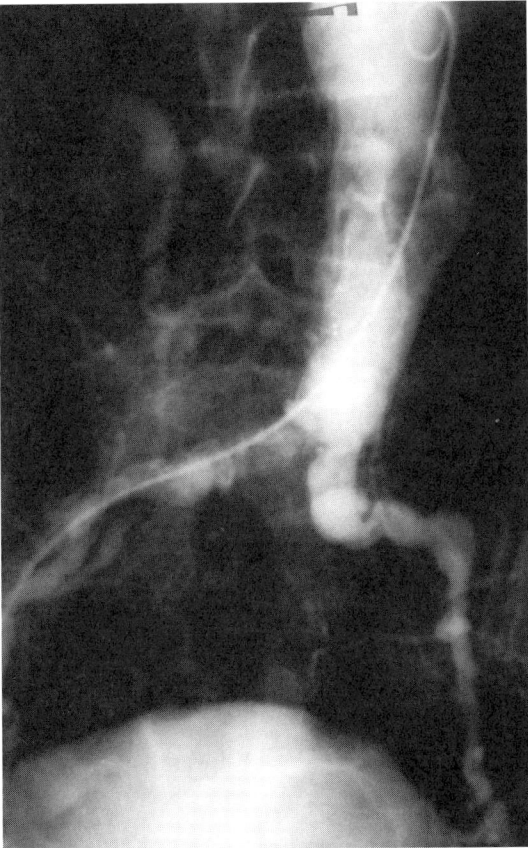

Figure 3-24. Computed tomography of the distal abdominal aorta shows rupture of a large abdominal aortic aneurysm with adjacent hematoma in the retroperitoneal space (arrow). Patient presented with a known abdominal aortic aneurysm and new onset of abdominal pain, but without syncope.

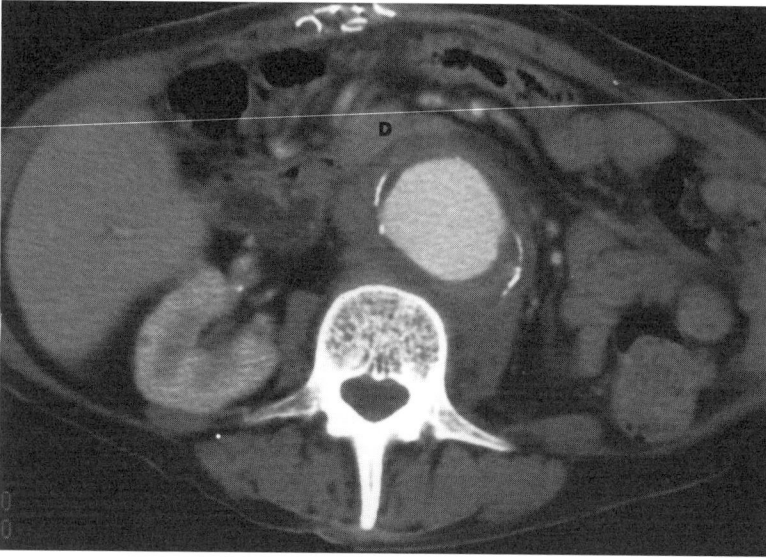

Figure 3-25. Inflammatory abdominal aortic aneurysm. Computed tomographic scan of the abdomen shows periaortitis (inflammatory aneurysm). Note the thick rind of tissue surrounding the aneurysm anteriorly, with adherence of the third portion of the duodenum (D).

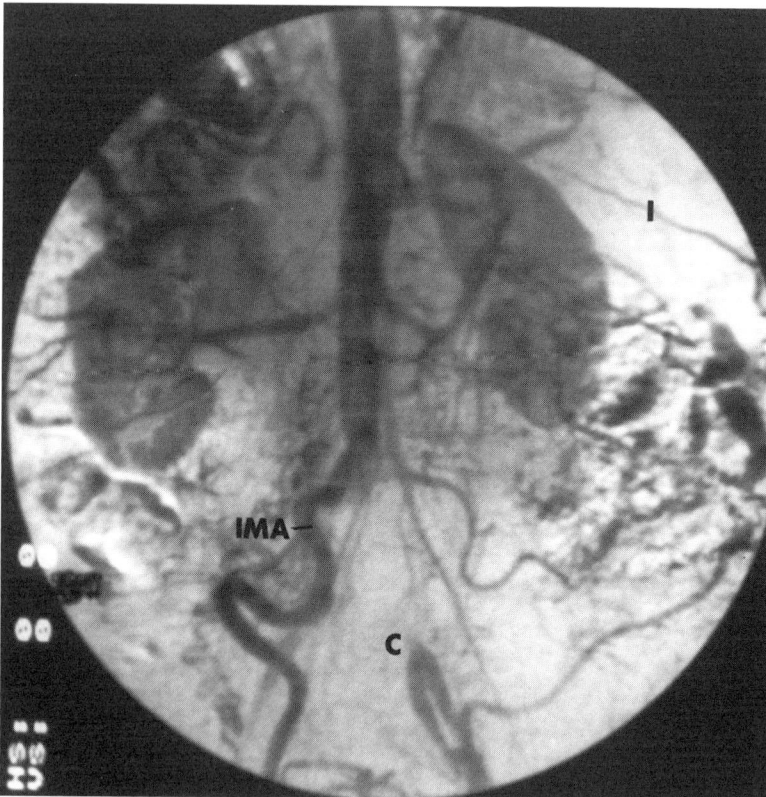

Figure 3-26. Translumbar aortogram shows atherosclerotic occlusion of the distal aorta with reconstitution of the common iliac (C) arteries via well-developed lumbar, intercostal (I), and retroperitoneal collaterals and the inferior mesenteric artery (IMA).

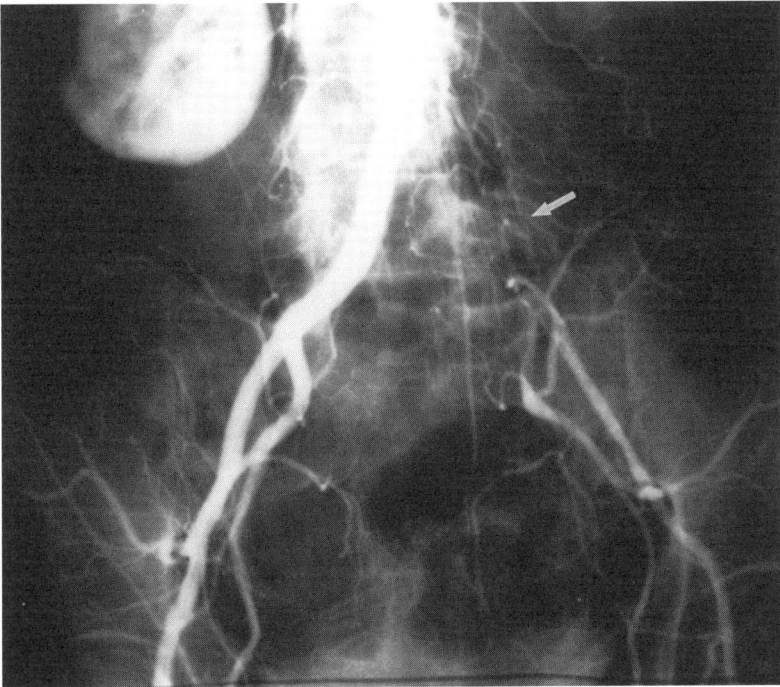

A

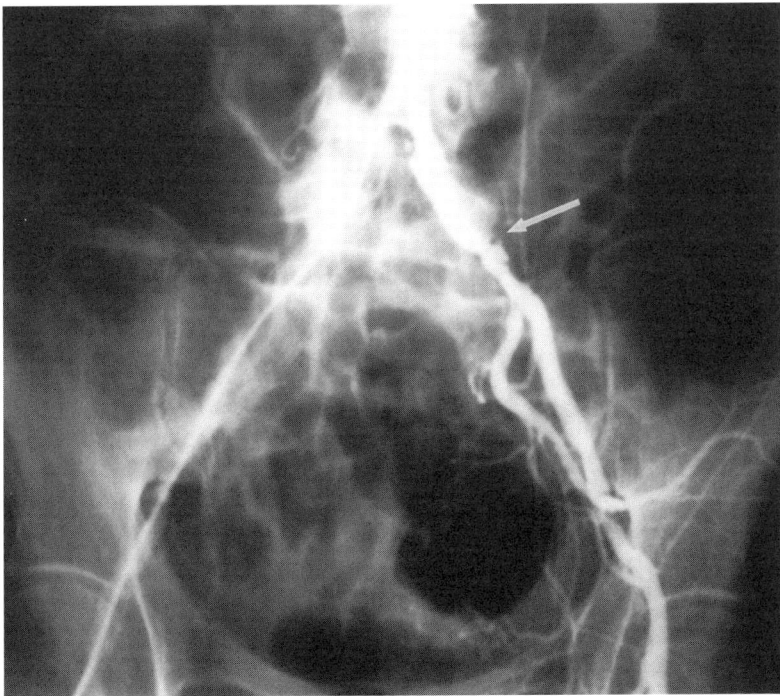

B

Figure 3-27. A. Acute thrombotic occlusion of the left common iliac artery (arrow) with prominent collaterals suggesting progressive atherosclerosis as the etiology. B. Pelvic arteriogram 24 hours after treatment with thrombolytic agent. Patency was restored, uncovering a left common iliac artery stenosis (arrow).

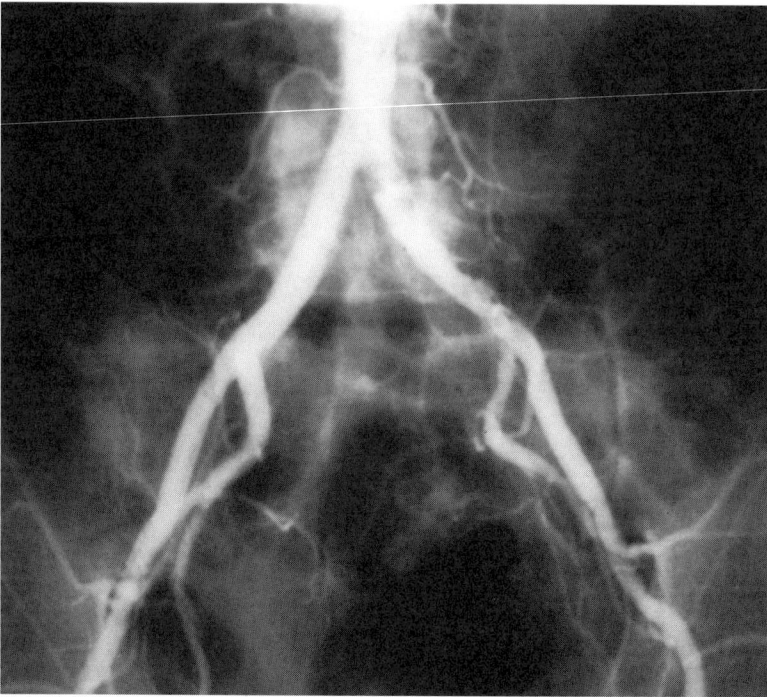

Figure 3-27. *(continued)* C. Left common iliac artery stenosis was treated with percutaneous transluminal angioplasty, which resolved the patient's symptoms.

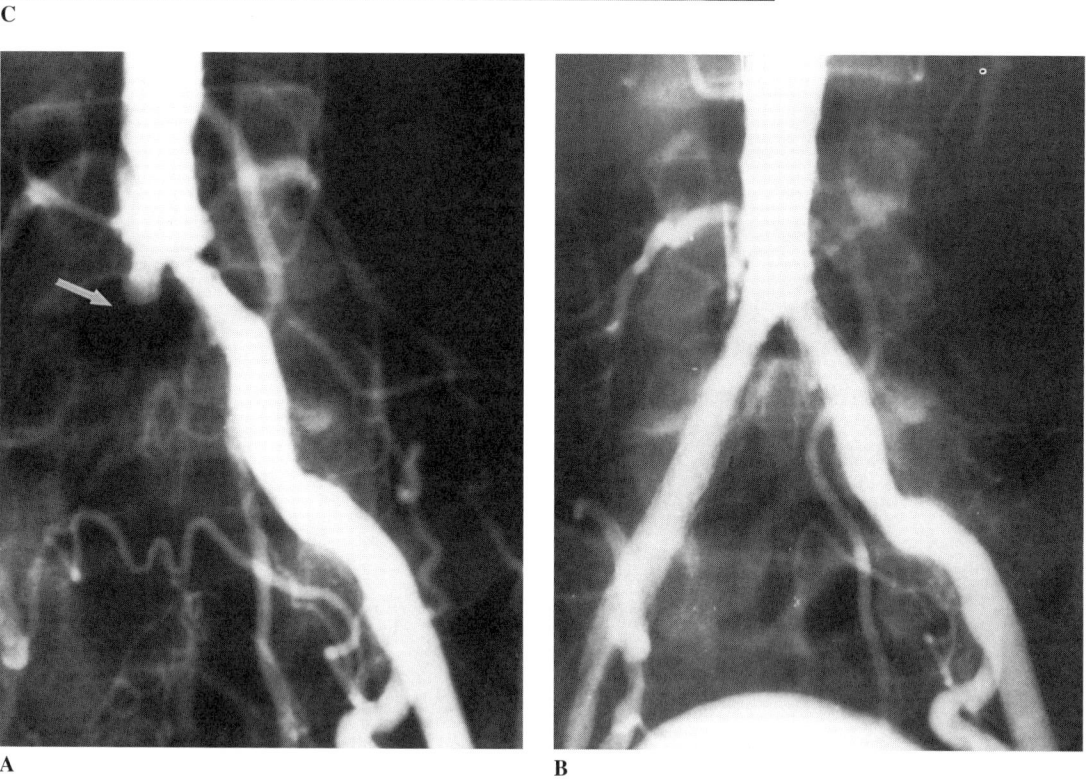

C

A

B

Figure 3-28. A. Pelvic arteriogram demonstrating a chronic occlusion of the right common iliac artery and stenosis of the proximal left common iliac (arrow). B. Repeat arteriogram after the right common iliac was primarily stented, as well as balloon angioplasty and stent placement of the left common iliac artery. Arteriogram shows an excellent percutaneous iliac reconstruction.

References

1. Shuford WH, Sybers RG. The Aortic Arch and Its Malformations. Springfield, IL: Thomas, 1974.
2. Khan S, Haust MD. Variations in the aortic origin of intercostal arteries in man. Anat Rec 1979;195:545.
3. Mirvis SE, Pais SO, Gens DR. Thoracic aortic rupture: advantages of intra-arterial digital subtraction angiography. AJR Am J Roentgenol 1986;146:987.
4. Stark P, Cook M, Vincent A, et al. Traumatic rupture of the thoracic aorta: a review of 49 cases. Radiology 1987;27:402.
5. Lundell CJ, Quinn MF, Finck EJ. Traumatic laceration of the ascending aorta: angiographic assessment. AJR Am J Roentgenol 1985;145:715.
6. Heystraten FM, Rosenbusch G, Kingma LM, et al. Chronic post-traumatic aneurysm of the thoracic aorta: surgically correctable occult threat. AJR Am J Roentgenol 1986;146:303.
7. Earnest F, Muhm JR, Sheedy PF Jr. Roentgenographic findings in thoracic aortic dissection. Mayo Clin Proc 1979;54:43.
8. Schnitker MA, Bayer CA. Dissecting aneurysm of the aorta in young individuals, particularly in association with pregnancy, with report of a case. Ann Intern Med 1944;20:486.
9. Abbott ME. Coarctation of the aorta of the adult type. II. A statistical study and historical retrospect of 200 recorded cases, with autopsy, of stenosis or obstruction of the descending arch in subjects above the age of 2 years. Am Heart J 1928;3:392, 574.
10. Harris PD, Malm JR, Bigger JT Jr, et al. Follow up studies of acute dissecting aortic aneurysms managed with antihypertensive agents. Circulation 1967;35(Suppl 1):183.
11. Shuford WH, Sybers RG, Weens HS. Problems in the aortographic diagnosis of dissecting aneurysm of the aorta. N Engl J Med 1969;280:225.
12. Siegelman SS, Sprayregen S, Strasberg Z, et al. Aortic dissection and the left renal artery. Radiology 1970;95:73.
13. DeBakey ME, Henly WS, Cooley DA, et al. Surgical management of dissecting aneurysm involving the ascending aorta. J Cardiovasc Surg 1964;5:200.
14. Daily PO, Trueblood HW, Stinson EB, et al. Management of acute aortic dissection. Ann Thorac Surg 1970;10:237.
15. Thorsen MK, SanDretto MA, Lawson TL, et al. Dissecting aortic aneurysms: accuracy of computed tomographic diagnosis. Radiology 1983;148:773.
16. DeSanctis RW, Doroghazi RM, Austen WG, et al. Aortic dissection. N Engl J Med 1987;317:1060.
17. Dee P, Martin R, Oudkerk M, et al. The diagnosis of aortic dissection. Curr Probl Diagn Radiol 1983;12:1.
18. Spittell JA Jr, Wallace RB. Aneurysms. In JL Juergens, JA Spittell Jr, JF Fairbairn II (eds), Peripheral Vascular Diseases. Philadelphia: Saunders, 1980;415.
19. Dinsmore RE, Jang GC. Roentgen diagnosis of aortic disease. Prog Cardiovasc Dis 1973;16:151.
20. Estes JR Jr. Abdominal aortic aneurysm: a study of one hundred and two cases. Circulation 1950;2:258.
21. Rösch J, Keller FS, Porter JM, et al. Value of angiography in the management of abdominal aortic aneurysm. Cardiovasc Radiol 1978;1:83.
22. Steinberg I. Isolated arteriosclerotic aneurysm of a common iliac artery. Report of three cases. AJR Am J Roentgenol 1963;90:166.
23. McCready RA, Pairolero PC, Gilmore JC, et al. Isolated iliac artery aneurysms. Surgery 1983;93:688.
24. Kasulke RJ, Clifford A, Nichols WK, et al. Isolated atherosclerotic aneurysms of the internal iliac arteries. Report of two cases and review of the literature. Arch Surg 1982;117:73.
25. Brewster DC, Retana A, Waltman AC, et al. Angiography in the management of aneurysms of the abdominal aorta. Its value and safety. N Engl J Med 1975;292:822.
26. Darling RC, Messina CR, Brewster DC, et al. Autopsy study of unoperated abdominal aortic aneurysms. Circulation 1977;56(Suppl 2):161.
27. Ottinger LW. Ruptured arteriosclerotic aneurysms of the abdominal aorta. Reducing mortality. JAMA 1975;233:147.
28. Edwards EA, LeMay M. Occlusion patterns and collaterals in arteriosclerosis of the lower aorta and iliac arteries. Surgery 1955;38:950.
29. Muller RF, Figley MM. The arteries of the abdomen, pelvis and thigh. I. Normal roentgenographic anatomy. II. Collateral circulation in obstructive arterial disease. AJR Am J Roentgenol 1957;77:296.
30. Raaf JH, Shannon J. Atherosclerotic coarctation of the abdominal aorta in women. Surg Gynecol Obstet 1980;150:715.
31. Holmes DR Jr, Burbank MK, Fulton RE, et al. Arteriosclerosis obliterans in young women. Am J Med 1979;66:997.
32. Veith FJ, Gupta SK, Wengerter KR, et al. Changing arteriosclerotic disease patterns and management strategies in lower-limb threatening ischemia. Ann Surg 1990;212:402.
33. Lammer J, Pilger E, Neumeyer K, Schreyer H. Intra-arterial fibrinolysis: long-term results. Radiology 1986;161:159.
34. Yedicka JW, Ferral H, Bjarnagen H, et al. Chronic iliac artery occlusions: primary recanalization with endovascular stents. J Vasc Interv Radiol 1994;5:843.
35. Parodi JC. Endovascular repair of abdominal aortic aneurysms. Adv Vasc Surg 1993;1:85.
36. Chuter TAM, Green RM, Ouriel K, et al. Transfemoral endovascular aortic graft placement. J Vasc Surg 1993;18:185.
37. Marin ML, Veith FJ. Transfemoral retrograde stent-graft repair of abdominal aortic aneurysms: the Parodi procedure. N Engl J Med (in press).
38. Parodi JC, Palmaz JC, Barone HD. Transfemoral intraluminal graft implantation for abdominal aortic aneurysms. Ann Vasc Surg 1991;5:491.

39. Marin ML, Veith FJ, Panetta TF, et al. Transluminally placed endovascular stented graft repair for arterial trauma. J Vasc Surg 1994;20:466.
40. Marin ML, Veith FJ, Cynamon J, et al. Transfemoral endoluminal repair of a penetrating vascular injury. J Vasc Interv Radiol 1994;5:592.
41. Marin ML, Veith FJ, Panetta TF, et al. Percutaneous transfemoral stented graft repair of a traumatic femoral arteriovenous fistula. J Vasc Surg 1993;18:298.
42. Marin ML, Veith FJ, Panetta TF, et al. Transfemoral stented graft treatment of occlusive arterial disease for limb salvage: a preliminary report [abstract]. Circulation 1993;88(Suppl 1):11.
43. Marin ML, Veith FJ, Cynamon J, et al. Transfemoral endovascular stented graft treatment of aortoiliac and femoropopliteal occlusive disease for limb salvage. Am J Surg 1994;168:156,
44. Dake MD, Miller DC, Semba CP. Transluminal placement of endovascular stent-grafts for the treatment of descending thoracic aortic aneurysms. N Engl J Med 1994;331:1729.

Chapter 4
Monitoring for Aortic Surgery

Steven B. Schulman and David S. Weiss

Patients arriving for aortic surgery present one of the most challenging medical scenarios facing the anesthesiologist, surgeon, and intensivist. It is crucial that the anesthesiologist caring for the patient in the perioperative period understands and is comfortable with all appropriate monitors to ensure the most favorable outcome. To determine the appropriate monitors for these patients, it is important to address what is being monitored and thereby what complications should be avoided. All patients undergoing surgery on the aorta are at risk for damage to the myocardium. Those undergoing surgery on the ascending aorta, the aortic arch, or both are also at risk for a cerebrovascular event. The repair of pathology affecting the descending aorta risks spinal cord ischemia, renal failure, and often gastrointestinal hypoperfusion. In addition, the desire to avoid severe hypothermia (or conversely the occasional need for extreme levels of hypothermia) mandate the requirement for accurate temperature assessment. This chapter discusses and compares the various monitors available based on the physiologic index requiring regulation.

Cardiac Monitoring

Concurrent Cardiac Disease

Nearly all patients undergoing surgery on their aorta have coexisting coronary artery disease. The incidence of significant coronary atherosclerosis (at least 75% occlusion of at least one vessel) in the patient with an abdominal aortic aneurysm (AAA) has been found to be 22–75%.[1–4] As many as one in four patients undergoing AAA repair will have a cardiac event (e.g., death, myocardial infarction [MI], congestive heart failure, unstable angina).[5,6] Fifty percent of the deaths following elective AAA repairs are of cardiac origin.[7–9] Nearly 90% of patients with thoracic aneurysmal disease have documented cardiovascular disease.[10] Aortic dissections are more common in patients with hypertension[11] and with prior cardiac surgery.[12] The risk of a cardiac event is multiplied when these patients are faced with the multitude of metabolic and hemodynamic derangements that can occur during aortic surgery. These events include (but are not limited to) washout acidosis, large fluid shifts, and cardiovascular instability complicating anesthetic induction, aortic cross clamping and aortic cross clamp release.[13–17] The cardiovascular indices that need to be monitored and oftentimes manipulated intraoperatively include the heart rate, the blood pressure (BP), cardiac arrhythmias, preload, myocardial ischemia, and left ventricular contractility.

Heart Rate

It is crucial to continuously assess the heart rate in the patient undergoing aortic surgery. Tachycardia increases myocardial oxygen demand and decreases oxygen supply (by limiting diastolic filling time), thereby tipping the patient toward myocardial ischemia. In addition, an increasing heart rate may be the first (and possibly the only) indication of light anesthesia.

The various monitors available to measure heart rate include electrocardiography (ECG), pulse oximetry, and invasive hemodynamic modalities (e.g., arterial line and pulmonary artery catheter [PAC]). The ECG is the simplest method and is most often very reliable. It may be substituted by one of the other aforementioned monitors in the presence of artifact from electrocautery or if the measured heart rate is erroneous due to peaked T waves or pacemaker spikes.

Arrhythmias

The presence of coexisting cardiac disease likely increases the risk of perioperative cardiac arrhythmias. When combined with the potential wide fluctuation in systemic vascular resistance, acid-base balance, electrolytes, temperature, oxygenation, and the ability to ventilate and the need for direct cardiac manipulation (i.e., "mugging the heart"), which occurs often, the risk of arrhythmias increases exponentially. If the operative procedure involves the ascending aorta, the transverse aorta, or both, it is important to be able to confirm asystole throughout the procedure and the return of an acceptable rhythm following cardiopulmonary bypass (CPB). The ECG is presently the best (and only) monitor routinely available for the continuous assessment of cardiac rhythm.

It is important to monitor the correct ECG lead to not only detect the arrhythmia, but also to correctly identify it so that the proper treatment can be employed. In one study of cardiac surgical patients,[18] lead V_5 led to a correct diagnosis of atrial arrhythmias in only 42% of cases, and lead II led to a correct diagnosis in 54% of cases, but an esophageal ECG led to a correct diagnosis in 100% of cases. Esophageal ECGs display a prominent P wave during atrial depolarization, often making arrhythmia identification more obvious.[19] Other ECG sites that may be used for the detection of intraoperative arrhythmias are the intracardiac ECG[20] and the tracheal ECG.[21] Although attractive for arrhythmia detection, their added cost and the fear of thermal burns have limited their use. ECG lead placement is discussed further in the section on monitoring for myocardial ischemia.

Blood Pressure

By monitoring the BP during anesthesia one is able to maintain end-organ perfusion, prevent catastrophic episodes of hypertension, and obtain information regarding ventricular afterload and contractility. The heart, brain, kidneys, and most vital organs are able to maintain constant perfusion throughout a wide range of mean arterial pressures; this is called *autoregulation*. By ensuring an adequate pressure inflow, one decreases the likelihood of ischemia or infarction. Aside from greatly increasing afterload and wall tension, severe hypertension may be blamed for difficulty with surgical anastamosis. As with heart rate, BP monitoring provides a relatively insensitive and nonspecific monitor for light anesthesia and hypovolemia.

Arterial Pressure Monitoring

All patients undergoing aortic surgery must have an intra-arterial catheter (a-line) during their operation. The a-line is necessary not only for continuous BP monitoring, but also for repeated measurement of arterial blood gases, electrolytes, hematocrit, and ongoing coagulation assessment. The only exception to this is the patient with a ruptured AAA in whom fluid resuscitation and control of the proximal aorta becomes the first priority. In this scenario a-line placement should be accomplished immediately following volume repletion and aortic cross clamping.

The major concern regarding a-line placement in these patients is the site to be used. More so than with any other type of surgical procedure, the site of the a-line is dependent on the site of the primary aortic pathology (Table 4-1). For surgery on the abdominal aorta, the a-line should be inserted in either upper extremity, preferably in the radial artery.

Descending Thoracic Aortic Surgery. Patients undergoing descending thoracic aortic surgery require two arterial lines, one proximal to the lesion and one distal to the lesion. The proximal a-line corresponds to perfusion to the brain and myocardium, and the distal relates perfusion to the spinal cord, kidneys, and viscera. Monitoring must include a right upper extremity a-line (in

Table 4-1. Sites for Arterial Cannulation

Aortic Pathology	Arterial Site
Ascending aorta	Left upper extremity
Aortic arch	Left upper extremity
Abdominal aorta	Left or right upper extremity
Descending aorta	Femoral and right upper extremity

case of any compromise of flow to the left sub-clavian artery). Either femoral artery is acceptable for the distal monitor. If partial bypass is to be employed, the surgical team should be consulted regarding which femoral artery will be used for monitoring and which for arterial cannulation (see Chapter 8).

Aortic Arch Surgery.   Patients with disease of the aortic arch (in whom arch replacement is planned) require deep hypothermic circulatory arrest with interruption of all blood flow. A left radial artery catheter should be placed as part of the standard monitoring. A left-sided a-line allows for the assessment of BP following completion of the first anastomosis and reestablishment of flow (see Chapters 6 and 7).

Ascending Aortic Surgery.   For patients with ascending aortic disease (with or without aortic insufficiency) there is the possibility of dissection or aneurysm involving the innominate artery. In addition, the innominate artery is often cross clamped during repair. Therefore, in these patients the a-line should be placed in the left radial artery. These patients require CPB, and due to the nature of the pathology, one of the femoral arteries will be used for arterial cannulation (see Chapter 6).

Complications.   The placement of invasive arterial monitoring is generally free of complications. Risks include direct peripheral neurologic trauma, infection, cerebral embolization,[22] pseudoaneurysm formation, and thrombosis with distal ischemia (especially in the case of end arteries lacking adequate collateral supply). Radial artery thrombosis is not generally a problem as most will recannulate within 2 weeks.[23]

Myocardial Ischemia

Anesthesiologists seek to avoid intraoperative myocardial ischemia through the maintenance of oxygen supply and the simultaneous minimization of oxygen demand. It was not until recently that evidence emerged indicating that perioperative ischemia portends a poor cardiac outcome. Slogoff and Keats[24] showed that in patients undergoing coronary artery bypass grafting (CABG), intraoperative ECG evidence of myocardial ischemia correlated with a threefold increase in the incidence of perioperative myocardial infarctions. Recently Pasternack and colleagues[25] confirmed that intraoperative ischemia in patients undergoing major vascular reconstruction often leads to perioperative MIs. Patients undergoing AAA repair are most likely to become ischemic during aortic clamping and unclamping.[15,26,27] Higher aortic cross clamping increases the likelihood of myocardial ischemia due to the reduction in systemic collateral circulation and the resulting greater increase in systemic vascular resistance.[28] Thus, in addition to avoiding myocardial ischemia through heart rate and BP regulation, it is important to diagnose the ischemia as early as possible to minimize complications.

Electrocardiography

Diagnosis of Ischemia.   The most common monitor used to diagnose myocardial ischemia is the ECG. The ECG changes that represent true myocardial ischemia have been studied in patients via correlation with pulmonary and left ventricular pressure changes,[29] regional left ventricular dysfunction,[30] and abnormalities of myocardial perfusion.[31] ECG evidence of ischemia is evaluated at the ST segment. A depressed ST segment is generally measured at the J point + 60–80 ms, depending on the heart rate (Figure 4-1). Horizontal and downsloping ST depression greater than or equal to 0.1 mV (1 mm) are both indicative of myocardial ischemia.[32] Upsloping ST depression is also considered significant,[32] although it may occasionally be seen in normal patients with tachycardia.[33] ST-segment elevation is measured at the J point and is considered significant if there is an increase greater than or equal to 0.2 mV (2 mm).[34,35] Symmetrical T-wave inversions may also indicate significant myocardial ischemia.[36] In order for an episode to be classified as significant

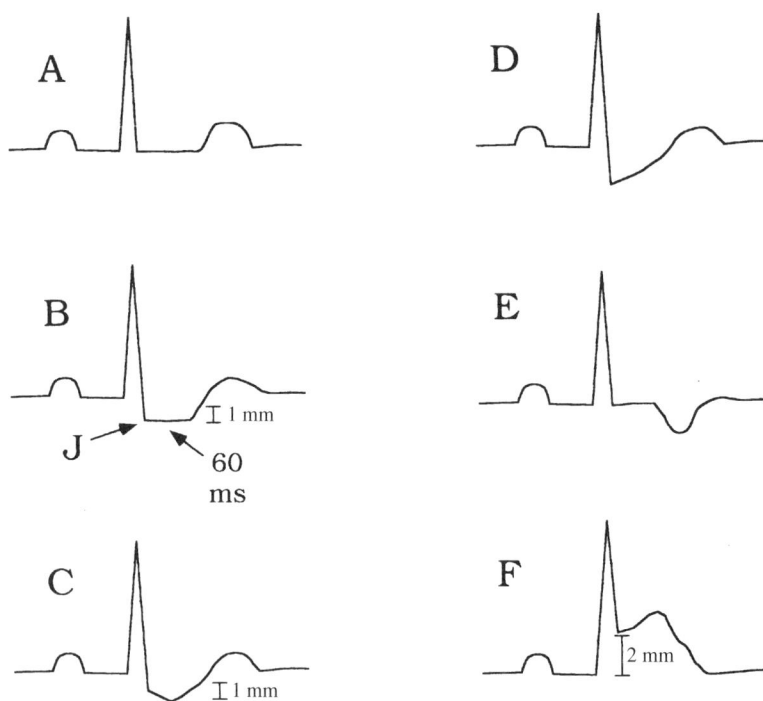

Figure 4-1. A. Normal electro-cardiogram. B. One-millimeter ST depression. C. One-millimeter downsloping ST depression. D. Upsloping ST depression. E. Symmetric T-wave inversions. F. ST elevation. ST-segment depression is measured at the J point + 60–80 ms. ST-segment elevation is measured at the J point. Complexes B, C, E, and F are all suggestive of myocardial ischemia. Complex D may represent myocardial ischemia but may also represent normal J point depression during tachycardia. (Reprinted with permission from S Schulman. The Diagnostic Workup of the Cardiac Patient for Non-Cardiac Surgery. Progress in Anesthesiology 1995;9(6). San Antonio, TX: Dannemiller Memorial Educational Foundation, 1995.)

it must continue for at least 1 minute and must be separated from other discrete episodes by at least 1 minute of normal baseline.[37]

Automated ST-Segment Trending.   The ability to continuously monitor the ST-segment height may allow for early intraoperative recognition and treatment of myocardial ischemia. Most intraoperative monitors with automated ST-segment trending (ASTST) ability generate an initial ECG template against which ongoing ECG complexes are compared. Newer monitors, which allow the user to set the isoelectric point and J point, are likely more accurate than older models, which relied on automated assessment of baseline.[38] ST-segment changes are averaged over a number of beats and the monitor updates the value over a periodic interval. It is also possible to have ST-segment trending as a table or graph display with alarm capabilities.

Computerized ST-segment analysis detects significant ST-segment changes often missed by an anesthesiologist[39] and greatly improves the anesthesiologist's ability to detect ischemia.[40] Jain and colleagues[41] found that in CABG patients, ST elevation of as little as 1.0 mm detected via ASTST correlated

with a 90% sensitivity and 100% specificity of evolving MI. Also in CABG patients, Kotter and coworkers[42] found that with the increased sensitivity to myocardial ischemia afforded by ASTST, the incidence of perioperative MI was significantly reduced. ASTST is therefore a helpful tool in the diagnosis of perioperative myocardial ischemia providing certain criteria are met.

According to American Heart Association criteria for ST-segment analysis, the frequency-response characteristics of the system must be in the range of 0.05–100.00 Hz.[43] This wide bandwidth yields tracings of a high resolution that allow for evaluation of QRS morphology (high frequency limit)[44] as well as ST-segment analysis (low frequency limit).[45] It is important to ensure that the ECG monitor used is calibrated to allow for a wide frequency response. For example, the Spacelabs Alpha 14 cardule (Spacelabs, Inc., Redmon, WA) has a frequency response bandwidth of 0.5–40.0 Hz in the monitoring mode, versus 0.05–70.00 Hz in the extended mode. In the monitoring mode, lower frequencies are filtered to reduce noise, thereby distorting the ST-segment data (Figure 4-2).[43] Whenever ST segments are being evaluated (with ASTST and visually), it is important that the

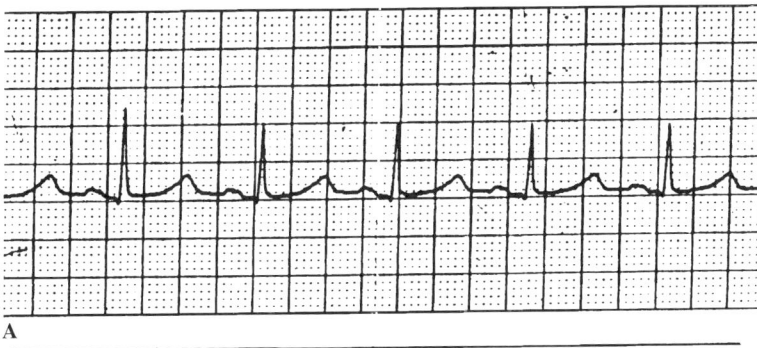

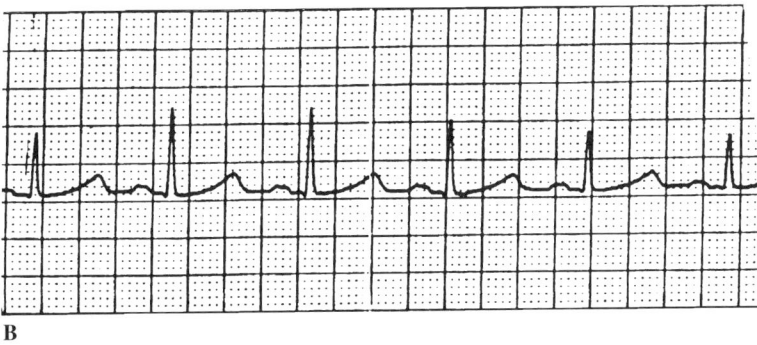

Figure 4-2. A. The electrocardiographic frequency response in the tracing is 0.05–70.00 mHz (extended). B. This is contrasted with a range of 0.5–40.0 mHz in this tracing (monitoring). Although there is somewhat less artifact in the tracing shown in B, it is apparently "flattened out," and misleading ST-segment changes may be obtained.

monitor have a wide frequency response (i.e., be in the extended mode). The aforementioned Spacelabs cardule circumvents this problem by automatically analyzing the ST segment at 0.05 Hz during ASTST.

Lead Positioning. Most anesthesia monitors only allow for the continuous assessment of two simultaneous ECG leads. Kaplan and King performed a study to determine which leads should be monitored.[46] They found that in patients undergoing CABG the precordial V_5 lead (anterior axillary line in the fifth intercostal interspace) was the best choice for the detection of intraoperative ischemia. London and colleagues[47] expanded on Kaplan and King's work in their study of high-risk patients undergoing noncardiac surgery. They confirmed that lead V_5 was the most sensitive for intraoperative myocardial ischemia (75%) (Figure 4-3). When combined with lead II, the sensitivity only increased to 80%. Leads V_4, V_5, and II when examined simultaneously yielded a sensitivity of 98%.

Surgical procedures on the thoracic aorta often render standard lead placement impossible due to interference with the operative field. Patients undergoing surgery of the descending aorta usually undergo a left thoracotomy for surgical access. The lateral position and open chest may alter the normal patterns of the ST-segment response. In these situations alternate ECG sites must be employed. If the lateral precordial leads are eliminated, almost 70% of ischemic changes may be missed if the ECG is the sole monitor for ischemia.[47]

There are a number of preexisting patient factors that may make ST-segment changes unreliable indicators of myocardial ischemia. Among these are the presence of a permanent pacemaker, left bundle branch block, left ventricular hypertrophy with strain pattern, and changes related to digoxin.[34,48–51] Intraoperative factors that may cause misleading ST-segment changes include alterations in body temperature, serum electrolytes, body position, or ventilatory pattern.[52] In this high-risk group of aortic surgery patients, additional monitors for myocardial ischemia must be employed that are more sensitive and reliable in a diverse group of patients.

Pulmonary Artery Catheterization

Since first introduced by Swan in 1970, the flotation of a fluid-filled catheter into the pulmonary

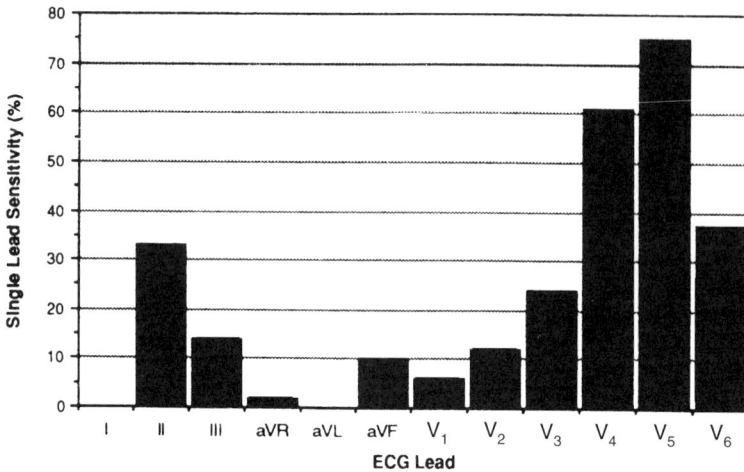

Figure 4-3. The distribution of ischemic ST-segment changes in each of the 12 leads for cardiac patients undergoing noncardiac surgery. Sensitivity is highest (75%) in lead V_5. (Reprinted with permission from M London, M Hollenberg, M Wong. Intraoperative myocardial ischemia: localization by continuous 12 lead electrocardiography. Anesthesiology 1988;69:232.)

artery has become commonplace when caring for the patient with cardiac disease undergoing cardiac surgery. Swan has estimated that over 2 million PACs are "floated" annually.[53] One of the indications for intraoperative use of a PAC is for the detection of myocardial ischemia.

It has been known since 1958 that an increase in the left ventricular end-diastolic pressure (LVEDP) often precedes clinical angina.[54] Müller and Rørvik[54] reported that myocardial ischemia causes an altered diastolic filling that manifests prior to clinical symptomatology. These same investigators concluded that the early use of nitroglycerin could interrupt the ischemic process. The PAC provides a means of indirectly measuring LVEDP with the goal of early recognition and treatment of myocardial ischemia.

When properly inserted, inflating the balloon on the PAC causes a distal migration and wedging in the distal pulmonary arteries. Theoretically, the pulmonary capillary wedge pressure (PCWP) correlates with the LVEDP. A decrease in compliance (as occurs with myocardial ischemia) may manifest as an elevation of PCWP (as a correlate of LVEDP) for a given preload. Thus, an increase in the wedge might serve as an indicator of myocardial ischemia. Another indicator of myocardial ischemia is the new onset of V waves in the PCWP tracing. Left ventricular ischemia can produce V waves via papillary muscle ischemia or by increasing LVEDP and thereby increasing the amount of blood in the left atrium at the onset of filling.[55] Additionally, the new onset of V waves in the pul-

monary artery waveform has also been reported to be indicative of myocardial ischemia.[56, 57]

Kaplan and Wells[58] were among the first to study the PAC as an intraoperative monitor for myocardial ischemia. In a study of 40 patients arriving for CABG surgery, they reported that 18 developed myocardial ischemia prior to CPB. Of these ischemic patients, three manifested solely as ST-segment depression, five as ST depression with an abnormal AC (early elevation in the PCWP tracing concordant with atrial and ventricular systole) or V wave, and ten had only an abnormal AC or V wave. They attributed the change in the wedge tracing to an abnormal myocardial relaxation yielding reduced left ventricular diastolic function (lusitropy). Decreased lusitropy caused an accentuation of left atrial pressure waveforms.[59] In addition, subendocardial ischemia may cause abnormal papillary muscle function and resultant mitral regurgitation.[58] They concluded that perioperative myocardial ischemia causes changes in the wedge pressure that occur before ECG changes, and with treatment the PCWP is reduced before the ECG returns to baseline.

Nevertheless, not all elevations in PCWP represent ischemic changes. In the aforementioned study there is no independent measure of myocardial ischemia, no discussion of perioperative fluid management, nor is there a confirmed absence of valvular disease. By assessing regional wall motion abnormalities (via echocardiography), or measuring myocardial lactate to confirm true ischemia, it would be more possible to state that the abnormal wedge tracing represents true ischemia. In addition, congestive heart failure, increased afterload, sympathetic stimulation, mitral stenosis, or mitral regurgitation may yield similarly abnormal tracings.[60] Thus, while the use of nitroglycerin may "flatten out" the wedge tracing, an elevation does not necessarily indicate myocardial ischemia.

Complications.   The placement of a PAC is not a benign procedure and any of a number of complications may occur from its use. Complications are related to the initial vascular cannulation, flotation of the catheter, and, finally, long-standing use. Cannulation of a major vein (e.g., internal jugular or subclavian) may cause pneumothorax, inadvertent arterial damage (or cannulation), hemothorax, or chylothorax. Flotation of the catheter has been associated with pulmonary artery rupture, ventricular arrhythmia, valvular damage, and heart block. PACs that remain in place for extended periods of time can become a nidus for thrombus, infection, or both.

Transesophageal Echocardiography

Method.   The most recently introduced intraoperative myocardial ischemia monitor is transesophageal echocardiography (TEE).[61] Two-dimensional TEE may be used to detect myocardial ischemia via evaluation of wall motion, wall thickening, or diastolic function.

Left ventricular systole is characterized by a contraction and thickening of the chamber walls, causing an ejection of the end-diastolic volume. It has been known since 1935[62] that an interruption in coronary blood flow causes specific myocardial regional wall motion abnormalities (RWMAs). These RWMAs follow a predictable course, with early ischemia causing hypokinesis (decreased wall motion), followed by akinesis (absent wall motion), and finally dyskinesis (paradoxical wall motion).[63] Patients undergoing aortic surgery are at high risk for the development of new RWMAs. Those having very proximal cross clamping (i.e., descending thoracic aneurysms and abdominal aortic supraceliac lesions) are especially vulnerable due to a limitation of collateral circulation,[64] and possibly higher wall stress (see Chapter 10).[15]

Percutaneous transluminal coronary angioplasty studies have shown that following coronary occlusion, systolic wall motion abnormalities begin within 10–19 seconds of balloon inflation and reach a maximum at approximately 30 seconds.[63,65] RWMAs have been shown to occur simultaneously with regional lactate production.[66] Transient occlusion followed by reperfusion yielded return of normokinesis within 43 seconds. Balloon inflation for longer than 5 minutes produced a longer recovery time (from 45 minutes to several weeks). This delay may represent "stunned" myocardium. Stunned myocardium represents regions that are akinetic or severely hypokinetic without being infarcted.[67] This may be contrasted with the term *hibernating myocardium,* which is used when referring to chronically hypoperfused regions of myocardium that develop RWMAs. Both conditions are characterized by a significant improvement in wall motion following a restoration of coronary blood flow (especially following coronary artery revascularization).

When using TEE to assess myocardial ischemia, the view most commonly evaluated is the left ventricular short axis at the level of the midpapillary muscles (Figure 4-4). This section shows the inferoposterior, lateral, anterior, and septal walls and represents myocardium supplied by all three coronary arteries. It is important not to neglect the left ventricular apex. Studies have shown that many episodes of missed ischemia occur in the apex.[68,69] New TEE-probe technology has made evaluation of the apex more reliable. Early TEE probes only allowed for a monoplane visualization of the heart and surrounding structures. With only a transverse "cut" through the myocardium it is likely that areas of ischemia may be missed. Newer probes allow for the visualization of both a transverse and longitudinal plane ("biplane") or a multitude of planes ("omniplane"). Figure 4-5 shows a left ventricular apical aneurysm that would have been missed if only the short axis view had been examined.

A number of studies have evaluated the sensitivity and specificity of new intraoperative RWMAs as predictors of adverse cardiac outcomes (generally defined as postoperative MI).[70–72] Smith and coworkers[71] studied 50 patients undergoing cardiac or vascular surgery. They found that new RWMAs that persisted significantly increased the chance of having a postoperative MI. No patient without a new RWMA had an immediate postoperative infarction. They also noted that in those patients with known coronary artery disease (demonstrated by preoperative coronary angiography), RWMAs occurred only in the areas of myocardium at

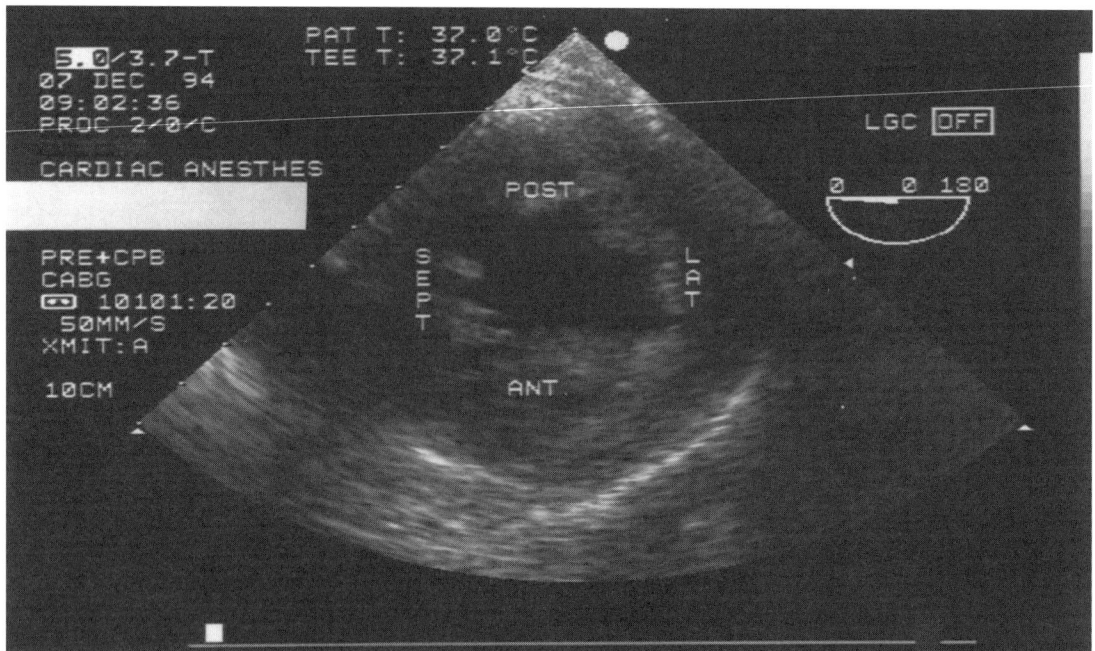

Figure 4-4. The left ventricular transgastric short-axis view at the midpapillary level displays myocardium supplied by all three coronary arteries. (LAT = lateral wall; ANT = anterior wall; SEPT = septum; POST = posterior/inferior wall.)

risk. This study was followed by Gewertz and coworkers,[70] who reported that persistent RWMAs detected on intraoperative TEE had a sensitivity of 100% for postoperative infarction.

However, London and coworkers[72] studied 175 patients with known cardiac disease undergoing noncardiac surgery. Surprisingly, they found that 57% of wall motion abnormalities were unassociated with an obvious clinical event (e.g., skin incision or aortic cross clamping), 43% occurred in the absence of any significant hemodynamic change, and most occurred randomly throughout the anesthesia. Although they found that RWMAs were much more common in those patients undergoing aortic vascular surgery as compared with other surgery (38% compared with 17%), most resolved without evidence of myocardial infarction. There were only four cardiac complications (three had MIs, one had an unstable angina), three of which occurred in patients without any TEE or ECG changes. They concluded that most intraoperative RWMAs are hypokinetic in nature and do not represent true myocardial ischemia. They also concluded that TEE is of limited value as an intraoperative monitor. In this study patients were followed and cardiac en-

zymes measured for up to 15 days postoperatively. More recent data from the same institution suggest that the only significant predictor of postoperative cardiac morbidity is immediate postoperative cardiac ischemia.[73] Without an examination of postoperative factors (that may have contributed to late myocardial events), it is not necessarily valid to extrapolate the findings of intraoperative monitoring for long-term postoperative events.

There are a number of reasons why apparent RWMAs may not be indicative of myocardial ischemia. The heart rotates and translates significantly during systole; therefore, it may be difficult at times to precisely evaluate segmental contraction.[74] Discoordinated contraction may occur due to artificial pacemaker activity or bundle branch block. Changes in preload, afterload, contractility, or any combination of these factors may also result in RWMAs not associated with myocardial ischemia.[71,75]

Ventricular wall thickening (with systole) is another measure of myocardial function. Subendocardial ischemia causes a decreased wall thickening that may also be evaluated via TEE. Canine studies[76–78] suggest that abnormalities in wall thickening may more closely reflect areas of myocardium

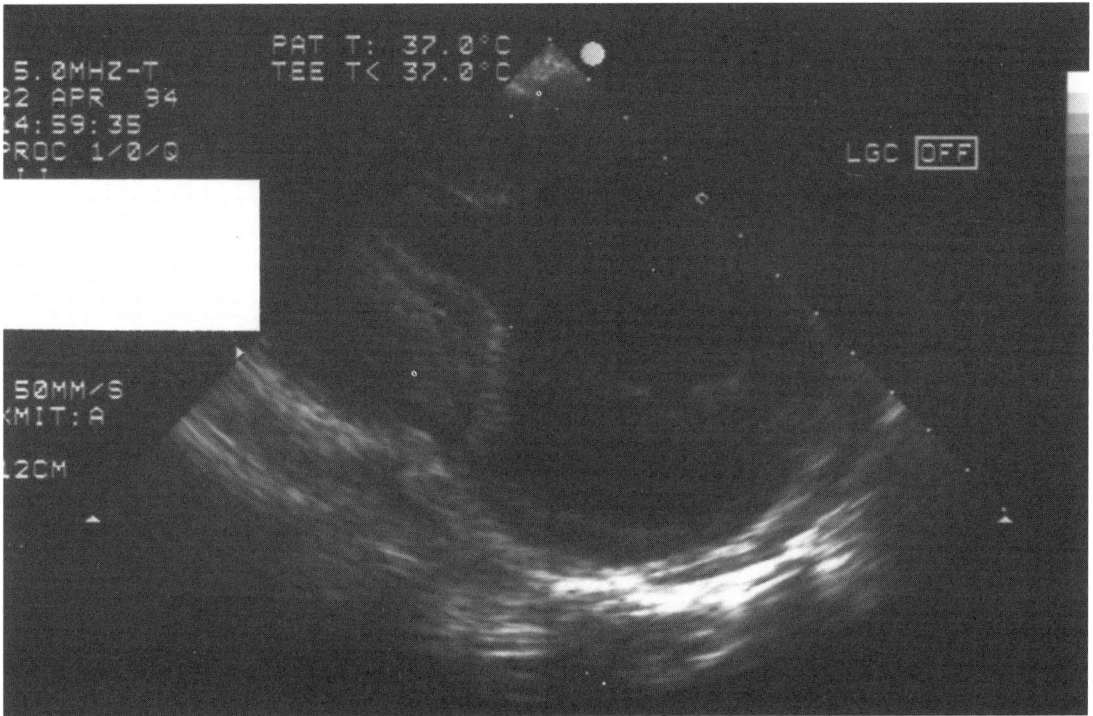

Figure 4-5. A left ventricular apical aneurysm as seen in the transgastric longitudinal view. This pathology would have been missed if the ventricle had only been scanned in the transverse plane.

at risk of infarction when compared with wall motion abnormalities (which tended to overestimate the true area of ischemia). Wall thickening measurements have also been found to be reproducible between multiple observers.[79]

Myocardial ischemia causes a decrease in diastolic function, which may be apparent through use of Doppler echocardiography.[80] By evaluating the inflow into the left ventricle (LV) through the mitral valve, it is possible to generate an E-to-A wave velocity ratio on a spectral display (Figure 4-6). The E wave represents normal diastolic filling of the left ventricle, and the A wave corresponds to filling that is secondary to atrial contraction. With normal compliance, the E wave peak velocity is greater than the A wave peak velocity. With decreasing compliance (as with early myocardial ischemia), the ratio is reversed. Alternatively, the area under the E wave or A waves may also be compared.

Limitations and Complications. Contraindications to the use of TEE include all pathology that

may contribute to esophageal rupture during probe insertion. Examples include esophageal varices, esophageal carcinoma, Zenker's diverticulum, esophageal stricture, Mallory-Weiss tear, and dysphagia of unknown etiology.

The risk of complications is small. In a series of 10,419 (awake) TEE examinations, Daniel and coworkers[81] reported a complication rate of only 0.18%. Complications included bronchospasm, hypoxemia, nonsustained ventricular tachycardia, complete heart block, and minor pharyngeal bleeding. They also reported the only case of esophageal perforation secondary to TEE (in a patient with unsuspected lung carcinoma). A recent case report from Spahn and coworkers[82] related the first incidence of intraoperative hypopharyngeal perforation by a TEE probe. The patient had an unrecognized esophageal stricture and long-term swallowing difficulties that were not elucidated during the preoperative interview. Another series from the Mayo Clinic,[83] including 1,110 patients, reported a 0.3% incidence of nonsustained ventricular tachycardia,

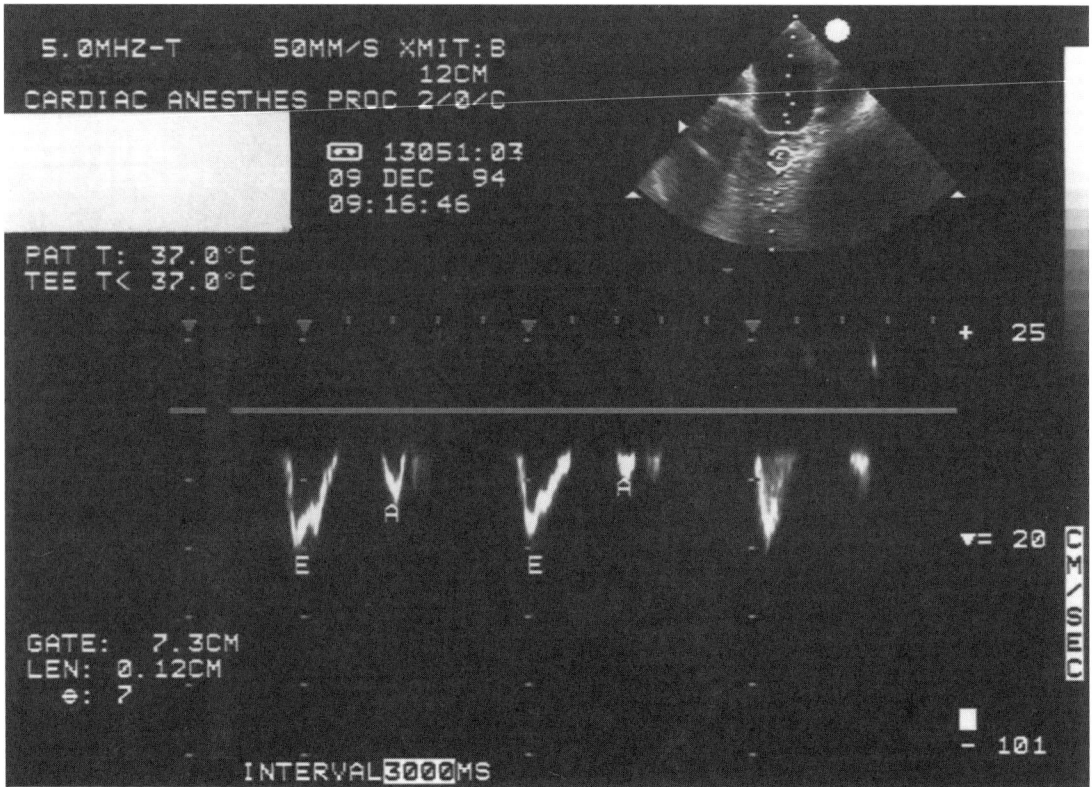

A

Figure 4-6. Via spectral analysis of pulsed waved Doppler frequency shifts during left ventricular inflow through the mitral valve one may determine diastolic function. The pulsed waved Doppler cursor must be positioned precisely at the level of the mitral valve. A. Normal diastolic function with the E wave (normal diastolic inflow) greater than the A wave (atrial contribution to ventricular filling). B. Poor diastolic function (myocardial ischemia, left ventricular hypertrophy) with the E wave less than the A wave. This indicates a greater contribution of the atrial kick to left ventricular filling.

0.3% nonsustained atrial arrhythmias, 0.2% congestive heart failure, and one episode of parotid swelling. The incidence of many of these complications is assumed to decrease under general anesthesia, but as yet there are no large-scale studies confirming its safety.

Comparisons of Electrocardiography, Pulmonary Artery Catheters, and Transesophageal Echocardiography for the Detection of Intraoperative Ischemia

Animal studies have shown that changes in RWMAs and wall thickness provide the earliest measure of myocardial ischemia.[84] Whereas changes in wall motion were generally obvious 15–30 seconds following coronary occlusion, ST-segment changes often lagged for 3–5 minutes and occasionally did not appear at all (Figure 4-7).[84]

Coronary angioplasty has provided a unique means of assessing the hemodynamic and clinical effects of acute myocardial ischemia in humans. Serruys and coworkers[85] found that ventricular diastolic relaxation was the index most sensitive to acute balloon-induced ischemia. This was followed by local systolic mechanical dysfunction (RWMAs) and then, much later, by changes in LVEDP.

Numerous human studies have confirmed that the appearance of RWMAs precede changes in the ST segment.[63,65,85,86] Hauser and coworkers[65] studied 18 patients undergoing coronary angioplasty. While monitoring all six limb leads (and V$_5$ for left anterior descending coronary angioplasty), they found that the onset of ST-segment changes began

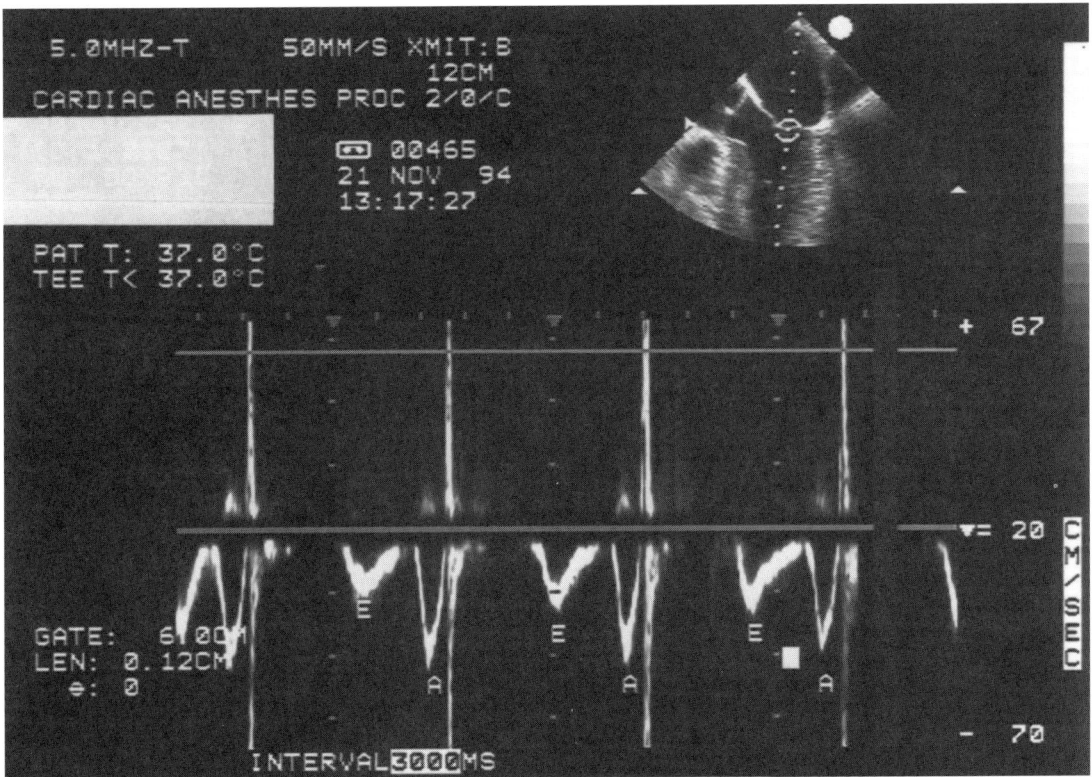

B

Figure 4-6. *(continued)*

approximately 11 seconds after the onset of dyssynergy. All patients exhibited RWMAs; only 8 of 18 had significant ECG changes (Figure 4-8). At no time were there ST-segment shifts without left ventricular wall motion abnormalities. In a similar study (using a 12-lead ECG), Wohlgelernter and colleagues[63] found that ST-segment changes lagged behind by up to 40 seconds and 2 of 14 patients did not have ECG changes at all with balloon inflation.

van Daele and colleagues[87] recently compared ST segments, wedge tracings, and TEE as monitors for perioperative myocardial ischemia in patients undergoing coronary artery surgery. While studying nearly 100 patients they found that TEE identified 14 patients with pre-CPB ischemia. Ten of these patients had concomitant ST-segment changes and all had an elevation of the PCWP. A significant number of patients had similar elevations in PCWP without myocardial ischemia. In this study, an increase in PCWP of 3 mm Hg was associated with a sensitivity of 33% and a positive predictive value of

only 15% for detection of myocardial ischemia. They concluded that the PCWP is a nonspecific indicator of myocardial ischemia because it is influenced by many factors that affect myocardial function and invite contradicting conclusions (e.g., an elevated PCWP may indicate fluid overload instead of myocardial ischemia or intraoperative blood loss may mask an ischemia-induced elevation in the PCWP). Similarly, Leung and colleagues[88] found that new post-CPB RWMAs (but not electrocardiographic changes) were associated with adverse outcome. Most episodes of TEE abnormalities (82%) were associated with unchanged ECGs. Only 10% of all RWMAs were associated with a concurrent increase in PCWP.

Smith and coworkers[71] studied patients with coronary disease undergoing major vascular surgery. New or more severe RWMAs appeared in 24 of 50 patients, whereas only 6 of these patients had significant ST-segment changes (multilead ECG system used). At no time was there ECG evidence of ischemia with-

Coronary
Flow
(% normal)

Time of onset of ECG changes and regional wall
motion abnormalities

20-80%

20%

0%
(complete
coronary
occlusion)

15 sec   30sec   1 min   2 min   10 min

Begin coronary   Time ——→
constriction

☐ = ECG changes (ST depression or elevation)

■ = Regional wall motion abnormalities
     (hypokinesia, akinesia, dyskinesia)

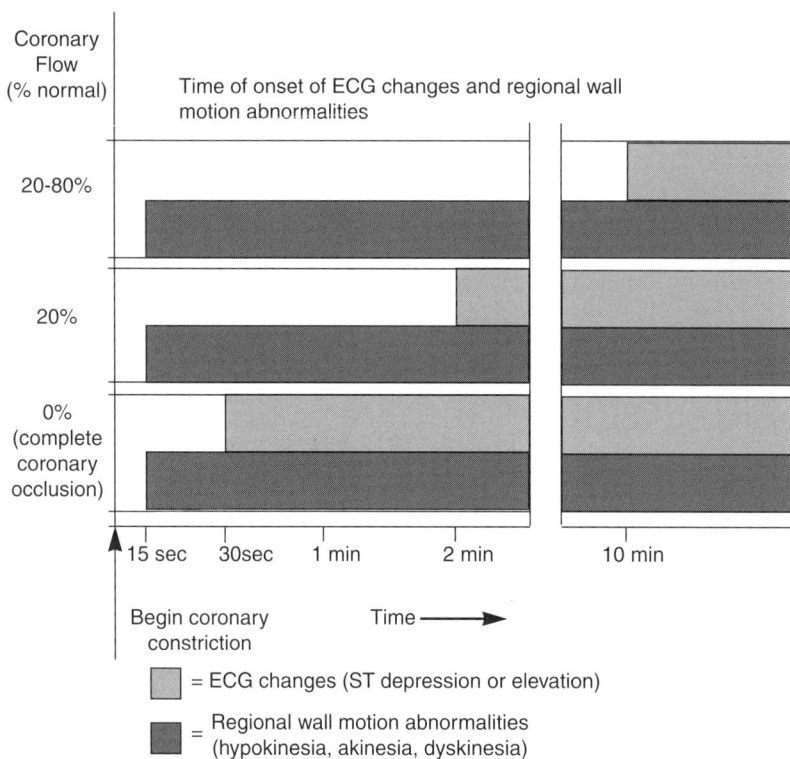

Figure 4-7. Temporal relationship between acute coronary constriction and onset of electrocardiogram and regional wall motion abnormalities. Electrocardiographic changes always lag behind regional wall motion abnormalities and oftentimes do not occur at all. (Reprinted with permission from F Clements, N Bruijn. Perioperative evaluation of regional wall motion by transesophageal two-dimensional echocardiography. Anesth Analg 1987;66:246.)

out ECG abnormalities. Of the four patients with perioperative MIs, three had TEE evidence of ischemia and only one had significant ECG changes. Koolen and coworkers[64] compared TEE with ECG in 51 patients undergoing AAA resection. There was an overall 16% rate of myocardial infarction by enzymes. They reported that the sensitivity of new or more severe RWMAs (which persist for 3 hours after unclamping) predicted perioperative infarction with a sensitivity of 88%, whereas ECG predicted infarction with a sensitivity of only 13%. The specificities were 72% and 95%, respectively. They attribute the low specificity of TEE to stunned myocardium. A significant limitation to this study is that only ECG lead II was continuously monitored. One would expect a significant amount of myocardial ischemia to be missed given this restriction.

Roizen and colleagues[15] compared the hemodynamic effects of aortic cross clamping at the supraceliac, suprarenal-infraceliac, and infrarenal levels. Patients were monitored with modified V_5 ECGs, PACs, and TEEs. When compared with lower cross clamping, supraceliac occlusion caused significant increases in left ventricular end-systolic

and end-diastolic areas, decreases in ejection fraction, and frequent RWMAs. The pulmonary artery wedge pressures were almost invariably unchanged. Even though systemic and pulmonary capillary wedge pressures were maintained at normal levels in 10 of 12 of these patients, 11 of 12 developed new RWMAs suggestive of myocardial ischemia. Electrocardiographic changes were not reported. They concluded that myocardial dysfunction (i.e., ischemia) varies with the level of occlusion and that most episodes of myocardial ischemia would be missed if not for intraoperative echocardiography. Unfortunately, this was not a blinded study and episodes of ischemia were immediately treated. Therefore, it is impossible to comment on whether the TEE changes were predictive and whether the treatment thereof improved patient outcome.

Slogoff and coworkers[89] have theorized that if the diagnostic criteria for ischemia via ECG were decreased from 0.100–0.025 mV the sensitivity for ischemia would equal that of TEE. Although this is an interesting hypothesis, one would expect a loss in specificity with such a decreased threshold.

II	III	V_1	V_2	V_3	V_5

Baseline

Ischemia

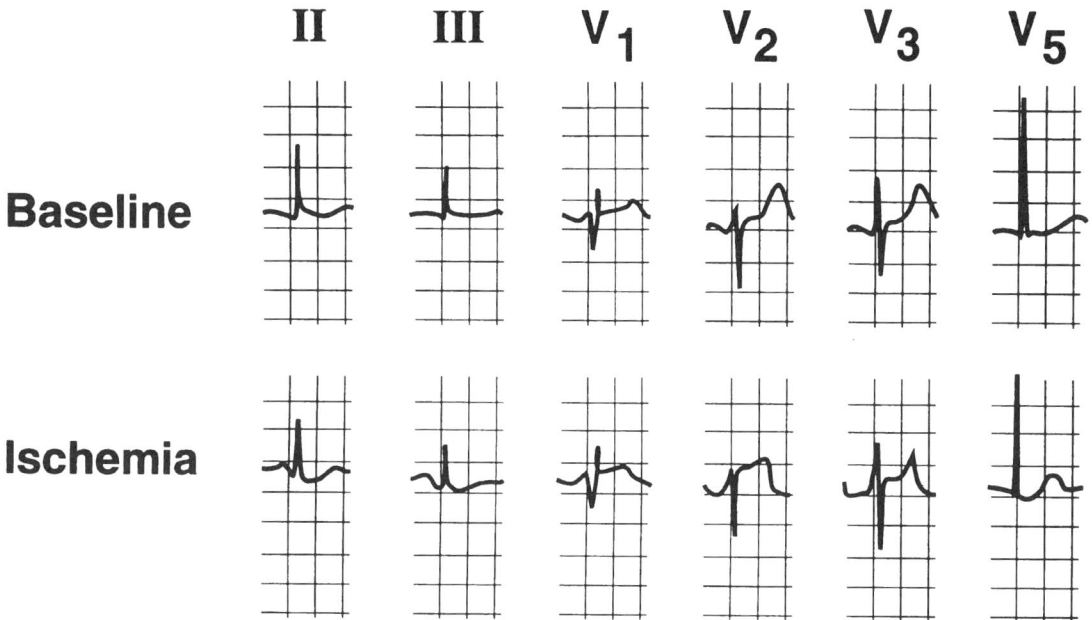

Figure 4-8. During aortic cross clamping for abdominal aortic aneurysm resection, this patient had relatively minor electrocardiographic changes in leads II and V_5. The precordial leads (which are not usually monitored) exhibited greater than 2-mm ST-segment elevation. This episode was accompanied by new dyskinesia on the transesophageal echocardiogram. (Reprinted with permission from M London, M Hollenberg, M Wong. Intraoperative myocardial ischemia: localization by continuous 12 lead electrocardiography. Anesthesiology 1988;69:232.)

Preload

Clinically preload is determined by estimating left ventricular end-diastolic volume (LVEDV). There are several methods for approximating LVEDV in the intraoperative period. In many clinical scenarios an ongoing measurement of the urine output will suffice. In the patient with aortic disease who is on diuretics preoperatively, who will be receiving diuretics intraoperatively, or who will be undergoing suprarenal aortic cross clamping, this becomes an unreliable and often inconsistent monitor. As was previously mentioned, the heart rate and BP also aid in the diagnosis of hypovolemia. The frequent presence of beta-blockers, vasodilators, and inotropes can cloud the picture and dictate the need for a more reliable monitor of preload.

Central Venous Pressure

The insertion of a fluid-filled catheter into a major vein allows for the transduction of central venous pressure (CVP). Common sites include the external jugular, internal jugular, subclavian, or femoral veins. The information generated from the CVP provides information about the right side of the heart. In patients with normal right-sided heart function without pulmonary hypertension, who are not receiving continuous positive airway pressure or positive end-expiratory pressure, and who have normal left heart diastolic function, the CVP also provides data relative to the left ventricular preload (Figure 4-9). Unfortunately, many patients undergoing aortic surgery do not fit these criteria.

Pulmonary Artery Diastolic Pressure

The continuous transduction of the pulmonary arterial pressures provides a more reliable index of true preload. Pulmonary artery diastolic pressure will be only slightly higher than the pulmonary capillary pressure, except in cases of pulmonary hypertension. However, even if a patient is known not to have preexisting pulmonary hypertension, oftentimes intraoperative acidosis and hypoxemia, hypercarbia, or

CVP------>PAD------>PCWP------>LAP------>LVEDP------>LVEDV

↑   ↑   ↑   ↑   ↑

R heart fn   PVR   Intra-alveolar   MV   LV diastolic fn
                         pressure

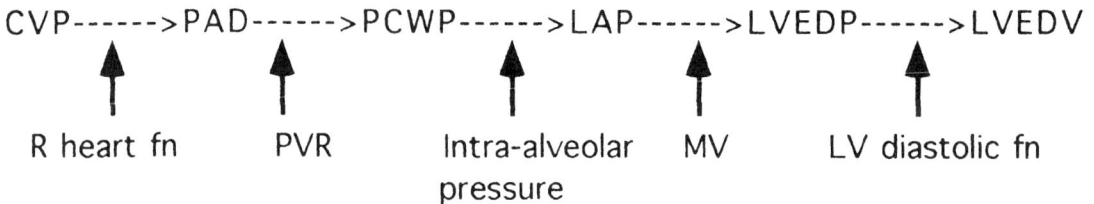

Figure 4-9. The central venous pressure (CVP) may be used as a measure of left ventricular end-diastolic volume (LVEDV) provided there is no right-sided heart pathology, pulmonary hypertension, high intra-alveolar pressures, mitral valve (MV) disease, or left ventricular diastolic dysfunction. (fn = function; PAD = pulmonary artery diastolic pressure; PCWP = pulmonary capillary wedge pressure; LAP = left atrial pressure; LVEDP = left ventricular end-diastolic pressure; PVR = pulmonary vascular resistance.) (Modified with permission from D Reich, J Kaplan. Hemodynamic Monitoring. In J Kaplan [ed], Cardiac Anesthesia [3rd ed]. Philadelphia: Saunders, 1993;261.)

both cause a constriction of the pulmonary vasculature and thus can make the pulmonary artery diastolic pressure an unreliable measure of LVEDV.

Pulmonary Capillary Wedge Pressure

A wedged PAC provides a PCWP that is often proportional to the LV filling pressures. However, there are a number of factors that alter the relationship between the PCWP and the true preload (see Figure 4-9). High intra-alveolar pressure generated with positive end-expiratory pressure and continuous positive airway pressure is transmitted through the pulmonary vasculature, causing a compression of the pulmonary veins and a distortion of the PCWP.[90] Patients with mitral valve stenosis require high left atrial pressures to allow for forward flow across a narrow orifice. Thus, the wedge may reflect left atrial pressures that are not proportional to left ventricular pressures.[91] Finally, and most significantly, when using a PAC to assess left ventricular preload, one assumes normal left ventricular diastolic function. The patient with a noncompliant left ventricle will have an altered pressure-volume relationship, and a small change in volume (LVEDV) may translate into a relatively large change in pressure (LVEDP) (Figure 4-10). Left ventricular hypertrophy and myocardial ischemia are examples of clinical scenarios that alter left ventricular compliance and thus shift the pressure-volume relationship. Clinically, this means that the PCWP overestimates true preload and is an unreliable monitor of volume status in these patients. Kalman and colleagues[92] reported 23 patients undergoing elective AAA resection in whom on unclamping the PCWP was unchanged with a simultaneous lowering of the LVEDV (evaluated using radionuclide assay). They point out that using the PCWP might result in inappropriate therapy, for example inotropic intervention may be used instead of volume resuscitation.

Recently, a number of authors have compared the use of CVP versus PAC in patients undergoing elective AAA resection. Isaacson and coworkers[93] studied 102 patients without coronary artery disease (i.e., no evidence via history, dipyridamole-thallium scan, or cardiac catheterization) who were undergoing elective AAA resection. Patients were randomly assigned to receive either CVP or PAC for perioperative monitoring. They found that there was no difference in outcome in this patient population. Additionally, hospital costs were approximately equal between groups. Joyce and coworkers[94] found that patients with ejection fractions (EFs) greater than 50% were at low perioperative risk and could be safely monitored during infrarenal aortic surgery with CVP monitoring. Adams and coworkers[95] studied patients without coronary artery disease and ejection fractions greater than 50%, and likewise concluded that CVP represented adequate monitoring.

Transesophageal Echocardiography

Whereas measurement of the CVP and PCWP provides pressure measurements from which vol-

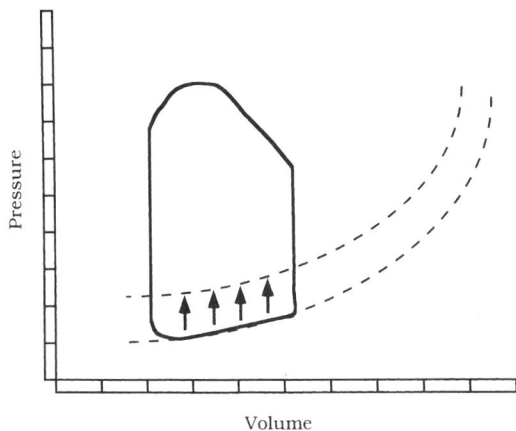

Figure 4-10. With decreasing diastolic function (upward arrows) a change in volume is manifested by a larger change in pressure. Thus, the left ventricular end-diastolic pressure is not always directly proportional to the left ventricular end-diastolic volume.

umes may often be inferred, two-dimensional TEE allows for the continuous calculation of actual end-diastolic areas from which volumes may be estimated.

Numerous studies have reported that the pulmonary artery diastolic and PCWPs do not accurately measure preload in patients undergoing AAA repair.[15,92,96,97] Changes in left ventricular compliance occurring after aortic cross clamping significantly affect the relationship between LVEDP and LVEDV. On the other hand, TEE has proven to accurately measure preload when compared with intraoperative radionuclide angiocardiograms (RNAs).[97] Reich and coworkers[98] confirmed the value of TEE to measure preload in a pediatric cardiac population. Cheung and colleagues[99] recently studied patients undergoing CABG to determine the value of TEE in the measurement of preload. Patients were rendered hypovolemic during a period of autologous blood collection and were simultaneously monitored with PACs and TEEs at the midpapillary short axis level. They confirmed that TEE is an accurate monitor for hypovolemia, even in the presence of abnormal LV function and RWMAs. They found that the PCWP correlated with LVEDV in those patients with normal LV function (i.e., r = 0.512, $P = 0.04$) and did not correlate in those patients with abnormal LV function (i.e., r = 0.327, $P = 0.28$).

Contractility and Left Ventricular Function

In some patient populations, with all other variables being equal, arterial BP provides a measure of myocardial contractility. With decreasing contractility one would normally expect a decline in arterial pressure, providing there has been no alteration in afterload. However, hypotension in and of itself may also be a marker for hypovolemia, peripheral vasodilation, or even bradycardia. The arterial pulse contour may provide a rough measure of contractility. It is most reliable with a central aortic waveform and is variable depending on changing the systemic vascular resistance,[100] as well as damping and resonance within the monitoring system.

Cardiac Output

Cardiac output (CO) is the most common methodology used to estimate contractility intraoperatively. The PAC allows for the intermittent assessment of CO via thermodilution. Usually 10 ml of saline (either iced or at room temperature) is injected into a central compartment (usually the right atrium), and a thermistor in the pulmonary artery measures the change in blood temperature over time. The cardiac output is then estimated with the following formula[101]:

$$CO = \frac{V_I \times (T_b - T_I) \times 60 \times 1.08}{A}$$

Provided:

V_I = the volume injected in milliliters
T_b = the blood temperature
T_I = the injectate temperature
1.08 = a correction factor taking into account the specific gravity and specific heat of the blood and indicator
60 = a conversion from liters per second to liters per minute
A = the area under the curve multiplied by the time required for the generation of the curve

In addition to the contractility, CO is also dependent on a number of physiologic variables including heart rate, preload, and afterload. When compared with nuclear ventriculography, it has failed to detect depression of systolic function during aortic clamping or decreased diastolic function during unclamping.[92] Patient factors that make the thermodilution CO invalid include tricuspid regurgitation,[102] intracardiac shunt,[103] and simultaneous volume infusion.[104] Other sources of error include inaccurate injectate volumes, slow injections (>2 seconds for 10 ml), poor mixing, and rapidly fluctuating hemodynamics.[105]

New PACs have been developed that allow for the continuous measurement of stroke volume (and a calculation of CO). With the Doppler principle, stroke volume is derived from the mean velocity of blood in the main pulmonary artery. Early studies have found the continuous CO reliable when compared with values calculated using the Fick method (in the catheterization laboratory),[106] and intraoperative intermittent thermodilution.[107,108]

CO may also be measured by TEE. Stroke volume is indirectly calculated from the product of the aortic valve cross-sectional area and the flow velocity-time integral derived via pulse wave Doppler through the main pulmonary artery or mitral valve. Aortic valve area is obtained from the transverse short axis plane. Multiplying the stroke volume by the heart rate will yield the CO. Although found to be reliable with transthoracic scanning,[109] it has had variable success with transesophageal views.[110,111] Darmon and colleagues[112] reported on CO values derived using the velocity-time integral obtained with continuous wave Doppler through the aortic valve. They also assumed a triangular (or "three-legged starfish") valvular shape. With these modifications, they found excellent correlation between thermodilution COs and COs obtained via TEE.

Hemoglobin Saturation of Venous Blood. Providing that oxygen consumption and arterial oxygen content remain constant, the mixed venous oxygen saturation will provide an indirect measure of the CO. This relationship is expressed with the Fick equation:

$$VO_2 = CO \times (CaO_2 - CvO_2)$$

or

$$\frac{SvO_2 = SaO_2 - VO_2}{(Hgb)(CO)}$$

Provided:

VO_2 = body oxygen consumption
CaO_2 = the oxygen content of arterial blood
CvO_2 = the oxygen content of venous blood

Hgb = the hemoglobin concentration
SvO_2 = the hemoglobin saturation of venous blood
SaO_2 = the hemoglobin saturation of arterial blood

Assuming that the Hgb, SaO_2, and VO_2 remain constant then:

$$SvO_2 = K - \frac{1}{CO}$$

and the SvO_2 provides an indirect measure of CO. A decrease in CO is manifested as a decrease in SvO_2. Likewise an increase in CO is seen as an increase in SvO_2. It provides an estimate of the CO relative to the oxygen demands of the body. The SvO_2 may be drawn intermittently from the distal port of a standard PAC or be continuously measured via a fiberoptic modification of a standard PAC.

Ejection Fraction

The EF represents the percentage of blood the heart ejects compared with the volume present at end diastole. It may be calculated as:

$$EF = \frac{LVEDV - LVESV}{LVEDV}$$

Using two-dimensional TEE it is only possible to measure cross-sectional areas during the cardiac cycle. With the probe positioned at the transgastric, midpapillary short-axis view, it is possible to calculate a fractional area of change (FAC):

$$FAC = \frac{LVEDA - LVESA}{LVEDA}$$

Provided:

LVEDA = the left ventricular end-diastolic area
LVESA = the left ventricular end-systolic area

This view provides the best estimation of EF because during systole the left ventricle contracts predominantly along its short axis.[113] Harpole and coworkers[97] confirmed the concordance of the FAC derived from intraoperative TEE with simultaneously derived EF from RNA.

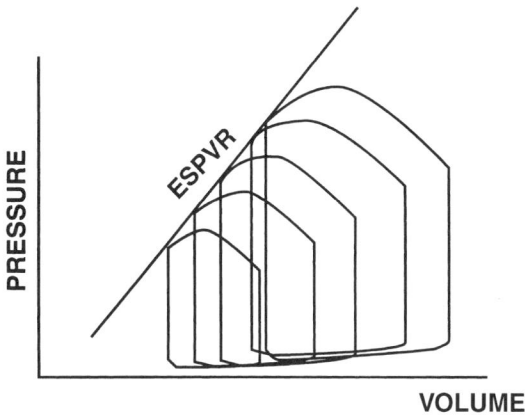

Figure 4-11. The end-systolic pressure volume relationship is obtained by connecting all the end-systolic points measured during a rapid decrease in preload. (Reprinted with permission from D Thys, P Dauchot. Advances in Cardiovascular Physiology. In J Kaplan [ed], Cardiac Anesthesia [3rd ed]. Philadelphia: Saunders, 1993;209.)

Two of the major problems with using EF as a monitor of LV function and contractility are its dependence on other hemodynamic variables and the assumption that the fractional area shortening derived at the midpapillary level represents the ejection of the entire left ventricle. The EF is not only a monitor of contractility but varies depending on preload and afterload.[114] For example, a patient with a high afterload (as with a very proximal aortic cross clamp) may appear to have a significantly diminished EF. However, that may not reflect the intrinsic contractility of the ventricle. Similarly, severe hypovolemia may give the appearance of false RWMAs that act to decrease the calculated EF.

New Transesophageal Echocardiographic Measures of Contractility

Investigators have recently conducted clinical studies using TEE to measure contractility in more innovative ways. One of the more promising is the automated pressure-area analysis (APAA). Whereas all previously discussed measures of contractility are variable based on preload and afterload, the APAA makes use of the preload independence of the left ventricular end-systolic pressure–volume relationship (end-systolic elastance) to describe left ventricular performance. The end-systolic pres-

sure–volume relationship is generated from a left ventricular-pressure loop (Figure 4-11). By varying the preload, one may construct a number of pressure-volume loops, all representative of the ventricle at different LVEDVs. The slope of a line drawn connecting the points of end systole will be proportional to the contractility. A greater slope corresponds to an increased contractility; a lesser slope to a decreased contractility (Figure 4-12).[115] This measure is thought to be independent of preload but still somewhat dependent on afterload.[116–118]

Automatic border detection (e.g., Acoustic Quantification, Hewlett Packard, Andover, MA) is a means of continuously evaluating the left ventricular cross-sectional area throughout the cardiac cycle. Through sophisticated real-time analysis of a raw echocardiographic signal, a border detection algorithm is able to distinguish between tissue and blood. The resultant picture on the screen combines the two-dimensional image with the generated endocardial border. The area within the border (the left ventricular area) is updated 32 times per second and may be expressed either numerically or graphically. Using automatic border detection simultaneously with a central aortic pressure monitor, Gorcsan and colleagues[119] performed canine experiments to generate pressure-area loops. Using inferior vena cava occlusion to vary preload, they were able to generate numerous

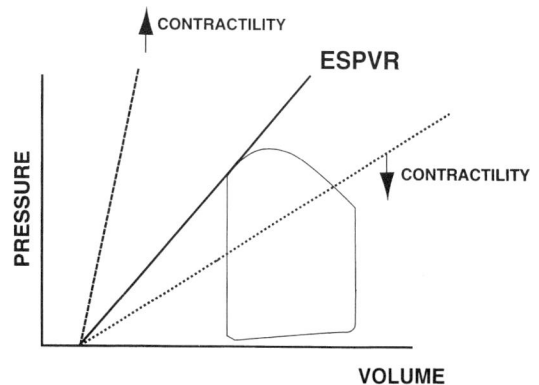

Figure 4-12. The slope of the end-systolic pressure volume relationship is directly proportional to contractility. A steeper slope represents greater contractility, a lesser slope decreased contractility. (Reprinted with permission from D Thys, P Dauchot. Advances in Cardiovascular Physiology. In J Kaplan [ed], Cardiac Anesthesia [3rd ed]. Philadelphia: Saunders, 1993;209.)

loops and thereby assess contractility. In the same study, they validated their model with positive and negative inotropes and by direct comparison with pressure-volume loops. More recently, Gorcsan and coworkers used APAA in patients undergoing CABG and concluded that it is a useful tool for measuring contractility after CPB.[120] The more recent data allow the use of a femoral arterial line instead of a central pressure monitor.[121]

Neurologic Monitoring

One of the most dreaded events in aortic surgery is a postoperative neurologic catastrophe. The incidence of paraplegia or paraparesis has been reported to be as high as 1.5% for coarctation of the aorta, 25% for traumatic aortic disruption, and 40% for repair of a descending aortic dissection.[122–133] These complications often occur despite appropriate surgical techniques and multiple attempts at prevention.[122–133] Cerebrovascular accidents remain a major complication of ascending and aortic arch surgery.

Spinal Cord Ischemia

Two patterns of neurologic complications related to spinal cord ischemia have been described.[123] Immediate complications result from perioperative acute spinal cord ischemia. Delayed complications occur from 1–21 days postoperatively. The incidence of immediate deficits can be limited because it is possible to identify and possibly prevent spinal cord ischemia.[123–125] A delayed deficit may result from prolonged subclinical ischemia or other postoperative complications that may cause a reduction in microcirculation.[123,126] Delayed complications are difficult to prevent.[123,127,128]

The goal of intraoperative neurologic monitoring is to detect changes in spinal cord function early enough to begin ameliorative measures to prevent postoperative paraplegia. As described in a following section, the evoked potential (EP) and other monitors of neurologic function are sensitive and selective indicators of ischemia in nervous tissue. Consequently, these modalities have been considered ideal for monitoring during aortic surgery.[122,129–133]

Monitoring Spinal Cord Function to Prevent Paraplegia

Blood Supply of the Spinal Cord

To understand the mechanics of spinal cord injury during aortic surgery, it is essential to understand the anatomy of spinal cord blood supply (Figure 4-13). The cord is supplied by one anterior and two posterior spinal arteries that originate from the vertebral arteries within the foramen magnum.[134–137] Venous drainage of the spinal cord is through the anterior and posterior spinal veins, which drain outward along the nerve roots.[126,134]

The anterior spinal artery runs in the anterior median sulcus along the entire length of the cord (see Figure 4-13B). It sends central and penetrating branches to supply the anterior two-thirds of the spinal cord. This region includes structure within the ventral and lateral portions of the cord such as the anterior horns, lateral spinothalamic tract, and pyramidal tract.[135] Motor functions are mediated via anterior spinal cord structures.[134,135] The posterior spinal arteries traverse either side of the cord to perfuse the posterior one-third of the spinal cord including the posterior funiculi and posterior horns.[135] Somatosensory information is conveyed from the periphery to the central nervous system through the dorsal columns of the posterior cord.[134,135] Thus, the motor and somatosensory systems receive a differential blood supply.[138] This important feature of spinal cord blood supply is discussed in the section on motor evoked potential.

The spinal arteries are supported by several radiculospinal branches of the vertebral artery and the aorta (see Figure 4-13A). From six to ten large anterior radicular arteries contribute to the anterior spinal artery throughout its length.[134,135,138] The large radiculospinals are distinguishable from smaller radicular arteries that enter through the intervertebral foramen to nourish nerve roots (see Figure 4-13B).[134] The radicular arteries arise from neighboring arteries at each level of the vertebral segments. Many small radicular arteries pass medially through the intervertebral foramina, together with the nerve roots. Most do not reach the cord; however, some of the larger arteries reach the dura mater where they give off meningeal branches and then divide into ascending and descending branches to join the spinal arteries.

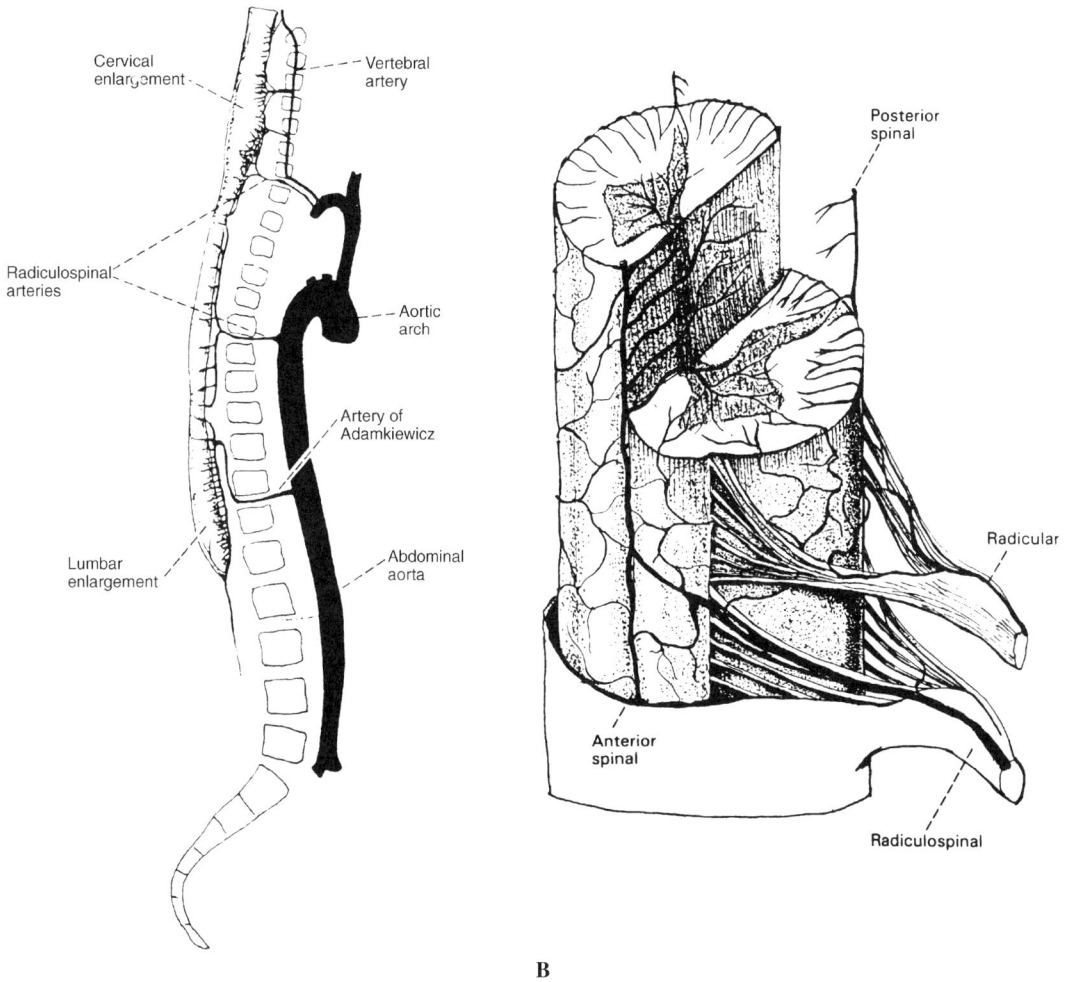

Figure 4-13. Blood supply of the spinal cord. A. Radiculospinal arteries. B. Arteries of the spinal cord and nerve roots. (Reprinted with permission from MJT FitzGerald. Neuroanatomy Basic and Applied. London: Bailliere Tindall, 1985.)

The spinal cord is well perfused at the cervical and upper thoracic regions. However, a general decrease in perfusion occurs in the mid to low thoracic regions.[138] The largest radiculospinal artery is the artery of Adamkiewicz (arteria medullaris magna), which, depending on individual anatomy, arises from the tenth to twelfth posterior intercostal artery of one side (see Figure 4-13A).[134,139] The artery of Adamkiewicz improves perfusion at these levels and descends to supply the lumbar enlargement and conus terminalis (see Chapters 1 and 8).[134,138] Depending on the origin of the artery of Adamkiewicz and the sufficiency of collateral circu-

lation, either aortic cross clamping, clamping of critical intercostal vessels, or both may interfere with the blood supply of the mid thoracic to lumbar regions of the spinal cord.[126,139–143] Moreover, although the artery of Adamkiewicz arises typically as a single branching of the aorta, it is not unusual for it to be a complex of arteries that are difficult to distinguish from segmental arteries perfusing the spinal cord.[138,144,145] As a result, it can be difficult to identify and preserve the vessels critical for spinal cord perfusion.[138,141,145,146]

The absence of adequate collateral blood flow to the distal aorta leads to spinal cord ischemia.

Factors that contribute to ischemia include interruption of critical intercostal arteries, aortic cross clamping, extended cross-clamp time, perioperative hypotension, increases in cerebrospinal fluid (CSF) pressure, and location and extent of the aortic pathology.[123,124,139,141,142,147–150] Obstruction of the venous outflow may produce spinal cord edema[134] and contribute to immediate and delayed neurologic deficits.[126]

Somatosensory Evoked Potential

In aortic surgery, somatosensory EPs (SSEPs) are monitored by stimulating the posterior tibial nerve at the ankle and recording the response of the somatosensory cortex at the scalp (Figure 4-14). An evoked response may also be recorded from the common peroneal nerve at the popliteal fossa and from the brain stem at the cervical spine. This may be advantageous because placing recording electrodes over the common peroneal nerve and the cerebral cortex allows simultaneous monitoring of both peripheral and central nervous system function. The brain stem response is more resistant to the effects of general anesthesia than the cortical potential and acts as a control measure for changes in the anesthetic profile.

Generation of the Evoked-Potential Signal

EPs represent the summed activity of large ensembles of pyramidal neurons in layers 3 and 5 of the cerebral cortex.[151,152] These neurons are arranged in a regular, vertical alignment relative to the cortical surface.[151–153] When a strong stimulus is presented to a peripheral sense organ, the normally rhythmic electroencephalogram (EEG) is replaced by low-voltage, fast potentials time-locked to the stimulus.[153] These potentials are called sensory EPs.[151] EPs may also be elicited by stimulating the somatosensory, visual, or auditory pathways.

Three species of neuronal activity may generate an evoked response: (1) activation of sensory neurons, (2) action potentials transmitted along axons, and (3) synaptic activity between neurons.[154] Accordingly, potentials evoked by peripheral stimulation may be recorded from a sensory nerve, from the dorsal columns of the spinal cord, and from the brain stem and cerebral cortex.[131,153,155,156]

Extraction of the Evoked Potential Signal

The electrical potential of an evoked response is minuscule when compared with other biologic signals such as the ECG or EEG. The electrical potential of a scalp recorded EP may range from only 0.02–5.00 µV.[151,157] This response is approximately one-tenth the amplitude of the EEG within which the signal is embedded.[151] Hence, a reliable method for extracting the EP signal from background noise is needed.[151,153,158,159]

Ensemble averaging is the most common method of signal extraction used in intraoperative monitoring. This procedure increases the signal-to-noise ratio of the EP by the square root of the number of single trials (stimulus repetitions).[159] Ensemble averaging assumes that the signal portion of the response is time-locked to each stimulus presentation ("property of stationarity"), and is of consistent shape from trial to trial ("property of nonrandomness"). Conversely, background noise is assumed to be nonstationary and random relative to the stimulus. Hence, noise tends to cancel, whereas the aggregate EP remains unchanged on average.[153,158,159]

Summated Potential

An important concern in monitoring SSEP function for aortic surgery is acquiring the data quickly enough to identify the onset of spinal cord ischemia. As a signal estimator of somatosensory function, the summated EP improves with an increasing number of trials.[158–160] Obviously, a large number of stimulus repetitions are required to detect and extract a weak signal. The number of averaged responses depends on the level of background noise and the strength of the EP, and may range from several hundred to several thousand single trials.[154,155,157,161,162]

Although it is desirable (and possible) to maximize the signal-to-noise ratio by collecting a large number of single trials, this may be entirely impractical in the operating room when a response is needed for analysis as soon as possible.[160] Consequently, a good rule of thumb is to continue averaging until the addition of further trials does little to change the overall morphology of the evoked response. In most cases, averages of 200–300 single trials will be sufficient to resolve a well-defined, intraoperative SSEP.

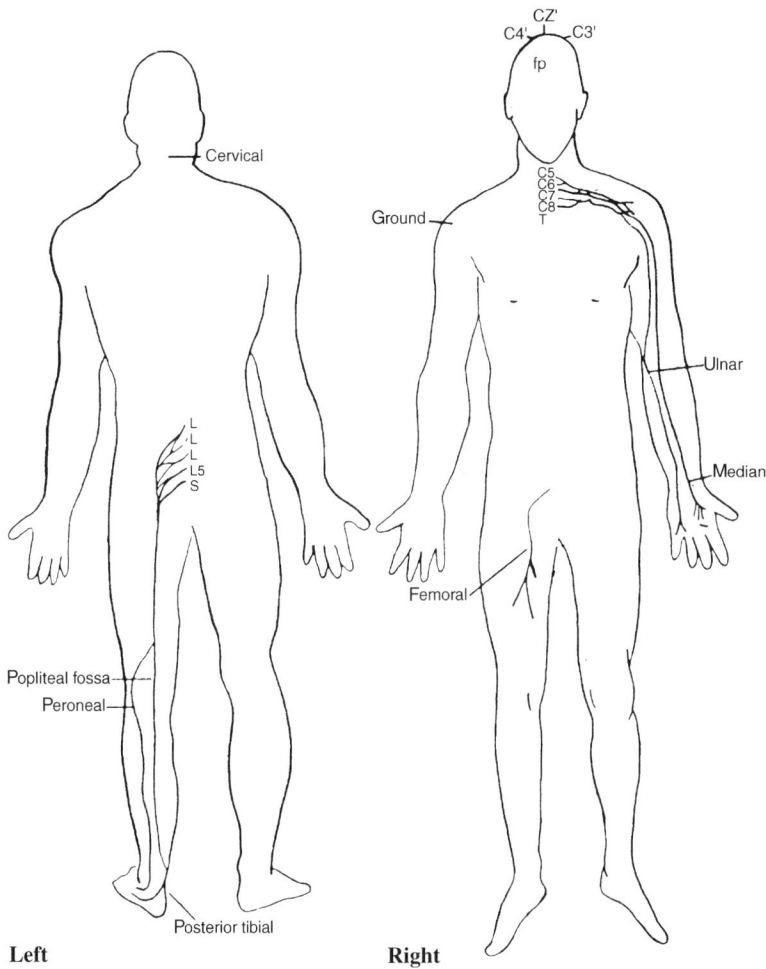

Figure 4-14. Stimulating and recording sites for the somatosensory evoked potential. Left. Dorsal aspect. Posterior tibial and common peroneal nerves. Right. Ventral aspect. Median and ulnar nerves. (Reprinted with permission from AM Padberg, LS Holland. Somatosensory Evoked Potentials. In DL Beck [ed], Handbook of Intraoperative Monitoring. San Diego: Singular Publishing Group, 1994.)

Evoking a Lower-Extremity Somatosensory Potential

Electrode Placement. A lower-extremity SSEP may be elicited by bipolar electrical stimulation applied to the posterior tibial nerve adjacent to the medial malleolus as it curves into the sole of the foot (see Figure 4-14). The posterior tibial nerve is a mixed nerve containing both sensory and motor components. Thus, direct stimulation of the nerve initiates movements about the ankle and activates the ascending dorsal column somatosensory system.[134,135,163] The cathode is placed midway between the median border of the Achilles tendon and the posterior border of the medial malleolus. The anode is placed 2–3 cm distal to the cathode. Stimu-

lating electrodes should be placed sufficiently apart so that a salt bridge between the anode and cathode does not develop during the procedure.[161] This occurs if electrolyte gel or patient sweat leaks between the electrodes forming a shunt, shorting them out.

Stimulating Electrodes. Various electrode types may be used for stimulus presentation. The most common and convenient are disposable pregelled silver and silver chloride disk electrodes. The skin should be cleaned thoroughly before applying the electrodes. Reducing the electrical resistance of the skin lowers the current necessary to elicit a response. Electrical stimulation may also be administered percutaneously using subdermal EEG needle electrodes.

*Recording a Lower Extremity
Somatosensory Potential*

Electrode Type.   The SSEP may be recorded with a variety of electrode types. Gold, silver, or silver chloride EEG cup electrodes are the most commonly used electrodes for recording from the surface of the scalp. Cup electrodes are fixed to the skin with standard electrode paste or with collodion. As an alternative to cup electrodes, sterilized subdermal needle electrodes are recommended in situations requiring a quick application of monitor leads. Prepasted electrodes or subdermal needles may be used to record the popliteal and cervical responses. All of the recording electrodes should be of the same metal.[164]

Isolating Sources of Artifact.   Identifying and removing sources of extraneous noise presents one of the most frustrating aspects of electrophysiologic monitoring in the operating room. Within the context of EP theory, background noise refers to any source of electrical activity other than the desired evoked response. Although background consists primarily of EEG or ECG signal, equipment and other extrinsic sources of interference may also be mixed into the noise factor. Ensemble averaging often fails to remove high-amplitude artifact.

Electromagnetic interference causes a spurious averaging at 60 Hz, generating a response with an interpeak latency of 16.6 ms.[160,164,165] Some common sources of electromagnetic interference encountered within the operating room include the fluid warmer, airway humidifier, cell saver, perfusion pump, and TEE. Additional sources of noise include overhead lights, motorized operating room tables, transcutaneous nerve simulators, beepers, watches, cardiac pacemakers, loose cables, and other related equipment. High-frequency artifact generated by electrocautery units is another ubiquitous source of noise in the operating room.[160,164,165]

Electrical noise can be intensified by an unwanted "antenna" effect, for example, by placing a fluid warmer with a strong magnetic field onto an intravenous pole. Braiding or wrapping the electrode wires together may help reduce the antenna effect. Stimulus artifact may become troublesome, especially if electrode contact impedances are too high or if wires leading from the stimulator to the stimulating electrodes run too close to the recording lines or preamplifier unit. ECG wires sometimes become tangled with the EP leads. The ECG signal may also be picked up by the EP equipment if the electrodes are improperly grounded or referenced. Likewise, the EP stimulus may be picked up on ECG monitoring. Other forms of interference are mechanical and may be caused by physical movement of the patient's head, movement of electrode wires, or accidental dislodgement of an electrode by the surgical team.

Tracking and eliminating electrical interference can often be frustrating.[164] The list of possible items that can cause artifact is constantly expanding. Nonetheless, whenever electrical noise is encountered, its source must be removed before EP monitoring can continue. Therefore, it is necessary to isolate all possible generators of noise by shutting off and turning back on in sequence all suspected culprits. These devices sometimes have to be unplugged as well.

*Components of the Somatosensory
Evoked Potential*

The EP, like the EEG, is a plot of voltage against time. By convention, the waveform components of an evoked response are designated positive (P) or negative (N) in relation to a reference electrode. In naming an EP waveform peak, the polarity of the component is followed by the ideal mean latency of the response.[157] For example, the P37 component consists of a positive response whose peak latency is expected to occur approximately 37 ms following stimulus presentation (Figure 4-15). Various elements of the lower extremity evoked response are now discussed.

Peripheral Nerve Response.   An evoked response from the sensory component of the posterior tibial nerve may be recorded directly at the central aspect of the popliteal fossa immediately below the division of the sciatic nerve into tibial and common peroneal branches (see Figure 4-14). Recording the afferent volley from the tibial nerve at the popliteal fossa may be used to demonstrate the adequacy of the peripheral stimulation.[155,166] Bipolar recordings are obtained using one electrode placed at the midline, approximately 2 cm superior to the popliteal crease. The second electrode is then placed 2 cm anterior or lateral to the first.

Spinal Potentials.   The roots of the sciatic nerve are found in the ventral rami of the fourth lumbar

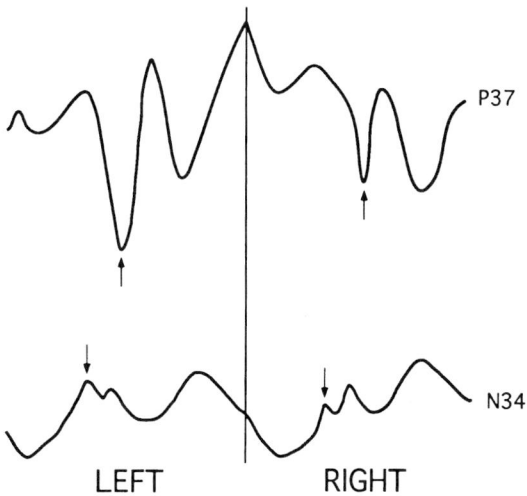

Figure 4-15. Examples of somatosensory evoked potentials elicited by stimulation of the posterior tibial nerve. Sequential left and right leg stimulation. Upper. P37 component recorded from the cerebral cortex. Lower. N34 component recorded from the brain stem.

to the third sacral nerves. The central processes of the dorsal root ganglia enter the posterior columns of the spinal cord where afferent fibers ascend ipsilaterally in a somatropic representation along the dorsal column-medial lemniscus system.[134,135,163] Evoked responses may be recorded directly from various levels of the sacral, lumbar, thoracic, and cervical spinal cord using needle electrodes placed by the surgeon into the appropriate interspinous ligaments or with subdermal needle electrodes placed adjacent to the vertebral interspace.[161] In this manner, the evoked response may be tracked as it ascends the spinal cord.[156,167]

Subcortical Potentials.   The ascending dorsal column fibers synapse in the dorsal column nuclei (nucleus gracilis) where postsynaptic elements decussate into the medial lemniscus and ascend to the ventral posterior thalamus.[134,135,163] The lemniscal-thalamic response is reflected in the P31 and N34 components of the lower extremity SSEP (see Figure 4-15).[155] The mean latency for the P31 component is 30.0 ± 2.2 ms.[131] The mean latency for the N34 component is 31.9 ± 1.7 ms.[131]

Although there is some controversy over specific origins for the P31 and N34 components, the general consensus suggests multiple sources within the

brain stem and thalamus.[131,154,155,168–176] The P31 and N34 components may be recorded at the upper cervical spine, mastoid process, or cervical-occipital juncture (see Figure 4-14).

Cortical Potentials.   The activation of the somatosensory cortex is reflected in the P37 component of the EP.[131,155,173,177] By convention, changes in the latency and amplitude of the P37 component are the primary monitors of SSEP function during aortic surgery. The mean latency for the P37 component is 38.6 ± 2.2 ms.[131]

There is considerable latitude in the electrode placement for the P37 component.[155] The P37 is usually recorded maximally somewhere between midline and central-parietal scalp locations. The typical recording site for the P37 is usually 1–2 cm posterior to the midsagittal vertex landmark. The recording electrode is referenced to the forehead.[155,161,178]

Monitoring Somatosensory Evoked Potential Changes in Aortic Surgery

Background.   Early studies demonstrated that SSEPs were a reliable measure of intraoperative spinal cord function.[131,132,179–181] The application of intraoperative SSEP monitoring to orthopedic procedures suggested a similar use in aortic surgery where spinal cord function was placed at risk. Three landmark papers published in 1982 proposed that changes in somatosensory function may warn of impending spinal cord ischemia.[122,129,133]

Experimental models of spinal cord ischemia were created in canines by proximal and distal occlusion of the thoracic aorta.[129,133] Aortic cross clamping proximal to the left subclavian artery resulted in the rapid onset of spinal cord ischemia. It was shown that changes to the SSEP correlated with the occlusion of spinal cord blood flow.[129,133] Cunningham and colleagues[122] described their initial clinical experiences with seven patients who underwent aortic surgery. These authors reported that increasing distal circulation (heparinized shunt, femoral-femoral bypass, reimplantation of intercostal arteries) following a loss of SSEP function resulted in a recovery of the potentials. No postoperative neurologic complications were observed.

Based on numerous human and canine studies,[129,133,182–186] several conclusions can be made. A significant deterioration in SSEP function marks the onset of spinal cord ischemia. The loss of the SSEP is prevented by maintaining an adequate level of perfusion to the spinal cord and periphery. Finally, a recovery of spinal cord function was reflected in the return of the evoked responses following surgical intervention.

Patterns of Change. The acquisition of preoperative baseline data is essential to successful monitoring of the somatosensory pathways. The onset of spinal cord ischemia is characterized by a significant increase in component latency followed by a reduction in signal amplitude. Relative to baseline measures, the conventionally accepted criteria for defining a significant change in intraoperative SSEP function during spinal cord surgery are (1) a 10% change in component latency and (2) a 50–60% attenuation in component amplitude.[140,143] The complete loss of an evoked response is the hallmark of spinal cord ischemia. Unilateral changes can occur during clamping of either left or right intercostal arteries.

One may observe either peripheral or central neurologic ischemia.[123] Peripheral nerve ischemia results when inadequate distal perfusion to the leg blocks the transmission of nerve impulses.[184] Spinal cord ischemia results as a consequence of an inadequate or interrupted perfusion to the cord itself.[148] Peripheral nerve ischemia mimics the effects of spinal cord ischemia and confounds the use of SSEPs to warn of impending spinal cord ischemia.[123,187] Direct, epidural stimulation of the spinal cord obviates the need for peripheral monitors and may be considered an alternative to posterior tibial nerve stimulation (while possible in major orthopedic and neurosurgery, this is not practiced in aortic surgery).[187–189]

Complete loss of the potential occurs approximately 20 minutes following hypoperfusion.[144] Recovery of the potentials is characterized by the reappearance of the response with prolonged latencies that eventually return to baseline.[123,190,191] It is not uncommon for the potentials to return to baseline levels considerably after wound closure. Hence, somatosensory monitoring may be continued postoperatively in the cardiac intensive care unit until a return to baseline is observed.

Four types of SSEP changes were initially described.[122,123,192] It is not unusual for an individual patient to exhibit multiple types of responses dur-

ing a single procedure. A type I event is characterized by a progressive deterioration of the SSEP following aortic cross clamping. A complete loss may be noted within 8–9 minutes. There is no attempt to provide distal aortic perfusion and, as a result, distal BP falls below 60 mm Hg. There is a high incidence of postoperative paraplegia following a type I event, especially if the EPs are absent for greater than 30 minutes and do not return within 50 minutes of reperfusion.

During a type II response there is essentially stable somatosensory function during the procedure. Adequate distal perfusion is provided using the appropriate bypass, shunt procedure, or both. Moreover, critical intercostal arteries are not located in the excluded aortic segment. Mean distal aortic BP is maintained above 60 mm Hg. This response suggests a good postoperative outcome for the patient.

A type III event is defined as a loss of EP following proximal and distal aortic cross clamping despite the use of appropriate bypass, shunt procedures, or both. Peripheral perfusion is adequate and distal aortic BP is above 60 mm Hg. A type III event suggests that vessels critical to spinal cord perfusion are located in the excluded aortic segment. The recommended surgical intervention is to identify and reimplant the excluded intercostal arteries.

A type IV response involves a gradual deterioration and loss of EPs despite appropriate bypass, shunt procedures, or both. The loss of potentials occurs within 30–50 minutes following proximal and distal aortic cross clamping. Unlike a type III response, the mean distal aortic BP decreases below 60 mm Hg. The recommended surgical intervention is rapid completion of the anastomoses.

The periods of high vigilance in which a change in SSEP function might occur include (1) patient positioning, (2) the placement of proximal and distal aortic cross clamps, (3) reimplantation of intercostal arteries, (4) beginning and ending partial bypass, (5) sewing proximal and distal ends of the graft, (6) testing anastomoses, and (7) reimplanting specific arteries to reperfuse organs. Aortic surgery can be unpredictable and the SSEP should be monitored not only during these high risk periods but continuously throughout the procedure.

Figure 4-16 illustrates stable cortical posterior tibial nerve SSEP function during a descending aortic procedure. The patient was placed on partial by-

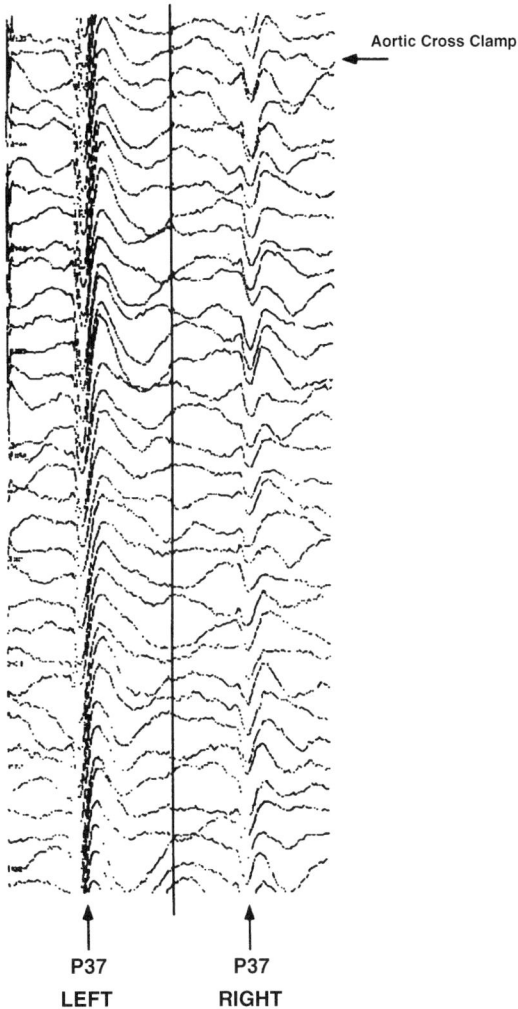

P37
LEFT

P37
RIGHT

Figure 4-16. An example of unchanged somatosensory evoked potential function during repair of descending aortic aneurysm. Somatosensory evoked potentials were recorded from the cerebral cortex in response to sequential left and right stimulation of the posterior tibial nerve. Somatosensory evoked potential functions remained stable throughout the procedure. The patient was placed on partial bypass and maintenance of spinal cord perfusion pressure was facilitated via withdrawal of cerebral spinal fluid.

pass and maintenance of spinal cord perfusion pressure was facilitated via withdrawal of cerebral spinal fluid. No changes in the P37 component were noted during the procedure.

Figure 4-17 depicts loss and recovery of the posterior tibial nerve SSEP following aortic cross clamping, release of the clamp, and reperfusion.

Effects of Anesthesia

Anesthetic drugs affect SSEP function in a dose-dependent manner.[143,172,176,193–195] This is due to the direct effects of anesthetic agents on the neuronal generators of the evoked response as well as the indirect effects of anesthesia on cerebral blood flow, cerebral metabolism, and cerebral perfusion pressure.[194] The effects of most anesthetic agents on EP waveform morphology resemble the effects of spinal cord injury—i.e., a reduction in amplitude and an increase in the latency of the evoked response. Consequently, anesthetic management may affect the reliability of SSEP monitoring. Moreover, the SSEP manifests a wide variability in response to anesthetic agents.[195] The effects of anesthesia on the SSEP are summarized in Table 4-2.

Inhalational Anesthetics. All inhalational anesthetics have profound depressant effects on SSEP function.[172,176,193–197] However, the literature is inconsistent as to which inhalant agent has a more potent effect on SSEP morphology.[193,195] It has been well documented that isoflurane levels in excess of 0.5% increase latency and decrease the amplitude of the somatosensory response (Figure 4-18).[143,172,194–196,198,199] Accordingly, in order to monitor reliable SSEPs, isoflurane levels are best maintained at concentrations of 0.3–0.5% inspired (T Sloan, personal communication, 1995).[172,193,194,199]

Nitrous oxide in excess of 60% inspired decreases SSEP amplitude (T Sloan, personal communication, 1995).[143,172,193,194,196,198,199] Nitrous oxide affects SSEP amplitude when coadministered with either narcotic or inhalational anesthetics.[193] This effect may be more pronounced in situations where preoperative SSEP data are abnormal.[193] Coadministration of nitrous oxide and isoflurane increase SSEP latency and decrease SSEP amplitude in a dose-dependent manner.[176,194,196,198] Wolfe and Drummond[176] reported that cortical SSEPs were substantially affected as end-tidal isoflurane levels in 60% nitrous oxide increased above 0.5% minimum alveolar concentration. These authors also noted a significant recovery in SSEP amplitude following removal of nitrous oxide from the anesthetic mixture.[176]

Halothane and enflurane also decrease the amplitude and increase the latency of the SSEP in a

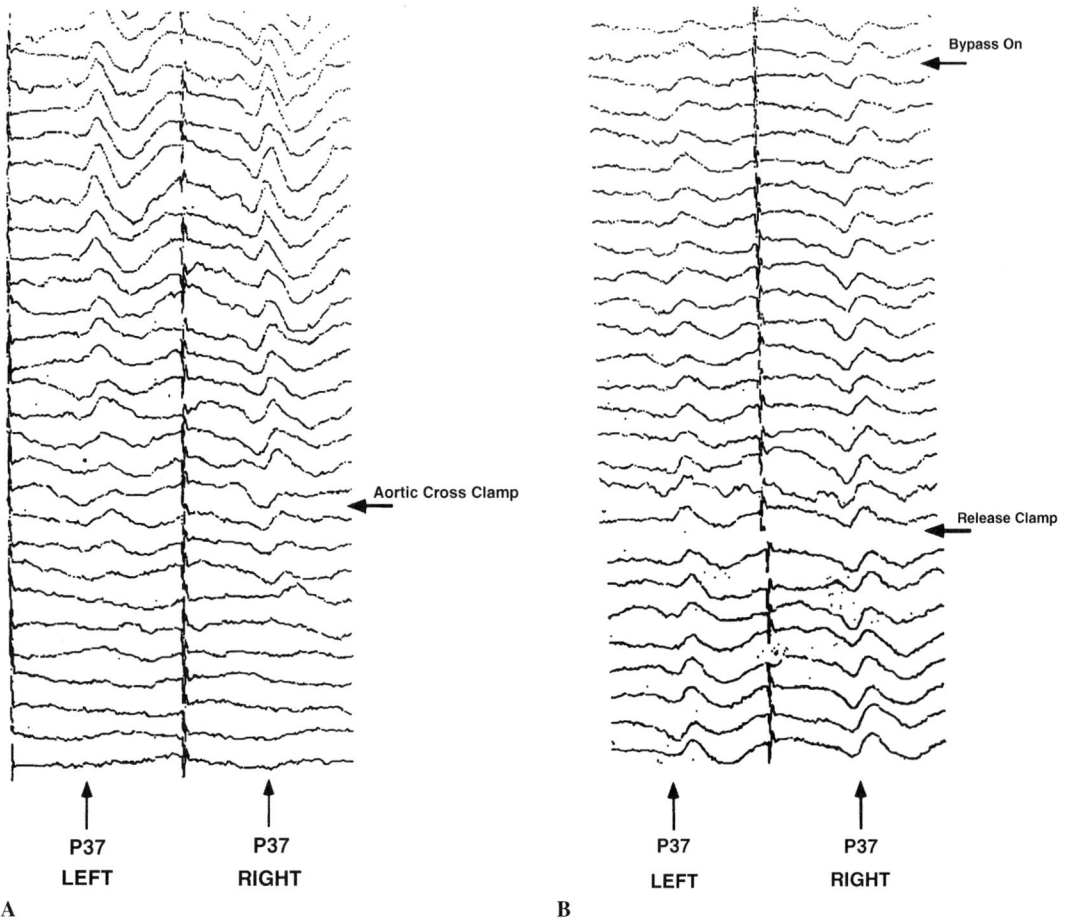

Figure 4-17. An example of changed somatosensory evoked potential function during repair of descending aortic aneurysm. Somatosensory evoked potentials were recorded from the cerebral cortex in response to sequential left and right stimulation of the posterior tibial nerve. A. Loss of somatosensory function following aortic cross clamping. B. Recovery of somatosensory function following reperfusion with partial bypass and release of clamp.

dose-dependent manner.[172,193,194] Desflurane and sevoflurane are relatively newer inhalant agents and have not been extensively studied. However, desflurane has been shown to affect SSEPs in a manner similar to other inhalational agents.[197]

Intravenous Agents.   Intravenous agents used for anesthetic induction cause transient changes in the SSEP.[194,195] The usual induction dose of thiopental will not affect the SSEP waveform.[193] Higher doses (20 mg/kg) will cause dose-dependent increases in latency and decreases in amplitude.[193,194] Thiopental infusion (2 mg/kg/hour) does not affect the somatosensory potential.[172] Conversely, etomidate

and ketamine increase the signal amplitude of the SSEP.[172,193–195]

Propofol (2.5 mg per kg) increases the latency of the cortical SSEP without affecting the amplitude of the response (Figure 4-19).[194] However, some studies have shown that propofol may potentiate SSEP amplitude.[172] Although the effects of midazolam are unclear, it produces a mild depression of cortical SSEP activity with slight increases in latency and a possible decrease in amplitude.[172,194,195]

The effects of narcotic analgesics on the SSEP are minimal and tend to be most prominent following repeat bolus administration (Sloan T, personal communication, 1995).[172,193] Narcotic-induced SSEP changes

Table 4-2. Effects of Anesthetic Agents on the Somatosensory and Transcranial Magnetic Motor Evoked Potential

Drug	Dose[a]	Effect on Somatosensory Evoked Potential		Effect on Transcranial Motor Evoked Potential	
		Latency	Amplitude	Latency	Amplitude
Inhalational agents					
Nitrous oxide	60%	No change	Decrease	Increase	Decrease
Isoflurane	0.5–1.5%	Increase	Decrease	Increase	Decrease
Enflurane	0.5–1.5 MAC	Increase	Decrease		
Halothane	0.5–1.5 MAC	Increase	Decrease	Increase	Decrease
Opiates (narcotics)					
Fentanyl	<75 µg/kg	Increase[b]	No change	No change?	No change?
Sufentanil	—	No change	Decrease[b]		
Alfentanil	—	No change	Decrease[b]		
Morphine	—	Decrease	Increase		
Meperidine	—	Increase	Increase or decrease		
Amnesic, sedative agents					
Ketamine	2 mg/kg	Increase	Increase	Increase	Decrease
Etomidate	0.05–0.30 mg/kg/min	Increase	Increase	Increase	No change
Propofol	2–6 mg/kg	Increase	No change		
Thiopental	4–6 mg/kg	No change	No change		
	>20 mg/kg	Increase	Decrease		
Pentobarbital	9–18 mg/kg	Increase	Increase		
Benzodiazepines	—				
Midazolam	0.2 mg/kg	No change	Decrease		
Diazepam	0.1 mg/kg	Increase	Decrease	Increase	Decrease
Droperidol	0.1 mg/kg	Increase	Decrease		
Muscle relaxants	—	No change	No change	c	c

[a]Doses applicable to somatosensory evoked potential function only.
[b]Indicates a modest change in somatosensory evoked potential function.
[c]All neuromuscular agents block the electromyographic motor potential. Conversely, neuromuscular block is required to record a neurogenic motor potential.
MAC = minimum alveolar concentration.
Source: Adapted from V Gugino, RJ Chabot. Somatosensory evoked potentials. Int Anesthesiol Clin 1990;28:154; SB Kinsella. Anesthesia and Intraoperative Monitoring. In DL Beck (ed), Handbook of Intraoperative Monitoring. San Diego: Singular Publishing Group, 1994; and RW McPherson. General Anesthetic Considerations in Intraoperative Monitoring: Effects of Anesthetic Agents and Neuromuscular Blockade on Evoked Potentials, EEG, and Cerebral Blood Flow. In CM Loftus, VC Traynelis (eds), Intraoperative Monitoring Techniques in Neurosurgery. New York: McGraw-Hill, 1994.

are less pronounced during continuous infusion.[172,194] Morphine and fentanyl have modest, dose-dependent effects on SSEP latency and amplitude.[172,193–195] Continuous infusion of sufentanil or alfentanil does not affect SSEP morphology.[193]

Neuromuscular Blockers. Neuromuscular blockers do not affect the SSEP.[195,200] An improved signal may be recorded from a relaxed patient due to the loss of muscle artifact at the electrode sites (Figure 4-20).[195] This is noted especially in potentials recorded from neck and occipital electrodes. The addition of muscle artifact to the subcortical SSEP waveform during the procedure may signify that neuromuscular paralysis is waning.

Cortical and Brain Stem Responses. Subcortical potentials are more resilient than cortical poten-

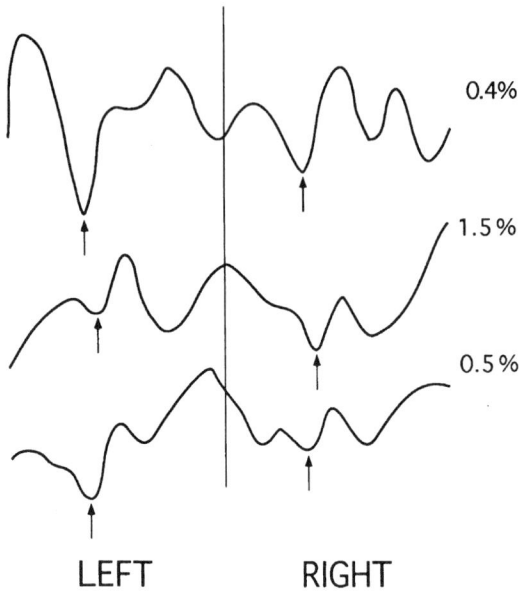

Figure 4-18. The effect of isoflurane on somatosensory evoked potential latency. Somatosensory evoked potentials were recorded from the cerebral cortex in response to sequential left and right stimulation of the posterior tibial nerve. Baseline latencies for the left and right P37 components were 35.0 and 32.0 ms, respectively (upper trace, 0.4% isoflurane). Latencies increased significantly to 40.0 ms, bilaterally (middle trace, 1.5% isoflurane). Latencies recovered following reduction in isoflurane anesthesia (bottom trace, 0.5% isoflurane).

tials to the effects of anesthesia[172,176,194,195,199,201] and may be a more reliable monitor when cortical potentials are affected by anesthetic management.[166,176] The resilience of the subcortical response may be related to the sequence of events in which anesthetic agents affect the central nervous system. Brain stem signs appear during the deeper stages of anesthesia.[195] Spinal cord, peripheral nerve, and motor EPs are relatively unaffected by anesthetic agents (T Sloan, personal communication, 1995).[143,172,193,199]

Concerns to Anesthesiologists. Anesthetic management during aortic procedures, especially involving inhalational agents, induces changes in EP amplitude or latency that mimic the effects of spinal cord ischemia. As a result, the effects of anesthesia must be accounted for to avoid false-positive interpretation errors during SSEP monitoring.

During patient setup, the surgical team should allow time for the acquisition of baseline SSEP data. Motor (movement) thresholds should be determined immediately following anesthetic induction before the muscle relaxant has taken effect.[155,161,172,202,203] If possible, inhalation anesthetic levels should not exceed 0.3–0.5% isoflurane in 50% nitrous oxide.

Communication between members of the surgical team (i.e., surgeon, anesthesiologist, and neurophysiologist) is crucial. Both the anesthesiologist and neurophysiologist should be aware of each stage in the surgical procedure. The anesthesiologist should inform the neurophysiologist about the patient's systemic and anesthetic status. The neurophysiologist should be familiar with the concerns of the anesthesiologist. It is possible to avoid false-positive interpretation errors by accounting systematically for anesthetic and physiologic variables prior to advising the surgical team of possible spinal cord ischemia.

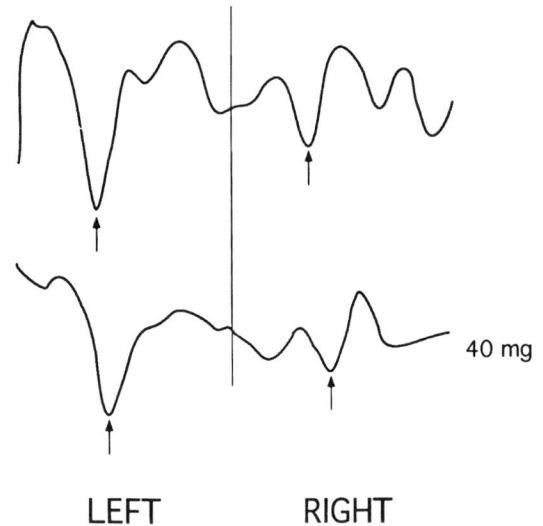

Figure 4-19. The effect of propofol on somatosensory evoked potential latency. Somatosensory evoked potentials were recorded from the cerebral cortex in response to sequential left and right stimulation of the posterior tibial nerve. Baseline latencies for the P37 component were 35.6 ms (left) and 33.0 ms (right) (upper trace). Latencies increased to 39.1 ms and 37.0 ms following a 40-mg bolus of propofol (lower trace).

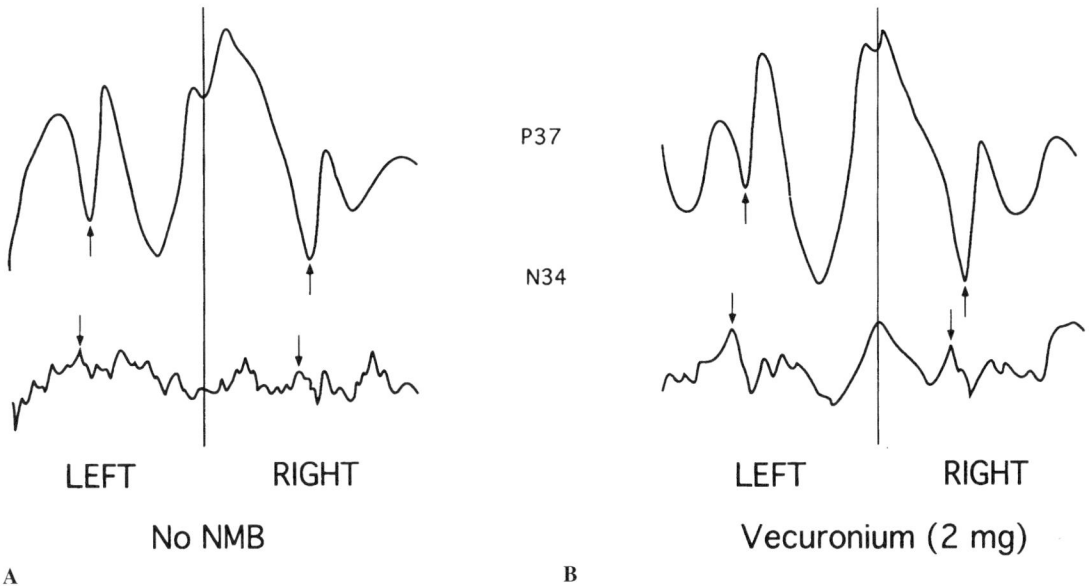

P37

N34

LEFT   RIGHT

No NMB

A

LEFT   RIGHT

Vecuronium (2 mg)

B

Figure 4-20. The effect of neuromuscular blockers on subcortical evoked potential morphology. Somatosensory evoked potentials were recorded from the cerebral cortex and brain stem in response to sequential left and right stimulation of the posterior tibial nerve. Cortical responses (P37) are shown in the upper traces. Subcortical potentials (N34) are shown in the lower traces. A. Electromyographic artifact appears bilaterally in the N34 component 30 minutes following a 2-mg bolus of vecuronium. The patient demonstrated loss of neuromuscular blockade (NMB). No change was noted in the P37 component. B. The electromyographic artifact was no longer present in the N34 component following a 2-mg bolus of vecuronium. The patient demonstrated full NMB.

Effects of Physiologic Factors

Physiologic variables that affect SSEP monitoring include body temperature, systemic BP, arterial oxygen and carbon dioxide tensions, hematocrit, and patient position.[193–195,200]

Hypothermia.   Hypothermia causes a linear increase in SSEP latency and an eventual loss of SSEP amplitude.[194,195,200,204] Hypothermia decreases the conduction velocity of nerve impulses along the axons and slows synaptic transmission by impairing the release of neurotransmitters.[195,205] The effects of hypothermia on SSEP amplitude are inconsistent in the literature. Some studies report decreases in amplitude,[194] whereas other studies report no change.[205] Cortical potentials are more sensitive to temperature changes than brain stem potentials.[195] SSEPs elicited by stimulation of the posterior tibial nerve are especially sensitive to hypothermia due to the length of the somatosensory pathway.[205] A decrease in nasopharyngeal tempera-ture of 2–3°C can prolong posterior tibial nerve latencies by more than 3 ms.[205] The effects of hypothermia on posterior tibial nerve SSEP latency are shown in Figure 4-21.

Hypothermia also affects peripheral and spinal SSEPs. Decreases in peripheral temperature decrease conduction velocity, leading to a gradual prolongation in SSEP latency.[200] Response amplitude is not usually affected by decreasing limb temperature.[200] Hypothermia often occurs during descending aortic surgery due to a limited ability to maintain normothermia. SSEP alteration under hypothermic conditions is often characterized by a slow deterioration followed by a rapid return to baseline.

SSEPs may be used to monitor central nervous system function during deep hypothermic circulatory arrest.[200,206] The disappearance of the SSEP may be used to determine the appropriate temperature for inducing hypothermic circulatory arrest.[206] Figure 4-22 shows the rapid loss and gradual return of the posterior tibial nerve SSEP during deep hypothermic circulatory arrest.

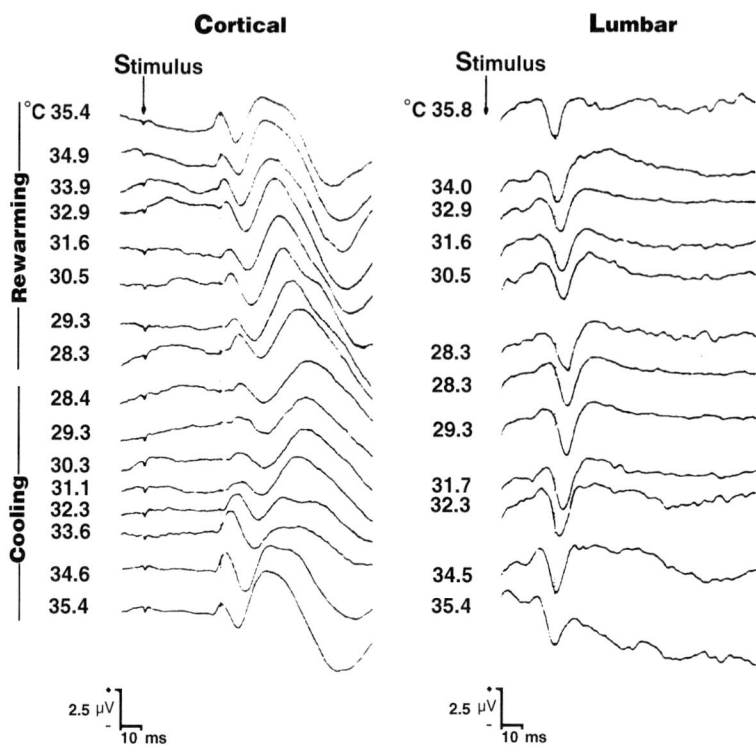

Figure 4-21. The effect of hypothermia on posterior tibial nerve somatosensory evoked potential function. Somatosensory evoked potentials were recorded from the cerebral cortex and lumbar spine during cardiopulmonary bypass. A prolongation in somatosensory evoked potential latency was noted with increased hypothermia. A recovery in somatosensory evoked potential latency occurred following return to normothermia. Left. Cortical somatosensory evoked potentials recorded from the scalp at the vertex. Right. Spinal cord potentials recorded at the T12–L1 interspace. (Reprinted with permission from AT van Rheineck Leyssius, CJ Kalkman, JG Bovill. Influence of moderate hypothermia on posterior tibial nerve somatosensory evoked potentials. Anesth Analg 1986;65:475.)

Hypotension. Hypotension causes decreased spinal cord perfusion and a reduction in neuronal function. This leads to prolonged SSEP latencies and attenuated SSEP amplitudes.[195,200] Cortical somatosensory function is noticeably altered when regional cerebral blood flow falls below 18 ml per 100 g per minute.[195] Significant SSEP changes occur when blood flow is within 10–15 ml per 100 g per minute.[207] The loss of SSEP function occurs within the range of synaptic transmission failure but above the threshold for total collapse of the neuronal membrane (10 ml per 100 g per minute). As a result, the cortical SSEP is a good indicator of cerebral ischemia.

An episode of acute hypotension might engender the loss of an already low amplitude SSEP signal.[200] A return to normotension should be followed by a return of the SSEP.[200] As with other physiologic and anesthetic factors, the cerebral cortex is more sensitive than brain stem structures to hemodynamic changes.[195] Because decreases in mean systemic BP to levels below cerebral autoregulation

result in a deterioration of the SSEP,[193] changes in the SSEP waveform can be used to infer the limits of an acceptable BP in a patient.[195]

Positioning. Changes in the SSEP waveform may occur following positioning of the patient.[208] These changes may be due to mechanical compression of nerves[195] or occlusion of blood vessels. Recovery of the SSEP follows patient repositioning. Compression of peripheral vessels due to positioning may cause a reversible ischemic neuropathy that can be monitored by peripheral SSEP function at Erb's point (median nerve) or at the popliteal fossa (posterior tibial nerve).[200] Partial compression may occur for a prolonged period with SSEP changes occurring several hours after the patient is initially positioned.[209]

Other. Alterations in hemoglobin concentration can cause changes in SSEP function.[195] Increases in SSEP latency have been reported with a hematocrit of 15% via hemodilution.[193] Hypocarbia (carbon dioxide tensions below 20 mm Hg) alters cerebral

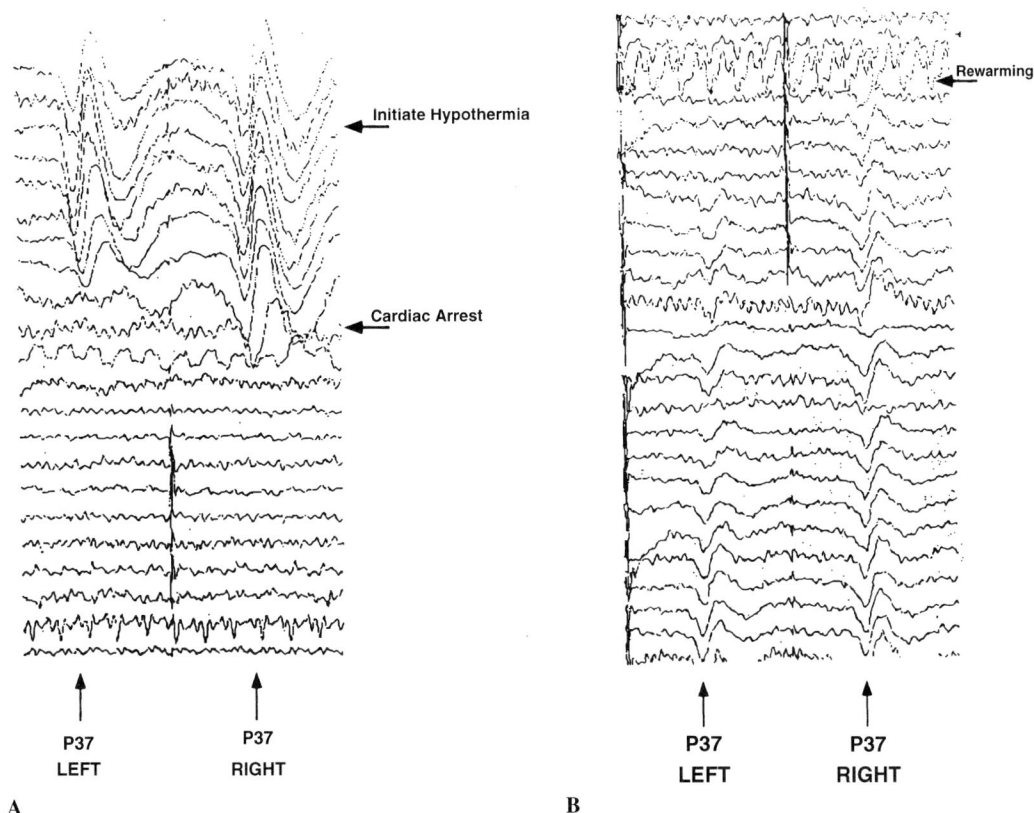

Figure 4-22. The effect of deep hypothermic cardiac arrest on somatosensory evoked potential function. Somatosensory evoked potentials were recorded from the cerebral cortex in response to sequential stimulation of the left and right posterior tibial nerves. A. As shown at the top of the figure, baseline latencies for the P37 component were 39.1 ms, bilaterally. A bilateral loss of evoked potential function occurred following deep hypothermic cardiac arrest. B. Recovery of evoked potential activity followed rewarming and resumption of cardiac function. However, evoked potential latencies were prolonged significantly following recovery (48.3 and 47.5 ms, left and right).

blood flow, leading to deterioration in the SSEP.[195] Increases in cerebral spinal fluid pressure, which reduce spinal cord perfusion pressure (SCPP), may lead to a reduction in SSEP amplitude and an increase in SSEP latency.[195]

Postoperative Monitoring

Postoperative somatosensory monitoring may be considered an adjunct to intraoperative monitoring of EP function. It is not uncommon for the evoked response to return to baseline levels postoperatively. Hence, monitoring the EPs in the intensive care unit may be used to document the return to baseline. The return to normothermia and nor-

motension in the intensive care unit may play a role in the recovery to baseline.

Motor Evoked Potential

Rationale

There are several reasons why SSEPs may not be the most appropriate neurophysiologic monitor for detecting intraoperative spinal cord ischemia. First, due to a more poorly collateralized arterial blood supply, the anterior spinal cord receives less perfusion than the posterior cord.[138,188,192,210] Experimental data have shown that spinal cord infarctions are characterized by degeneration of gray matter, hemorrhage, and anterior horn motor neuron death.[211] Therefore, a more sensitive modality for early detection of spinal cord ischemia should be a procedure that monitors preferentially anterior spinal cord function.[138,188,192,210,212–217] Animal and human studies have demonstrated the effectiveness of the motor EPs (MEP) in detecting spinal cord ischemia.[188,192,209,215–222]

Second, SSEPs are susceptible to false-negative errors. Monitoring sensory pathways via the SSEP assesses the functional integrity of the dorsal columns; however, paraplegia results from insult to the anterior columns (anterior spinal artery syndrome). Although there is a good correlation between a preserved somatosensory response and normal motor function,[161] an intact SSEP does not guarantee intact motor function.[199,212,223] Cases of postoperative paraplegia with unchanged intraoperative somatosensory function (false-negative error) have been reported in the literature.[161,192,199,215,224–227] The MEP has a much higher negative predictive value because it assesses the functional integrity of the motor pathway directly.

Finally, unlike the SSEP, the spinal cord MEP is resistant to the effects of anesthesia (Sloan T, personal communication, 1995).[143,193,199] As discussed earlier, anesthetic-induced changes in SSEP morphology represent a major cause of false-positive errors in SSEP monitoring.

Evoking a Motor Potential

Methods of Stimulation. MEPs are elicited by stimulating either the spinal cord or cerebral cortex. In the former, the descending motor pathways of the spinal cord are activated by either translaminar or percutaneous stimulation.[228] Translaminar stimulation is generally more appropriate for spinal cord surgery. In percutaneous stimulation, insulated needle electrodes are placed outside of the surgical field, rostral to the incision. The electrodes are passed lateral to the spinous process so that the electrode tip approaches the vertebral lamina. The anode is rostral to the cathode, placed typically in an adjacent vertebra.[228]

Direct stimulation of the cerebral cortex is achieved transcranially using a magnetic coil placed on the scalp over the motor cortex.[213,223,229,230] The resulting magnetic field stimulates the corticospinal tract and activates muscle groups contralateral to the stimula-

tion.[213,223,229,231] Although transcranial magnetic stimulation has been applied to aortic and other vascular surgeries,[139,218,221,232] the procedure is technically demanding[213] and the overall safety of delivering magnetic stimulation to the cerebral cortex is not clear at the present time.[143] Moreover, this technique is still in its experimental stage[143] and has restricted use in the operating room. For these reasons, magnetic stimulation of the motor cortex will not be discussed in this chapter. Interested readers should refer to the articles by Chiappa[229] and Owen[143] for concise reviews of the transcranial magnetic technique.

Types of Motor Responses

All limbs distal to the level of stimulation are activated by spinal cord stimulation. Stimulation of the cervical spine elicits movement of both upper and lower extremities. Midthoracic stimulation activates the lower extremities only.

Two types of MEPs are monitored depending on the location of the sampling electrodes and the depth of muscle relaxation. For this reason, a bipolar recording technique is required to sample the response from a specific nerve or muscle.[228] A neurogenic MEP (NMEP) is recorded using electrodes placed over a peripheral mixed nerve such as the common peroneal nerve as it traverses the popliteal fossa. An electromyographic (EMG) motor potential is measured with electrodes placed over the appropriate musculature for the stimulated nerve roots. EMG monitoring requires the preservation of neuromuscular function. As such, it is not a practical monitor for aortic surgery.

Stimulation Parameters

Caution must be exercised when setting stimulation levels.[228] Stimulus intensity should be close to the threshold necessary to evoke a response. If a motor response is not present at sufficiently high levels of stimulus intensity, the functional integrity of the stimulating and recording electrodes should be verified. The integrity of the stimulating electrodes may be checked by attempting to record a typical SSEP at the cervical and cortical electrode sites. The absence of a somatosensory response indicates an improper electrode placement or some other problem.[228] The integrity of the recording electrodes at the popliteal fossa may be tested by stimulating the posterior tibial nerve in the usual manner

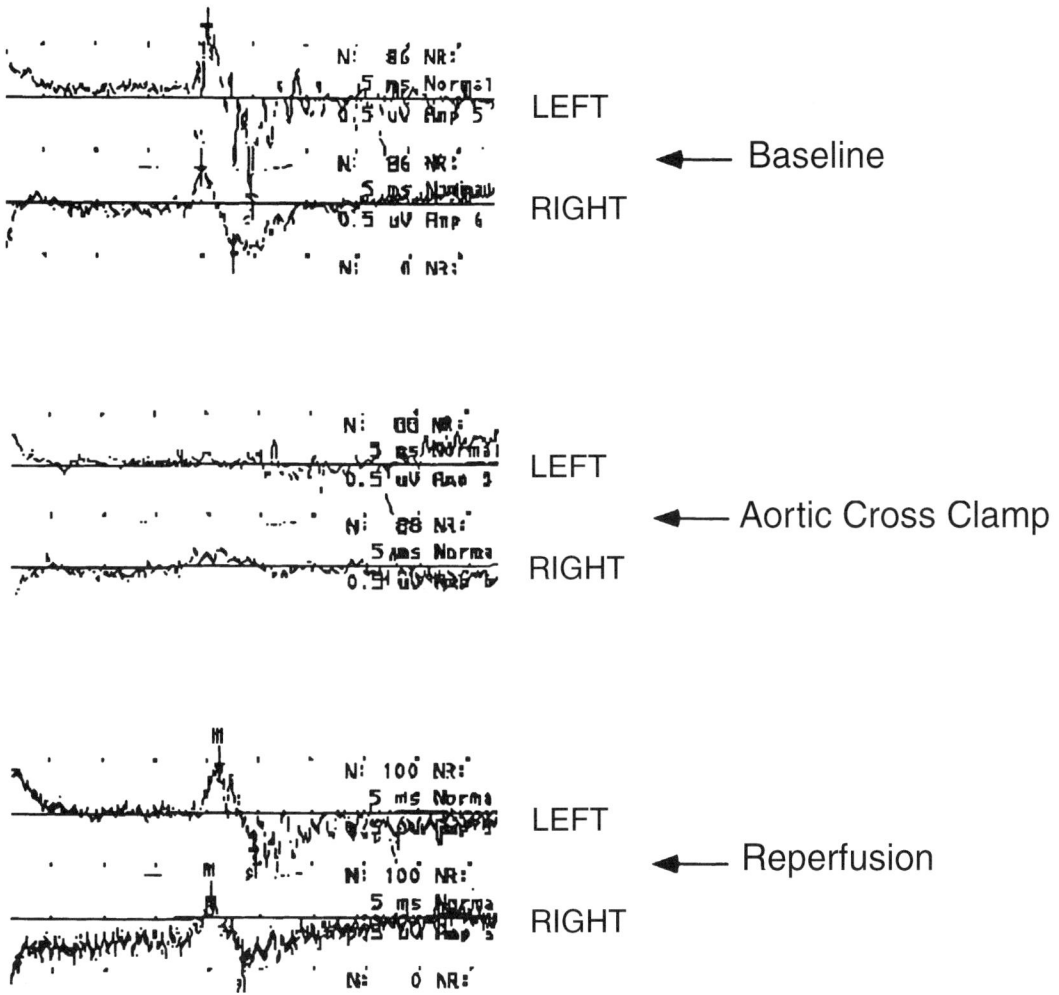

Figure 4-23. The effect of aortic cross clamping on the motor evoked potential. Neurogenic motor evoked potentials were recorded in response to left and right percutaneous stimulation of the spinal cord. Baseline motor evoked potentials recorded prior to application of clamp (upper trace). Loss of potential following aortic cross clamping (middle trace). Recovery of the motor evoked potential following reperfusion (lower trace).

for a lower extremity SSEP. If a response is detected at the common peroneal nerve, then the recording electrodes are viable.[228]

Criteria for Intraoperative Change

Amplitude is the primary waveform characteristic used to interpret a significant change in the NMEP response. Owen and colleagues[199] recommend a 60% attenuation in signal amplitude as the necessary condition for advising the surgeon of an impending change. The initiation of ameliorative measures should be undertaken with an amplitude change of 80%.[228] A 10% prolongation in latency marks a significant change in the NMEP.[199] Changes in the MEP during aortic surgery are illustrated in Figure 4-23.

Effects of Anesthesia

MEPs elicited by direct spinal cord stimulation are resistant to the effects of inhalational anesthesia.[143,199] Profound neuromuscular blockade should be maintained throughout the period of monitoring the NMEP.

On the other hand, MEPs elicited by transcranial magnetic stimulation are highly sensitive to inhalational,[143,199,233–235] intravenous,[143,199,236,237] and narcotic[230] anesthetic techniques (see Table 4-2). Thus, as with the SSEP, transcranial MEPs are susceptible to anesthetic related confounds and interpretation errors.

Recommendations

Owen and colleagues recommend the NMEP for monitoring the integrity of anterior column function.[228] Although the NMEP is not a true motor response,[228] it is the neurologic precursor to muscle contraction and provides a direct measure of anterior column function. Moreover, the neurogenic response is more reliable than the EMG potential,[228] and as previously mentioned, the ability to monitor is independent of neuromuscular activity.

The NMEP is recorded from a mixed peripheral nerve with both motor and sensory fibers. Direct stimulation of the spinal cord activates the entire nerve; hence, the neurogenic response contains both orthodromic (motor) and antidromic (sensory) components. These components may be distinguished easily from one another. The orthodromic response occurs at an earlier latency than the sensory component.[228] As a result, interpretation of the NMEP should not be confounded by the presence of a sensory component.

Conclusions

Although SSEPs are accurate predictors of spinal cord injury, they do not differentiate between anterior and posterior cord insult.[217] SSEPs do not monitor motor function directly. Conversely, MEPs do not monitor the posterior and lateral columns of the spinal cord[217] and fail to monitor somatosensory function.[238] Consequently, proponents of MEP monitoring suggest concurrent use with SSEPs in order to provide a "complete" monitor of both sensory and motor spinal cord function.[228,230] No false-negative results are expected when both modalities are monitored.[199] A comparison of motor and SSEPs is summarized in Table 4-3.

Spinal Cord Perfusion Pressure

SCPP is approximated as the difference between mean distal aortic pressure and mean CSF pressure (see Chapter 8).[147,150] Cross clamping the de-

scending thoracic aorta leads to an elevated BP proximal to the clamp, a decrease in BP distal to the clamp, an increase in CSF pressure, and a corresponding decrease in SCPP.[123,147,150,211] The elevation in CSF pressure may occur within 15 minutes after aortic cross clamping.[211] Hence, it has been suggested that withdrawing CSF prior to cross clamping the aorta may augment SCPP by increasing the pressure gradient between distal aortic BP and the spinal cord[123] and thereby protect the cord from an ischemic event.[150,211,239-242]

A decrease in SCPP below 40–50 mm Hg may result in temporary spinal cord ischemia.[147,149] In the presence of significant change in EP response, the maintenance of an adequate SCPP may prolong the period of "safe" ischemia before the spinal cord is irreversibly damaged.[123,147,211] Figure 4-24 shows the relationship between the onset of a significant increase (10%) in SSEP latency (L-10 time) and SCPP in a canine model of aortic cross clamping, spinal cord ischemia, and postoperative paraplegia.[123,147]

Electroencephalography

Methods of Recording

The EEG provides a noninvasive monitor of cortical function.[243] Similar to the SSEP, the EEG is recorded from the surface of the scalp using cup or subdermal needle electrodes. Various electrode montages, derived from the standardized international 10/20 system for EEG measurements, are used to localize underlying brain structures for EEG monitoring (Figure 4-25). The literature is inconclusive as to the most efficient number of channels and the most appropriate electrode configuration for monitoring EEG.[244,245] Nonetheless, in most situations, electrodes are arrayed over the frontal, parietal, and temporal lobes.[207,245] A typical frontotemporal EEG montage might include electrodes placed over the F4–C4, F3–C3, and F8–T4, F7–T3 (or T4–T6, T3–T5) electrode sites.[244] An alternative montage for coverage of the frontoparietal region might add the C3–P3 and C4–P4 electrode placements (see Figure 4-25).[244]

Electroencephalogram Frequencies

The frequency bandwidth of the EEG is from 1 to 30 Hz.[151,162] Although the waveform characteristics

Table 4-3. A Comparison of Neurogenic Motor and Somatosensory Evoked Potentials

	Neurogenic Motor Evoked Potential	Somatosensory Evoked Potential
Sensitivity to		
Severe structural damage to cord	Same	Same
Moderate structural damage to cord	Same	Same
Mild structural damage to cord	More	Less
Onset of spinal cord ischemia	More	Less
Effects of muscle relaxant	More	Less
Effects of halogenated anesthesia	Less	More
Reliable measure of		
Anterior spinal cord function	More	Less
Postoperative motor function	More	Less
Posterolateral spinal cord function	Less	More
Postoperative somatosensory function	Less	More
Dependent on		
Peripheral nerve function	Yes	Yes
Cortical/brain stem function	No	Yes
Spinal cord function	Yes	Yes
Other		
Loss of potential following spinal cord ischemia	Same or sooner	Same or later
Methodologic or technical difficulty	More	Less
Criteria for change	Amplitude	Latency and amplitude
Predict spinal cord ischemia	Yes	Yes

Source: Adapted from JH Owen. Update on evoked potentials during spinal surgery. Curr Opin Orthoped 1993;4:12.

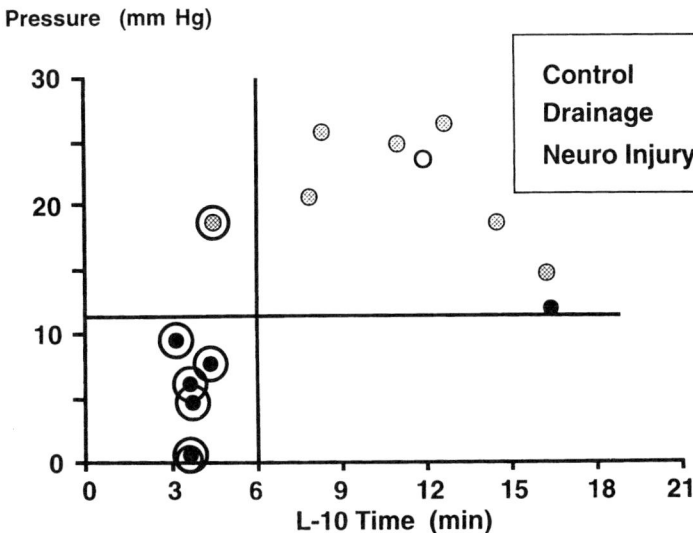

Figure 4-24. The relationship between spinal cord perfusion pressure and significant increases in somatosensory evoked potential latency is shown. Data were taken from a canine model of spinal cord ischemia. The horizontal and vertical lines indicate critical perfusion pressure (11.5 mm Hg) and time of onset (6 minutes) to a 10% increase (L-10 time) in somatosensory evoked potential latency. (Reprinted with permission from CP Marini, JN Cunningham. Issues Surrounding Spinal Cord Protection. Advances in Cardiac Surgery [Vol 4]. Chicago: Mosby–Year Book, 1993;89.)

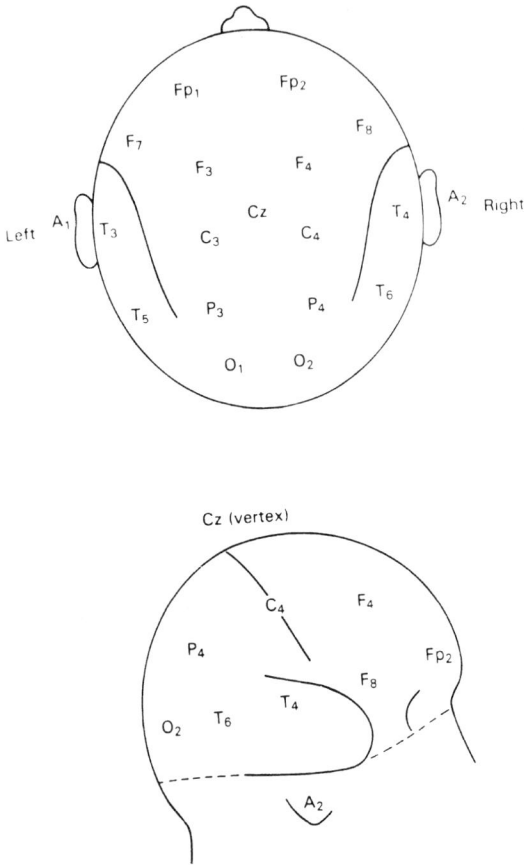

Figure 4-25. The international 10/20 system of electrode placement. Abbreviations for electrode sites are as follows: A = auricle; C = central; Cz = vertex; F = frontal; Fp = frontal pole; O = occipital; P = parietal; T = temporal. Odd numerical subscripts indicate left hemisphere sites. Even numerical subscripts indicate right hemisphere sites. (Reprinted with permission from JH Martin. The Collective Electrical Behavior of Cortical Neurons: The Electroencephalogram and the Mechanisms of Epilepsy. In ER Kandel, JH Schwartz, TM Jessell [eds], Principles of Neural Science [3rd ed]. East Norwalk, CT: Appleton & Lange, 1991.)

of the EEG signal are often complex, four dominant bandwidths are used to describe EEG activity.[151,162] The alpha rhythm (8–13 Hz) is recorded from a normal resting adult brain.[151,162,243] It reflects a state of relaxed wakefulness.[151] Alpha is generated by thalamocortical pacemaker activity at approximately 10 Hz.[162] Alpha waves are best recorded over the parietal and occipital lobes.[151,162,243] Beta waves (13–30 Hz) are associated with cerebral arousal and intense mental activity.[151,162] Beta activity is best recorded

from the frontal cortex.[151,162,243] The beta rhythm is generated by asynchronous activity within many regions of the cerebral cortex.[162] Theta activity occurs at 4–7 Hz and is observed during drowsiness and stage 1 sleep.[151,162,243] Delta occurs at 0.5–4.0 Hz and is a characteristic of slow-wave sleep.[151,162,243]

Electroencephalogram Analysis

EEG is analyzed by qualitative and quantitative methods.[243,246] Qualitative analysis requires visual inspection of EEG data as it appears in real-time display either on paper or computer. This method of analysis is somewhat cumbersome in the operating room where changes in ongoing EEG activity must be assessed quickly and without undue difficulty.[243]

In quantitative analysis, a short epoch of EEG data is processed and reduced to a single distribution that describes activity within the EEG bandwidths.[246] The data are sampled digitally and the complex EEG waveform is broken down mathematically into a series of sine waves that taken together represent the original waveform. The amplitude of each frequency in the EEG is calculated using the fast Fourier transform (FFT).[243,246] The output from the FFT is a histogram of frequency (Hz) by amplitude (mV^2). The area under the FFT histogram may be summed to reflect the energy contained within each of the four EEG bandwidths. This distribution is easy to interpret and provides an instantaneous assessment of ongoing EEG function.

The compressed spectral array (CSA) is a common methodology used intraoperatively to describe the power spectra of an EEG epoch. The CSA is a plot of frequency (bandwidth) by amplitude (power). In order to represent changing CSA distributions over time, individual histograms for each epoch are stacked vertically creating a pseudo–three-dimensional graphic.[243] The process of constructing a CSA histogram is illustrated in Figure 4-26.

Another common histogram is the density spectral array (DSA). In the DSA frequency is plotted against time, with changes in amplitude represented by graduations in the gray scale or color of a shaded dot (Figure 4-27).[243] The selection of a particular display is often a question of personal preference. However, regardless of the graphic depiction, each variation of the FFT histogram shows essentially

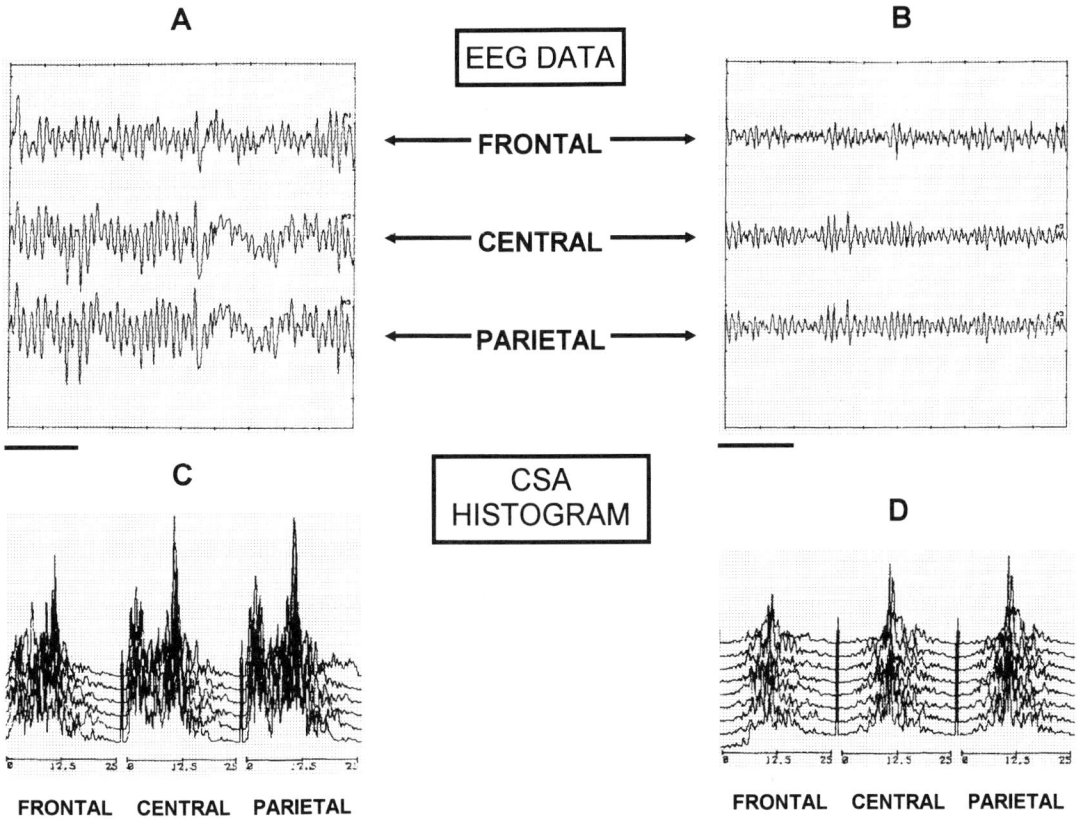

Figure 4-26. Examples of compressed spectral array (CSA) histograms derived from EEG data. Each epoch of the EEG is decomposed into basic frequencies using a Fourier transform. Output power spectra are displayed as a histogram of frequency (Hertz) by amplitude (power in millivolts squared). The area under the histogram may be organized to represent specific EEG bandwidths. Individual CSA histograms are stacked vertically to create a pseudo–three-dimensional representation of ongoing EEG function over time. In the examples depicted, 5-second samples of EEG activity were recorded from midline frontal, central, and parietal electrode sites. The raw EEG data were filtered to illustrate specific EEG bandwidths. A. EEG filtered (1–10 Hz) to emphasize high-amplitude, slow-frequency activity within delta, theta, and low-alpha bandwidths. B. EEG filtered (10–30 Hz) to emphasize low-amplitude fast activity within high-alpha and beta bandwidths. C. CSA histograms calculated from EEG activity depicted in panel A. The power spectra reflects high-amplitude, slow-wave activity. D. CSA histograms calculated from EEG activity depicted in panel B. The power spectra reflects lower amplitude alpha and beta activity. (The solid line underneath each EEG sample represents 1 second.)

the same data, i.e., the spectral content of EEG (frequency by amplitude) as it changes over time.

Electroencephalogram Applications

In the setting of aortic surgery, the EEG may be used to confirm adequate brain temperature for deep hypothermic circulatory arrest (DHCA) or to measure cerebral ischemia. Changes in cortical metabolism secondary to ischemic or hypothermic events are reflected in shifts in the patterning of

the EEG frequency and amplitude distribution over time.[194,207,247,248]

Hypothermia. The surgical repair of ascending and aortic arch aneurysms is performed under DHCA (see Chapters 6 and 7). Deep hypothermia is induced in order to decrease the metabolic requirements of the brain and protect the central nervous system.[195,206] Brain metabolism decreases about 55% per each 10°C change in body temperature.[194] The EEG may be used during DHCA to

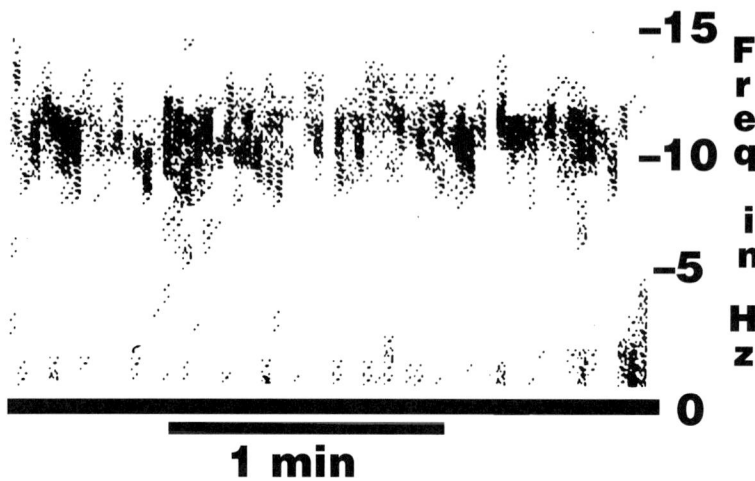

Figure 4-27. An example of a density spectral array showing ongoing electroencephalogram activity within the alpha bandwidth (8–13 Hz). Electroencephalogram spectra are displayed as a function of frequency over time with changes in amplitude represented by gradations in the gray or color scale. (Reprinted with permission from WJ Levy. Intraoperative EEG patterns: implications for EEG monitoring. Anesthesiology 1984;60:430.)

confirm electrical silence (maximum cerebral protection from hypothermia).

As shown in Figure 4-28, EEG frequency and amplitude decrease linearly with temperature.[194,247,249] As illustrated by a DSA histogram in Figure 4-29, an abrupt change in the baseline EEG pattern occurs following initiation of hypothermic CPB.[194,247] Patterns of burst suppression are common during hypothermic bypass.[194,247] The DSA pattern for burst suppression is shown in Figure 4-30. Rewarming is characterized by a gradual increase in the amplitude of higher frequency EEG (Figure 4-31).

Cerebral Ischemia.   The EEG may be used during CPB as a monitor of cerebral hypoxemia. In response to cerebral ischemia, synaptic activity between cortical neurons fails before cell membrane integrity. Thus, the loss of electrophysiologic activity between cortical neurons may predict impending and irreversible cerebral ischemia.[207] Intraoperative EEG changes are characterized by attenuation or loss in the high-frequency beta and alpha bandwidths, and the appearance or increase in low frequency delta and theta activity.[207] With prolonged ischemia this may progress to an isoelectric state (Figure 4-32).[207,248] If ischemia were due to global hypoperfusion during CPB, it is conceivable that EEG monitoring may allow for an improvement in neurologic outcome by signaling a need for higher pump flows. It may be useful as a monitor of cerebral circulation during retrograde perfusion (see Chapter 7), but at the present time studies confirming its utility are lacking. Unfortunately, many episodes of stroke during proximal aortic surgery are likely due to

macroemboli (particulate matter) or microemboli (microgaseous bubbles) and thus outcome may be predicted, but not necessarily altered.

Both hypothermia and cerebral hypoxemia cause a generalized slowing of the EEG that may progress to isoelectric acitivity. Thus, in the presence of hypothermia, cerebral ischemia may be masked. Conversely, true ischemia may masquerade as hypothermia.

Effects of Anesthesia

The effects of anesthetic agents on the EEG are dose dependent (Table 4-4). On anesthetic induction, rhythmic beta activity appears over the anterior hemisphere. The amplitude of the beta activity increases and the activity spreads over a larger cortical area. As consciousness is lost, the beta rhythm slows to within the alpha range. The lighter stages of steady-state anesthesia are characterized by alpha and low beta activity. This pattern may resemble sleep spindles, but the spindles appear continuously rather than in bursts. Transient delta activity may also be observed over the frontal cortex. More persistent delta may be seen with the use of enflurane and isoflurane. At deeper levels of anesthesia, increasing power in the delta range occurs. Burst suppression and isoelectric EEG occur at deep levels of anesthesia.[194,207,250]

Temperature

Depending on the site of aortic surgery, it may be necessary to monitor temperature to either prevent or con-

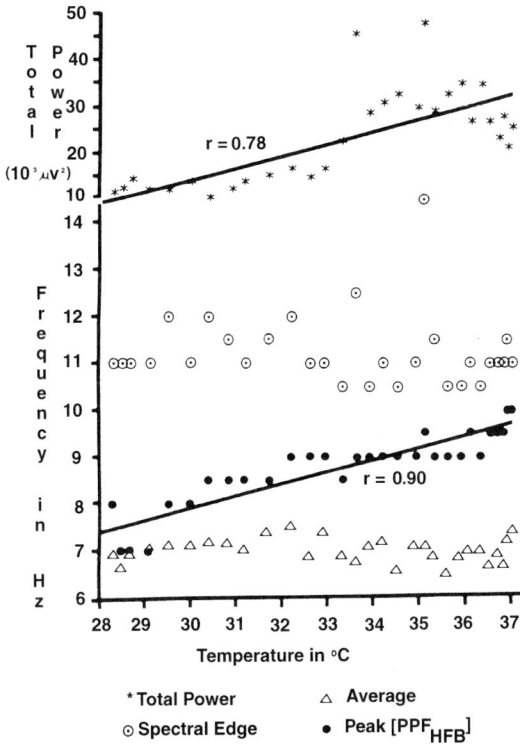

Figure 4-28. The relation between features of the electroencephalogram and hypothermia. Electroencephalogram (EEG) amplitude (total power) and temperature (upper function). EEG bandwidth and temperature (lower function). Note the decrease in power and the slowing of frequency with increasing hypothermia. (PPF = peak power frequency; HFB = high-frequency band.) (Reprinted with permission from WJ Levy. Quantitative analysis of EEG changes during hypothermia. Anesthesiology 1984;60:291.)

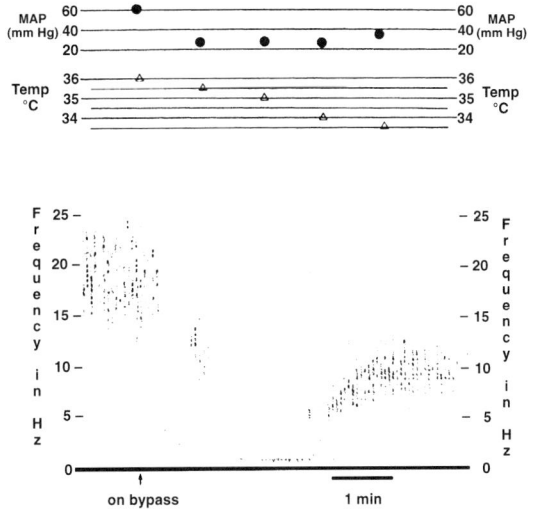

Figure 4-29. An example of a density spectral array showing the effects of hypothermia on electroencephalogram (EEG) frequency. Note the transient loss of EEG power followed by a slowing in EEG frequency. (MAP = mean arterial pressure.) (Reprinted with permission from WJ Levy. Quantitative analysis of EEG changes during hypothermia. Anesthesiology 1984;60:291.)

firm hypothermia. Patients undergoing ascending or arch surgery usually require DHCA (see Chapter 7). Profound hypothermia (15–18°C core temperature) significantly decreases brain and myocardial oxygen demand and allows for an arrest of the circulation with a relative degree of safety.[251,252] Prior to arrest it is important to accurately document adequate hypothermia in an attempt to minimize neurologic damage.

Surgery on the abdominal and descending thoracic aorta may be associated with significant hypothermia secondary to heat loss to the environment as well as unwarmed fluid replacement. Whereas hypothermia of only 2–3°C is associated with significant protection against tissue ischemia[253] and hypoxemia,[254] hypothermia below 33°C may be associated with significant sequelae. A hypothermic

drift to 34–35°C has been shown to double the duration of spinal cord ischemia that can be sustained without neurologic insult (see Chapter 8).[255,256] However, in addition to prolonging emergence, this decrease in body temperature may be associated with coagulopathy,[257] decreased drug metabolism,[258] and potential postoperative shivering. Hypothermia below 30°C increases the likelihood of spontaneous ventricular fibrillation.

Therefore, it is important to accurately monitor temperature in aortic surgery. The site chosen to monitor core temperature must be accurate. Core temperature reflects the temperature of blood perfusing the hypothalamus (the control center for body temperature regulation).[259] Accurate locations while on CPB (where blood temperature is being regulated) include the nasopharynx, tympanic membrane, and distal esophagus.[260,261] The latter may prove to be relatively difficult if TEE is being used concurrently. If CPB is not being used, then the pulmonary artery thermistor provides an excellent measure of core temperature.[262] If inspired gases are not being actively warmed, tracheal temperatures have been shown to correlate with aortic and jugular vein

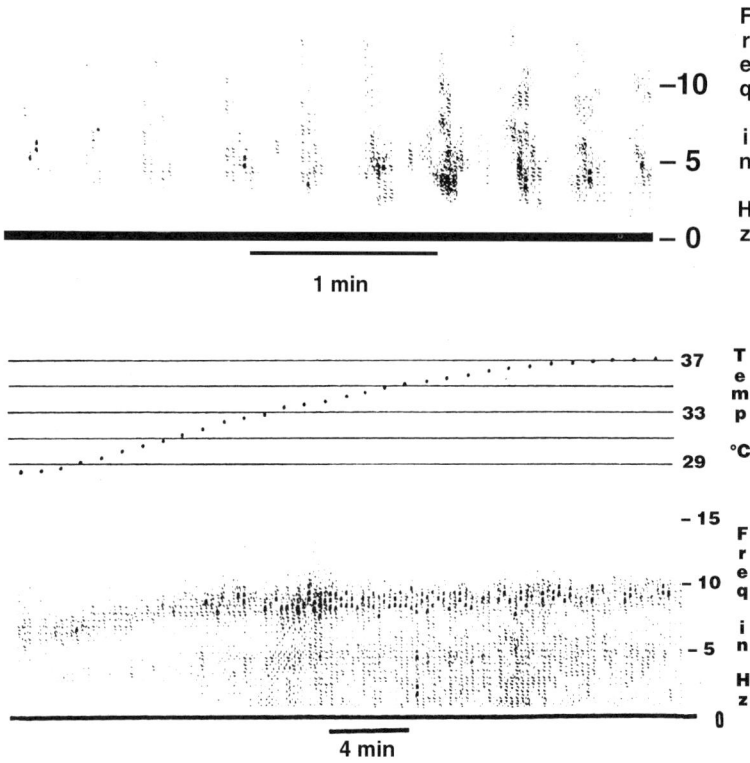

Figure 4-30. An example of a density spectral array showing the typical pattern of hypothermic-induced burst suppression. (Reprinted with permission from WJ Levy. Quantitative analysis of EEG changes during hypothermia. Anesthesiology 1984;60:291.)

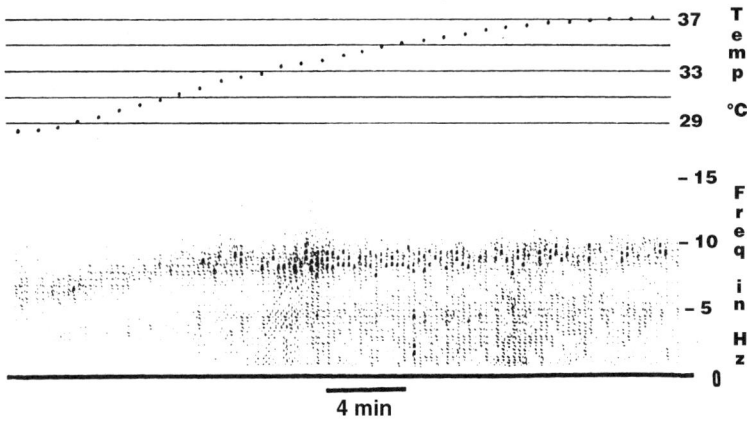

Figure 4-31. An example of a density spectral array showing the effects of rewarming on electroencephalogram (EEG) activity. Note the increase in EEG power and return to activity within the alpha bandwidth. (Reprinted with permission from WJ Levy. Quantitative analysis of EEG changes during hypothermia. Anesthesiology 1984;60:291.)

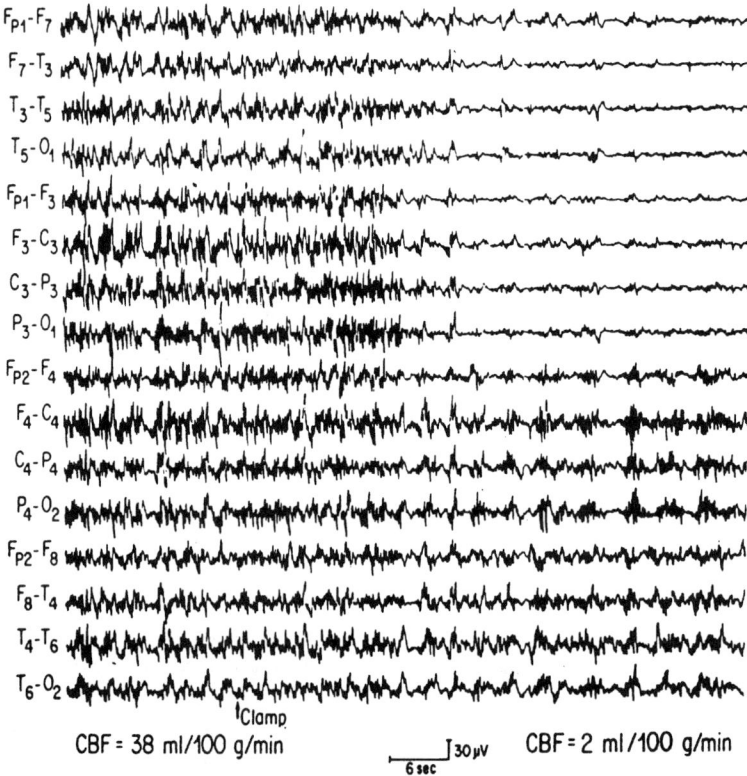

Figure 4-32. An example of isoelectric electroencephalogram (EEG) secondary to cortical ischemia. Brain activity was recorded during a left carotid endarterectomy. Note the dramatic and rapid attenuation in EEG power over the left hemisphere associated with severe and sudden unilateral cerebral ischemia. (CBF = cerebral blood flow.) (Reprinted with permission from ON Markland. Continuous Assessment of Cerebral Function with Electroencephalogram and Somatosensory Evoked Potential Techniques During Extracranial Vascular Reconstruction. In CM Loftus, UC Traynelis [eds], Intraoperative Monitoring Techniques in Neurosurgery. New York: McGraw-Hill, 1994.)

Table 4-4. The Effects of Anesthetic Agents and Physiologic Factors on the Electroencephalogram

Increased frequency
  Barbiturates (low doses)
  Benzodiazepines (low doses)
  Etomidate (low doses)
  Nitrous oxide (30–70%)
  Volatile agents (<1 MAC)
  Ketamine
  Arterial hypoxemia (initially)
  Hypercarbia (mild)
  Seizures
Electrical silence
  Barbiturates (coma doses)
  Etomidate (high doses)
  Isoflurane (2 MAC)
  Arterial hypoxemia (severe)
  Hypothermia (<20°C)
  Brain death
Decreased frequency with increased amplitude
  Barbiturates (moderate doses)
  Etomidate (moderate doses)
  Opioids
  Volatile agents (>1 MAC)
  Arterial hypoxemia (mild)
  Hypocarbia (moderate to extreme)
  Hypothermia
Decreased frequency with decreased amplitude
  Barbiturates (high doses)
  Arterial hypoxemia (mild)
  Hypocarbia (severe)
  Hypothermia (<35°C)

MAC = minimum alveolar concentration.
Source: Reprinted with permission from AA Bendo, IS Kass, J Hartung, JE Cottrell. Neurophysiology and Neuroanesthesia. In PG Barash, BF Cullen, RK Stoelting (eds), Clinical Anesthesia. Philadelphia: Lippincott, 1992;882.

temperatures.[263] Rectal, bladder, oral, and axillary temperatures generally reflect core temperature but with significantly greater variability (and often with a significant lag time) than those sites previously discussed.[262,263] Kern and colleagues[264] have suggested that due to nonhomogenous brain cooling, tympanic membrane temperature was not a valid indicator of brain temperature. Rather, they suggested that infants undergoing DHCA should be cooled until the jugular venous blood saturation is maximal. In a study of 27 patients undergoing giant cerebral aneurysm clipping with CPB and DHCA, Stone and colleagues[265] compared brain temperature with na-

sopharyngeal, esophageal, pulmonary artery, tympanic membrane, bladder, rectal, axillary, and sole of the foot temperatures. They concluded that at circulatory arrest, the nasopharyngeal, esophageal, and pulmonary artery temperatures best approximated brain temperature. However, there was significant variability and discordance. Thus, they recommend monitoring all three sites when accurate brain temperature is critical.

Acknowledgments

The authors acknowledge the kind assistance of Richard Austin, M.D., The Long Island Jewish Medical Center, New Hyde Park, NY; Nick Grasso, M.T., Mt. Sinai Hospital, New York, NY; Jeffrey Owen, Ph.D., Surgical Monitoring Services, Denver, CO; Tod Sloan, M.D., Ph.D., University of Texas Health Science Center, San Antonio, TX; and Joseph Danto, Ph.D., Physiologic Assessment Services, Englewood, NJ.

References

1. Brown OW, Hollier LH, Pairolero PC, et al. Abdominal aortic aneurysm and coronary artery disease: a reassessment. Arch Surg 1981;116:1484.
2. Hertzer NR, Young JR, Kramer JR, et al. Routine coronary angiography prior to elective aortic reconstruction. Arch Surg 1979;114:1336.
3. Hertzer N. Clinical experience with preoperative coronary angiography. J Vasc Surg 1985;3:510.
4. Tomatis LA, Fierens EE, Verbrugge GP. Evaluation of surgical risk in peripheral vascular disease by coronary arteriography: a series of 100 cases. Surgery 1971;71:429.
5. Johnston K. Multicenter prospective study of nonruptured abdominal aortic aneurysm. Part II. Variables predicting morbidity and mortality. J Vasc Surg 1989;9:437.
6. Golden M, Whittemore A, Donaldson M, Mannick J. Selective evaluation and management of coronary artery disease in patients undergoing repair of abdominal aortic aneurysms. A 16-year experience. Ann Surg 1990;212:415.
7. Beaupré P, Cahalan M, Kremer P, et al. Does pulmonary artery occlusion pressure adequately reflect left ventricular filling during anesthesia and surgery? Anesthesiology 1983;59:3.
8. Ellis J, Mangano E, van Dyke D. Relationship of wedge pressure to end-diastolic volume in patients undergoing myocardial revascularization. J Thorac Cardiovasc Surg 1979;78:605.

9. Hertzer N. Fatal myocardial infarction following abdominal aortic aneurysm resection: three hundred forty three patients followed 6–11 years postoperatively. Ann Surg 1980;192:667.

10. Pressler V, McNamara J. Thoracic aortic aneurysm: natural history and treatment. J Thorac Cardiovasc Surg 1980;79:489.

11. Crawford E, Svensson L, Coselli J, et al. Aortic dissection and dissecting aortic aneurysms. Ann Surg 1988;208:254.

12. Murphy D, Craver J, Jones E, et al. Recognition and management of ascending aortic dissection complicating cardiac surgical operations. J Thorac Cardiovasc Surg 1983;85:247.

13. Falk J, Rackow E, Blumenberg R, et al. Hemodynamic and metabolic effects of abdominal aortic cross clamping. Am J Surg 1981;142:174.

14. Hudson R, Wurm W, O'Donnell T, et al. Hemodynamics and prostacyclin release in the early phases of aortic surgery: comparison of transabdominal and retroperitoneal approaches. J Vasc Surg 1988;7:190.

15. Roizen M, Beaupré P, Alpert R. Monitoring with two dimensional transesophageal echocardiography: comparison of myocardial function in patients undergoing supraceliac, suprarenal-infraceliac, or infrarenal aortic occlusion. J Vasc Surg 1984;1:300.

16. Longo T, Marchetti G, Vercellio G. Coronary hemodynamic changes induced by aortic cross clamping. J Cardiovasc Surg 1969;10:36.

17. Reiz S, Peter T, Rais O. Hemodynamic and cardiometabolic effects of infrarenal aortic and common iliac artery declamping in man—an approach to optimal volume loading. Acta Anaesthesiol Scand 1979;23:579.

18. Kates R, Zaidan J, Kaplan J. Esophageal lead for intraoperative monitoring. Anesth Analg 1982;61:781.

19. Narang J, Thys D. Electrocardiographic Monitoring. In J Ehrenwerth, J Eisenkraft (eds), Anesthesia Equipment: Principles and Applications. St. Louis: Mosby–Year Book, 1993;287.

20. Chatterjee K, Swan H, Ganz W. Use of a balloon-tipped flotation electrode catheter for cardiac monitoring. Am J Cardiol 1975;36:56.

21. Mylrea K, Calking J, Carlson J. ECG lead with the endotracheal tube. Crit Care Med 1983;11:199.

22. Chang C, Dughi J, Shitabata P. Air embolus and the radial arterial line. Crit Care Med 1988;16:141.

23. Kim J, Arakawa K, Bliss J. Arterial cannulation: factors in the development of occlusion. Anesth Analg 1975;54:836.

24. Slogoff S, Keats AS. Does perioperative myocardial ischemia lead to postoperative myocardial infarction? Anesthesiology 1984;62:107.

25. Pasternak PF, Grossi EA, Baumann FG, et al. The value of silent myocardial ischemia monitoring in the prediction of perioperative myocardial infarction in patients undergoing peripheral vascular surgery. J Vasc Surg 1989;10:617.

26. Reiz S, Balfors E, Bredgaard-Sorenson M, et al. Coronary hemodynamic effects of general anesthesia and

surgery. Modification by epidural analgesia in patients with ischemic heart disease. Reg Anesth 1982;7:8.

27. Catoire P, Saada M, Liu N, et al. Effect of preoperative normovolemic hemodilution of left ventricular segmental wall motion during abdominal aortic surgery. Anesth Analg 1992;75:654.

28. Johnston W, Balestrieri F, Plonk G. The influence of periaortic collateral vessels on the intraoperative hemodynamic effects of acute aortic occlusion in patients with aorto-occlusive disease or abdominal aortic aneurysm. Anesthesiology 1987;66:386.

29. Levy R, Shapiro L, Wright C. The haemodynamic significance of asymptomatic ST segment depression assessed by ambulatory pulmonary pressure monitoring. Br Heart J 1986;56:526.

30. Cohn P, Brown E, Wynne J. Global and regional left ventricular ejection fraction abnormalities during exercise in patients with silent myocardial ischemia. J Am Coll Cardiol 1983;1:931.

31. Deanfield J, Shea M, Ribiero P. Transient S-T segment depression as a marker of myocardial ischemia during daily life. Am J Cardiol 1984;54:1195.

32. Stuart R, Ellestad M. Upsloping S-T segments in exercise stress testing. Am J Cardiol 1976;37:19.

33. Fletcher G, Froelicher V, Hartley L. Exercise standards: a statement for health professionals from the American Heart Association. Circulation 1990;82:2286.

34. Mangano DT, Hollenberg M, Fegert G, et al. Perioperative myocardial ischemia in patients undergoing noncardiac surgery—I: incidence and severity during the 4 day perioperative period. J Am Coll Cardiol 1991;17:843.

35. Stoelting R, Dierdorf S, McCammon R (eds). Anesthesia and Co-Existing Disease, Vol II. New York: Churchill Livingstone, 1988;10.

36. Castellanos A, Kessler KM, Myerburg RJ. The Resting Electrocardiogram. In RC Schlant, RW Alexander (eds), The Heart: Arteries and Veins (8th ed). New York: McGraw-Hill, 1994;326.

37. Gottlieb S. Detection of myocardial ischemia using continuous electrocardiography. Int Anesthesiol Clin 1992;30:19.

38. Partridge B, Barash P, London M, McCann H. Automated S-T segment trending: what does it mean? J Clin Monit 1991;8:66.

39. Kotrly K, Kotter G, Mortara D, et al. Intraoperative detection of myocardial ischemia with an S-T segment trend monitoring system. Anesth Analg 1984;63:343.

40. Griffin R, Kaplan J. Myocardial ischaemia during noncardiac surgery: a comparison of different lead systems using computerized ST segment analysis. Anaesthesia 1987;42:155.

41. Jain U, Wallis D, Moran J. Significance of electrocardiographic ST elevation during coronary artery bypass surgery. Anesth Analg 1994;78:638.

42. Kotter G, Kotrly K, Kalbfleisch J, et al. Myocardial ischemia during cardiovascular surgery as detected by an

ST segment trend monitoring system. J Cardiovasc Anesth 1987;1:190.

43. Pipberger H, Arzbaecher R, Berson A. AHA committee report: recommendations for standardization of leads and of specifications for instruments in electrocardiography and vectorcardiography. Circulation 1975;52:11.

44. Arbeit S, Rubin I, Gross H. Dangers in interpreting the electrocardiogram from the oscilloscope monitor. JAMA 1970;211:453.

45. Berson A, Pipberger H. The low-frequency response of electrocardiographs, a frequent source of recording errors. Am Heart J 1966;71:779.

46. Kaplan J, King S. The precordial electrocardiographic lead (V_5) in patients who have coronary artery disease. Anesthesiology 1976;45:570.

47. London M, Hollenberg M, Wong M. Intraoperative myocardial ischemia: localization by continuous 12 lead electrocardiography. Anesthesiology 1988;69:232.

48. Whinnery J, Froelicher V, Stewart A, et al. The electrocardiographic response to maximal treadmill exercise of asymptomatic men with left bundle branch block. Am Heart J 1977;94:316.

49. Orzan F, Garcia E, Mathur V, Hall R. Is the treadmill exercise test useful for evaluating coronary artery disease in patients with complete left bundle branch block? Am J Cardiol 1978;42:36.

50. Raby K, Goldman L, Creager M, et al. Correlation between perioperative ischemia and major cardiac events after peripheral vascular surgery. N Engl J Med 1989;321:1296.

51. Hollenberg M, Mangano D, Browner W, et al. Predictors of postoperative myocardial ischemia in patients undergoing noncardiac surgery. JAMA 1992;268:205.

52. Knight AA, Hollenberg M, London MJ, et al. Perioperative myocardial ischemia: importance of the preoperative ischemic pattern. Anesthesiology 1988;68:681.

53. Swan H. The pulmonary artery catheter. Dis Mon 1991;37:473.

54. Müller O, Rørvik K. Hemodynamic consequences of coronary heart disease with observation during anginal pain and on the effect of nitroglycerin. Br Heart J 1958;20:302.

55. Sigwart U, Grbic M, Goy J. Left atrial function in transient left ventricular ischemia produced during percutaneous transluminal coronary angioplasty of the left anterior descending coronary artery. Am J Cardiol 1990;65:282.

56. Dobson G, Horan B, Bradburn N. Significance of diastolic pulmonary artery pressure peaks. J Clin Monit 1992;8:62.

57. Reich D, Kaplan J. Hemodynamic Monitoring. In J Kaplan (ed), Cardiac Anesthesia. Philadelphia: Saunders, 1993;261.

58. Kaplan J, Wells P. Early diagnosis of myocardial ischemia using the pulmonary artery catheter. Anesth Analg 1981;60:789.

59. Sharma B, Hodges M, Asinger R, et al. Left ventricular function during spontaneous angina pectoris: effect of nitroglycerin. Am J Cardiol 1980;46:34.

60. Fuchs R, Heuser R, Yin F. Limitations of pulmonary V waves in diagnosing mitral regurgitation. Am J Cardiol 1982;49:849.

61. Clements F, Bruijn N. Perioperative evaluation of regional wall motion by transesophageal two-dimensional echocardiography. Anesth Analg 1987;66:246.

62. Tennant R, Wiggers C. The effect of coronary occlusion on myocardial contraction. Am J Physiol 1935;112:351.

63. Wohlgelernter D, Cleman M, Highman H, et al. Regional myocardial dysfunction during coronary angioplasty: evaluation by two-dimensional echocardiography and 12-lead electrocardiography. J Am Coll Cardiol 1986;7:1245.

64. Koolen J, Visser C, Reichert S, et al. Improved monitoring of myocardial ischaemia during major vascular surgery using transesophageal echocardiography. Eur Heart J 1992;13:1028.

65. Hauser A, Gangadharan V, Ramos R, et al. Sequence of mechanical, electrocardiographic and clinical effects of repeated coronary artery occlusion in human beings: echocardiographic observations during coronary angioplasty. J Am Coll Cardiol 1985;5:193.

66. Waters D, Luz P, Wyatt H, Swan H. Early changes in regional and global left ventricular function induced by graded reductions in regional coronary perfusion. Am J Cardiol 1977;39:537.

67. Kloner R, Przyklenk K, Patel B. Altered myocardial states. The stunned and hibernating myocardium. Am J Med 1989;86:14.

68. Shah P, Kyo S, Matsumara M, Omoto R. Utility of biplane transesophageal echocardiography in left ventricular wall motion analysis. J Cardiothorac Vasc Anesth 1991;5:316.

69. Chung F, Seyone C, Rakowski H. Transesophageal echocardiogram may fail to diagnose perioperative myocardial infarction. Can J Anaesth 1991;38:98.

70. Gewertz B, Kremser P, Zarins C, et al. Transesophageal echocardiographic monitoring of myocardial ischemia during vascular surgery. J Vasc Surg 1987;5:607.

71. Smith J, Cahalan M, Benefiel D, et al. Intraoperative detection of myocardial ischemia in high risk patients: electrocardiography versus two-dimensional echocardiography. Circulation 1985;72:1015.

72. London M, Tubau J, Wong M, et al. The "natural history" of segmental wall motion abnormalities in patients undergoing noncardiac surgery. Anesthesiology 1990;73:644.

73. Mangano D, Browner W, Hollenberg M, et al. Association of perioperative myocardial ischemia with cardiac

morbidity and mortality in men undergoing noncardiac surgery. N Engl J Med 1990;323:1781.

74. Sutton D, Cahalan M. Intraoperative assessment of left ventricular function with transesophageal echocardiography. Cardiol Clin 1993;11:389.

75. Ross J. Assessment of ischemic regional myocardial dysfunction and its reversibility. Circulation 1986;74:1186.

76. Buda A, Zotz R, Pace D, Krause L. Comparison of two-dimensional echocardiographic wall motion and wall thickening abnormalities in relation to the myocardium at risk. Am Heart J 1986;111:587.

77. Lieberman A, Weiss J, Jugdutt B, et al. Two-dimensional echocardiography and infarct size: relationship of regional wall motion and thickening to the extent of myocardial infarction in the dog. Circulation 1981;63:739.

78. O'Boyle J, Parisi A, Nieminen M, et al. Quantitative detection of regional left ventricular contraction abnormalities by 2-dimensional echocardiography. Comparison of myocardial thickening and thinning and endocardial motion in a canine model. Am J Cardiol 1983;51:1732.

79. Konstadt S, Abrahams H, Nejat M, Reich D. Are wall thickening measurements reproducible? Anesth Analg 1994;78:619.

80. Nishimura R, Abel M, Hatle L, et al. Assessment of diastolic function of the heart: background and current applications of Doppler echocardiography. Mayo Clin Proc 1989;64:181.

81. Daniel W, Erbel R, Kasper W, et al. Safety of transesophageal echocardiography: a multicenter survey of 10,419 examinations. Circulation 1991;83:817.

82. Spahn D, Schmid S, Carrel T, et al. Hypopharynx perforation by a transesophageal echocardiography probe. Anesthesiology 1995;82:581.

83. Khandheria B, Seward J, Tajik A. Transesophageal Echocardiography. In E Braunwald (ed), Heart Disease: A Textbook of Cardiovascular Medicine (3rd ed). Philadelphia: Saunders, 1992;290.

84. Battler A, Froelicher V, Gallagher K, et al. Dissociation between regional myocardial dysfunction and ECG changes during ischemia in the conscious dog. Circulation 1980;62:735.

85. Serruys P, Wijns W, van den Brand M, et al. Left ventricular performance, regional blood flow, wall motion and lactate metabolism during transluminal angioplasty. Circulation 1984;70:25.

86. Visser C, David G, Kan G, et al. Two-dimensional echocardiography during percutaneous transluminal coronary angioplasty. Am Heart J 1986;111:1035.

87. van Daele M, Sutherland G, Mitchell M, et al. Do changes in pulmonary capillary wedge pressure adequately reflect myocardial ischemia during anesthesia? A correlative preoperative hemodynamic, electrocardiographic and transesophageal echocardiographic study. Circulation 1990;81:865.

88. Leung J, O'Kelly B, Browner W, et al. Prognostic importance of postbypass regional wall motion abnormal-ities in patients undergoing coronary artery bypass graft surgery. Anesthesiology 1989;71:16.

89. Slogoff S, Keats A, David Y, Igo S. Incidence of perioperative myocardial ischemia detected by different electrocardiographic systems. Anesthesiology 1990;73:1074.

90. Lorman J, Powers S, Older T, et al. Correlation of pulmonary capillary wedge and left atrial pressure: a study in the patient receiving positive end-expiratory pressure ventilation. Arch Surg 1974;109:270.

91. Manjuran R, Agarwal J, Roy S. Relationship of pulmonary artery diastolic and pulmonary artery wedge pressures in mitral stenosis. Am Heart J 1975;89:207.

92. Kalman P, Wellwood M, Weisel R. Cardiac dysfunction during abdominal aortic operation: the limit of the pulmonary wedge pressures. J Vasc Surg 1986;3:773.

93. Isaacson I, Lowdon J, Berry A, et al. The value of pulmonary artery and central venous monitoring in patients undergoing abdominal aortic reconstructive surgery: a comparative study of two selected, randomized groups. J Vasc Surg 1990;12:754.

94. Joyce W, Provan J, Ameli F, et al. The role of central haemodynamic monitoring in abdominal aortic surgery. A prospective randomised study. Eur J Vasc Surg 1990;4:633.

95. Adams J, Clifford E, Henry R, Poulos E. Selective monitoring in abdominal aortic surgery. Am Surg 1993;59:559.

96. Bush H, LoGerfo F, Weisel R. Assessment of myocardial performance and optimal volume loading during elective abdominal aortic aneurysm resection. Arch Surg 1977;112:1301.

97. Harpole D, Clements F, Quill T, et al. Right and left ventricular performance during and after abdominal aortic aneurysm repair. Ann Surg 1989;209:356.

98. Reich D, Konstadt S, Nejat M, et al. Intraoperative transesophageal echocardiography for the detection of cardiac preload changes induced by transfusion and phlebotomy in pediatric patients. Anesthesiology 1993;79:10.

99. Cheung A, Savino J, Weiss S, et al. Echocardiographic and hemodynamic indexes of left ventricular preload in patients with normal and abnormal ventricular function. Anesthesiology 1994;81:376.

100. English J, Hodges M, Sentker C, et al. Comparison of aortic pulse-wave contour analysis and thermodilution methods of measuring cardiac output during anesthesia in the dog. Anesthesiology 1969;52:56.

101. Hamilton W, Moore J, Kinsman J. Studies on the circulation. IV. Further analysis of the injection method, and of changes in hemodynamics under physiological and pathological conditions. Am J Physiol 1932;99:534.

102. Hamilton M, Stevenson L, Woo M, et al. Effect of tricuspid regurgitation on the reliability of the thermodilution cardiac output technique in congestive heart failure. Am J Cardiol 1989;66:945.

103. Fischer A, Benis A, Jurado R, et al. Analysis of errors in measurement of cardiac output by simultaneous dye and thermal dilution in cardiothoracic surgical patients. Cardiovasc Res 1978;12:190.

104. Wetzel R, Latson T. Major errors in thermodilution cardiac output measurement during rapid volume infusion. Anesthesiology 1985;62:684.

105. Conway J, Lund J. Thermodilution method for measuring cardiac output. Eur Heart J 1990;11(Suppl 1):17.

106. Segal J, Nassi M, Ford A, Schuenemeyer T. Instantaneous and continuous cardiac output in humans obtained with a Doppler pulmonary artery catheter. J Am Coll Cardiol 1990;16:1398.

107. Segal J, Gaudiani V, Nishimura T. Continuous determination of cardiac output using a flow-directed Doppler pulmonary artery catheter. J Cardiothorac Vasc Anesth 1991;5:309.

108. Stoddard M, Prince C, Ammash N, et al. Pulsed Doppler transesophageal echocardiographic determination of cardiac output in human beings: comparison with thermodilution technique. Am Heart J 1993;126:956.

109. Lewis A, Kuo L, Nelson J, et al. Pulsed Doppler echocardiographic determination of stroke volume and cardiac output: clinical validation of two new methods using the apical window. Circulation 1984;70:425.

110. Muhiudeen I, Kuecherer H, Lee E. Intraoperative estimation of cardiac output by transesophageal pulsed Doppler echocardiography. Anesthesiology 1991;74:9.

111. Savino J, Troianos C, Aukburg S. Measurement of pulmonary blood flow with transesophageal two-dimensional and Doppler echocardiography. Anesthesiology 1991;75:445.

112. Darmon P-L, Hillel Z, Mogtader A, et al. Cardiac output by transesophageal echocardiography using continuous-wave Doppler across the aortic valve. Anesthesiology 1994;80:796.

113. Rankin J, McHale P, Arentzen C, et al. Three dimensional dynamic geometry of the left ventricle in the conscious dog. Circ Res 1976;39:304.

114. Robotham J, Takata M, Berman M. Ejection fraction revisited. Anesthesiology 1991;74:172.

115. Thys D, Dauchot P. Advances in Cardiovascular Physiology. In J Kaplan (ed), Cardiac Anesthesia (3rd ed). Philadelphia: Saunders, 1993;209.

116. Sagawa K, Suga H, Shoukas A. End-systolic pressure/volume ratio: a new index of ventricular contractility. Circulation 1981;63:1223.

117. Carbello B, Spann J. The uses and limitations of end-systolic indices of left ventricular function. Circulation 1984;69:1058.

118. Katz A. Influence of altered inotropy and lusitropy on ventricular pressure-volume loops. J Am Coll Cardiol 1988;11:438.

119. Gorcsan J, Romand J, Mandarino W, et al. Assessment of left ventricular performance by on-line pressure-area relations using echocardiographic automated border detection. J Am Coll Cardiol 1994;23:242.

120. Gorcsan J, Gasior T, Mandarino W, et al. Assessment of the immediate effects of cardiopulmonary bypass on left ventricular performance by on-line pressure-area relations. Circulation 1994;89:180.

121. Gorcsan J, Denault A, Gasior T, et al. Rapid estimation of left ventricular contractility from end-systolic relations using echocardiographic automated border detection and femoral arterial pressure. Anesthesiology 1994;81:553.

122. Cunningham J Jr, Laschinger JC, Merkin HA, et al. Measurement of spinal cord ischemia during operations upon the thoracic aorta: initial clinical experience. Ann Surg 1982;196:285.

123. Marini CP, Cunningham JN. Issues surrounding spinal cord protection. Adv Card Surg 1993;4:89.

124. Cunningham J Jr, Laschinger JC, Spencer FC. Monitoring of somatosensory evoked potentials during surgical procedures on the thoracoabdominal aorta. IV. Clinical observations and results. J Thorac Cardiovasc Surg 1987;94:275.

125. Dasmahapatra HK, Coles JG, Taylor MJ, et al. Identification of risk factors for spinal cord ischemia by the use of monitoring of somatosensory evoked potentials during coarctation repair. Circulation 1987;76:1114.

126. Piano G, Gewertz BL. Mechanism of increased cerebrospinal fluid pressure with thoracic aortic occlusion. J Vasc Surg 1990;11:695.

127. Crawford ES, Mizrahi EM, Hess KR, et al. The impact of distal aortic perfusion and somatosensory evoked potential monitoring on prevention of paraplegia after aortic aneurysm operation [published erratum appears in J Thorac Cardiovasc Surg 1989;97:665]. J Thorac Cardiovasc Surg 1988;95:357.

128. Crawford ES, Svensson LG, Hess KR, et al. A prospective randomized study of cerebrospinal fluid drainage to prevent paraplegia after high-risk surgery on the thoracoabdominal aorta. J Vasc Surg 1991;13:36.

129. Coles JG, Wilson GJ, Sima AF, et al. Intraoperative detection of spinal cord ischemia using somatosensory cortical evoked potentials during thoracic aortic occlusion. Ann Thorac Surg 1982;34:299.

130. Cracco RQ, Evans B. Spinal evoked potential in the cat: effects of asphyxia, strychnine, cord section and compression. Electroencephalogr Clin Neurophysiol 1978;44:187.

131. Eisen A. The somatosensory evoked potential. Can J Neurol Sci 1982;9:65.

132. Larson SJ, Walsh PR, Sances A Jr, et al. Evoked potentials in experimental myelopathy. Spine 1980;5:299.

133. Laschinger JC, Cunningham J Jr, Catinella FP, et al. Detection and prevention of intraoperative spinal cord ischemia after cross clamping of the thoracic aorta: use of somatosensory evoked potentials. Surgery 1982;92:1109.

134. FitzGerald MJT. Neuroanatomy: Basic and Applied. London: Bailliere Tindall, 1985.

135. Gatz AJ. Manter's Essentials of Clinical Neuroanatomy and Neurophysiology (4th ed). Philadelphia: Davis, 1970.

136. Gillilan LA. The arterial blood supply of the human spinal cord. J Comp Neurol 1958;75:75.

137. Rowland LP. Clinical Syndromes of the Spinal Cord and Brain Stem. In ER Kandel, JH Schwartz, TM Jessell (eds), Principles of Neural Science (3rd ed). New York: Elsevier, 1991;711.

138. Owen JH. Anatomy and Physiology of Peripheral and Spinal Cord Tracts Subserved by Somatosensory and Motor Evoked Potentials. Current Topics in Neurophysiological Intraoperative Monitoring. Baltimore: Nicolet Biomedical, 1994.

139. Murray MJ, Bower TC, Oliver W Jr, et al. Effects of cerebrospinal fluid drainage in patients undergoing thoracic and thoracoabdominal aortic surgery. J Cardiothorac Vasc Anesth 1993;7:266.

140. Apel DM, Marrero G, King J, et al. Avoiding paraplegia during anterior spinal surgery: the role of somatosensory evoked potential monitoring with temporary occlusion of segmental spinal arteries. Spine 1991;16:365.

141. Laschinger JC, Izumoto H, Kouchoukos NT. Evolving concepts in prevention of spinal cord injury during operations on the descending thoracic and thoracoabdominal aorta. Ann Thorac Surg 1987;44:667.

142. Okamoto Y, Murakami M, Nakagawa T, et al. Intraoperative spinal cord monitoring during surgery for aortic aneurysm: application of spinal cord evoked potential. Electroencephalogr Clin Neurophysiol 1992;84:315.

143. Owen JH. Update on evoked potentials during spinal surgery. Curr Opin Orthoped 1993;4:12.

144. Kaplan BJ, Friedman WA, Alexander JA, Hampson SR. Somatosensory evoked potential monitoring of spinal cord ischemia during aortic operations. Neurosurgery 1986;19:82.

145. Keen G. Spinal cord damage and operations for coarctation of the aorta: aetiology, practice, and prospects. Thorax 1987;42:11.

146. Wyss P, Stirnemann P, Mattle HP. Schaden des ruckenmarks bei eingriffen an der aorta. [Spinal lesions in surgery of the aorta]. Schweiz Rundsch Med Prax 1992;81:1105.

147. Grubbs PE, Marini C, Toporoff B, et al. Somatosensory evoked potentials and spinal cord perfusion pressure are significant predictors of postoperative neurologic dysfunction. Surgery 1988;104:216.

148. Laschinger JC, Cunningham J Jr, Isom OW, et al. Definition of the safe lower limits of aortic resection during surgical procedures on the thoracoabdominal aorta: use of somatosensory evoked potentials. J Am Coll Cardiol 1983;2:959.

149. Maeda S, Miyamoto T, Murata H, Yamashita K. Prevention of spinal cord ischemia by monitoring spinal cord perfusion pressure and somatosensory evoked potentials. J Cardiovasc Surg (Torino) 1989;30:565.

150. Oka Y, Miyamoto T. Prevention of spinal cord injury after cross clamping of the thoracic aorta. J Cardiovasc Surg 1987;28:398.

151. Martin JH. The Collective Electrical Behavior of Cortical Neurons: The Electroencephalogram and the Mechanisms of Epilepsy. In ER Kandel, JH Schwartz, TM Jessell (eds), Principles of Neural Science (3rd ed). New York: Elsevier, 1991;778.

152. Mitzdorf U. Properties of the evoked potential generators: current source-density analysis of visually evoked potentials in the cat cortex. Int J Neurosci 1987;33:33.

153. John ER, Ruchkin DS, Villegas J. Experimental background: signal analysis and behavioral correlates of evoked potential configurations in cats. Ann N Y Acad Sci 1964;112:362.

154. Ghigo J, Erwin AC, Erwin CW. Near-field vs. far-field evoked potentials. American Journal of Electroencephalogram Technology 1991;30:109.

155. AEEGS. Standards for short latency somatosensory evoked potentials. J Clin Neurophysiol 1994;11:66.

156. Cracco RQ, Cracco JB, Anziska BJ. Somatosensory evoked potentials in man: cerebral, subcortical, spinal, and peripheral nerve potentials. American Journal of Electroencephalogram Technology 1979;19:59.

157. Robertson SC, Traynelis VC, Yamada TT. Identification of the Sensorimotor Cortex with SSEP Phase Reversal. In CM Loftus, VC Traynelis (eds), Intraoperative Monitoring Techniques in Neurosurgery. New York: McGraw Hill, 1994;107.

158. Glaser EM, Ruchkin DS. Principles of neurobiological signal analysis. New York: Academic, 1976.

159. John ER. Neurometrics: Clinical Applications of Quantitative Electrophysiology. Hillsdale, NJ: Lawrence Erlbaum Associates, 1977.

160. Bamford CR, Graeme K, Steiner G, et al. The somatosensory evoked potential: solutions to some technical problems. Am J EEG Technol 1994;34:23.

161. AEEGS. Guideline eleven: guidelines for intraoperative monitoring of sensory evoked potentials. J Clin Neurophysiol 1994;11:77.

162. Epstein CM, Andriola MR. Introduction to EEG and Evoked Potentials. Philadelphia: Lippincott, 1983.

163. Kelly JP. The Neural Basis of Perception and Movement. In ER Kandel, JH Schwartz, TM Jessell (eds), Principles of Neural Science (3rd ed). New York: Elsevier, 1991;283.

164. Walcoff MR. Troubleshooting somatosensory evoked potentials. American Journal of Electroencephalogram Technology 1993;33:50.

165. Kalkman CJ, Romijn K, Denslagen W. Eliminating diathermy-induced artifacts during intraoperative monitoring of somatosensory-evoked potentials: a hardware solution. J Clin Monit 1991;7:320.

166. Dunne JW, Field CM. The value of noninvasive spinal cord monitoring during spinal surgery and interventional angiography. Clin Exp Neurol 1991;28:199.

167. Eggermont JJ. The somatosensory evoked potential and its maturation: toward a normative data set. Am J Electroenceph Tech 1989;29:235.

168. Abbruzzese M, Favale E, Leandri M, Ratto S. New subcortical components of the cerebral somatosensory evoked potential in man. Acta Neurol Scand 1978;58:325.

169. Buettner UW, Timmann D. Diagnostic significance of tibial nerve somatosensory evoked potentials (spinal and cortical components) with spinal cord lesions. Electroencephalogr Clin Neurophysiol 1990;41(Suppl):309.

170. Cracco RQ, Cracco JB. Somatosensory evoked potential in man: far field potentials. Electroencephalogr Clin Neurophysiol 1976;41:460.

171. Desmedt JE, Cheron G. Central somatosensory conduction in man: neural generators and interpeak latencies of the far-field components recorded from neck and right or left scalp and earlobes. Electroencephalogr Clin Neurophysiol 1980;50:382.

172. Gugino V, Chabot RJ. Somatosensory evoked potentials. Int Anesthesiol Clin 1990;28:154.

173. Ryu H, Uemura K. Origins of the short latency somatosensory evoked potentials in cats—with special reference to the sensory relay nuclei. Exp Neurol 1988;102:177.

174. Sances A Jr, Larson SJ, Cusick JF, et al. Early somatosensory evoked potentials. Electroencephalogr Clin Neurophysiol 1978;45:505.

175. Taylor MJ, Black SE. Lateral asymmetries and thalamic components in far-field somatosensory evoked potentials. Can J Neurol Sci 1984;11:252.

176. Wolfe DE, Drummond JC. Differential effects of isoflurane/nitrous oxide on posterior tibial somatosensory evoked responses of cortical and subcortical origin. Anesth Analg 1988;67:852.

177. Hayashi N, Nishijo H, Endo S, et al. Dipole tracing of monkey somatosensory evoked potentials. Brain Res Bull 1994;33:231.

178. Nuwer MR. Recording electrode site nomenclature. J Clin Neurophysiol 1987;4:121.

179. Engler GL, Spielholz NJ, Bernhard WN, et al. Somatosensory evoked potentials during Harrington instrumentation for scoliosis. J Bone Joint Surg [Am] 1978;60:528.

180. Hargadine JR, Snyder E. Brainstem and somatosensory evoked potentials: application in the operating room and intensive care unit. Bulletin of the Los Angeles Neurological Society 1982;47:62.

181. Spielholz NI, Benjamin MV, Engler GL, Ransohoff J. Somatosensory evoked potentials during decompression and stabilization of the spine. Methods and findings. Spine 1979;4:500.

182. Cheng MK, Robertson C, Grossman RG, et al. Neurological outcome correlated with spinal evoked potentials in a spinal cord ischemia model. J Neurosurg 1984;60:786.

183. Grabitz K, Freye E, Sandmann W. Somatosensory evoked potential, a prognostic tool for the recovery of motor function following malperfusion of the spinal cord: studies in dogs. J Clin Monit 1993;9:191.

184. Laschinger JC, Cunningham J Jr, Nathan IM, et al. Experimental and clinical assessment of the adequacy of partial bypass in maintenance of spinal cord blood flow during operations on the thoracic aorta. Ann Thorac Surg 1983;36:417.

185. Mongan PD, Peterson RE, Williams D. Spinal evoked potentials are predictive of neurologic function in a porcine model of aortic occlusion. Anesth Analg 1994;78:257.

186. Nuwer MR. Use of somatosensory evoked potentials for intraoperative monitoring of cerebral and spinal cord function. Neurol Clin 1988;6:881.

187. North RB, Drenger B, Beattie C, et al. Monitoring of spinal cord stimulation evoked potentials during thoracoabdominal aneurysm surgery. Neurosurgery 1991;28:325.

188. Drenger B, Parker SD, McPherson RW, et al. Spinal cord stimulation evoked potentials during thoracoabdominal aortic aneurysm surgery. Anesthesiology 1992;76:689.

189. Grossi EA, Laschinger JC, Krieger KH, et al. Epidural-evoked potentials: a more specific indicator of spinal cord ischemia. J Surg Res 1988;44:224.

190. de-Mol BA, Boezeman EH, Hamerlijnck RP, de-Geest R. Experimental and clinical use of somatosensory evoked potentials in surgery of aneurysms of the descending thoracic aorta. Thorac Cardiovasc Surg 1990;38:146.

191. Mizrahi EM, Crawford ES. Somatosensory evoked potentials during reversible spinal cord ischemia in man. Electroencephalogr Clin Neurophysiol 1984;58:120.

192. Laschinger JC, Owen J, Rosenbloom M, et al. Direct noninvasive monitoring of spinal cord motor function during thoracic aortic occlusion: use of motor evoked potentials. J Vasc Surg 1988;7:161.

193. Kinsella SB. Anesthesia and Intraoperative Monitoring. In DL Beck (ed), Handbook of Intraoperative Monitoring. San Diego: Singular Publishing Group, 1994;227.

194. McPherson RW. General Anesthetic Considerations in Intraoperative Monitoring: Effects of Anesthetic Agents and Neuromuscular Blockade on Evoked Potentials, EEG, and Cerebral Blood Flow. In CM Loftus, VC Traynelis (eds), Intraoperative Monitoring Techniques in Neurosurgery. New York: McGraw-Hill, 1994;97.

195. Sloan T. Anesthesia for Evoked Potential Monitoring. In Current Topics in Neurophysiological Intra-Operative Monitoring. Baltimore: Nicolet Biomedical, 1994.

196. McPherson RW, Mahla M, Johnson R, Traystman RH. Effects of enflurane, isoflurane, and nitrous oxide on somatosensory evoked potentials during fentanyl anesthesia. Anesthesiology 1985;62:626.

197. Sloan T, Rogers J, Sloan G, Rogers J. Desflurane Depresses Sensory Evoked Potentials in the Baboon. Presented at the Fifth Annual Meeting of the American Society of Neurophysiological Monitoring. Chicago: American Society of Neurophysiologic Monitoring, 1994.

198. Perlik SJ, VanEgeren R, Fisher MA. Somatosensory evoked potential surgical monitoring. Observations during combined isoflurane-nitrous oxide anesthesia. Spine 1992;17:273.

199. Owen JH, Bridwell KH, Grubb R, et al. The clinical application of neurogenic motor evoked potentials to monitor spinal cord function during surgery. Spine 1991;16:385.

200. Erwin AC, Erwin CW. Intraoperative Monitoring: Anesthetic and Physiologic Effects. In R Clark-Bash (ed), 1994 ASET Annual Courses. Course II: Intraoperative Monitoring. Chicago: American Society of Electrodiagnostic Technologists, 1994;29.

201. Kochs E, Schulte-am-Esch J. Evozierte potentiale und intravenose anasthetika [Evoked potentials and intravenous anesthetics]. Klin Wochenschr 1988;66(Suppl 14):1.

202. Nuwer MR, Dawson EC. Intraoperative evoked potential monitoring of the spinal cord. A restricted filter, scalp method during Harrington instrumentation for scoliosis. Clin Orthop 1984;183:42.

203. Picton TW, Hink RF. Evoked potentials: How? What? Why? Am J EEG Technol 1974;14:9.

204. Markand ON, Warren C, Mallik GS, Williams CJ. Temperature-dependent hysteresis in somatosensory and auditory evoked potentials. Electroencephalogr Clin Neurophysiol 1990;77:425.

205. van Rheineck Leyssius AT, Kalkman CJ, Bovill JG. Influence of moderate hypothermia on posterior tibial nerve somatosensory evoked potentials. Anesth Analg 1986;65:475.

206. Guerit JM, Baele P, de-Tourtchaninoff M, et al. [Somatosensory evoked potentials in patients undergoing circulatory arrest under profound hypothermia]. Neurophysiol Clin 1993;23:193.

207. Markland ON. Continuous Assessment of Cerebral Function with EEG and Somatosensory Evoked Potential Techniques During Extracranial Vascular Reconstruction. In CM Loftus, UC Traynelis (ed), Intraoperative Monitoring Techniques in Neurosurgery. New York: McGraw-Hill, 1994;19.

208. Grundy BL, Procopio PT, Jannetta PJ, et al. Evoked potential changes produced by positioning for retromastoid craniectomy. Neurosurgery 1982;10:766.

209. Simpson R Jr, Robertson CS, Goodman JC. Alterations in the corticomotor evoked potential following spinal cord ischemia. J Neurosci Methods 1989;28:171.

210. Levy WJ. Spinal evoked potentials from the motor tracts. J Neurosurg 1983;58:38.

211. McCullough JL, Hollier LH, Nugent M. Paraplegia after thoracic aortic occulusion: influence of cerebrospinal fluid drainage. J Vasc Surg 1988;7:153.

212. Levy W, McCaffrey M, York D. Motor evoked potential in cats with acute spinal cord injury. Neurosurgery 1986;19:9.

213. Levy WJ. Transcranial stimulation of the motor cortex to produce motor-evoked potentials. Medical Instrumentation 1987;21:248.

214. Machida M, Weinstein SL, Yamada T, et al. Monitoring of motor action potentials after stimulation of the spinal cord. J Bone Joint Surg Am 1988;70:911.

215. Machida M, Weinstein SL, Yamada T, et al. Dissociation of muscle action potentials and spinal somatosensory evoked potentials after ischemic damage of spinal cord. Spine 1988;13:1119.

216. Machida M, Yamada T, Ross M, et al. Effect of spinal cord ischemia on compound muscle action potentials and spinal evoked potentials following spinal cord stimulation in the dog. J Spinal Disord 1990;3:345.

217. Ueta T, Owen JH, Sugioka Y. Effects of compression on physiologic integrity of the spinal cord, on circulation, and clinical status in four different directions of compression: posterior, anterior, circumferential, and lateral. Spine 1992;8(Suppl):S217.

218. Kraus KH, Pope ER, O'Brien D, Hay BL. The effects of aortic occlusion on transcranially induced evoked potentials in the dog. Vet Surg 1990;19:341.

219. Osenbach RK, Hitchon PW, Mouw L, Yamada T. Effects of spinal cord ischemia on evoked potential recovery and postischemic regional spinal cord blood flow. J Spinal Disord 1993;6:146.

220. Reuter DG, Tacker W Jr, Badylak SF, et al. Correlation of motor-evoked potential response to ischemic spinal cord damage. J Thorac Cardiovasc Surg 1992;104:262.

221. Shokoku S, Uchida H, Teramoto S. An experimental study on spinal cord ischemia during cross clamping of the thoracic aorta: the monitoring of spinal cord ischemia with motor evoked potential by transcranial stimulation of the cerebral cortex in dogs. Surg Today 1993;23:1068.

222. Simpson R Jr, Contant CF, Robertson CS, Goodman JC. Spectral analysis of corticomotor evoked potentials in spinal cord injury. Part 1. Acute studies. Neurol Res 1993;15:367.

223. Levy WJ, York DH, McCaffrey M, Tanzer F. Motor evoked potentials from transcranial stimulation of the motor cortex in humans. Neurosurgery 1984;15:287.

224. Ginsburg HH, Shetter AG, Raudzens PA. Postoperative paraplegia with preserved intraoperative somatosensory evoked potentials: a case report. J Neurosurg 1985;62:296.

225. Lesser RP, Raudzens P, Luders H, et al. Postoperative neurological deficits may occur despite unchanged intraoperative somatosensory evoked potentials. Ann Neurol 1986;19:22.

226. Zornow MH, Drummond JC. Intraoperative somatosensory evoked responses recorded during onset of the anterior spinal artery syndrome [comments]. J Clin Monit 1989;5:243.

227. Zornow MH, Grafe MR, Tybor C, Swenson MR. Preservation of evoked potentials in a case of anterior spinal artery syndrome. Electroencephalogr Clin Neurophysiol 1990;77:137.

228. Owen JH. Protocol Manual: Motor Evoked Potentials. Current Topics in Neurophysiological Intra-Operative Monitoring. Baltimore: Nicolet Biomedical, 1994.

229. Chiappa KH. Transcranial motor evoked potentials. Electromyogr Clin Neurophysiol 1994;34:15.

230. Edmonds H Jr, Paloheimo MP, Backman MH, et al. Transcranial magnetic motor evoked potentials (tcM-MEP) for functional monitoring of motor pathways during scoliosis surgery. Spine 1989;14:683.

231. Burke D, Hicks R, Gandevia SC, et al. Direct comparison of corticospinal volleys in human subjects to transcranial magnetic and electrical stimulation. J Physiol (Lond) 1993;470:383.

232. Anderson LC, Hemler DE, Luethke JM, Latchaw RE. Transcranial magnetic evoked potentials used to monitor the spinal cord during neuroradiologic angiography of the spine. Spine 1994;19:613.

233. Calancie B, Klose KJ, Baier S, Green BA. Isoflurane-induced attenuation of motor evoked potentials caused by electrical motor cortex stimulation during surgery. J Neurosurg 1991;74:897.

234. Hicks RG, Woodforth IJ, Crawford MR, et al. Some effects of isoflurane on I waves of the motor evoked potential. Br J Anaesth 1992;69:130.

235. Sloan T, Rogers J, Sloan G, Rogers J. Desflurane Depresses Transcranial Motor Evoked Potentials in the Baboon. Presented at the Fifth Annual Meeting of the American Society of Neurophysiologic Monitoring. Chicago: American Society of Neurophysiologic Monitoring, 1994.

236. Herdmann J, Lumenta CB, Huse KO. Magnetic stimulation for monitoring of motor pathways in spinal procedures. Spine 1993;18:551.

237. Kawaguchi M, Sakamoto T, Shimizu K, et al. Effect of thiopentone on motor evoked potentials induced by transcranial magnetic stimulation in humans. Br J Anaesth 1993;71:849.

238. Kalkman CJ, Brink SA. Variability of somatosensory cortical evoked potentials during spinal surgery. Spine 1991;16:924.

239. Blaisdell FW, Cooley DA. The mechanism of paraplegia after temporary aortic occlusion and its relationship to spinal fluid pressure. Surgery 1962;51:351.

240. Dasmahapatra HK, Coles JG, Wilson GJ, et al. Relationship between cerebrospinal fluid dynamics and reversible spinal cord ischemia during experimental thoracic aortic occlusion. J Thorac Cardiovasc Surg 1988;95:920.

241. Elmore JR, Gloviczki P, Harper CM, et al. Failure of motor evoked potentials to predict neurologic outcome in experimental thoracic aortic occlusion. J Vasc Surg 1991;14:131.

242. Miyamoto K, Ueno A, Wada T. A new and simple method of preventing spinal cord damage following temporary occlusion of the thoracic aorta by draining the cerebrospinal fluid. J Cardiovasc Surg (Torino) 1960;16:188.

243. Schwartz DM, Bloom MJ, Pratt RE. Intraoperative monitoring of the processed electroencephalogram. Seminars in Hearing 1988;9:153.

244. Craft RM, Losasso TJ, Perkins WJ, et al. EEG monitoring for cerebral ischemia during carotid endarterectomy (CEA): how much is enough? Abstract presented at the 22nd Annual Meeting of the Society of Neuroanesthesia and Critical Care, October 14, 1994.

245. Mahla ME. Basics of Intraoperative EEG Monitoring. Presented at the Fifth Annual Meeting of the American Society of Neurophysiologic Monitoring. Chicago: American Society of Neurophysiologic Monitoring, 1994.

246. Levy WJ. Intraoperative EEG patterns: implications for EEG monitoring. Anesthesiology 1984;60:430.

247. Levy WJ. Quantitative analysis of EEG changes during hypothermia. Anesthesiology 1984;60:291.

248. Levy W, Shapiro H, Maruchak G, Meathe M. Automated EEG processing for intraoperative monitoring. Anesthesiology 1980;53:231.

249. Russ W, Sticher J, Scheld H, Hempelmann G. Effects of hypothermia on somatosensory evoked responses in man. Br J Anaesth 1987;59:1484.

250. Miller C. A Drug Reference for EEG Technologists. American Society of EEG Technologists, 1985.

251. Griepp R, Stinson E, Hollingsworth J, et al. Prosthetic replacement of the aortic arch. J Thorac Cardiovasc Surg 1975;70:1051.

252. O'Connor J, Wilding T, Farmer C, et al. The protective effect of profound hypothermia on the canine central nervous system during one hour of circulatory arrest. Ann Thorac Surg 1986;41:255.

253. Chopp M, Welch K, Tidwell C, et al. Effect of mild hypothermia on recovery of metabolic function after global cerebral ischemia in cats. Stroke 1988;19:1521.

254. Carlsson C, Hägerdal M, Siesjö B. Effect of mild hypothermia in cerebral oxygen deficiency caused by arterial hypoxia. Anesthesiology 1976;44:27.

255. Vacanti F, Ames A. Mild hypothermia and Mg^{++} protect against irreversible damage during CNS ischemia. Stroke 1984;15:695.

256. Coles J, Wilson G, Sima A, et al. Intraoperative management of thoracic aortic aneurysm, experimental evaluation of perfusion cooling of the spinal cord. J Thorac Cardiovasc Surg 1983;85:292.

257. Valeri R, Cassidy G, Khuri S, et al. Hypothermia-induced reversible platelet dysfunction. Ann Surg 1987;205:175.

258. Heier T, Caldwell J, Sessler D, Miller R. Mild intraoperative hypothermia increases action and spontaneous recovery of vecuronium blockade during nitrous oxide-isoflurane anesthesia in humans. Anesthesiology 1991;74:815.

259. Hensel H. Neural processes in thermoregulation. Physiol Rev 1973;53:954.
260. Webb G. Comparison of esophageal and tympanic temperature monitoring during cardiopulmonary bypass. Anesth Analg 1973;52:729.
261. Kern F, Ungerleider R, Schulman S. Comparison of two strategies of CPB cooling on jugular venous oxygen saturation. Anesthesiology 1992;77:1136.
262. Cork R, Vaughan R, Humphrey L. Precision and accuracy of intraoperative temperature monitoring. Anesth Analg 1983;62:211.
263. Yamakage M, Kawana S, Watanabe H, Namiki A. The utility of tracheal temperature monitoring. Anesth Analg 1993;76:795.
264. Kern F, Jonas R, Mayer J. Temperature monitoring during CPB in infants: does it predict efficient brain cooling. Ann Thorac Surg 1992;54:749.
265. Stone J, Young W, Smith C, et al. Do standard monitoring sites reflect true brain temperature when profound hypothermia is rapidly induced and reversed? Anesthesiology 1995;82:344.

Chapter 5

Bleeding and Transfusion in the Patient Undergoing Aortic Surgery

Sarojini Rao, Nabil Ghabrial, and Ketan Shevde

Hemostasis and Coagulation

There are various causes of coagulation abnormalities during aortic surgery. These include the effects of cardiopulmonary bypass, massive hemorrhage, dilutional effects on coagulation factors, platelet abnormalities, profound hypothermia, fibrinolysis, and disseminated intravascular coagulation (DIC).

Hemostasis

Normal hemostasis is dependent on the interaction between blood and its circulating cellular elements within the blood vessel. A series of steps known as the coagulation cascade is responsible for the formation of a clot.[1] When a blood vessel is injured, the following sequence of events occurs (Figure 5-1).

A primary hemostatic plug (platelet plug) is the initial response to vessel injury and occurs within a few minutes after the injury. This response is a result of the interaction between the injured vessel and platelets and depends on proper functioning of platelets with regard to their activation, adhesion, and aggregation. The platelet plug releases vasoactive substances that cause vasoconstriction of the injured vessel, thus decreasing the amount of bleeding.

A definitive hemostatic plug is formed within 1–2 hours. Its formation involves the following two steps: (1) a loose fibrin clot is formed through activation of the coagulation mechanism, and (2) a definitive plug is formed by activation of factor XIII, which cross-polymerizes the loose fibrin clot to form an insoluble hemostatic clot.[2]

Factors Affecting Hemostasis and Coagulation

When the endothelium is injured, platelets come in contact with the von Willebrand factor (vWF), which is bound to the exposed endothelium. Glycoprotein Ib, a platelet membrane component, attaches to vWF, thus anchoring the platelets to the vessel wall. Platelet membrane glycoprotein Ia and IIb may also attach the platelet directly to the exposed collagen. On contact with collagen, platelets release the contents of cytoplasmic granules extracellularly. The released substances include adenosine diphosphate (ADP), serotonin, platelet factor IV (PF-IV), and catecholamines. ADP is a potent aggregating agent that causes platelets to be activated and at the same time stimulates platelet G protein and thromboxane A_2 (TxA_2). Serotonin and TxA_2 are potent vasoconstrictors.[3] ADP and TxA_2 activate glycoproteins on the platelets (GPIIb and GPIIIa),[4] which are rendered capable of binding circulatory proteins (fibrinogen). Several platelets bind tightly and interface with fibrinogen to form a platelet plug.

Blood Vessels

The vascular endothelium provides an excellent nonthrombogenic surface. This is due to the negatively charged membrane proteins, which actively repel circulating coagulant proteins. In addition, the endothelial cells synthesize multiple cell surface

CONTACT PHASE
Damaged vascular surface
Endothelial basement membrane
Collagen

PLATELET ACTIVATION

Resting platelet

F VIII:vWF
Fibronectin
Fibrinogen
Thrombin

Platelet adhesion

TxA_2
ADP

Aggregation

TxA_2 synthesis
and granule release

TxA_2
ADP
Ca^{++}
Fibrinogen
F V
F VIII

PLATELET PLUG

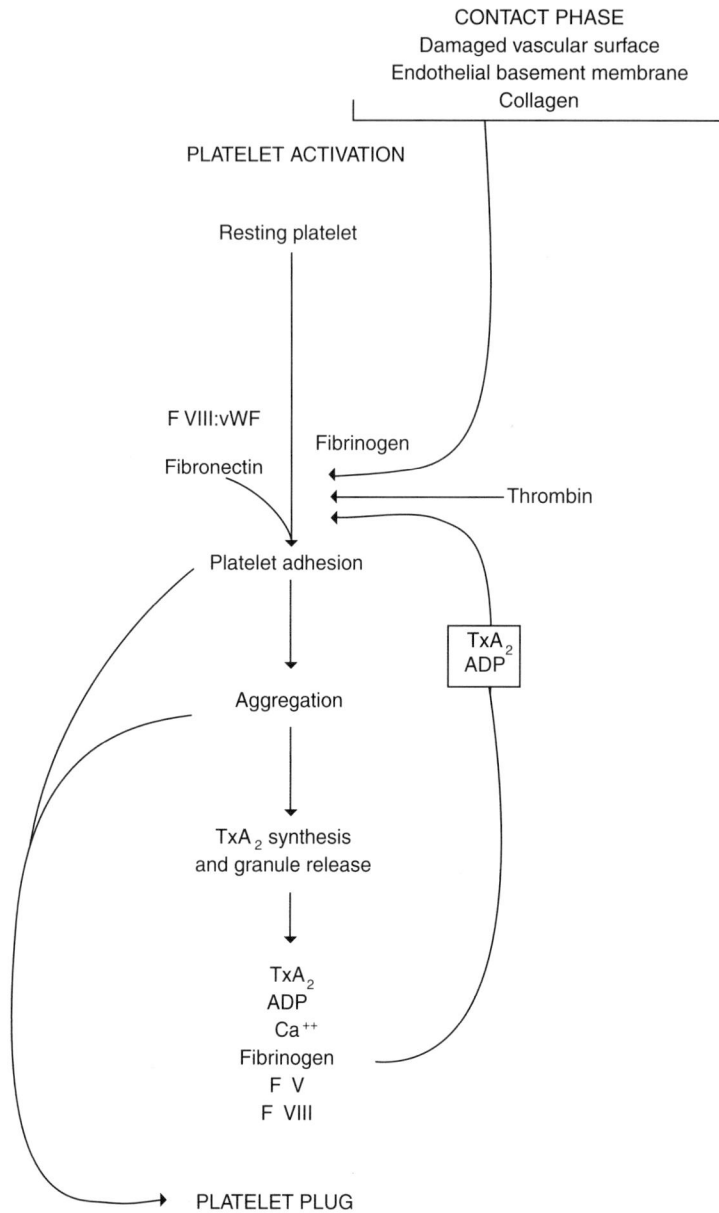

Figure 5-1. Schematic representation of the hemostatic system depicting the vascular and platelet components. The physiologic hemostatic process is initiated on contact of blood with subendothelial basement membrane and collagen in traumatized vessels during the contact phase. Exposure to the vascular subendothelial surface triggers activation of platelet function and production of activated factor XII (F XII → F XIIa). Synthetic surfaces in the extracorporeal circuit also induce platelet and factor XII activation. Platelet activation results in a sequence of events beginning with cell adhesion to the subendothelial surface (or extracorporeal circuit). Platelet aggregation to form the hemostatic platelet plug, thromboxane A_2 (TxA_2) synthesis, and secretion of platelet granule products (adenosine diphosphate [ADP], fibrinogen, factor V, and calcium) then occur. TxA_2 and adenosine diphosphate stimulate continuing platelet aggregation. Fibrinogen and factors V and VIII, which are secreted from the activated platelet, and platelet factor III (PF3), a phospholipid in the platelet cell membrane, play important roles in the coagulation cascade. (Reprinted with permission from FW Campbell. In FA Hensley [ed], The Practice of Cardiac Anesthesia [5th ed]. Boston: Little, Brown, 1990.)

components that are specifically antithrombotic, such as prostacyclin, adenosine, and protease inhibitors. These cells also incorporate heparin sulfate on the luminal surface of the blood vessel that can stimulate antithrombin III (AT-III), the most important inhibitor of blood coagulation. In addition, the vascular endothelium contains a receptor called thrombomodulin, which forms a complex with thrombin that stimulates fibrinolysis by synthesiz-

ing tissue plasminogen activators (Figure 5-2). The vascular endothelium also synthesizes proteins such as factor VIII, fibronectin, vWF, lipoprotein lipase, and prostacyclin,[5] which are potent vasodilators and inhibitors of the hemostatic function of platelets.

Thrombomodulin. The vascular endothelium contains receptors called thrombomodulins that form a complex with thrombin to alter its activity

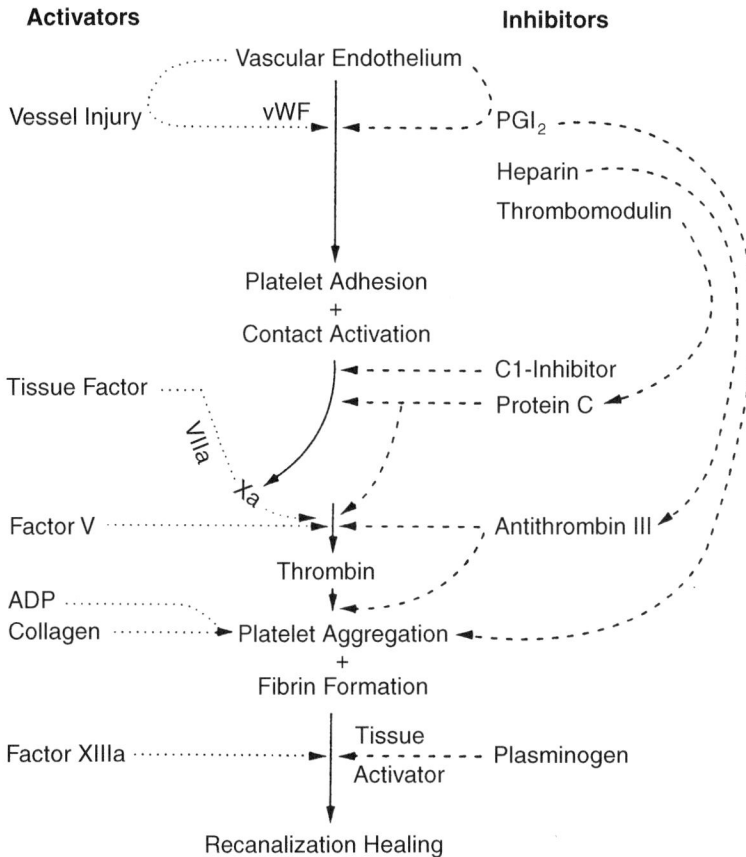

Figure 5-2. A synopsis of hemostasis. The sequential events that make up the process of hemostasis are shown in the center following the central solid arrows. At each step activators (dotted arrows on the left) and inhibitors (dashed arrows on the right) interact to provide a finely controlled process. (vWF = von Willebrand factor; PGI_2 = prostaglandin I_2; ADP = adenosine diphosphate.) (Reprinted with permission from RW Colman. Hemostasis and Thrombosis: Basic Principles and Clinical Practice. Philadelphia: Lippincott, 1987.)

radically in such a way as to prevent thrombin from activating protein C, factor V, and factor VIII, thus preventing factor VIII from activating factor Xa or converting fibrinogen to fibrin. The thrombin-thrombomodulin complex converts protein C to an active form that is capable of inactivating factors V and VIII and also regulating the release of tissue plasminogen activators.

Control of Bleeding. The blood vessel has an important role to play in the control of bleeding. This role includes vasoconstriction of the main vessel and dilation of anastomotic vessels that help to shunt the blood away from the bleeding site. Bleeding into adjacent tissues exerts external pressure on the bleeding vessels and helps decrease the amount of blood loss. Finally, if bleeding continues, hypotension ensues and decreases further bleeding.

Coagulation System

Coagulation Factors

The coagulation factors[6] (Table 5-1) are either enzymes or protein cofactors that circulate in the blood. These factors exist in an inactive form, and when they are activated, the suffix *a* is added to signify the state of activation. The suffix is not used for factors I, V, and VIII, which exist in their enzymatically active form. All coagulation factors are synthesized in the liver except factor VIII, which is synthesized by the reticuloendothelial system, and factor III (tissue thromboplastin), which is present in the subendothelial layer of blood vessels. Vitamin K–dependent factors II, VII, IX, and X require vitamin K, which is required for synthesis of specific amino acids that enable them to bind calcium. Factors V and VIII have the shortest half-life (8–12

Table 5-1. List of Coagulation Factors with Some of Their Eponyms

Factor	Synonym
I	Fibrinogen
II	Prothrombin, prethrombin
III	Tissue factor, tissue thromboplastin
IV	Calcium
V	Labile factor, proaccelerin, plasma accelerator globulin (acG)
VI	No factor assigned to this numeral
VII	Stable factor, proconvertin, autoprothrombin I, serum prothrombin conversion acceleration (SPCA)
VIII	Antihemophilic globulin (AHG), antihemophilic factor (AHF), thromboplastinogen, platelet cofactor I, antihemophilic factor A
IX	Plasma thromboplastin component (PTC), Christmas factor, autothrombin II, antihemophilic factor B, platelet cofactor 2
X	Stuart-Prower factor, autoprothrombin C (or auto prothrombin III)
XI	Plasma thromboplastin antecedent (PTA), Rosenthal's syndrome, antihemophilic factor C
XII	Hageman's factor, glass factor
XIII	Fibrin stabilizing factor (FSF), Laki-Lorand factor, fibrinase serum factor, urea-insolubility factor

hours) and are therefore known as labile factors because they are quickly lost from stored blood. Factor VIII exists as a complex with vWF (VIII:vWF) and coagulant factor VIII:C. Factor VIII:C is missing in patients with hemophilia. Factor VIII:vWF has two functions: (1) it mediates platelet adhesion to foreign surfaces such as collagen during the formation of the primary hemostatic plug, and (2) it regulates the production and release of factor VIII:C. These two factors are the products of two different genes and possess two different immunologic properties, yet they are closely associated in the plasma.

Coagulation Pathways

The main purpose of the coagulation pathway is to activate thrombin so the reaction may proceed toward formation of a stable, insoluble fibrin clot. This is achieved via the intrinsic or extrinsic coagulation pathway (Figure 5-3). It should be pointed out that the rigid separation of the coagulation cascades into two separate systems is no longer valid

because the pathways are interrelated and interactive. For example, factor VIIa can activate factor IX and in addition factors IXa, Xa, XIIa, and thrombin can probably activate factor VII.[7]

Coagulation is initiated by the disruption of the endothelial cell layer exposing a negatively charged collagen matrix that autoactivates factor XII to XIIa. High molecular weight kininogen (HMWK) binds prekallikrein (PK) and factor XI to this surface. Factor XIIa cleaves factor XI and PK to form kallikrein.

In the intrinsic pathway, activated factor XII converts factor IX to IXa, which, in the presence of factor VIII, platelet phospholipid, and calcium, activates factor X to Xa.

The extrinsic pathways begin with tissue thromboplastin, which is a substance released from damaged tissue that in the presence of factor VIIa activates factor X to Xa with the help of platelet phospholipid and Ca^{++}.

The common pathway involves factor Xa, which splits prothrombin (factor II) to thrombin (factor IIa), using platelet phospholipid, Ca^{++}, and factor V. Thrombin cleaves fibrinogen to form a soluble fibrin monomer and also activates factor XIII. Activated factor XIII cross-links the soluble fibrin monomer strands to form an insoluble, stable clot (see Figure 5-3).

Modulators of Coagulation

Thrombin. Thrombin is the most important coagulation modulator. It causes a positive feedback of the coagulation pathway by activating factors V, VIII, and XIII. It cleaves fibrinogen to fibrin, stimulates platelet recruitment, and releases tissue plasminogen activator (t-PA) from activating protein C, which inactivates factors Va and VIIIa.

Anticoagulant Proteins. A number of circulating proteins may slow the speed with which coagulation factors are activated or inhibit their activity after activation has taken place. Among these are protein C, alpha$_1$-antitrypsin, alpha$_2$-macro globulin, antithrombin III (AT-III), and protein S. AT-III enhances the anticoagulant effect of heparin 100-fold by increasing the sensitivity of heparin to thrombin. AT-III is the most important inhibitor of blood coagulation because it binds to the active site of thrombin, inhibiting its

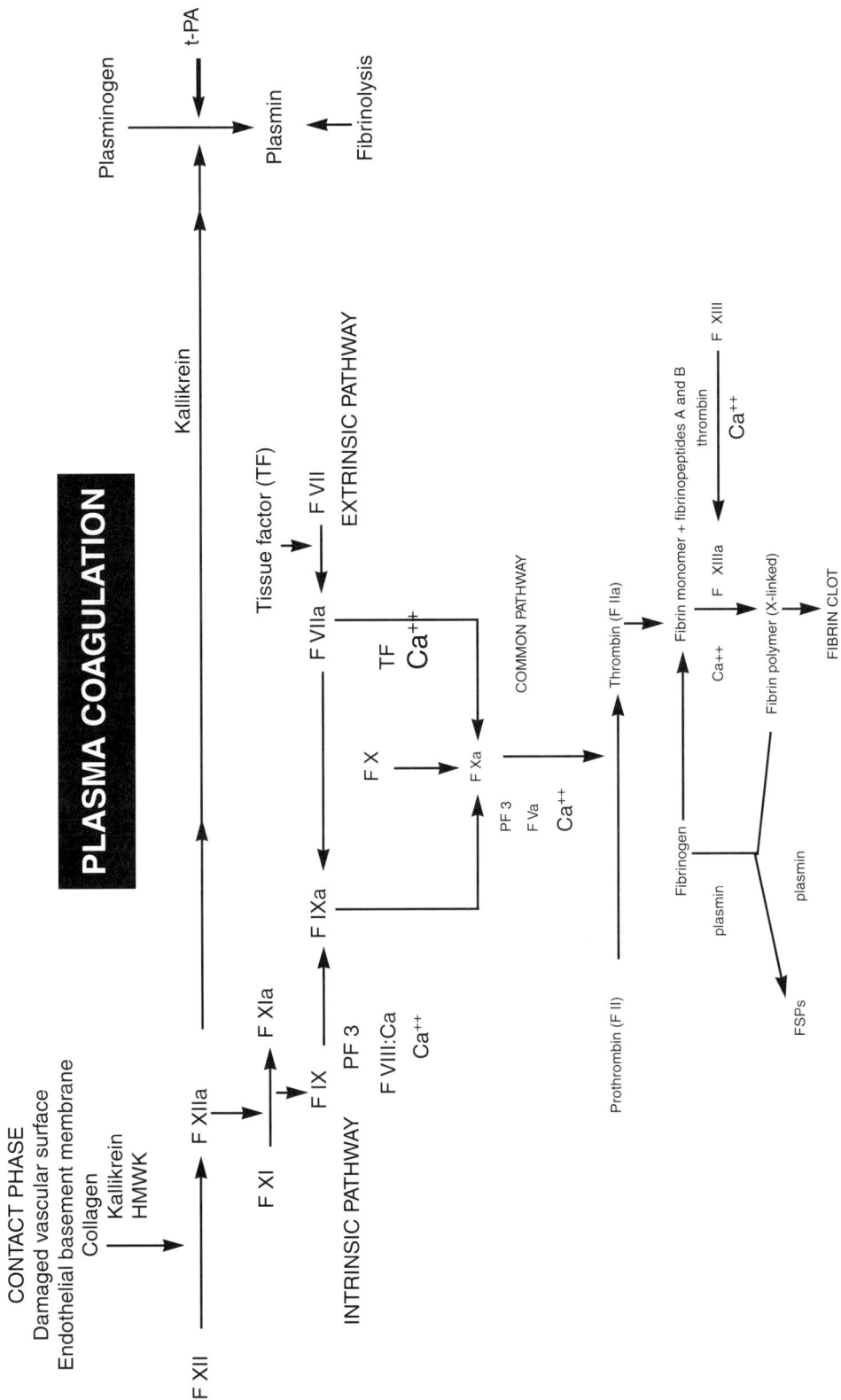

PLASMA COAGULATION

Figure 5-3. Schematic diagram of the plasma coagulation pathway divided into intrinsic, extrinsic, and common component pathways. (F = factor; a = activated coagulation factor; Ca++ = ionized calcium; HMWK = high-molecular-weight kininogen; PF 3 = platelet factor 3. Roman numerals indicate different coagulation factors by numbers.)

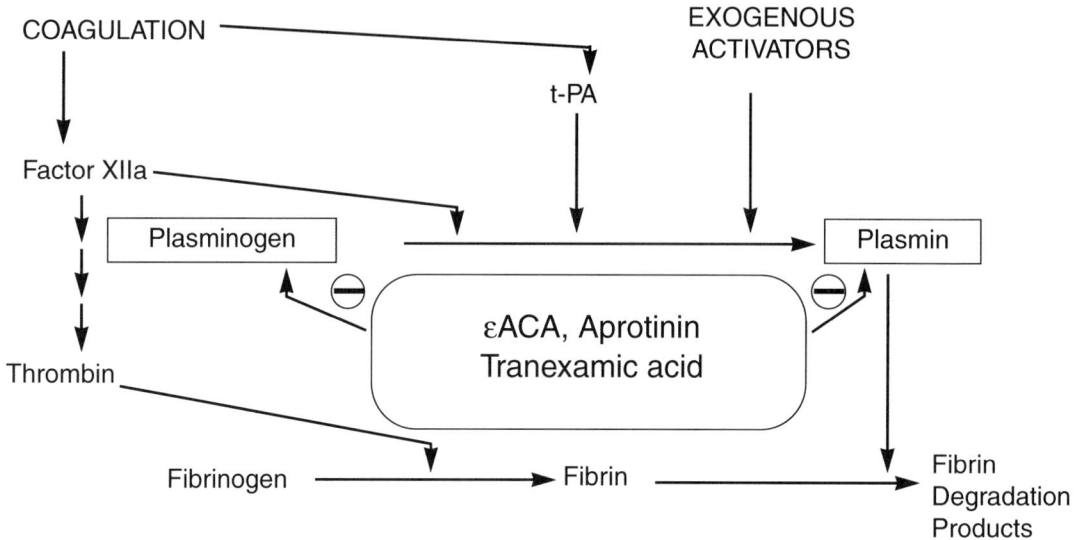

Figure 5-4. The fibrinolytic pathway. Coagulation results in formation of thrombin, which yields fibrin, t-PA, or both and factor XIIa, which convert plasminogen to plasmin in the vicinity of clot. Plasmin splits fibrin. Antifibrinolytic drugs inhibit plasminogen and plasmin. Exogenous activators of fibrinolysis, such as streptokinase, may also convert plasminogen to plasmin. (εACA = epsilon aminocaproic acid; t-PA = tissue plasminogen activator.) (Reprinted with permission from GP Gravlee. Cardiopulmonary Bypass: Principles and Practice. Baltimore: Williams & Wilkins, 1993.)

action. It also inhibits factors XIIa, XIa, IXa, Xa, and kallikrein.

Fibrinolytic System

The fibrinolytic system helps to keep thrombus formation localized to the region of hemorrhage and prevents the process from continuing to the point of extensive intravascular thrombosis by remodeling and dissolving clots that are formed at the site of injury. Fibrinolysis depends on the activation of a cleaving enzyme called plasminogen. Activation of plasminogen may occur within the intrinsic, extrinsic, or the common pathway. Plasminogen is stimulated by several activators to form plasmin, which then splits fibrin, liberating fibrin-degradation products (FDP). FDPs possess an anticoagulant property of their own and help limit the clot size. Fibrinolysis is normally limited to the site of clot formation by the scavenging protein alpha$_2$-antiplasmin, which quickly con-

sumes any formed plasmin[8] to prevent systemic fibrinolysis (Figure 5-4).

Extrinsic Fibrinolysis

t-PA is probably the primary plasminogen activator. It is a serine protease that is synthesized by endothelial cells and released by exercise, stress, venous occlusion, and heparin therapy. t-PA enhances the formation of plasmin from plasminogen. Its activity is increased 1,000-fold in the presence of fibrin, thus setting up a positive feedback mechanism localizing fibrinolysis to the area of clot formation. The circulating plasminogen is quickly rendered inactive, therefore limiting widespread fibrinolysis.

Intrinsic Fibrinolysis

Factor XIIa and thrombin formed during the first phase of coagulation can activate plasminogen to plasmin, thus lysing fibrin.

Exogenous Activators

Exogenous activators include streptokinase (derived from group C beta-hemolytic streptococci), urokinase (derived from purified human urine), anisoylated plasminogen streptokinase activator, single chain urokinase activator, and recombinant t-PA.[9] These activators cleave plasminogen to plasmin, but do so with a low fibrin affinity and therefore require large doses of activators at the site of thrombosis. The ideal thrombolytic agent is one that achieves rapid clot lysis without causing bleeding or rethrombosis and is inexpensive. Such an ideal agent is not currently available.

Abnormalities of Coagulation Associated with Surgery of the Aorta

Cardiopulmonary Bypass

In addition to the effects of heparin and protamine on the coagulation system, the components of the cardiopulmonary bypass (CPB) system also alter all aspects of the hemostatic system. This is particularly true if CPB lasts for more than 2 hours. In addition, hypothermia during CPB also adversely affects hemostasis.

Platelets

Both platelet function and number are altered adversely during CPB and constitute the most common causes of post-CPB coagulopathy; however, platelet dysfunction plays a larger role than thrombocytopenia.[10–12] Thrombocytopenia occurs as a result of a multitude of factors. Among them are hemodilution, hypothermia-induced splenic sequestration of platelets,[13] and sequestration of platelets in the reticuloendothelial system following protamine administration, which can cause a transient but significant (40%) decrease in platelet counts for up to 2 hours.[14] Mechanical destruction of platelets can occur as a result of interaction between blood and the components of the extracorporeal perfusion system. Components that contribute most to such destruction are the oxygenator, the cardiotomy suction device, and the pump heads. Rheologic factors that affect blood in the pump cause shear stress, turbulence, and stagnation. There is evidence to suggest that these may affect red cells more than platelets. Platelet counts may drop as much as 20% within the first 2 minutes after commencement of CPB.[15] However, the impact of thrombocytopenia on post-CPB bleeding is usually small because the platelet count usually remains above 100,000 per µl, and the inverse relationship between bleeding time and platelet count exists only when the count drops to below 100,000 per µl. More important is the effect on platelet dysfunction that occurs when platelets come in contact with nonendothelial surfaces, such as CPB tubing, and suction devices.[16] The deposition of fibrinogen on these synthetic surfaces acts as a nidus for platelet adhesion, aggregation, and activation. When these platelets are released back into the circulation, they have a decreased amount of binding glycoprotein receptors Ib and IIb/IIIa. These platelets also have a depleted quantity of intracellular granules. These abnormalities give rise to impaired activity and lack of adhesiveness during and in the immediate period following CPB.[17–20]

CPB also activates the fibrinolytic system that causes platelet dysfunction due to the local formation of plasmin, which affects platelets' membrane receptors.[21–24] Thus, antifibrinolytic medications such as epsilon aminocaproic acid, tranexamic acid, and aprotinin can prevent some of the platelet dysfunction seen with CPB.

Hypothermia

Hypothermia contributes to organ preservation during CPB but also impairs coagulation in the postbypass period. Most enzymatic reactions, including those controlling the coagulation cascade,[25–27] are attenuated by 7% for each 1°C decrease in temperature. Hypothermia also causes decreased aggregation of platelets due to inhibition of ADP, thromboxane, and prostacyclin.[28] In addition, it causes sequestration of platelets in the splanchnic circulation, which usually reverses 1 hour after rewarming.[25,26,29,30]

Hypothermia also enhances the activity of a specific heparin-like inhibitor of factor Xa.[31] Hypothermia activates fibrinolysis by increasing thromboplastin secretion from the injured vascular endothelium.[32]

Coagulation Factors

Dilution of coagulation protein can be a factor contributing to post-CPB coagulopathy. A 30%

dilution of coagulation proteins below normal routinely occurs with the CPB priming solution. However, the remaining levels of coagulation factors are still above the threshold required for adequate coagulation (20–30% of normal in adult patients during surgery). This may not, however, be applicable to pediatric patients, in whom there is relatively large pump priming volume in relation to blood volume. Consumption of coagulation proteins induced by CPB might cause further reduction and impairment of hemostasis. This involves several mechanisms. The extrinsic pathway may be activated by blood-synthetic surface contact. The intrinsic pathway may be activated by thromboplastin released from damaged leukocytes and platelets or by platelet aggregation. During CPB the turbulent flow through the cardiotomy suction may cause protein denaturation and inactivation of the enzymes of the coagulation system.

Fibrinolysis

Fibrinolysis can occur during CPB despite adequate heparinization.[33,34] Thrombin formation and an increase in its activity may continue in the extracorporeal circuit as demonstrated by the appearance of fibrinopeptide fragments and thrombin-antithrombin complexes.[35] This leads to an increase in the level of plasminogen activators, especially t-PA, while the levels of its inhibitors remain unchanged. Activation of fibrinolysis and the formation of FSPs further impair hemostasis.[36,37] The severity of fibrinolysis increases with longer pump time or when the patient is inadequately heparinized. In most cases a mild fibrinolytic state occurs during CPB and resolves spontaneously with little clinical impact. This type of fibrinolysis does not constitute DIC since it is neither disseminated nor intravascular.

Disseminated Intravascular Coagulation

DIC is a pathologic syndrome characterized by uncontrolled disseminated activation of the coagulation system, leading to the formation of fibrin thrombi and activation of the fibrinolytic system in the systemic circulation.[38] DIC can occur in aortic surgery whether or not CPB is used. It can be triggered by CPB, massive blood loss, massive transfusion, and hypothermia. DIC leads to the consumption of platelets and procoagulants, especially

factors V and VIII.[39] Patients with DIC have a wide spectrum of clinical manifestations, ranging from significant hemorrhage, disseminated thrombosis, or both, to the presence of laboratory findings of DIC without clinical manifestations. There is no one pathognomonic test for DIC. Colman and Robboy[40] have established the following criteria. In the absence of hepatic disease or a history of acute blood transfusion, they used a screening triad of prothrombin time greater than 15 seconds, fibrinogen level less than 160 mg/dl, and a platelet count of less than 150,000 per μl. In the presence of these three findings DIC is diagnosed with a great deal of certainty, but if only two of these test results are positive, either thrombin time or FDP should be measured. It is also helpful to perform the more specific D-Dimer test, which measures degradation products only related to cross-linked fibrin as opposed to those of fibrin and fibrinogen as measured by the regular FDP test.

The initial treatment of DIC is to correct the primary disorder. This may be all that is necessary. If the initial treatment is not successful, some recommend heparin therapy. Heparin therapy may be started to stop clot formation and to inhibit the consumption of coagulation factors and platelets. Heparin doses of 40–80 U/kg are administered every 4–6 hours, the objective being to prolong the whole blood clotting time to two to three times normal.[41] Monitoring heparin therapy is recommended with whole blood clotting time rather than with partial prothrombin time. Partial prothrombin time is more sensitive when the coagulation factors are depleted in the presence of FDP and is therefore less specific in DIC. The addition of cryoprecipitate to the therapeutic regimen of DIC has been recommended because it is rich in fibrinogen and factor VIII, both of which are decreased in DIC.[42]

Heparin

Heparin is frequently used in aortic surgery. The standard heparin preparations consist of a mixture of polyionic mucopolysaccharides with a molecular weight ranging from 2,000–30,000 daltons. Heparin is found mostly in the lungs, intestines, and liver, with skin, lymph nodes, and thymus providing less plentiful sources. Most commercial preparations of heparin are derived from pig intestines. Some commercial heparin is prepared from bovine lung,[43,44] which is highly sulfated and therefore requires more protamine for neutralization. Bovine lung heparin also causes more thrombocytopenia,[45,46] has a shorter anticoagulant effect, and is more expensive.

Heparin exerts its anticoagulant activity via antithrombin III, which is the major inhibitor of thrombin, factor IXa, and factor Xa. Unfractionated heparin accelerates thrombin antithrombin binding by 2,000-fold.[47,48] In contrast, low molecular weight heparin preferentially inhibits factor Xa. The heparin–AT-III complex also binds to platelets, inhibiting platelet aggregation.

Heparin is water soluble and has a volume of distribution that appears to be the same as plasma volume. It is metabolized by the liver and has a half-life of between 90 and 120 minutes. A history of cigarette smoking is associated with more rapid heparin clearance, whereas hypothermia, hypoxia, and decreased hepatic blood flow slow heparin clearance. The resistance of patients with deep vein thrombosis or pulmonary embolism to heparin therapy may be due to the release from thrombi of platelet factor 4, which is a known heparin antagonist. Chronic renal failure prolongs elimination of high- but not low-molecular-weight heparin. Chronic liver disease does not change elimination.

Patients receiving heparin may develop an idiosyncratic thrombocytopenia [49] due to immunologically induced antiplatelet antibodies that cause platelet aggregation. These aggregates might cause platelet emboli, called white clots, composed of platelets and fibrin. Thrombocytopenia generally resolves several days after heparin is stopped but can return if it is readministered. These patients may be treated with an alternative to heparin on CPB called ancrod. Ancrod is an enzyme obtained from snake venom that degrades fibrinogen. Ancrod must be administered 12–24 hours prior to surgery and can only be reversed with fibrinogen-containing transfusion products.[50]

The individual anticoagulant response to heparin varies greatly and some presumed cases of heparin resistance may represent nothing more than this normal variation.[51,52] Some cases of heparin resistance can occur in patients with a congenital lack of functional AT-III or in patients with liver disease or those with poor nutritional status who may be chronically AT-III deficient. In these patients either the administration of supernormal doses of heparin or the use of

fresh frozen plasma may be necessary to provide adequate amounts of AT-III for anticoagulation.[53]

Heparin rebound occurs several hours after protamine neutralization and these patients develop clinical bleeding associated with prolongation of clotting times. This phenomenon is often attributed to the reappearance of circulating heparin, which might be due to the late release of heparin sequestered in tissues, delayed return of heparin to the circulation from the extracellular space via lymphatics, or rapid clearance of protamine relative to heparin. If heparin rebound is accompanied by clinical bleeding it can be treated by the administration of supplemental doses of protamine.[54,55]

Low-molecular-weight heparin consists of certain fragments (approximately 1–2%) of standard heparin, whose molecular weight is approximately 6,000–7,000 daltons, and is prepared either by fractionation of the standard heparin or by de novo synthesis.[56] Low-molecular-weight heparin has at least double the half-life of unfractionated heparin,[57] and it is believed that it prevents thrombus formation without increasing the incidence of clinical bleeding.[58–64]

Protamine

Protamine, a polycationic protein derived from salmon sperm, possesses strong alkalinity because of an amino acid composition consisting of 67% arginine.[65] Heparin, a polyanion, binds ionically to protamine to produce a stable precipitate. Protamine contains two active sites, one that neutralizes heparin and another that exerts a mild anticoagulant effect independent of heparin. The alkaline protamine forms a tight ionic bond with the acidic sulfhydryl groups of the heparin molecule on the basis of 1 to 1 mg ratio. When bound to protamine, heparin is unable to form a complex with AT-III. The protamine heparin complex is removed from the circulation by the reticuloendothelial system, the liver, or both. Protamine is more lipophilic than heparin and has a larger volume of distribution. Its half-life (30–60 minutes) is shorter than that of heparin. The difference in half-lives is partially responsible for the phenomenon of heparin rebound.

Protamine Reaction.   Protamine administration has been associated with several patterns of hemodynamic reactions. These reactions are classified

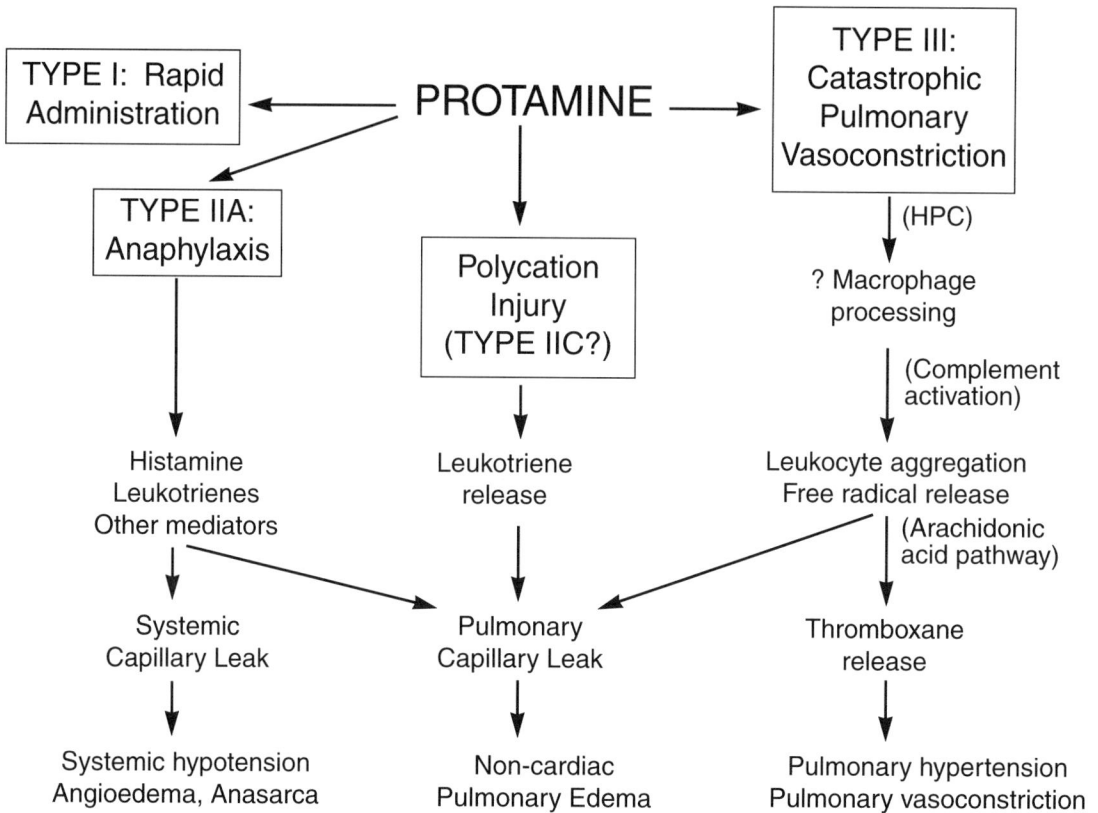

Figure 5-5. Speculative mechanisms of some protamine reactions. (HPC = heparin-protamine complex.) (Reprinted with permission from J Harrow. Management of Coagulation and Bleeding Disorders. In J Kaplan [ed], Cardiac Anesthesia [3rd ed]. Philadelphia: Saunders, 1993.)

into three major categories according to Harrow's classification (Figure 5-5).[66]

TYPE I REACTION.   The occurrence of transient systemic hypotension is due to rapid administration. This is presumably due to histamine release causing peripheral vasodilation. The prophylactic administration of H_1 and H_2 antihistaminics[67] have been advocated to prevent this type of reaction. The reactions can be considerably tempered by infusing protamine at rates slower than 5 mg per minute.[68]

TYPE II REACTION.   This is either a true immunoglobulin E–mediated anaphylaxis or an anaphylactoid reaction presumably due to prior sensitization to protamine. This may occasionally occur in patients with allergies to fish (not shellfish), in diabetic patients receiving NPH or prota-

mine zinc insulin,[69] or in patients who have had previous vasectomies.[70]

TYPE III REACTION.   Delayed anaphylactoid reactions can occur with the administration of protamine. These are mediated by complement activation with secondary release of thromboxane and other vasoactive substances,[66,71–73] causing increased pulmonary vascular resistance, right-sided heart failure, decreased left ventricular preload causing low stroke volume, and systemic hypotension.

Site of Protamine Administration.   This site of protamine administration has been studied as a triggering factor for protamine reactions. It had been suggested that vasoactive substances are released on exposure of the pulmonary vasculature to protamine.[74] Because of this, it has been recommended that protamine be given in the left side of the circulation (such as in the aortic root or left atrial line) or via a peripheral vein.[75]

Transfusion and Volume Therapy

One of the major problems during aortic surgery can be extensive blood loss. It is advisable to have sufficient large-bore intravenous access. Blood warmers are necessary to warm blood, fluids, and blood components. Replacement of large volumes of blood can be accomplished with rapid infusion systems. These are essential for the resuscitation of hypovolemic trauma patients and particularly useful in aortic aneurysm surgery, especially descending thoracic aneurysm surgery. The Level I fluid warmer system (Level One, Rockland, MA) is designed for safe and rapid warming of intravenous fluids administered to patients. This system warms fluids to a minimum delivery temperature of 36°C at flow rates of up to 700 ml per minute.

Currently, packed red cells are used routinely instead of whole blood for transfusion therapy. The primary advantages of blood component therapy are that the specific portions of the blood that patients require can be administered, allowing several patients to benefit from a single donation and avoid administration of unnecessary or unwanted components. Separation also permits each to be stored under optimal conditions and for varying lengths of time.

With rapid blood loss it is often impossible to follow the hematocrit in determining the level at which packed red blood cells should be transfused. Rather, rapid transfusion continues as loss continues, with final hematocrit adjustments made later.

Replacement of Coagulation Factors

The Baylor surgical group reported that the average blood component use during descending thoracic aorta repair is 10 units of packed red cells, 7.2 units of fresh frozen plasma (FFP), and 13 units of platelets.[76]

The routine use of blood components is no longer an acceptable practice. While there is no one single test that will provide a complete profile of the coagulation function during massive transfusion or CPB, increasing the availability and rapidity of perioperative coagulation tests can identify coagulation deficiencies in a timely manner. Tests of gross clotting, as measured by a thromboelastograph, can guide component therapy. Activated coagulation time, platelet count, prothrombin time, activated partial thromboplastin time, and fibrinogen level also provide important information that can be used to transfuse only those components specifically required in a given patient (Tables 5-2 and 5-3 and Figure 5-6) (see also Chapter 12).

Fresh Frozen Plasma

Plasma separated from whole blood soon after its collection and frozen promptly at –18°C may be stored up to 1 year. Plasma treated in this manner retains most coagulation factor activity. Each unit of FFP has a volume of 200–250 ml. Transfusion of FFP is indicated for the replacement of deficient coagulation factors. Coagulation factor activity greater than 20% of normal is usually sufficient for surgical hemostasis. Some have questioned the benefit of FFP transfusion to correct deficiency of factors V and VIII in massively transfused patients.[77,78] Although a decrease in factors V and VIII appears to be an unlikely primary cause of bleeding during massive blood transfusion, such deficiencies may intensify bleeding from other causes, such as dilutional thrombocytopenia. There is no documentation that FFP has a beneficial effect when used as a part of the transfusion management of patients with massive hemorrhage in the absence of a documented clotting factor deficiency.[79]

Even when packed erythrocytes are used to replace blood loss equivalent to one blood volume, clotting factors in the form of FFP may not be necessary to maintain the prothrombin time or plasma thromboplastin time at normal levels.[80]

Platelet Concentrates

CPB-related platelet dysfunction and dilutional thrombocytopenia with massive blood loss are the usual indications for platelet transfusion in aortic surgery. It is misleading to use the platelet count as the sole criteria in deciding whether to transfuse platelets because significant platelet dysfunction may result in bleeding despite a normal count. Bleeding

Table 5-2. A Treatment Plan for Excessive Bleeding After Cardiopulmonary Bypass

Action	Amount	Suggested by
1. Rule out surgical cause	—	Inspection of puncture sites Chest radiograph
2. More protamine	0.5–1.0 mg/kg	Activated coagulation time >150 seconds or a partial thromboplastin time >1.5 times control
3. Warm the patient	—	Core temperature <34°C
4. Apply positive-end expiratory pressure	5–10 cm H_2O	—
5. Desmopressin	0.3 μg/kg IV	Prolonged bleeding time
6. Aminocaproic acid or tranexamic acid	150 mg/kg 10–20 mg/kg	Fibrin split products >10 μg/ml
7. Platelet transfusion	1 unit/10 kg	Platelet count <100,000/ml
8. Fresh frozen plasma	15 ml/kg	Prothrombin time or a partial thromboplastin time >1.5 times control
9. Cryoprecipitate	1 unit/4 kg	Fibrinogen <100 g/l

Source: Reprinted with permission from J Harrow. Management of Coagulation and Bleeding Disorders. In J Kaplan (ed), Cardiac Anesthesia (3rd ed). Philadelphia: Saunders, 1993

time begins to increase when the platelet count decreases to less than 100,000 per μl. Thromboelastography is a qualitative test used to measure platelet dysfunction. This test measures alterations in shear elasticity and mechanical impedance, produced by the changing viscoelastic properties of forming clot.

Pooled platelets increase a patient's exposure to transfusion-associated infections. Single donor platelets, collected from a single donor by plateletpheresis will substantially decrease the patient exposure. Platelet concentrates are prepared by centrifugation of citrated whole blood within 4 hours after collection. One unit of (pooled) platelet concentrate will increase the platelet count between 5,000 and 10,000 per μl, one unit of single donor platelets will increase the platelet count four to five times as much.

Cryoprecipitate

Cryoprecipitated antihemophilic factor (factor VIII) is that fraction of plasma that precipitates when FFP is thawed at 1–6°C. This fraction can then be stored for future use. Cryoprecipitate is rich in fibrinogen and the labile coagulation factors V and VIII, vWF, and factor XIII. It is indicated in patients with fibrinolysis whose plasma fibrinogen level is less than 100 mg per dl. The usual adult dose would be 10 units. Commercial factor VIII concentrates, in con-

Table 5-3. A Dozen Ways to Stop Bleeding

S	Suction—limit cardiotomy
T	Temperature—rewarm sufficiently
O	Oxygenator—choose membranes for long cases
P	Preoperative problems—diagnose and treat first
B	Blood pressure—avoid hypertension after aortotomy
L	Ligatures—repair all vascular trespass
E	Extracorporeal circuit—minimize its volume
E	Epsilon aminocaproic acid, etc.—antifibrinolytic prophylaxis
D	Drugs—cease platelet-inhibiting drugs in advance
I	IV fluids—limit fluids, hemoconcentrate, and diurese
N	Neutralize heparin fully
G	Go with deliberate speed (tardiness begets bleeding)

Source: Reprinted with permission from J Harrow. Management of Coagulation and Bleeding Disorders. In J Kaplan (ed), Cardiac Anesthesia (3rd ed). Philadelphia: Saunders, 1993.

trast to single donor cryoprecipitate, contain a standardized amount of antihemophilic factor. These preparations, however, are more expensive than cryoprecipitated antihemophilic factor and have a potentially greater risk for transmitting viral diseases because they are prepared from pooled plasma derived from a large number of donors. Hepatitis is the most common adverse side effect of pooled plasma products, reflecting the multiple donor source of the fibrinogen.

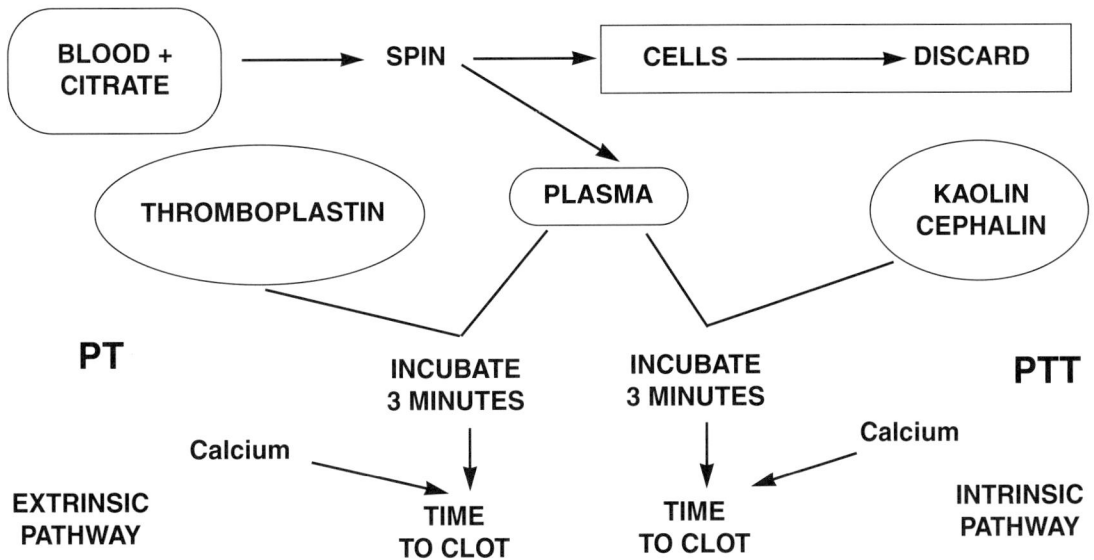

Figure 5-6. Elements of the prothrombin time (PT) and the activated partial thromboplastin (PTT): Citrated plasma is incubated with either thromboplastin or a phospholipid (cephalin or equivalent) and activator (kaolin or equivalent). Following a 3-minute incubation period, the recalcification time is measured. (Reprinted with permission from J Harrow. Management of Coagulation and Bleeding Disorders. In J Kaplan [ed], Cardiac Anesthesia [3rd ed]. Philadelphia: Saunders, 1993.)

Hemostasis-Altering Drugs

Desmopressin Acetate

Desmopressin acetate (DDAVP) is a synthetic analogue of endogenous arginine. The mechanism of procoagulant effect of desmopressin is believed to be due primarily to release of vWF and factor VIII. vWF plays a major role in platelet function by serving as a mediator for the adhesion of platelets to vascular endothelium and to other platelets. Effects of DDAVP administration following CPB on platelet dysfunction and prevention of blood loss in cardiac surgical patients have been studied and the results are contradictory. Nevertheless, when massive blood loss and platelet dysfunction are expected, prophylactic DDAVP may be helpful. The dose of DDAVP is 0.3 μg/kg by intravenous infusion over 15–20 minutes. The peak effect of DDAVP occurs at 90–120 minutes.

A decrease in arterial blood pressure due to peripheral vasodilation may occur in association with the infusion of desmopressin.[81] Desmopressin has

demonstrated hemostatic efficacy in patients with uremia, cirrhosis, and other platelet disorders. There are also some data to indicate that desmopressin may correct aspirin-induced prolongation of bleeding time.

Antifibrinolytic Agents

Antifibrinolytic agents inhibit plasminogen activation and fibrinolysis. Plasminogen activation is theorized to occur after the skin incisions are made. While increased plasmin activity can cause many coagulation maladies concomitantly, prevention of increased plasminogen activation would theoretically decrease the bleeding associated with the perioperative consumptive coagulopathy, which can occur due to decreased coagulation factors compounded by increased bleeding (Figure 5-7).

Epsilon aminocaproic acid and tranexamic acid are the two synthetic antifibrinolytic agents that have been investigated.[82,83] Studies done on patients undergoing CPB showed that the fibrinolytic system is activated at the time of sternotomy because

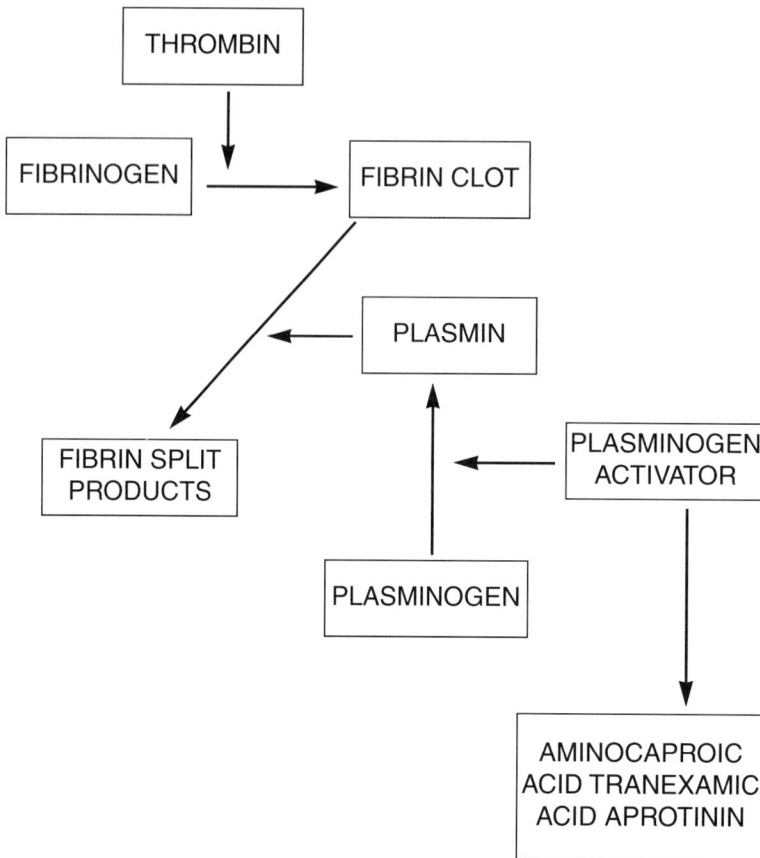

Figure 5-7. Stimulation of coagulation proteins and fibrinolysis.

of increased plasminogen activity and continues until the end of the procedure. Both these drugs were shown to significantly decrease postoperative bleeding when used prophylactically. Epsilon aminocaproic acid (5 g) is given intravenously at a slow rate over 30 minutes before the skin incision is made; thereafter 1 g of epsilon aminocaproic acid is given every hour. Tranexamic acid is approximately seven times more potent than epsilon aminocaproic acid and has fewer side effects.[84]

Aprotinin

Aprotinin is a naturally occurring protease inhibitor that inhibits plasmin, kallikrein, trypsin, and other proteolytic enzymes, leading to direct inhibition of fibrinolysis. Royston and colleagues reported that high-dose aprotinin decreased blood loss in patients undergoing repeat cardiac surgery from 1,500 ml in the control group to 280 ml in the aprotinin-treated group.[85,86] Aprotinin's effectiveness in reducing

blood loss and transfusion requirement in surgery requiring CPB is well established and it has been used in over 100,000 patients undergoing CPB worldwide. Its effectiveness is best seen in repeat cardiac procedures and in patients treated with aspirin.

In 1993 aprotinin was approved by the Food and Drug Administration for clinical use; however, its use is likely to be limited because of its expense. Anaphylaxis occurs in 0.5% of patients. Therefore, it is important to give a test dose prior to administering this drug. The dose of aprotinin is 280 mg given intravenously prior to sternotomy, followed by a 70-mg/hour infusion, with an additional 280 mg added to the pump prime. Infusion is continued until the termination of surgery. Aprotinin can affect the activated clotting time as measured by diatomaceous earth. Therefore, the standard activated coagulation time should be maintained above 700 seconds. The kaolin-activated coagulation time is unaffected by aprotinin and can be maintained in the usual range. Used prophylactically, aprotinin can reduce perioperative blood loss and the need for transfusions.[85,86]

Other Volume Therapy

Hetastarch

Hetastarch is a mixture of synthetic polysaccharides with a molecular weight of 450,000 daltons. There is no risk of disease transmission with its use because it is not a biologic product. It is indicated in the treatment of hypovolemia when plasma volume expansion is desired. Hetastarch is not a substitute for blood or plasma. Coagulopathy associated with hetastarch has been studied. Gold and colleagues randomized 40 patients undergoing elective repair of abdominal aortic aneurysms to receive either 5% albumin or 6% hetastarch in a dose of 1 g/kg (approximately 1,200 ml of 5% albumin or 1,100 ml of 6% hetastarch).[87] They found no increase in the incidence of clinical bleeding. Boldt and colleagues administered 7.2% saline in 6% hetastarch before CPB and found that it provided improved hemodynamics, gas exchange, and decreased perioperative fluid requirements compared with patients receiving conventional 6% hetastarch.[88,89]

Pentastarch

Low-molecular-weight hydroxyethyl starch is a new synthetic starch solution of low molar substitution and low molecular weight. Due to lower molar substitution ratio, pentastarch is more rapidly and completely degraded by circulating amylase than is the chemically similar hetastarch. Pentastarch induces plasma volume expansion of about one to five times the administered volume, whereas hetastarch produces expansion approximately equal to the volume administered.[90] Thus, pentastarch may be a more potent volume expander with shorter duration of action than either hetastarch or albumin.

Chemical characteristics of pentastarch and hetastarch suggest that coagulation disturbances associated with pentastarch would be similar to those of hetastarch. Infusion of 1,000 ml of 6% hetastarch into healthy human subjects has been reported to result in the prolongation in activated prothrombin time and the reduction in factor VIII coagulant levels when compared with 5% albumin.[90] This study also reported that the effects of pentastarch infusion on coagulation were not significantly different from those after albumin infusion, except that factor VIII decreased by nearly 50% (of baseline preinfusion levels) in pentastarch patients. However, no evidence of clinical bleeding was associated with either of these solutions.[90] In general 10% pentastarch as a colloid volume expander is as safe and effective as 5% albumin.

Albumin

Albumin is a naturally occurring plasma protein that makes up part of plasma. It is used to treat patients who have lost a large volume of blood and those with low blood albumin levels. Blood group testing is not required before giving an albumin transfusion. It is available as a 5% or 25% solution and has been widely used for its oncotic properties. The 25% albumin solution has an oncotic equivalent five times that of plasma. Albumin is prepared from pooled human plasma and is heat treated to eliminate viral and bacterial contamination.

Administration of plasma protein fraction or serum albumin should be restricted to the treatment of documented hypoproteinemia or when oncotic pressure is low. These solutions expand the vascular space for a longer period of time than balanced salt solutions.

Crystalloids

Ringer's lactate, 0.9% NaCl, or plasmalyte solutions are frequently used during aortic surgery. Infusions of large quantities of crystalloid may lower colloid oncotic pressure significantly, thereby allowing pulmonary edema to occur at lower pulmonary capillary wedge pressures. Lowering colloid oncotic pressure may also aggravate a pulmonary capillary leak.

Many aortic surgery patients have associated heart disease or congestive heart failure, and capillary leak may be a problem. There is much information in the literature to suggest that patients who are given colloid are resuscitated more quickly, require less fluid for resuscitation, have a lower incidence of adult respiratory distress syndrome, less weight gain, and require shorter periods of mechanical ventilation.[91,92] However, there is also a great deal of information regarding the use of crystalloid that shows no difference in morbidity and mortality.[93–95] Large volumes of crystalloid have been used safely in prospective studies involving moderate hemorrhage in vascular surgery. It is evident that considerable controversy still surrounds this subject.

Blood Salvage and Conservation Techniques

Preoperative Donation

Preoperative collection of blood is suitable for most patients scheduled for elective surgical procedures in which the need for transfusion is anticipated. Its use promotes conservation of resources by the blood bank. The limitations of this technique are the patient's ability to generate red blood cells and to tolerate the anemia caused by phlebotomy.

The American Association of Blood Banks' standards require that self-donors have a hemoglobin level of greater than or equal to 10 g per dl or hematocrit of more than 33% prior to each phlebotomy and that there be no evidence of bacteremia. Donations are usually scheduled weekly, with the last phlebotomy performed at least 72 hours prior to surgery to permit restoration of plasma volume. Withdrawal of 4 or more units of blood is possible if iron therapy is administered in addition to recombinant human erythropoietin. Debilitated patients who are given iron and recombinant erythropoietin can also tolerate preoperative phlebotomy and can donate up to 4 units of blood within 10 days before the planned surgical procedure with maintenance of hemoglobin over 10 g/dl.[96,97]

Erythropoietin

Erythropoietin, a naturally occurring protein hormone produced and released by renal cells, stimulates stem cells to develop red blood cells.

Epogen is human recombinant erythropoietin, which is identical to human erythropoietin. This drug is now available and is currently being used to treat patients with renal failure and other diseases that result in chronic anemia. Erythropoietin treatment has also been used to increase the volume of red cells obtained during preoperative autologous donation before elective surgery.[98] This drug is also useful postoperatively to improve the hematocrit

level. The efficacy of preoperative erythropoietin treatment in general is being evaluated for patients who are to undergo procedures with significant anticipated blood loss.[99]

Hemodilution

Acute normovolemic hemodilution is achieved by means of exchange of blood for crystalloid or colloid solution. The purpose is to lower the hematocrit, but not the intravascular volume prior to surgical blood loss and then reinfuse patients with fresh whole blood after major blood loss has occurred. The major advantage is that platelet function and coagulant factor function are maintained. Other advantages include the fact that the technique is easy, inexpensive, and takes less planning than preoperative autologous donation. But this can only be done in patients whose hematocrit is greater than 33%. Blood is collected in standard blood bags containing an anticoagulant, such as heparin or citrate. Collection of blood is done using large-bore intravenous lines or through a central vein.

Hemodilution has been used to decrease blood transfusion requirements for various surgical procedures, including thoracic, cardiac, and vascular procedures. However, one must be careful because of the high incidence of coronary artery disease in aortic surgical patients. Hemodilution may cause a greater incidence of myocardial ischemia during periods of increased myocardial oxygen requirement or decreased myocardial oxygen delivery. On the other hand, hemodilution may have some benefit because of decreased viscosity and improved coronary and tissue blood flow.

The volume of blood to be removed is calculated on the basis of the patient's estimated blood volume (EBV), initial hematocrit (H original), desired hematocrit (H final), and the average of H original and H final (H average).

Volume to be removed =

$$\frac{EBV \times (H\ original - H\ final)}{H\ average}$$

Cell Saver

Intraoperative blood salvage is indicated for autotransfusion in a variety of surgical procedures in which major blood loss is anticipated. Intraoperative blood salvage is often acceptable to Jehovah's witnesses, provided the salvaged blood remains in continuity with the circuit. Intraoperative salvage is usually accomplished with a semicontinuous flow centrifugation device that washes cells as they are collected. Alternatively, economical canister-based collection systems can be combined with washing and concentration by standard blood bank instruments outside the operating room. Centrifuge-based cell salvage devices are ideal when hemorrhage is substantial. Canister collection systems are usually chosen when smaller volumes of blood loss are anticipated. Postoperative blood loss can also be collected with canister systems and reinfused following washing or only filtration. An example of a centrifuge-based device is the Haemonetics Cell Saver, (Haemonetics Corp., Braintree, MA). The disposable equipment consists of an aspiration and anticoagulation assembly, reservoir with filter, centrifuge bowl, waste bag, and tubing. The double-lumen aspiration set incorporates an anticoagulant line through which heparin is administered at a controlled rate. The salvage blood, mixed with the anticoagulant solution, collects in the disposable reservoir containing a filter. The filtered blood is then pumped into a wash bowl that has a centrifugation speed of approximately 5,000 rpm. Once the bowl is filled, the contents are washed with saline. Most of the white blood cells, platelets, activated clotting factors, free plasma hemoglobin, cell fragments, and other debris are eliminated into the waste bag along with the excess saline wash solution. The red cells suspended in saline have a hematocrit of up to 60%. These are pumped into the reinfusion bag. The entire washing and concentrating process requires 3–10 minutes, depending on the apparatus and degree of automation used (Figures 5-8 and 5-9).

Complications of Massive Transfusion

Acute Complications

Citrate Toxicity. Rapid infusion of citrate in stored blood may produce sequestration of serum calcium resulting in decreased myocardial contractility, low cardiac output, and hypotension. Patients with normal liver function can metabolize citrate without a problem. If ionized calcium is

low, calcium chloride, 5–10 mg/kg intravenously, can be given.

Hypothermia. Hypothermia can be caused by the rapid infusion of cold blood products. Hypothermia of less than 30°C in surgical patients may increase ventricular irritability and predispose the patient to cardiac arrhythmias including ventricular fibrillation. This complication can be avoided by using blood warmers. Rapid infusion blood warmers such as the Level I (Level One, Rockland, MA) are available and highly effective.

Transfusion Reactions

Immediate intravascular hemolytic reactions are caused by red cell antibodies that bind to complement. Most often (but not always), these are caused by anti-A or anti-B reactions during a blood group–incompatible transfusion. Most are caused by clerical or system errors in which patients receive the wrong blood.

Classic signs and symptoms include chills, fever, and chest and flank pain. During general anesthesia one should be aware of hemoglobinuria, unexplained hypotension, and bleeding diathesis. When acute reaction is suspected, transfusion must be stopped immediately. The blood bank should be notified and all units cross-matched should be rechecked. Treatment usually consists of hydration, alkalinization of urine, mannitol, and intravenous infusion of dopamine for improved renal perfusion.

Delayed Complications of Massive Transfusion

Hepatitis C. Hepatitis C probably represents greater than 95% of what was previously called transfusion-associated non-A, non-B hepatitis. The risk of non-A, non-B hepatitis is about 1 in 3,300 units transfused, a marked improvement from 1 in 10 transfusion recipients contracting posttransfusion non-A, non-B hepatitis just 10 years ago.[100] This is because of better serologic tests to detect antibodies to hepatitis C. Forty to 50% of patients with hepatitis C have evidence of chronic active or persistent hepatitis on liver biopsy, and of these, 25% may develop carcinoma of the liver.

Hepatitis B. The risk of hepatitis B following transfusion is about 1 in 200,000 units. By routinely

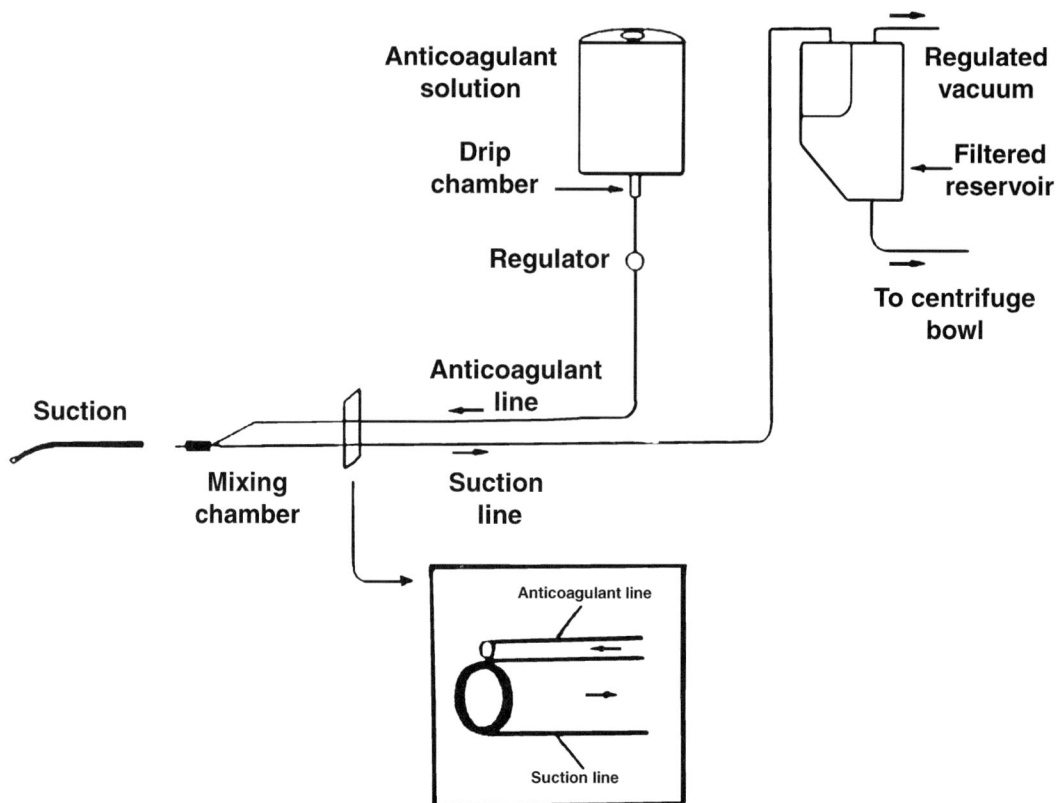

Figure 5-8. The typical blood collection system includes a suction apparatus that aspirates blood into a filtered reservoir. As blood is drawn from the surgical field, it enters a small mixing chamber to which an anticoagulation solution is added. Following mixing, the anticoagulation blood is carried to a reservoir where it is filtered and stored until centrifugation is desired. A closeup of the double-lumen suction tubing shows a small tube providing the anticoagulant solution to the mixing chamber, and a large tube serving to transport the aspirated blood. (Reprinted with permission from GP Gravlee. Cardiopulmonary Bypass: Principles and Practice. Baltimore: Williams & Wilkins, 1993.)

screening and eliminating those donors who are positive for Hbs Ag, an 80–90% reduction in the incidence of hepatitis B has resulted.

Acquired Immunodeficiency Syndrome.   Data from the American Red Cross HIV blood donor study was used in 1992 to estimate the likelihood of HIV-1 transmission via blood transfusion to be 1 in 225,000 units transfused. It is clearly a low incidence and is getting lower. With the diligent application of epidemiologic data to remove high-risk donors from the donor pool, public education programs, and the development and implementation of tests to screen donated units for anti–HIV-1 antibodies, there has been a marked reduction of the risk of transmitting HIV-1 through a blood transfusion.

Conclusion

Conservation of homologous blood and blood products is an important part of an anesthesiologist's responsibility while taking care of patients undergoing aortic surgery. With adequate knowledge of the intricacies of the coagulation system and appropriate use of all available means of conserving extraneous blood and blood products, it is possible to limit transfusion to a minimum, without jeopardizing patient care and surgical outcome. Preoperative autologous blood deposits are generally underused and many blood bank facilities can augment self-donation programs and help maximize blood conservation. In most operating rooms cell-saver devices are commonly used and

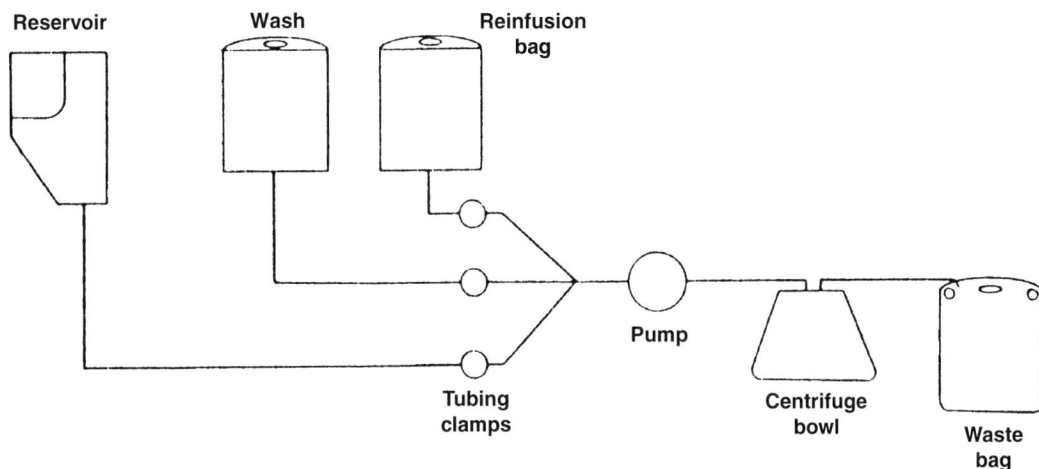

Figure 5-9. Schematic for a typical cell separator showing the reservoir bag into which aspirated anticoagulated blood is accumulated. Other portions of the apparatus include a reservoir for saline wash solution, a bag for collecting the washed blood, serial tubing clamps operated by a microprocessor, a pump head that allows flow in either direction (depending on which tubing clamps are open or shut), a centrifuge bowl for cell separation, and a waste bag for discarding supernatant during the washing process. (Reprinted with permission from GP Gravlee. Cardiopulmonary Bypass: Principles and Practice. Baltimore: Williams & Wilkins, 1993.)

provide valuable assistance to the anesthesiologist. Use of pharmacologic agents such as epsilon aminocaproic acid and aprotinin should be considered in appropriate clinical settings. Equipment to assess coagulation, platelet function, and oncotic pressure in or in close proximity to the operating room will greatly facilitate patient care.

References

1. Colman RW, Hirsch J, Marder VJ, Salzman EW (eds), Hemostasis and Thrombosis: Basic Principles and Clinical Practice (2nd ed). Philadelphia: Lippincott, 1987.
2. Colman RW, Marder VJ, Salzman EW, Hirsch J. Overview of Hemostasis. In RW Colman, J Hirsch, VJ Marder, EW Salzman (eds), Hemostasis and Thrombosis: Basic Principles and Clinical Practice (2nd ed). Philadelphia: Lippincott, 1987;3.
3. Kessler CM. The pharmacology of aspirin, heparin, coumarin and thrombolytic agents. Chest 1991;99:97.
4. Triplett DA. Overview of Hemostasis. In JE Menitove, LJ McCarthy (eds), Hemostatic Disorders and the Blood Bank. Arlington, VA: American Association of Blood Banks, 1984;1.
5. Thorup OA Jr. Fundamentals of Clinical Hematology (5th ed). Philadelphia: Saunders, 1987;778.
6. Pittiglia HD. Introduction to Hemostasis: An Overview of Hemostatic Mechanisms, Platelet Structure and Function and Extrinsic and Intrinsive Systems. In HD Pittiglio, RA Saches (eds), Introduction to Hemostasis. Philadelphia: FA Davis, 1987;325.
7. Furie B, Furie BC. Molecular and cellular biology of blood coagulation. N Engl J Med 1992;326:800.
8. Francis RB, Feinstein DI. Clinical significance of accelerated fibrinolysis in liver disease. Hemostasis 1984;14:460.
9. Goldberg M, Colonna-Rimano P, Babin N. Emergency coronary artery bypass surgery following intracoronary streptokinase. Anesthesiology 1984;61:601.
10. McFarlane RG. Symposium No. 27. Zoological Society of London. The Hemostatic Mechanism in Man and Other Animals. London: Academic, 1970.
11. Barrer MJ, Ellison N. Platelet function. Anesthesiology 1977;46:202.
12. Tomasullo BA, Lenes BA. Platelet Transfusion Therapy. In JE Menitove, LJ McCarthy (eds), Hemostatic Disorders in the Blood Bank. Arlington, VA: American Association of Blood Banks, 1984;63.
13. Heyns AD, Lotter MG, Badenhorst PN, et al. Kinetics and in vivo redistribution of III indium labeled human platelets after intravenous protamine sulphate. Thromb Haemost 1980;44:65.
14. Kirklin JK, Chenoweth DE, Naftel DC, et al. Effects of protamine administration after cardiopulmonary bypass on complement, blood elements, and the hemodynamic state. Ann Thorac Surg 1986;41:193.
15. Bick RI. Alterations of hemostasis associated with cardiopulmonary bypass surgery. Semin Thromb Hemost 1985;11:281.

16. Edmunds LH, Ellison N, Colman RW, et al. Platelet function during open heart surgery: comparison of membrane and bubble oxygenators. J Thorac Cardiovac Surg 1982;83:805.

17. Harker LA, Malpass TW, Branson HE. Mechanism of abnormal bleeding in patients undergoing cardiopulmonary bypass. Acquired transient platelet dysfunction associated with selective granule release. Blood 1980;56:824.

18. Rinder CS, Bohnert J, Rinder II, et al. Platelet activation and aggregation during cardiopulmonary bypass. Anesthesiology 1991;75:388.

19. Rinder CS, Matthew JP, Rinder HM, et al. Modulation of platelet surface adhesion receptors during cardiopulmonary bypass. Anesthesiology 1991;75:563.

20. Rinder CS, Bohnert J, Rinder HM, et al. Platelet activation and aggregation during cardiopulmonary bypass. Ann Surg 1981;1993:105.

21. Adelman B, Rizk A, Hanners E. Plasminogen interactions with platelets in plasma. Blood 1988;72:1530.

22. van Oeveren W, Eijsman I, Roosendaal KJ, et al. Platelet preservation by aprotinin during cardiopulmonary bypass. Lancet 1988;1:644.

23. van Oeveren W, Harder MP, Roosendaal KJ, et al. Aprotinin protects platelets against the initial effect of cardiopulmonary bypass. J Thorac Cardiovasc Surg 1990;99:788.

24. Havel M, Teufelsbauer H, Knobel P, et al. Effect of intraoperative aprotinin administration on postoperative bleeding in patients undergoing cardiopulmonary bypass operation. J Thorac Cardiovasc Surg 1991;101:968.

25. Michenfelder JD, Theye RA. Hypothermia: effects on canine brain and whole-body metabolism. Anesthesiology 1968;29:1107.

26. Villalobos TJ, Aderson E, Barila TG. Hematologic changes in hypothermic dogs. Proc Soc Exp Biol Med 1985;89:192.

27. Hessel EA, Scher G, Dillard DH. Platelet kinetics during deep hypothermia. J Surg Res 1980;28:23.

28. Soslau G, Harrow J, Brodsky I. The effect of tranexamic acid on platelet ADP during extracorpeal circulation. Am J Hematol 1991;38:113.

29. Khuri SF, Wolfe JA, Josa M, et al. Hematologic changes during and after bypass and their relationship to bleeding time and nonsurgical blood loss. J Thorac Cardiovasc Surg 1992;104:94.

30. Valeri CR, Khabbaz K, Khuri SF, et al. Effects of skin temperature on platelet function in patients undergoing extracorporeal bypass. J Thorac Cardiovasc Surg 1988;104:108.

31. Cornillon B, Mzazorana M, Dureau G, et al. Characterization of a heparin-like activity released in dogs during deep hypothermia. Eur J Clin Invest 1988;18:460.

32. Yoshihara H, Yamamoto T, Mihara H. Changes in coagulation and fibrinolysis occuring in dogs during hypothermia. Thromb Res 1985;37:503.

33. Jobes DR, Ellison N, Campbell RW. Limitations for ACT [Letter]. Anesth Analg 1989;69:142.

34. Addonizio VP Jr, Macarak EJ, Niewarowski S, et al. Preservation of human platelets with prostaglandin E, during in vitro cardiopulmonary bypass. Circ Res 1979;44:350.

35. Mammen EF, Koets MH, Washington BC, et al. Hemostasis changes during cardiopulmonary bypass surgery. Semin Thromb Hemost 1985;11:281.

36. Marengo-Rowe AJ, Leveson JE. Fibrinolysis: A Frequent Cause of Bleeding. In N Ellison, DR Jobes (eds), Effective Hemostasis in Cardiac Surgery. Philadelphia: Saunders, 1988;41.

37. Umlas J. Fibrinolysis and disseminated intravascular coagulation in open heart surgery. Transfusion 1976;16:460.

38. Davis GC, Sobel M, Salzman EW. Elevated plasma fibrinopeptide A and thromboxane B levels during cardiopulmonary bypass. Circulation 1980;61:808.

39. Miller RD. Problems in massive transfusion. Anesthesiology 1973;39:82.

40. Colman RW, Robboy SJ. Postoperative disseminated intravascular coagulation. Urol Clin North Am 1976;3:379.

41. Culliford AT, Gitel SG, Starr N, et al. Lack of correlation between activated clotting time and plasma heparin during cardiopulmonary bypass. Ann Surg 1981;193:105.

42. Hattersley PG, Kunkel M. Cryoprecipitate as a source of fibrinogen in treatment of disseminated intravascular coagulation. Transfusion 1976;16:641.

43. Rodriguez HJ, Vanderwielen N. Molecular weight determination of commercial heparin sodium USP and its sterile solutions. J Pharm Sci 1979;68:588.

44. Racanelli A, Fareed J, Walenga JM, et al. Biochemical and pharmacological studies on the protamine interactions with heparin, its fractions and fragments. Semin Thromb Hemost 1985;11:176.

45. Saekema JCJ. Heparin and its biocompatibility. Clin Nephrol 1986;26(Suppl 1):3.

46. Hirsh J. Heparin. N Engl J Med 1991;324:1565.

47. Rosenberg RD. Biochemistry of heparin antithrombin reactions and the physiologic role of this natural anticoagulant mechanism. Am J Med 1989;87:2.

48. Villanueva GB, Danishelfsky I. Evidence for a heparin induced conformational change on antithrombin III. Biochem Biophys Res Comm 1977;74:803.

49. Godal HC. Heparin Induced Thrombocytopenia. In DA Lane, U Lindhal (eds), Heparin. Boca Raton, FL: CRC Press, 1989.

50. Zulys VJ, Teasdale SJ, Michel ER, et al. Ancrod as an alternative to heparin anticoagulation for cardiopulmonary bypass. Anesthesiology 1989;71:870.

51. Gravlee GP, Haddon WS, Rothberger HK, et al. Heparin dosing and monitoring for cardiopulmonary bypass. J Thorac Cardiovasc Surg 1990;99:518.

52. Young JA, Kisker T, Doty DB. Adequate anticoagulation during cardiopulmonary bypass determined by activated clotting time and the appearance of fibrin monomer. Ann Thorac Surg 1978;26:231.

53. Soloway HB, Christansen IW. Heparin anticoagulation during cardiopulmonary bypass in an antithrombin III deficient patient. Implications relative to the etiology of heparin. Am J Clin Pathol 1980;73:723.

54. Perkins A, Acra DJ, Rolls MR. Estimation of heparin levels in stored and traumatized blood. Blood 1961;18:807.

55. Frick PG, Broxlli H. The mechanism of heparin rebound after extracorporeal circulation for open cardiac surgery. Surgery 1966;59:721.

56. Hanson LA. Heparin Sulfate Proteoglycans: Structure and Properties. In DA Lane, U Lindahl (eds), Heparin. Boca Raton, FL: CRC Press, 1989.

57. Nader HB, Dietrich CP. Natural Occurrence and Possible Biological Role of Heparin. In DA Lane, U Lindahl (eds), Heparin. Boca Raton, FL: CRC Press, 1989.

58. Planes A, Vochell N, Fagola M, et al. Efficacy and safety of a perioperative enoxaparin regimen in total hip replacement under various anesthesia. Am J Surg 1991;161:525.

59. Lassen MR, Borril C, Christansen HM, et al. Prevention of thromboembolism in 190 hip arthroplasties. Acta Orthop Scand 1991;62:33.

60. Torholm C, Broeng L, Jorgesen PS, et al. Thromboprophylaxis by low molecular weight heparin in elective hip surgery. J Bone Joint Surg Am 1991;73:434.

61. Turpie AG. Efficacy of a postoperative regime of enoxaparin in deep vein thrombosis prophylaxis. Am J Surg 1991;161:532.

62. Massonnet-Castel S, Pelissier E, Dreyfus G, et al. Rationale for development of low molecular weight heparin in extracorporeal circulation. Lancet 1984;1:1182.

63. Massonnet-Castel S, Pelissier E, Dreyfus G, et al. Low molecular heparin and their clinical potential in the prevention of postoperative venous thrombosis. Am J Surg 1991;161:512.

64. Massonnet-Castel S, Pelissier E, Bara L, et al. Partial reversal of low molecular weight heparin (PK 10169) anti Xa activity by protamine sulfate. In vitro and in vivo study during cardiac surgery with extracorporeal circulation. Haemostasis 1986;16:139.

65. Ando T, Yamasaki M, Suzuki K. Protamine. In A Kleinzeller, GF Springer, HG Wittman (eds), Molecular Biology, Biochemistry and Biophysics (Vol. 12). Berlin: Springer-Verlag, 1973;12:1.

66. Harrow JC. Protamine allergy. J Cardiothorac Anesth 1988;2:225.

67. Parsons RS, Mohandas K. The effect of histamine receptor blockade on the hemodynamic response to protamine. J Cardiothorac Anesthes 1989;3:37.

68. Morel DR, Zopol WM, Thomas SJ, et al. C_SA and thromboxane generation associated with pulmonary vaso- and bronchoconstriction during protamine reversal of heparin. Anesthesiology 1987;66:597.

69. Stoelting RK, Henry DP, Verbur KM, et al. Hemodynamic changes and circulating histamine concentration following protamine administration to patients and dogs. Can Aneasth Soc J 1984;31:535.

70. Sheridan P, Blain R, Vezina D, Bleau G. Prospective Evaluation of the Safety of Heparin Reversal with Protamine in Vasectomized Patients after Cardiopulmonary Bypass. Presented at the Proceedings of the 10th Annual Meeting of the Society of Cardiovascular Anesthesiologists, New Orleans, April 1988.

71. Levy J, Schwieger IA, Zaiden JR, et al. Evaluation of patients at risk for protamine reactions. J Thorac Cardiovasc Surg 1989;98:200.

72. Watson RA, Ansbacher R, Barry M, et al. Allergic reaction to protamine. A late complication of elective vasectomy. Urology 1983;22:493.

73. Best N, Teisner B, Grudzinkas JG, Fisher MM. Classical pathway activation during an adverse response to protamine sulfate. Br J Anaesth 1983;55:1149.

74. Goldman BS, Joison J, Austen WG. Cardiovascular effects of protamine sulfate. Ann Thorac Surg 1969;7:459.

75. Casthely PA, Goodman K, Fyman PN, et al. Hemodynamic changes after the administration of protamine. Anesth Analg 1986;65:78.

76. Crawford ES, Fenstermacher JM, Richardson W. Reappraisal of adjuncts to avoid ischemia in the treatment of thoracic aortic aneurysms. Surgery 1970;67:182.

77. Miller RD, Robbins TO, Tong MJ, Barton SL. Coagulation defects associated with massive transfusions. Ann Surg 1971;174:794.

78. Counts RB, Haisch C, Simon TL, et al. Hemostasis in massively transfused trauma patients. Ann Surg 1979;190:91.

79. Bove JR. Fresh frozen plasma: too few indications—too much use [editorial]. Anesth Analg 1985;64:849.

80. Murray DJ, Olson J, Strauss R, Tinker JH. Coagulation changes during packed red cell replacement of major blood loss. Anesthesiology 1988;69:839.

81. D'Alauro F, John RA. Hypotension related to desmopressin administration following cardiopulmonary bypass. Anesthesiology 1988;69:962.

82. Hardy JF, Derocher J. Natural and synthetic antifibrinolytics in cardiac surgery. Can J Anaesth 1992;39:353.

83. Del Rossi AJ, Ceraianu AC, Botros S, et al. Prophylactic treatment of post perfusion bleeding using EACA. Chest 1989;96:27.

84. Horrow JC, Hlavacek J, et al. Prophylactic tranexamic acid decreases bleeding after cardiac operation. J Thorac Cardiovasc Surg 1990;99:70.

85. Royston D. High dose aprotinin therapy: a review of the first five years experience. J Cardiothorac Vasc Anesth 1992;6:76.

86. Royston D. High dose aprotinin therapy. Cardiothoracic Vascular Anesthesia Update 1993;3:Chapter 12.

87. Gold MS, Russo J, Tissot M, et al. Comparison of hetastarch to albumin for perioperative bleeding in patients undergoing abdominal aortic aneurysm surgery. A prospective, randomized study. Ann Surg 1990;211:482.

88. Boldt J, Ling D, Weidler B, et al. Acute preoperative hemodilution in cardiac surgery: volume replacement

with a hypertonic saline–hydroxyethyl starch solution. J Cardiothorac Vasc Anesth 1991;5:23.

89. Boldt J, Zickmann B, Ballesteros M, et al. Cardio-respiratory responses to hypertonic saline solution in cardiac operations. Ann Thorac Surg 1991;51:610.

90. Stump DC, Strauss RG, Henriksen RA, et al. Effects of hydroxyethyl starch on blood coagulation particularly factor VIII. Transfusion 1985;25:349.

91. Skillman JJ, Restall DS, Salzman EW. Randomized trial of albumin vs electrolyte solutions during abdominal aortic operations. Surgery 1975;78:291.

92. Boutros AR, Ruess R, Olsen L, et al. Comparison of hemodynamic, pulmonary and renal effects of use of three types of fluids after major surgical procedures on the abdominal aorta. Crit Care Med 1979;7:9.

93. Virgilio RW, Rice CL, Smith DE, et al. Crystalloid vs colloid resuscitation: is one better ? A randomized clinical study. Surgery 1979;85:129.

94. Lowe RJ, Moss GS, Jilek J, Levine HD. Crystalloid vs colloid in the etiology of pulmonary failure after trauma: a randomized trial in man. Surgery 1977;81:676.

95. Metildi LA, Shackford SR, Virilio RW, Peters RM. Crystalloid vs colloid in fluid resuscitation of patients with severe pulmonary insufficiency. Surg Gynecol Obstet 1984;158:207.

96. Spiess BD, Sassatti RJ, McCarthy RF, et al. Autologous blood donation: hemodynamics in a high risk patient population. Transfusion 1992;32:17.

97. Newman MM, Hamstra R, Block M. Use of banked autologous blood in elective surgery. JAMA 1971;218:861.

98. Goodnough LT, Rednick S, Price TH, et al. Increased preoperative collection of autologous blood with recombinant human erythropoietin therapy. N Engl J Med 1989;321:1163.

99. D'Ambra MN. The effect of perioperative administration of recombinant human erythropoietin in CABG patients: a double blind, placebo controlled trial. Anesthesiology 1992;77:159.

100. Donahue JG, Munoz A, Ness PM, et al. The declining risk of post hepatitis C virus infection. N Engl J Med 1992;327:369.

Chapter 6

Anesthesia for Surgery
of the Ascending Aorta

Gerald A. Schiff

History

The first known description of aortic disease is attributed to Galen who wrote, "when the arteries are enlarged, the disease is called an aneurysm."[1] In the second century, the Roman physician and surgeon, Antyllus described proximal and distal ligations of an aneurysm, with excision and removal of the contents.[2] Little more was described of the clinical manifestations of the disease until 1555, when Vesalius diagnosed a pulsating tumor near the vertebrae in a patient's back and called it "a dilatation of the aorta."[3] Morgagni, in 1761, reported the first description of both the clinical and the pathologic findings of aortic dissection.[4] In 1804, Moore and Morchison inserted lengths of silver wire in a thoracic aneurysm in order to induce clot formation,[5] and in 1879 Corradi added to this method the passage of a galvanic current through the wire.[2] In 1976 Altman and Voorhees reported a patient with a 38-year survival following aneurysmal wiring.[6]

In 1940 Pearse called attention to the irritating properties of cellophane as a means of gradual occlusion of larger arteries.[7] By 1948, surgical techniques had advanced to allow resection and end-to-end anastamosis of a coarctation of the aorta by Shumacker.[8] In 1951, Oudot of France first used a homograft to replace a thrombosed aortic bifurcation,[9] and in 1952 DeBakey and colleagues described the successful resection of a thoracic aortic aneurysm and replacement with a homograft.[10] A year later, Blakemore and Voorhees[11] and Shumacker and King[12] reported the use of a synthetic prosthesis for aortic replacement. The current surgical technique of leaving the aneurysmal sac intact and restoring flow with an indwelling permanent graft has been popularized by the group at Baylor University and at the Texas Heart Institute.[13]

Anatomy

The aorta is the largest artery in the human body, consisting of a thoracic and an abdominal portion. The thoracic aorta is further subdivided into three segments: the ascending aorta, the aortic arch, and the descending thoracic aorta (Figure 6-1) (see Chapter 1).

The ascending aorta in a normal adult is about 3 cm wide at its origin at the base of the heart and extends 5–6 cm cephalad to join the aortic arch. Normally, the ascending aorta lies just to the right of the midline, with its proximal portion within the pericardial cavity. Nearby structures include the pulmonary trunk (anteriorly), left atrium, right pulmonary artery, and right main stem bronchus (posteriorly). The only vessels that normally arise from the ascending aorta are the right and left coronary arteries, which originate in Valsalva's sinus just above the aortic valve (see Chapter 1).

The arch of the aorta gives rise to all the brachiocephalic vessels. It courses slightly leftward in front of the trachea and then proceeds dorsally and inferiorly above the left main stem bronchus to the

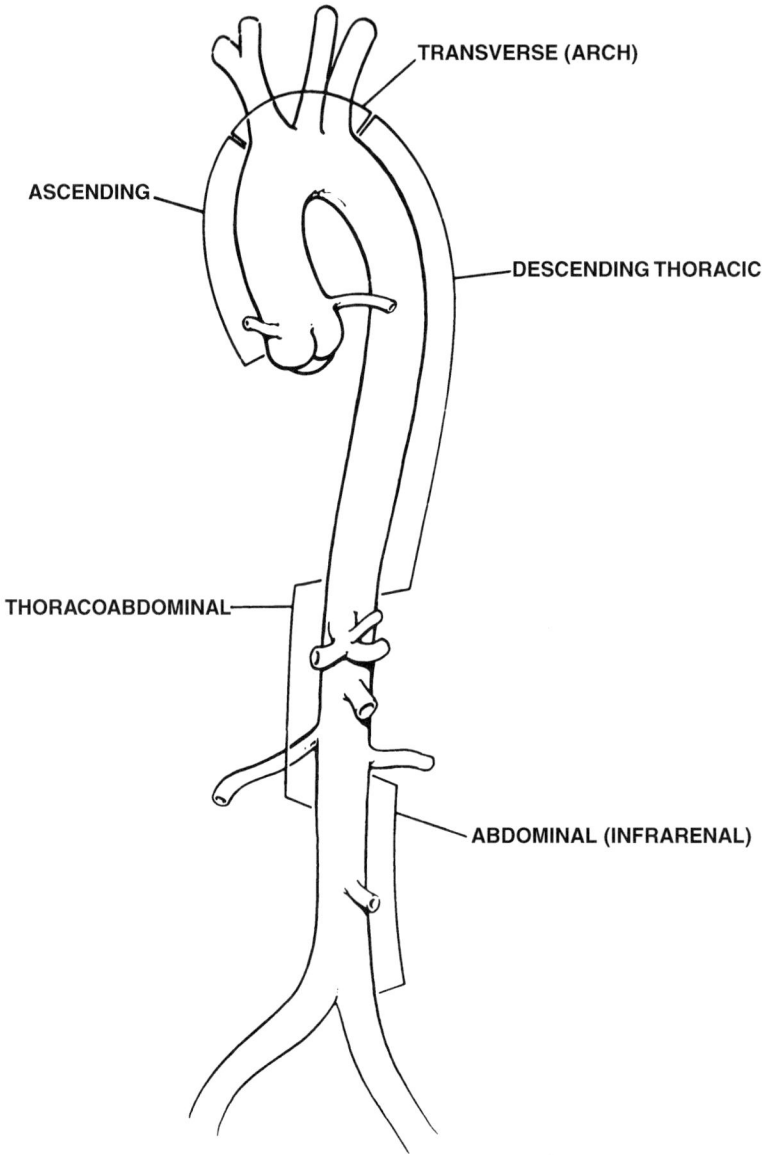

Figure 6-1. Anatomic divisions of the aorta used for classification of aortic aneurysms according to location. (Reprinted with permission from DA Cooley. Surgical Treatment of Aortic Aneurysms. Philadelphia: Saunders, 1986;2.)

left of the trachea and the esophagus. Other closely related structures include the left phrenic and vagus nerves to the left of the arch, and, inferiorly, the bifurcation of the pulmonary trunk and most of the left lung. The left recurrent laryngeal nerve also loops underneath the arch of the aorta.

The descending thoracic aorta is the continuation of the aorta beyond the arch. It lies in the posterior mediastinum to the left of the vertebral column, gradually courses in front of the vertebral column as it descends behind the esophagus and passes through the diaphragm, usually at the level of the twelfth thoracic vertebra.

Thoracic Aortic Aneurysms

There are many causes of thoracic aortic aneurysms and the nomenclature is confusing at best. One can differentiate the acute aortic dissection or "acute dissecting aortic aneurysm" from aneurysmal dilatation of the thoracic aorta, or atherosclerotic aneurysms as distinct entities in terms of origin, structure and prognosis; however, the clinical presentation between the two is sometimes difficult, if not impossible to differentiate (see Chapter 1).[14]

During the first part of the twentieth century, syphilis was by far the leading cause of thoracic aortic aneurysms. In Boyd's review of 4,000 aortic aneurysms, syphilis was implicated in 92% of patients.[15] Syphilis typically results in luetic aortitis and ascending aortic aneurysm. During the past 50 years, with the arrival of antibiotic therapy and the general decline of syphilis worldwide, tertiary syphilis is no longer a significant factor in the etiology of aneurysm.[16]

Another misperception is the common belief that most thoracic aortic aneurysms are due to atherosclerosis.[17,18] Crawford[19] believes that most aneurysms in the thoracic aorta are not due to atherosclerosis. He believes they are due primarily to a number of medial degenerative diseases, including cystic medial necrosis, the type of pathology that is seen in Marfan's syndrome, intimal dissection, and fusiform dilatation. The underlying disease involves a medial degeneration. It is true that atherosclerosis can be present in many patients with associated disease of the branch vessels, and it is often severe, but it is unusual as an etiologic agent in the ascending aorta. Atherosclerosis is superimposed on the underlying connective tissue abnormality, much like a scar on an injury. This is the primary subtlety in the concept of aneurysmal disease of the thoracic aorta. Atherosclerosis is common, but it is not usually the cause of aneurysmal disease.[19]

Laas et al., in 1991, reported a series of 124 surgical patients who presented with aneurysms of the ascending aorta, the aortic arch, or both.[18] The etiology of the aneurysms was confirmed by histologic examination. While almost 100% of cases of nondissecting aneurysmal medial degeneration involve the ascending aorta, atherosclerotic aneurysms tend to be variable in location. Atherosclerotic aneurysms involve the ascending aorta in 50% of patients, the aortic arch in 30% of patients, and portions of the descending thoracic aorta in 20% of the patients.[18] The atherosclerotic process leads to a weakening of the aortic wall and localized dilatation. Cholesterol deposits weaken the strength of the aortic wall. This weakness can contribute to the expansion of the aneurysm, especially in the presence of hypertension.

The natural history of thoracic aortic aneurysms differs somewhat from that of abdominal aortic aneurysms. Spontaneous rupture is less common in thoracic aortic aneurysms because a growing thoracic aneurysm usually results in earlier symptoms related to the compression of the surrounding structures. Pain is usually steady but occasionally pulsates and may be extremely severe. The sternum and right thoracic cage may be eroded by large aneurysms of the ascending aorta, and the vertebral column and left ribs may be eroded by descending thoracic aortic aneurysms. Wheezing, dyspnea, cough, hemoptysis, and recurrent pneumonia can result from compression of the tracheobronchial tree. Hoarseness may follow compression of the recurrent laryngeal nerve, and dysphagia can arise from pressure against the esophagus.[20–24]

The male to female ratio of cases of thoracic aortic aneurysms is 1.7 to 1.0, and the mean age at diagnosis is 69 years.[25] Therefore, coexisting medical problems are common, with preexisting hypertension occurring in the majority of patients.

Marfan's Syndrome

An important cause of ascending aortic enlargement is Marfan's syndrome. Marfan's syndrome is an autosomal dominant disorder of connective tissue.[26] The genetic basis of the condition has recently been elucidated, at least in part, with a mutation of the fibrillin-1 gene being responsible for 25–30% of cases.[27] The noncardiovascular manifestations include generalized skeletal abnormalities and ectopia lentis (displacement of the lens of the eye.) The cardiovascular manifestations include aortic root dilatation, aortic valvular insufficiency, mitral valve prolapse, mitral regurgitation, aortic dissection, and aortic rupture. Although the cardiovascular complications of Marfan's syndrome are not necessarily the most disabling, they are the most frequent cause of death.[28] The occurrence of both dissection and regurgitation is directly related to the relative size of the aortic root. Dilatation, usually confined to the proximal ascending aorta, is progressive as medial degeneration continues. By reducing the rate of pressure change (dp/dt) in the aortic root, beta-adrenergic blockade is effective in slowing the rate of aortic dilatation and reducing the development of aortic complications.[29] Beta-blockade is also beneficial because it controls some of the rhythm disorders associated with mitral valve prolapse, a condition that affects 60% or more of patients with Marfan's syndrome.

Because of the poor long-term prognosis for patients with Marfan's syndrome, general recommendations have been made regarding prophylactic aortic root replacement for aortic dilatation in symptomatic Marfan's syndrome patients. The Johns Hopkins group initially recommended surgical intervention when the aortic root diameter exceeded 5.5 cm.[30] Subsequently, this threshold diameter was increased to 6 cm to facilitate coronary ostial reimplantation.[31] Improved surgical techniques, the low operative risk for prophylactic composite valve graft (<1%), and the occurrence of dissection in Marfan's syndrome patients with aortic root diameters of less than 5 cm has prompted Smith et al.,[32] Crawford et al.,[33] and Pyeritz[34] to recommend prophylactic composite valve graft replacement whenever the diameter of the aortic root exceeds twice the normal caliber of the distal ascending aorta. The use of composite valve graft replacement is warranted in patients with Marfan's syndrome even in the presence of a competent aortic valve because of the high propensity for the subsequent development of aortic insufficiency of the native aortic valve.[18]

Aneurysm of Valsalva's Sinus

Although most aneurysms of Valsalva's sinus are thought to be congenital, they may be secondary to medionecrosis, atherosclerosis, ankylosing spondylitis, Marfan's syndrome, endocarditis, penetrating injuries, and, rarely, syphilis.[35] The primary lesion appears to result from either congenital absence or thinning of the aortic media in the wall of the aortic sinus. High aortic pressure over the course of time on this weak area of the wall ultimately leads to aneurysm formation. These aneurysms are commonly associated with an intracardiac fistula and can rupture into an adjacent low-pressure cardiac chamber. Additionally, ventricular septal defects are present in 30–50% of patients with congenital Valsalva's sinus aneurysm.[36] As many as 10% of patients may have significant valvular or subvalvular pulmonary stenosis.

Aneurysms arising from the right coronary sinus are most common and account for 72% of lesions.

They frequently project into the adjacent right ventricular outflow tract. Noncoronary sinus aneurysms are the second most common and account for 25–30% of Valsalva's sinus aneurysms. These usually project into the right atrium and rarely into the right ventricle. Conduction abnormalities including complete heart block, and right bundle-branch block may occur when rupture occurs in areas adjacent to the tricuspid valve (due to the close proximity of the atrioventricular node and the conduction pathways). Aneurysms arising from the left coronary sinus are rare; they can rupture into the left atrium or pericardium, which may be catastrophic. Anesthetic technique and surgical approaches are consistent with elective surgery for ascending aortic aneurysm (see following section).

Aortic Arteritis Syndromes

Rare causes of ascending aortic aneurysm include infections that can cause mycotic aneurysms requiring surgery.[37] Granulomatous arteritis involves the aorta in approximately 15% of cases.[38] This aortitis can coexist with the more classic and prevalent syndromes of temporal arteritis and polymyalgia rheumatica or, rarely, the aorta may serve as the primary target of this disease. The granulomatous inflammation of the aortic wall may lead to localized aneurysm formation, aortic annular dilatation, and aortic regurgitation.

Takayasu's disease[39] can involve the aorta with areas of marked intimal proliferation and fibrosis causing scarring and degeneration of the elastic fibers of the aorta (see Chapter 1). This can lead to obliterative luminal changes of the aorta, localized aneurysm formation, poststenotic dilatation, and calcification in the aortic and arterial walls. Hypertension develops secondary to coarctation of the aorta and renal artery stenosis. The ostia and proximal segments of the coronary arteries can be affected resulting in angina or myocardial infarction.[40]

Isolated aortic regurgitation due to dilatation of the aortic valve ring with associated aortic root involvement can occur during the course of ankylosing spondylitis,[41] arthritis associated with ulcerative colitis,[42] relapsing polychondritis,[43] Reiter's syndrome,[44] psoriatic arthritis,[45] and Behçet's syndrome.[46] Reported instances of aortitis complicating each of these diseases are rare. Nevertheless, the symptoms of aortic regurgitation and resultant heart failure can eventually dominate the clinical picture. Aortic valve replacement should be performed when indicated; however, in contrast to Marfan's syndrome, replacement of the ascending aorta is almost never necessary (see Chapter 1).

Acute Ascending Aortic Dissection

Acute dissection of the aorta is the most frequent catastrophic disease involving the aorta and remains the leading cause of death from aortic pathology.[47] It is characterized by the separation of the layers of the aortic media by a column of circulating blood, thereby creating a false lumen. Pulsatile flow within the false lumen may extend proximally or distally, causing compression of the true lumen, resulting in occlusion or disruption of the major tributaries of the aorta and ultimately death due to ischemia or rupture. This acute event is not associated with the presence of an aneurysm. The widely used misnomer *dissecting aortic aneurysm* is inappropriate. *Acute dissection of the aorta* is a better term for describing the acute process. Aortic dissection has been recognized only recently as a common aortic problem.[48] It occurs at an incidence of approximately 5–10 patients per million of the population per year, which is at least two to three times the incidence of ruptured abdominal aortic aneurysm.[49] It is seen in all age groups, although it is rare in the extremes of life. Seventy-five percent of aortic dissections occur between the fourth and the seventh decades of life, and the peak incidence is in the 50- to 69-year-old age group.[50,51] Aortic dissection is relatively rare in patients under 40 years of age, except in those with familial predisposition,[52] Marfan's syndrome,[53] or congenital heart lesions, such as coarctation of the aorta[54] or bicuspid aortic valve.[55] Although dissection is predominate in men, with a male-to-female ratio of 3 to 1, an unexplained relationship exists between pregnancy and aortic dissections, with about half of all dissections in women under the age of 40 occurring during pregnancy.[56,57] It is rare among Asians, and there is a slight apparent increase among blacks. This probably is associated with a higher predisposition to hypertension, rather than an increased predisposition to aortic dissection.[50]

Classifications

Many classifications have been described to categorize aortic dissections. The original classification of dissections by DeBakey and colleagues[58] was subsequently simplified into three basic types in accordance with the origin and the extent of the dissection.[59] In type I, the dissection starts with an intimal tear in the ascending aorta within several centimeters of the aortic valve and extends distally for a variable distance, usually throughout the remaining aorta. Aortic valvular insufficiency is frequently present. Type II is characterized by a dissection that is limited to the ascending aorta. There is usually a transverse tear in the intima beginning just above the aortic valve that terminates just proximal to the origin of the innominate artery. It is seen almost exclusively in dissections with aneurysmal dilatation of the ascending aorta, such as those that result from Marfan's syndrome.[60] It is also often associated with aortic valvular insufficiency. Type III is characterized by the fact that the dissecting process arises in the descending thoracic aorta, usually at the origin of the left subclavian artery or distal to it at the site of the ligamentum arteriosum and extends distally for a varying distance. The type III dissection has been subdivided into IIIA and IIIB. Type IIIA is limited to the descending thoracic aorta, whereas type IIIB extends into the abdominal aorta (Figure 6-2) (see Chapter 8).

Cooley described a classification based on the site of origin of the dissection.[2] Type A dissections have intimal tears occurring above the level of the coronary ostia. There may be extension of the dissection into the descending and abdominal aorta or beyond. Aortic valvular regurgitation frequently results, and injuries to the coronary arteries can also occur. In type B dissections, the site of origin is distal to the aortic arch and the dissection proceeds distally. In some instances, however, the dissection may also extend proximally into the ascending aorta (Figure 6-3).

The Stanford classification, proposed by Daily et al.[61] is based on the clinical approach to therapy. Type A includes all proximal dissections and those distal dissections that extend retrograde to the arch and to the ascending aorta, requiring urgent surgical therapy. Type B refers to all other distal dissections without proximal extension. Approximately

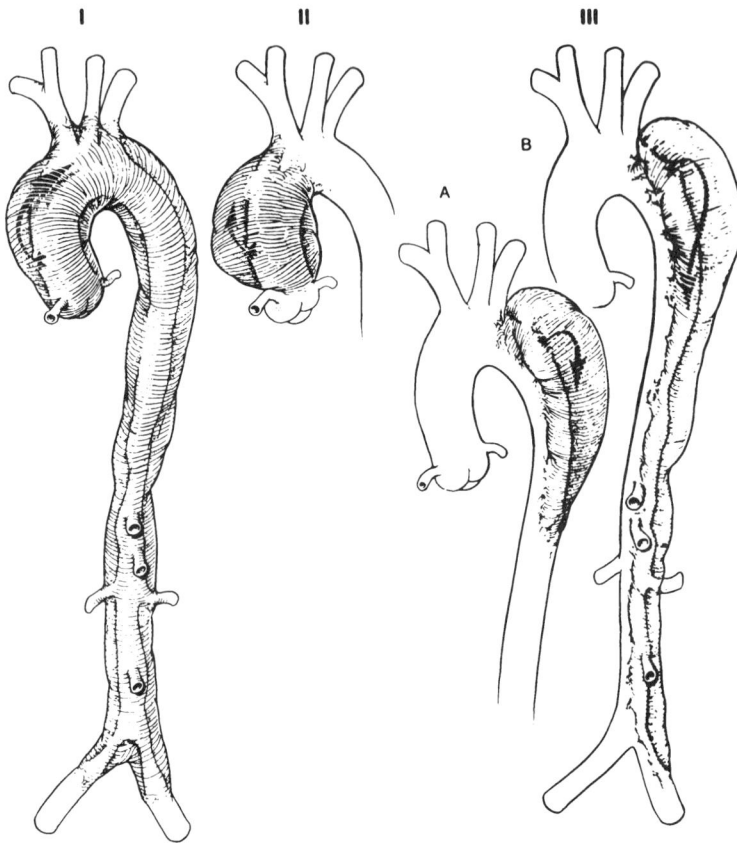

Figure 6-2. DeBakey classification of dissecting aneurysms of the thoracic aorta. Type I: The dissection and the intimal tear arises in the ascending aorta and extends distally for a variable distance. Type II: The dissection is limited to the ascending aorta. Type III: The dissection arises in the descending thoracic aorta and extends distally for a variable distance. (A) Limited to the descending thoracic aorta. (B) The dissection extends into the abdominal aorta. (Reprinted with permission from DA Cooley. Surgical Treatment of Aortic Aneurysms. Philadelphia: Saunders, 1986;44.)

75% of untreated patients with type A dissection die within the first 2 weeks of onset, twice the mortality seen with type B dissections during the same time period.[49]

Pathophysiology of Ascending Aortic Dissections

The process of aortic dissection involves an initial phase in which the intimal tear occurs and a subsequent phase in which the dissection propagates. The intimal tear is a consistent feature of aortic dissection. The majority of intimal tears are located within the first few centimeters of the ascending aorta, at the initial portion of the descending aorta and the aortic isthmus. These are fixed points along the aorta that are subject to the most pronounced hydrodynamic forces. It is uncertain whether the primary event in aortic dissection is rupture of the intima with secondary dissection into the media or hemor-

rhage within a diseased media followed by disruption of the adjacent intima and subsequent propagation of the dissection.[62] This second process, termed *cystic medial necrosis*, most often is the result of chronic stress against the aortic wall, as can occur with long-standing hypertension.[63] Cystic medial necrosis also appears to be an intrinsic feature in the formation of aortic disease in patients with Marfan's syndrome[64] and Ehlers-Danlos syndrome.[65] The injury in these patients is more severe at an earlier age because it is caused by a connective tissue disorder. The aortic wall of these patients with Marfan's and Ehlers-Danlos syndromes is intrinsically weakened and is therefore easily damaged (see Chapter 1).

Once initiated through the intimal tear, the dissecting process progresses rapidly along the length of the aorta, usually in the outer third of the media; hence the incidence of rupture into the pleural or pericardial spaces through the thinner outer wall is

A   B

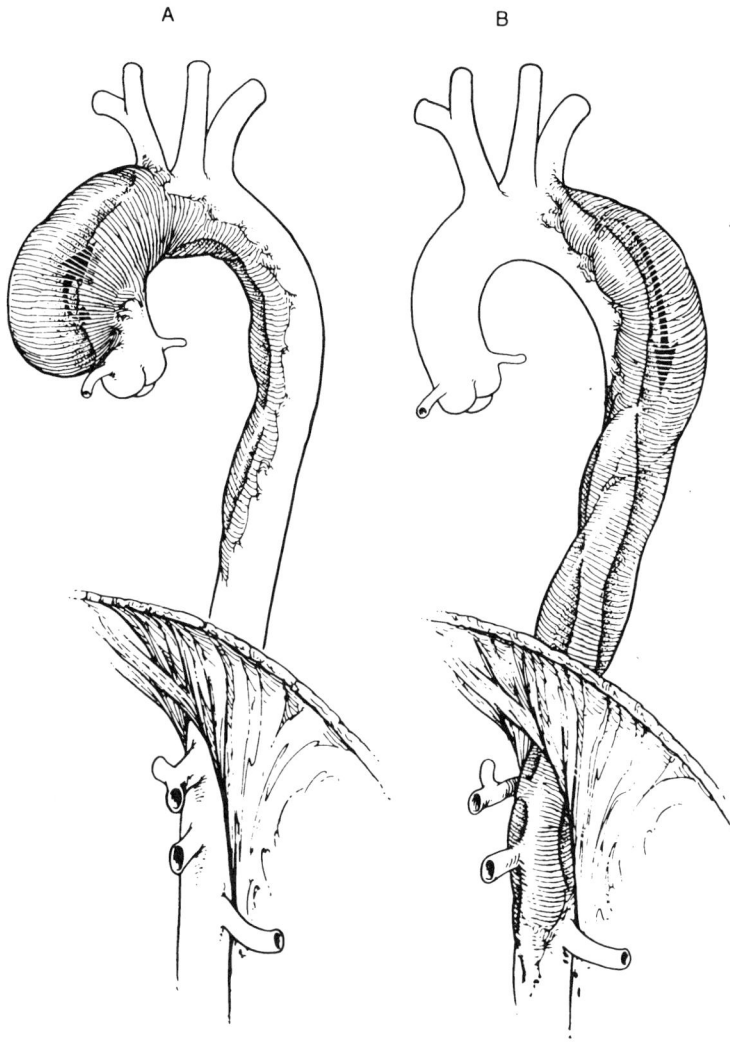

Figure 6-3. Cooley classification of dissecting aneurysms based on the site of origin. Indications for surgical intervention vary between the two types, especially in acute cases. A. In type A aneurysms the intimal tear occurs transversely above the level of the coronary orifices. Type A cases may have extension of the dissection into the descending and abdominal aorta or beyond. B. In type B aneurysms the site of origin is distal to the aortic arch, and the dissection proceeds distally. In some instances, the dissection may extend proximally into the ascending aorta. (Reprinted with permission from DA Cooley. Surgical Treatment of Aortic Aneurysms. Philadelphia: Saunders, 1986;45.)

more common than the occurrence of a reentry tear downstream back into the true lumen. The major hydrodynamic forces contributing to the separation of the layers of the media are the velocity of the blood ejected from the heart and the rate of myocardial fiber shortening (dp/dt).[66] Treatment aimed at decreasing these forces is the main focus of intensive medical treatment of aortic dissections: decreasing contractility, controlling blood pressure, and reducing heart rate.[67,68]

The progress of the dissecting process in the false lumen has several major pathologic, as well as clinical, consequences. The dissection can interrupt the blood supply to the major branches of the aorta by extrinsic compression from the false lumen or by actually shearing off the branches from the true lumen. Either process could result in major end-organ or limb ischemia. Proximal extension of the dissection toward the aortic root causes detachment of the aortic commissures, leading to prolapse of the leaflets and acute aortic insufficiency. Proximal dissection can also cause dissection of the coronary arteries, usually the right, leading to myocardial ischemia and infarction. Retrograde extension of the false lumen can readily rupture into the pericardial or the pleural spaces. Rupture into the pericardium is the most common cause of death in the first 2 weeks following dissection.[50] In patients who survive the acute episode, the false lumen either thromboses and heals or remains patent and continues to enlarge, forming an aneurysmal dilatation. This dilatation, when subjected to sudden increases in hydrodynamic forces, can result in either sudden rupture of the aorta or symptoms caused by local compression from the expanding aorta.

Clinical Presentation

By far, the most common presenting symptom of aortic dissection is severe pain, which is found in over 90% of cases.[69] In fact, those patients without pain usually have suffered some disturbance of consciousness as a result of the dissection interfering with cerebral blood flow. The pain, which is often described as tearing or ripping, is frequently most severe at its inception, which contrasts with the pain of myocardial ischemia and infarction, which often increases in a crescendo pattern described as a squeezing or crushing pain.

Vasovagal manifestations, such as diaphoresis, pallor, apprehension, nausea, vomiting, and lightheadedness, are common at the outset. The patient often appears pale and sweaty, as in shock, but may have moderate or even severe hypertension that may prove difficult to control. This response in dissection is thought to be related to renal ischemia.[70] The presence of hypotension is an ominous sign indicating either cardiac tamponade or hypovolemia due to rupture into the pleural cavity. Occasionally hypotension may be due to disruption of the coronary circulation and resultant myocardial ischemia or infarction.

The location of the pain also aids the diagnosis. Although pain may be felt simultaneously in the anterior and posterior chest with both proximal and distal dissection, pain in the neck, throat, and arm are more common in ascending aortic or aortic arch dissections. Also, the absence of posterior interscapular pain strongly suggests against a distal aortic dissection.

Syncope is the second most common presenting symptom of dissection. It is usually transient and is related to temporary ischemia of the central nervous system. Syncope without focal neurologic signs may signify rupture of the dissection into the pericardial cavity with cardiac tamponade.[71]

Other less common modes of presentation include congestive heart failure with or without associated chest pain, cerebrovascular accidents, and paraplegia.

Heart failure usually results from severe acute aortic regurgitation, secondary to the dissection, or from disruption of the origin of a coronary artery.

Diminution or absence of pulses in one or more extremities may be noted. Slater and DeSanctis[71] found that almost half of all the patients with type A dissection and one-sixth of those with type B dissection had loss or decrease of one or more pulses. With proximal dissection, pulse deficits were evenly distributed along the arterial tree, while distal dissections typically involved the left subclavian and other distal arteries.

New cardiac murmurs may also be heard; they may be systolic, diastolic, or both. A diastolic murmur of aortic regurgitation indicates involvement of the ascending aorta and is present in two-thirds of these cases. There are three mechanisms of aortic regurgitation in proximal dissections: (1) the dissection may dilate the aortic root, widening the annulus so that the aortic leaflets are unable to coapt in diastole; (2) in an asymptomatic dissection, pressure from the dissecting hematoma may depress one leaflet below the line of closure of the others; and (3) the annular support of the leaflets or the leaflets themselves may be torn so as to render the valve incompetent.

A pericardial rub is infrequent, but when present, is an ominous sign indicating involvement of the root of the aorta with leakage of blood into the pericardial sac.[72] Neurologic deficits associated with aortic dissection include cerebrovascular accidents, ischemic peripheral neuropathy, ischemic paraparesis, and disturbances of consciousness.[73] Each of these is more common with proximal dissection, but deficits in the lower extremities are equally frequent in proximal and distal dissection.

Other associated clinical manifestations include Horner's syndrome[74] due to compression of the superior cervical sympathetic ganglion, vocal cord paralysis, and hoarseness from pressure against the left recurrent laryngeal nerve. Superior mediastinal syndrome from superior vena caval compression,[75] tracheal or bronchial compression with bronchospasm,[76] hemorrhage into the tracheobronchial tree with hemoptysis,[77] hematemesis due to erosion into the esophagus,[78] spontaneous hemothorax[79] from rupture of the dissection into one of the pleural spaces, and heart block from retrograde burrowing of a dissection into the interatrial septum and then down into the atrioventricular node can all be seen.[80]

Table 6-1. Characteristics of Type A and Type B Aortic Dissections

	Type A	Type B
Frequency (%)	65–70	30–35
Average age (yrs)	50–55	60–70
Associated hypertension (%)	50	80
Arterial pressure on admission	50% normal or elevated; 50% hypotensive	80% normal or elevated; 20% hypotensive
Pain	Anterior substernal	Posterior, midscapular
Associated atherosclerosis	±	++
Aortic regurgitation (%)	50	10
Diastolic murmur (%)	50	10
Pericardial effusion	++	±
Pleural effusion	±	++ (left pleura)
Syncope	++	Rare
Hemiparesis or hemiplegia	+	–
Paraparesis or paraplegia	±	+
Acute mortality (%)	90–95	40
Renal-intestinal infarction	+	+
Myocardial infarction	+	Rare

+ = frequently present; ± = sometimes present, sometimes absent; – = usually absent.
Source: Adapted with permission from MA Ergin, JD Galla, S Lansman, RB Griepp. Acute dissections of the aorta: current surgical treatment. Surg Clin North Am 1985;65:721.

Additional complications can result from occlusion of important arteries by the dissection; mesenteric infarction, renal infarction, and myocardial infarction are among the most serious occlusive events (Table 6-1).

Diagnostic Techniques

Routine laboratory studies are not specific in making the diagnosis of aortic dissection. Anemia may result from significant hemorrhage. A mild-to-moderate polymorphonuclear leukocytosis, (10,000–14,000 per ml) is common. Lactic acid dehydrogenase and bilirubin levels are sometimes elevated because of blood sequestered within the false lumen. Tencate et al.[81] have described a consumptive coagulopathy in patients with ruptured or dissected aortic aneurysms. They report that a prolonged prothrombin time due to a decrease of one or more clotting factors and formation of fibrin degradation products can be used to differentiate a rupture or dissecting aortic aneurysm from other conditions with a similar acute onset. This may also be associated with a decrease in platelet count.

The most common electrocardiographic finding is a reflection of preexisting hypertension with left ventricular hypertrophy and left ventricular strain.[50] The presence of electrocardiographic evidence of ischemia does not rule out dissection; however, the absence of an ischemic pattern makes the diagnosis of acute myocardial ischemia less likely and may lead one to consider an acute aortic dissection. Occasionally, heart block may be seen with involvement of the interatrial and membranous septum by the dissecting hematoma.[82]

Transthoracic echocardiography was first used to diagnose aortic dissection in 1972.[83] M-mode in combination with cross-sectional (two-dimensional) echocardiography can be used to reveal a widened aortic root with delineation of the dissecting hematoma, acute aortic regurgitation, pericardial effusion, an oscillating aortic flap, and the presence of a more echodense outer aortic wall.[84] However, transthoracic echocardiography is not capable of ruling out an acute dissection with certainty.

Computed tomography (CT) with contrast injection is quite accurate in defining both ascending and descending thoracic aortic dissections provided there is identification of a false lumen to distinguish the dissection from a fusiform aneurysm.[85,86] Although quite reliable for demonstrating the dissection, CT scanning has the limitations of not showing the site of entry and not documenting aortic insufficiency (see Chapter 3).

The chest roentgenogram has the ability to provide much substantiative data to corroborate the diagnosis of aortic dissection. These are all based on the distortion created by the false lumen and the leakage of blood into the pleural spaces. Chest radiography almost always reveals an abnormally widened mediastinum with blurring or obliteration of the aortic knob (see Chapter 3).[87]

The most important study in the diagnosis of aortic dissection has been aortic angiography.[88] Although it is an invasive procedure with some risk, one can demonstrate the entire aorta from the aortic annulus to the aortic bifurcation in a short time. The main points of interest relevant for the surgeon are the presence of ascending aortic involvement, location of the intimal tear, extent of the false lumen, state of the major branches of the aorta, presence of aortic regurgitation, presence of a reentry tear, and patency of the false lumen.

Transesophageal echocardiography (TEE) has recently appeared as the new standard for diagnosing aortic dissections.[89,90] Due to the close anatomic relationship between the esophagus and the thoracic aorta, TEE allows visualization of the entire thoracic aorta, including most of the aortic arch. An intimal flap within the aorta separating the true and false lumens can easily be seen. In most cases the true lumen is compressed by the false lumen. The true and false lumens can be differentiated using the TEE by the following:

1. The systolic enlargement of the true lumen on M-mode.
2. The demonstration of systolic forward flow in the true lumen and delayed flow or no flow in the false lumen using pulsed wave Doppler echocardiography.
3. The demonstration of entry jets during systole at the entry tear using color flow Doppler (Figure 6-4).

TEE has an additional advantage in that in critically ill patients with a 2% mortality per hour[91] and associated poor hemodynamic status, diminished renal function, or both, the examination can be performed quickly and safely at the bedside, in the in-tensive care unit, or in the emergency department without radiologic dye.

A study by Nienaber et al.[92] has shown that there is approximately a 15% incidence of false-positive findings in the ascending aorta using TEE. They note that magnetic resonance imaging (MRI) is capable of noninvasively examining most thoracic aortic abnormalities with few limitations and with a high degree of specificity and sensitivity. Details of aortic dissection, including its size, extent, and involvement of major arch and abdominal branch vessels, are often seen clearly with MRI. The limitations of MRI stem from the long scan time and strong magnetic field used. The relatively long scan time implies a sensitivity to motion artifact, which makes MRI less applicable in uncooperative, unstable, or claustrophobic patients. Also, patients who depend on devices with ferromagnetic properties, such as pacemakers, pulmonary artery catheters, cerebral aneurysm clips, and ventilators, cannot be examined by MRI.[93] A noninvasive diagnostic strategy using MRI in all hemodynamically stable patients and TEE in patients who are too unstable to be moved or are not candidates for MRI should be considered the optimal approach to detecting dissection of the thoracic aorta. Comprehensive and detailed evaluation can thus be reduced to a single noninvasive diagnostic test in the investigation of suspected dissections of the thoracic aorta.

Aortic Dissection Following Cardiac Surgery

Traumatic deceleration-type injury to the aorta usually results in aortic rupture of the descending thoracic aorta and is addressed in Chapter 8. However, iatrogenic aortic injuries sometimes occur in the ascending aorta and require emergent surgical repair. Ascending aortic dissection is a rare, but often catastrophic, complication of cardiac surgical procedures. The initiating event is an intimal injury from surgical manipulation of the ascending aorta, usually in patients predisposed to aortic injury by cystic medial degeneration, long-standing hypertension, or advanced atherosclerosis of the aortic wall[94–99] (Figure 6-5A).

In a retrospective review of 14 patients who developed ascending aortic dissection during or after cardiac surgery, Murphy and colleagues[100] ascribed the development of aortic dissection to direct aortic ma-

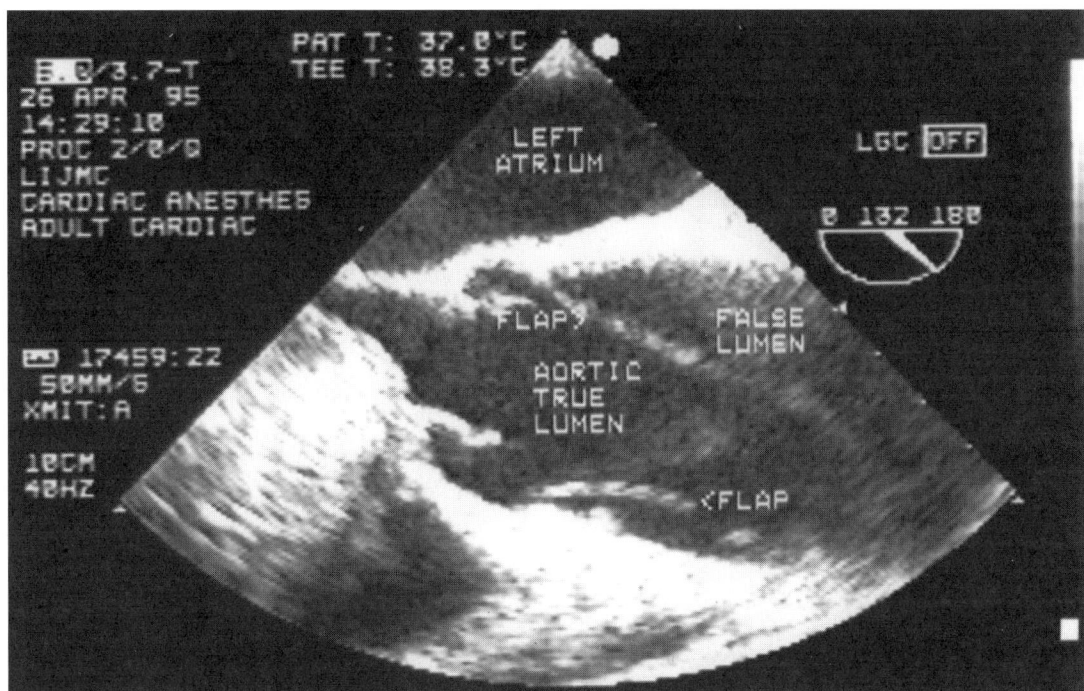

Figure 6-4. Two-dimensional transesophageal echocardiographic image of an aortic dissection. The intimal flap is clearly visible separating the true and false lumens within the aorta.

nipulation. These manipulations include the aortic cross clamp, the side-biting clamp, proximal vein graft anastamosis, aortotomy suture line, aortic cannulation site, and the inadvertent injection of cardioplegia solution between the layers of the aorta. Prompt diagnosis is the most important factor in the successful management of both intraoperative and postoperative ascending aortic dissections. Early recognition of an aortic dissection developing intraoperatively requires a high index of suspicion whenever any area of discoloration develops on the surface of the ascending aorta. Dissection must be differentiated from the commonly occurring subadventitial hematoma. Dissection in the postoperative period is usually delayed until the development of the hydrodynamic forces necessary for propagation of the dissection process (e.g., the patient emerging from anesthesia with subsequent tachycardia and hypertension).[66]

The signs and symptoms of postoperative aortic dissection, although similar to those occurring with spontaneous dissection, may be difficult to recognize following cardiac surgical procedures. The typical ripping or tearing pain of aortic dissection may be mis-

interpreted as incisional, pericardial, or myocardial pain in the medicated postoperative patient. Hemorrhage from the aorta, presenting as either excessive mediastinal drainage from the chest tubes or hemopericardium or hemothorax following removal of the mediastinal chest tube, can play a significant role in the postoperative presentation of aortic dissection. Echocardiography may play a role in the reevaluation of a suspected postoperative aortic dissection.[101–103]

In patients with persistent mediastinal hemorrhage, cardiac tamponade, new onset aortic regurgitation, or loss of a carotid or upper extremity pulse, prompt mediastinal exploration is the most expeditious way to establish the diagnosis and avoid costly delays in definitive therapy. Prompt efforts to reduce the aortic blood pressure, heart rate, and dp/dt can prevent further extension of the dissection process or rupture of the aorta. With intraoperative dissections, these hemodynamic parameters may be altered by arterial vasodilation and beta-adrenergic blockers, as well as by adjustments to cardiopulmonary bypass blood flow. The physician must exercise caution to avoid myocardial ischemia by prolonged reduction

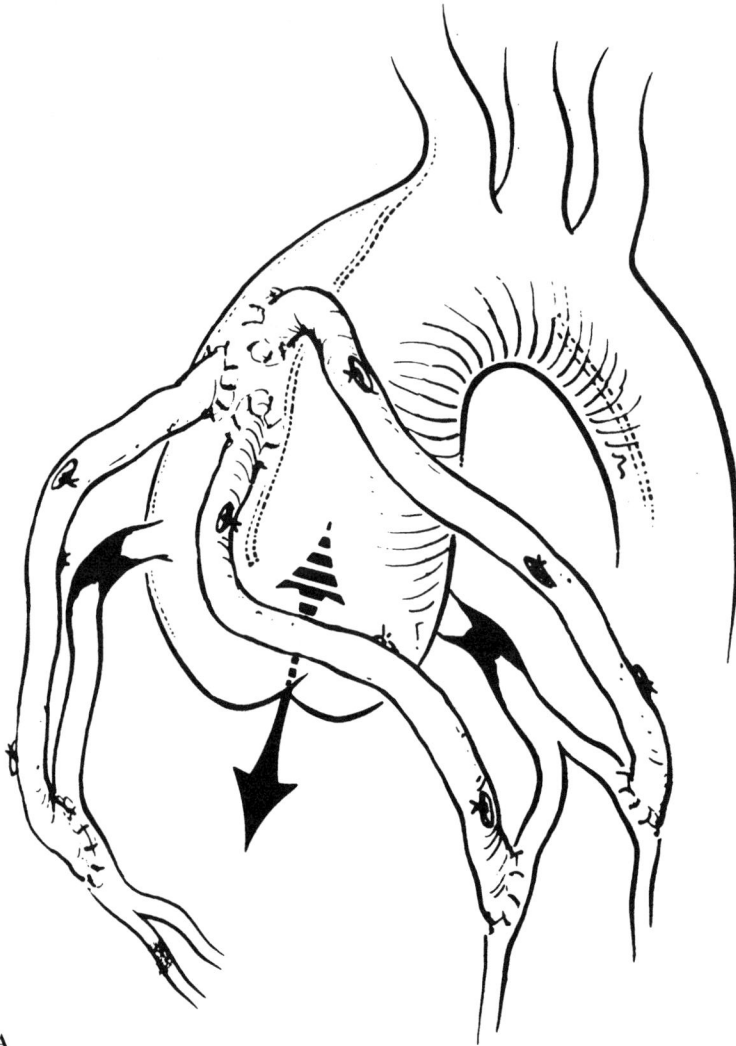

Figure 6-5. A. Dilated ascending aorta from dissection occurring after coronary artery bypass grafting. The true lumen is indicated by the arrows. B. Method of treatment using composite valve graft and reattaching native coronary artery ostia and bypass grafts. (Reprinted with permission from ES Crawford, JL Crawford, HJ Saft, et al. Redo operations for recurrent aneurysmal disease of the ascending aorta and transverse aortic arch. Ann Thorac Surg 1985;40:439.)

A

in arterial blood flow and coronary perfusion pressure. Techniques in surgical management of ascending aortic dissection complicating cardiac surgical procedures are similar to those used in spontaneous ascending aortic dissection. The morbidity and mortality of this lesion can best be reduced by early diagnosis and definitive surgical repair before a fatal rupture or extension (Figure 6-5B).

Intramural Hematoma

Intramural hematoma of the thoracic aorta[104] is a diagnosis of exclusion and represents spontaneous, localized hemorrhage into the wall of the thoracic aorta in the absence of bona fide aortic dissection, intimal tear, or penetrating atherosclerotic ulcer. This syndrome has also been called *mediastinal apoplexy*. Intramural hematoma can occur as a result of bleeding within the aortic media from the vasa vasorum of the aortic wall, or from disruption of an atherosclerotic plaque. The clinical presentation of patients with intramural hematoma can mimic that of acute aortic dissection. Furthermore, standard radiologic imaging techniques are frequently inconclusive. A CT scan may not show evidence of intramural disruption or false lumen, and aortography and

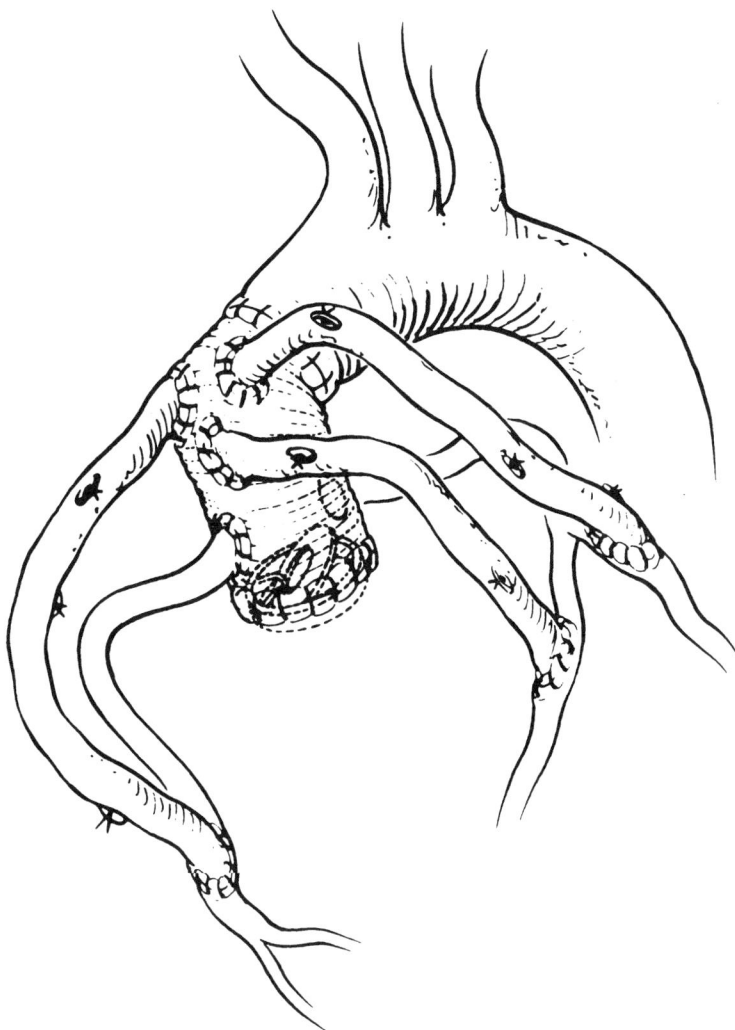

B

MRI also may not show signs of an intramural hematoma. The optimal mode of therapy for these patients, whether it is medical or medical and surgical, remains problematic because of the lack of information available.

One should remember that intramural hematoma of the thoracic aorta is a distinct pathologic entity. All patients with an intramural hematoma should have their hemodynamic status monitored carefully and treated with aggressive antihypertensive therapy. Frequent serial assessment is necessary using TEE or MRI and CT scans. Patients with ascending aortic or aortic arch intramural hematoma or ongoing pain or expansion of the intramural

hematoma should probably undergo early graft replacement. Patients with intramural hematoma involving the descending thoracic aorta who have no evidence of progression and become pain-free can probably be treated conservatively, but require antihypertensive therapy and serial aortic imaging surveillance indefinitely.

Initial Acute Medical Management

All patients with acute ascending aortic dissection, regardless of the type of dissection, or with symptomatic or expanding thoracic aortic aneurysm should be started on aggressive medical therapy to control pain and prevent rupture or extension as soon as the diagnosis is suspected.[72] The goals of medical therapy are to decrease the velocity of the left ventricular contraction, dp/dt,[66] and to reduce the systolic blood pressure to the lowest acceptable level to maintain adequate cardiac, cerebral, and renal perfusion. Patients are usually treated with intravenous morphine to control the pain caused by the dissection, as well as to decrease anxiety levels and resultant catecholamine surges that could cause an extension of the pathologic process. In addition, a combination of beta-adrenergic blocking agents and vasodilators are used to control blood pressure. It is important to note that beta-blockade should be established prior to the introduction of vasodilators, otherwise, any sudden decrease in afterload would trigger an increase in left ventricular contractility and an increase in shearing force (dp/dt) to the aortic wall. Beta-blockade can be induced with intravenous doses of propranolol, 0.5 mg, labetalol, 5–10 mg, or esmolol, 0.5–1.0 mg/kg followed by a continuous infusion of esmolol to reduce the heart rate to 60–70 beats per minute. In patients with asthma or severe chronic obstructive pulmonary disease, the beta$_1$ selective esmolol or metoprolol or the calcium channel blocker verapamil can be used to decrease heart rate and contractility.[105]

Vasodilator therapy is usually started with sodium nitroprusside titrated to reduce systolic blood pressure to 100–120 mm Hg, provided the patient continues to maintain an adequate urinary output and myocardial ischemia does not develop. Maintaining urinary output will also help delay a buildup of cyanide through the excretion of the metabolite sodium thiocyanate.[106] Again, it is important to reiterate that sodium nitroprusside alone can cause an increase in dp/dt that can potentially contribute to an extension of the disease, and therefore adequate simultaneous beta-adrenergic blockade is essential when this drug is used in this setting.

If nitroprusside is ineffective or poorly tolerated, the ganglionic blocking agent trimethaphan can be used. The dosage should be titrated to the arterial blood pressure. Limitations to the use of trimethaphan include hypotension, tachyphylaxis, urinary retention, and ileus. In contrast to nitroprusside, trimethaphan reduces dp/dt. This reduc-

tion should provide a relative advantage in the treatment of aortic dissection and obviate the need for beta-adrenergic blockade.

An alternate agent for reducing both blood pressure and dp/dt is reserpine, administered at 1–2 mg every 4–6 hours. Side effects include drowsiness, depression, and peptic ulceration.

Anesthetic Management of Ascending Aortic Surgery

Monitoring

A radial arterial catheter should be placed to accurately and continuously monitor arterial blood pressure and to obtain blood specimens for laboratory analysis. A left radial, femoral, or other distal site should be used in patients with ascending aortic pathology, because the innominate artery is frequently obstructed by the aortic cross clamp, may be involved in the surgical repair, or both.

Continuous electrocardiographic monitoring should begin with simultaneous leads II and V$_5$ to detect arrhythmias and myocardial ischemia. A central venous catheter is inserted to measure central venous pressure, as well as to rapidly administer fluids and drugs into the central circulation. An internal jugular vein or median cephalic vein approach is frequently chosen because the subclavian vein can be distorted or compressed by the enlarging aneurysm and there is the possibility of accidental puncture of the aneurysm when using the subclavian approach. A pulmonary artery catheter should be inserted to measure hemodynamics and filling pressures and to aid in diagnosing pericardial tamponade resulting from retrograde dissections. Occasionally, the right atrium is so compressed by the aortic dissection that one may not be able to pass the pulmonary artery catheter into the right ventricle until after the chest has been opened. If a Ross procedure is planned (see section on Surgical Considerations), a pulmonary artery catheter should probably not be used. An indwelling bladder catheter should be inserted to measure hourly urine output. This is also helpful in diagnosing an extension of the dissection to the abdominal aorta involving the renal arteries because disrupting renal perfusion would decrease or eliminate urine output. Proper judgement as to the appropriate balance between preoperative preparation and patient risk is extremely critical (see Chapter 4).

On arrival in the operating room additional large-bore intravenous catheters for rapid fluid transfusion with fluid warming capability are used. Pulse oximetry for continuous arterial oxygen saturation monitoring, as well as end-tidal carbon dioxide analysis, is also used. Intraoperative TEE should be used to monitor cardiac function and evaluate continuing aortic pathology. Core temperature monitoring to evaluate the effect of induced hypothermia is used for all cardiothoracic procedures, and arterial blood gas, electrolyte, hematocrit, and coagulation studies should be rapidly available to the operating room team (see Chapter 5).

Anesthetic Management

Pharmacologic premedication should be given to patients to reduce anxiety and apprehension (thereby preventing a sudden increase in circulating catecholamines), to provide analgesia for potentially painful events prior to induction (e.g., vascular cannulation), and to produce some degree of amnesia. Regardless of the drug combination chosen, one must be prepared to give additional intravenous medication when the patient arrives in the operating room to supplement inadequate sedation. Similarly, elderly and debilitated patients require less premedication to achieve a desired level of sedation. All patients should receive supplemental oxygen with the premedication.

The induction of anesthesia should be tailored to the patient's pathology and physical condition, with the following principles in mind.

- One should avoid sudden increases in heart rate or blood pressure because this can increase dp/dt and cause a sudden expansion or extension of the aortic injury.
- Aortic rupture is always a possibility with hypotension from sudden hypovolemia and exsanguination.
- During anesthetic induction, the aorta can dissect retrograde into the pericardium, causing acute pericardial tamponade and hypotension.
- Retrograde dissection can also cause hypotension by obstructing or disrupting coronary

blood flow, leading to acute myocardial ischemia, or cause hypotension by disrupting the aortic valve leaflets, leading to acute aortic insufficiency requiring afterload reduction to control hemodynamics.

The presentation may range from the elective repair of a dilated ascending aortic aneurysm without evidence of aortic valvular disease or dissection to a patient rushed to the emergency room 30 minutes after eating a full dinner in cardiogenic shock from acute aortic valvular insufficiency secondary to a large proximal aortic dissection. In the acute emergent setting, the induction should be smooth and rapid but controlled with the aim to prevent tachycardia, increases in dp/dt, hypertension, or hypotension. Small-to-moderate doses of narcotics, benzodiazepines, etomidate, thiopental, lidocaine, or some combination of these drugs can be used depending on the patient's hemodynamic and volume status. Ketamine may be a useful adjunct in the acute hypovolemic patient. Ketamine, however, may increase dp/dt and should only be used in small doses with constant hemodynamic vigilance. Increases in dp/dt should be promptly treated. This should be followed by a high-dose muscle relaxant, cricoid pressure, and rapid endotracheal intubation. The standard practices of airway evaluation, management of the difficult airway, and full stomach precautions should be followed.

If the patient has severe tracheobronchial compression or occlusion,[107,108] significant risk of aortic rupture, or presents with severe aortic regurgitation with pericardial tamponade,[109] hemodynamics should be managed with femoral arterial–femoral venous bypass instituted under local anesthesia prior to the induction of general anesthesia. For elective aneurysm repair, higher induction doses of anesthetics are used and a slower and more controlled increase in the depth of anesthesia is achieved. Any of the standard intravenous or inhalation anesthetic techniques can be safely employed. The addition of intravenous esmolol, sodium nitroprusside, further intravenous anesthetics, or potent inhalation agents can be used for more precise control of arterial blood pressure. The treatment of hypotension can include the infusion of fluids or the administration of a vasopressor such as phenylephrine. The use of ephedrine or epinephrine should be avoided as any beta-agonist can increase dp/dt and cause an extension of the aortic injury. Multiple units of packed red blood cells should be available in the operating room prior to the induction of anesthesia, as well as a cell saver to process and transfuse blood to the patient in the event of a sudden aortic rupture.

Procedures on the ascending thoracic aorta are complicated by the potential for long bypass and aortic cross-clamp times. Bypass time in a series by Mayer et al.[110] was 115 minutes for elective repair, and Kouchoukos et al.[111] reported a similar bypass time of 116 minutes. These procedures can therefore be associated with pump-induced coagulation disorders including platelet dysfunction, dilution of clotting factors, and primary or secondary fibrinolysis (see Chapter 5). Occasionally, procedures originally thought only to involve the ascending aorta require aortic arch surgery as well. The management of aortic arch surgery and deep hypothermic circulatory arrest is discussed in Chapter 7.

Other complications of these procedures include hemorrhage from the multiple suture lines and coagulopathy, renal failure, myocardial infarction, acute left ventricular failure, and focal neurologic deficits.[111] Acute left ventricular dysfunction can result from inadequate myocardial protection or myocardial edema following a long aortic cross-clamp time and resultant myocardial ischemia. Additionally, ventricular arrhythmias are common.

The physician should consider the possibility of an air or particulate embolism to the coronary arteries in patients who suddenly develop signs of myocardial ischemia or left ventricular dysfunction after removal of the aortic cross clamp. Increasing the coronary perfusion pressure can usually purge the air from the coronary circulation; however, one must be careful not to disrupt the aortic suture lines as a result of the increased pressure. Inotropic support may be necessary to maintain cardiac output until left ventricular function recovers from the embolic and cross clamp–induced ischemia.

Patients with aortic valve regurgitation and volume overloaded ventricles often require inotropic support to discontinue cardiopulmonary bypass. One possible explanation is that intramyocardial catecholamines are depleted in patients with chronic aortic valve insufficiency.[112]

Sudden hemodynamic decompensation after chest wall closure may result from compression or kinking of the aortic graft by the chest wall and may even necessitate surgical repositioning of the aortic graft on cardiopulmonary bypass. It has been reported that patients with Marfan's syndrome are the most susceptible to late bleeding problems, usually along the suture lines.[110]

Surgical Considerations

Many surgical techniques have been developed to correct life-threatening pathology in the ascending aorta. In 1956, Cooley and DeBakey[113] reported on the successful resection of an ascending aortic aneurysm. They used a homograft to replace the aorta from just above the coronary ostia proximally to the base of the innominate artery distally. They were able to successfully cross clamp the ascending aorta for a prolonged period of time because of Gibbon's development of the cardiopulmonary bypass pump.[114] Subsequently, direct coronary perfusion[115] and the use of myocardial cooling[116] were introduced as methods of myocardial protection during cross clamping of the ascending aorta. This was a satisfactory approach for resection of an isolated ascending aortic aneurysm.

In 1964, Wheat and colleagues[117] reported on the first successful replacement of the entire ascending aorta with reimplantation of the coronary ostia and simultaneous replacement of the aortic valve in a patient with a dilated ascending aorta and aortic valvular insufficiency. In that procedure the coronary ostia were left attached to the rim of the aortic wall. A prosthetic aortic valve was inserted and a Teflon aortic graft was used to replace the ascending aorta. The anastomosis of the tube graft to the skirt of the prosthetic aortic valve allowed for inclusion of the two small tongues of the aortic wall that contained the coronary ostia.

In 1968, Bentall and DeBono[118] described the technique in which the ascending aorta and aortic valve are replaced with a composite unit of tubular graft sewn to the aortic annulus with anastomosis of the coronary ostia directly into the sides of the graft. This technique of direct implantation of the coronary arteries can lead to traction on the aortic wall at the level of the reimplanted ostia and become a source of significant postbypass hemorrhage, which is difficult to control because of its inaccessibility (especially the left coronary artery).[111,119] These same mechanisms have been blamed for the occurrence of

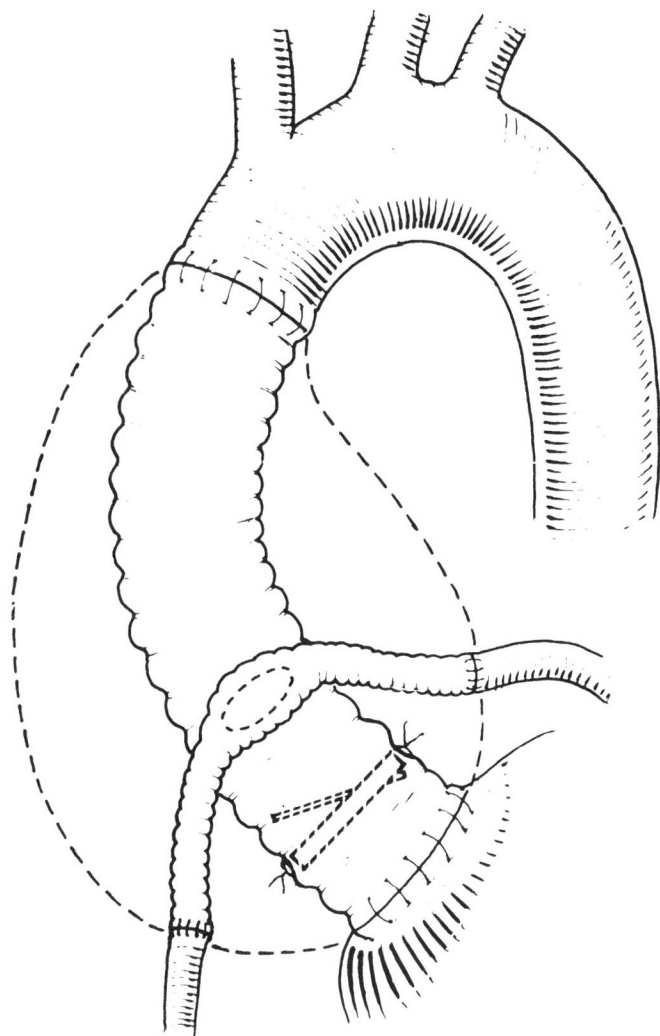

Figure 6-6. Replacement of the ascending aorta using a tube graft containing a prosthetic aortic valve and reimplantation of the coronary arteries by an intermediate tube graft. (Reprinted with permission from C Cabrol, A Pavie, P Mesuitdrey, et al. Long-term results with total replacement of the ascending aorta and reimplantation of the coronary arteries. J Thorac Cardiovasc Surg 1986;91:17.)

false aneurysms demonstrated later at the zone of coronary reimplantation.[120]

To eliminate these risks, Cabrol and coworkers in 1978[121] and 1981[122] introduced a technically easier procedure of connecting the right and left coronary ostia to a tubular graft and then creating a side-to-side anastomosis with the valve conduit to reestablish coronary blood flow. This allowed for easier control of bleeding at the coronary suture lines. Additionally, intermittent coronary perfusion with cold cardioplegia can easily be given through the tubular graft for added myocardial protection.

Acute left ventricular dysfunction and myocardial ischemia can occur, however, during chest closure as a result of compression of the coronary tubular graft. Immediate reopening of the chest and surgical reposition of the tube graft may be necessary to correct this problem (Figure 6-6).

Cooley[123] made a strong argument for employing hypothermic circulatory arrest during the repair of the ascending aorta. He notes that frequently the aneurysm and the pathologic process extend to the proximal transverse aortic arch and into the adjacent tributaries and the bra-

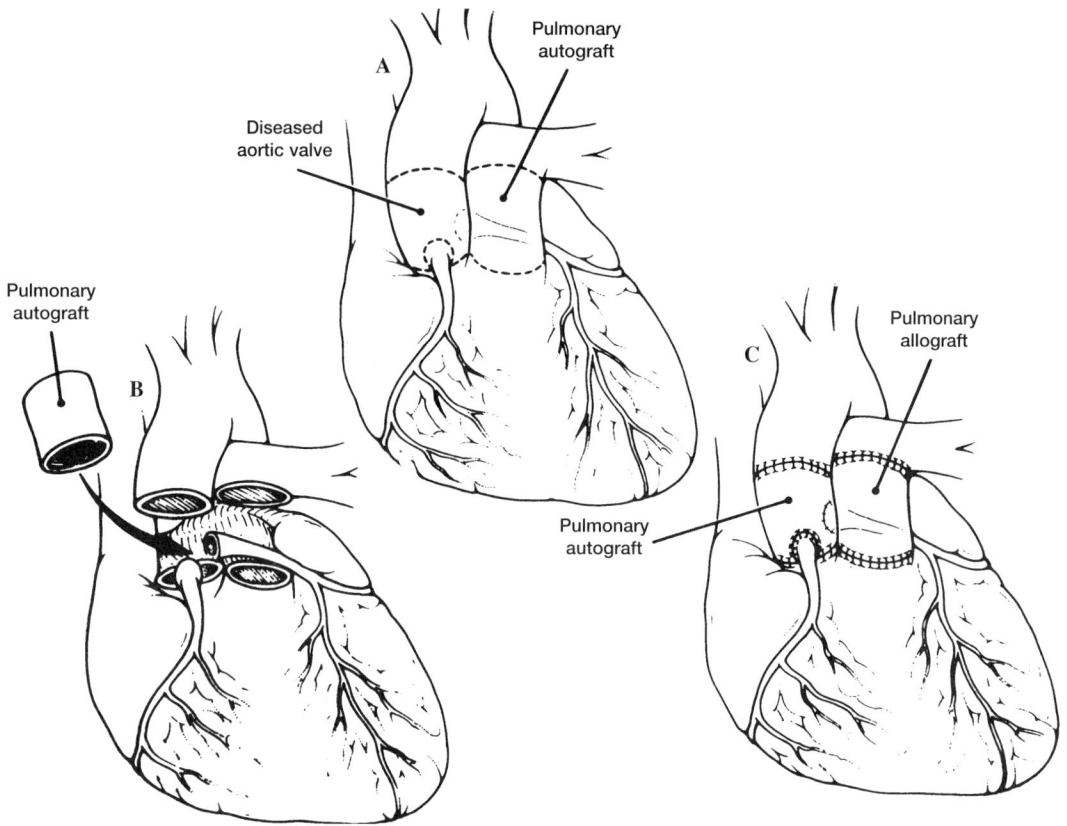

Figure 6-7. Schematic representation of the operative procedure. A. The aortic valve and the adjacent aorta are excised, leaving buttons of the aortic tissue surrounding the coronary arteries. B. The pulmonary valve, with a small rim of right ventricular muscle and the main pulmonary artery, is also excised. Next, the pulmonary autograft is sutured to the aortic annulus and to the distal aorta, and the coronary arteries are attached to openings in the pulmonary artery. C. A pulmonary-root allograft is then sutured into the right ventricular outflow tract. (Reprinted with permission from NT Kouchoukos, VG Davila-Roman, TL Spray, et al. Replacement of the aortic root with a pulmonary autograft in children and young adults with aortic valve disease. N Engl J Med 1994;330:1.)

chiocephalic vessels. Under these circumstances, cannulation of the transverse aorta should be avoided. The ascending aorta should not be cross clamped, because atherosclerotic particles and debris can embolize into the cerebral circulation from manipulation of the diseased ascending aorta. Induction of profound hypothermia permits total circulatory arrest for periods of usually less than 60 minutes.[124]

Once the distal anastomosis has been accomplished, the clamp is placed on the woven Dacron tube and circulation is restored using the femoral arterial cannula. Additionally, in patients who present with type A aortic dissections, the aorta sometimes has its distal true lumen crushed or malaligned dur-

ing aortic cross clamping. This makes for a less than satisfactory distal repair. For these reasons, Cooley advocates incorporating the use of hypothermic circulatory arrest for repair of the ascending aorta based on the disease process in each individual patient (see Chapter 7).

In 1994, Kouchoukos et al.[125] reported on the successful replacement of the aortic root with a pulmonary autograft in 33 patients. This procedure was initially described by Ross in 1967.[126] The aortic valve and a portion of the ascending aorta are removed, leaving buttons of aortic tissue surrounding the coronary arteries. The pulmonary valve and the main pulmonary artery are excised. The pulmonary autograft is then sutured to the aortic annulus and

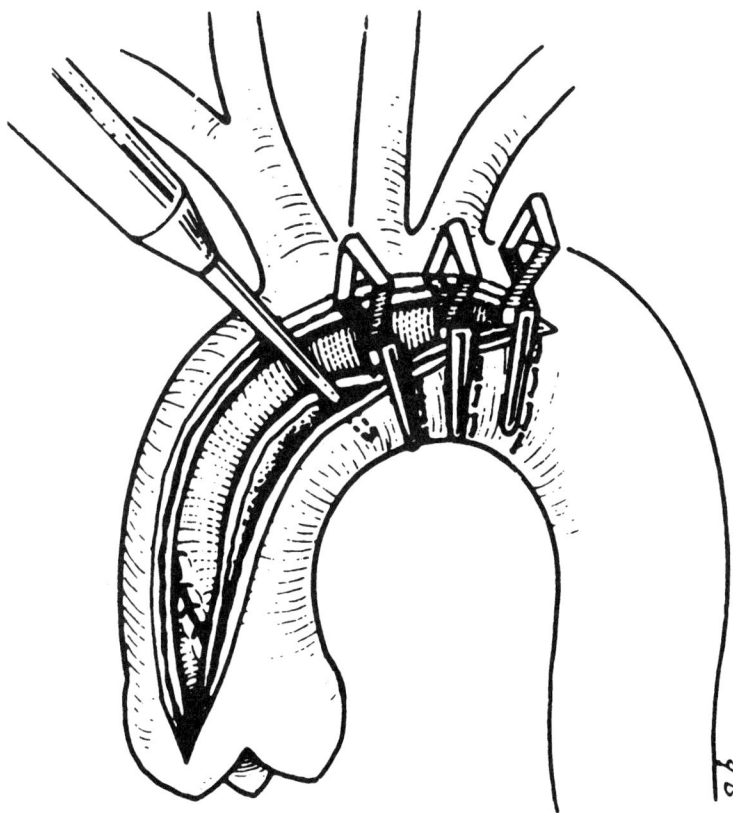

Figure 6-8. Illustration of glue aortoplasty. Glue is injected into the space separating the layers (false lumen), and the intimal tear is sutured. (Reprinted with permission from A Carpentier. "Glue aortoplasty" as an alternative to resection and grafting for the treatment of aortic dissection. Semin Thorac Cardiovasc Surg 1991;3:213.)

to the distal aorta, and the coronary arteries are attached to openings in the pulmonary artery. A pulmonary root allograft is then sutured into the right ventricular outflow tract. This procedure can serve as an alternative to the replacement of the aortic valve with a mechanical or bioprosthetic valve or an allograft. The advantages include the use of autologous tissue with documented long-term viability,[127] the optimal or near optimal alignment and function of the valve leaflets, and the absence of substantial transvalvular pressure gradients, the lack of thromboembolism, and the absence of the need for anticoagulant therapy.[128] The physician must be careful to avoid elevated right-sided pressures following this repair. Direct pressure measurements may not be available because many anesthesiologists elect not to float a pulmonary artery catheter through the pulmonary allograft. Although replacement of the aortic root with a pulmonary root is a more complex operation, it may prove to be the optimal substitute in children and young adults[129] (Figure 6-7).

Finally, there has been recent interest in glue aortoplasty as an alternative to resection and grafting for the treatment of aortic dissections.[130] In 1979, Guilmet et al.[131] proposed reinforcing the aortic layers remaining after resection of the ascending aorta with resorcinol glue. Resorcinol glue is a mixture of gelatin and resorcin, which can be polymerized by adding formaldehyde and glutaraldehyde. After application of the glue, the tissue is four to five times stronger than the original tissue.

In 1989, Fabiani et al.[132] suggested the use of surgical glue to stick the aortic layers together as the primary treatment of a type A aortic dissection. This technique would allow reconstruction rather than replacement of the dissected aorta (Figure 6-8).

References

1. Galen J. Observations on Aneurysm (Translated by JE Erickson). London: Sydenham Society, 1944.
2. Cooley DA. Surgical Treatment of Aortic Aneurysms. Philadelphia: Saunders, 1986;1:43.

3. Osler W. Aneurysm of the abdominal aorta. Lancet 1905;2:1089.

4. Morgagni GB. DeSedibus et Causes Morborum per Anatomen Indagitis. Veneties, 1761. In A Alexander (translation), The Seats and Causes of Diseases Investigated by Anatomy. London: Miller and Cedele, 1769.

5. Moore CH, Morchison C. On a method of procuring consolidation of fibrin in certain incurable aneurysms. Med Chir Trans 1864;47:129.

6. Altman P, Voorhees AB Jr. Aneurysm of the aorta treated by wiring: case report of a 38-year survival. Ann Surg 1976;184:738.

7. Pearse HE. Experimental studies on the gradual occlusion of large arteries. Ann Surg 1940;112:923.

8. Shumacker HB Jr. Coarctation and aneurysm of the aorta: report of a case treated by excision and end-to-end suture of the aorta. Ann Surg 1948;127:655.

9. Oudot J. La Greffe vasculaire dans les thromboses du carrefour aortique. Resse Med 1951;59:234.

10. DeBakey ME, Cooley DA. Successful resection of aneurysm of thoracic aorta and replacement by graft. JAMA 1953;152:673.

11. Blakemore AH, Voorhees AB Jr. The use of tubes constructed from vinyon "N" cloth in bridging arterial defects—experimental and clinical. Ann Surg 1954;140:324.

12. Shumacker HB Jr, King H. The use of pliable plastic tubes as aortic substitutes in man. Surg Gynecol Obstet 1954;99:287.

13. DeBakey ME, Cooley DA, Crawford ES, Morris GC. Aneurysms of the thoracic aorta: analyses of 179 cases treated by resection. J Thorac Cardiovasc Surg 1958;36:393.

14. McNamara JJ, Pressler VM. Natural history of arteriosclerotic thoracic aortic aneurysms. Ann Thorac Surg 1978;26:468.

15. Boyd LJ. A study of four thousand reported cases of aneurysm of the thoracic aorta. Am J Med Sci 1924;168:654.

16. Rockwell DH, Yobs AR, Moore MB. The Tuskegee study of untreated syphilis: the 30th year of observation. Arch Intern Med 1946;114:792.

17. Joyce JW, Fairbairrn JF II, Kincaid OW, Juergons JL. Aneurysms of the thoracic aorta, a clinical study with special reference to prognosis. Circulation 1964;29:176.

18. Laas J, Jurmann M, Heinemann M, Borst HG. Management and follow-up of proximal aortic aneurysms. Semin Thorac Cardiovasc Surg 1991;3:266.

19. Crawford ES. Operative indications and follow-up of aneurysms. Semin Thorac Cardiovasc Surg 1991;3:277.

20. Duke RT, Barrett MR II, Payne SD, et al. Compression of left main bronchus and pulmonary artery by thoracic aortic aneurysm. AJR Am J Roentgenol 1987;149:261.

21. Charrette EJP, Winton TL, Salerno TA. Acute respiratory insufficiency from an aneurysm of the descending thoracic aorta. J Thorac Cardiovasc Surg 1983;85:467.

22. Cramer M, Foley WD, Palmer TE, et al. Compression of right pulmonary artery by aortic aneurysms: CT demonstration. J Comput Assist Tomogr 1985;9:310.

23. MacGillivray RG. Tracheal compression caused by aneurysms of the aortic arch. Implication for the anaesthetist. Anaesthesia 1985;40:270.

24. Tominaga R, Tanaka J, Kawachi Y, et al. Surgical treatment of respiratory insufficiency due to tracheobronchial compression by aneurysms of the ascending aorta and innominate artery. J Cardiovasc Surg 1988;29:413.

25. Pressler V, McNamara JJ. Thoracic aortic aneurysm: natural history and treatment. J Thorac Cardiovasc Surg 1980;79:489.

26. Pyeritz RE, McKusick VA. The Marfan syndrome: diagnosis and management. N Engl J Med 1979;300:772.

27. Tsipouras P, Del Mastro R, Sarfarazi M, et al., and the International Marfan Syndrome Collaborative Study. Genetic linkage of the Marfan syndrome, ectopia lentis, and congenital structural arachnodactyly to the fibrillin gene on chromosomes 15 and 5. N Engl J Med 1992;326:905.

28. Marsalese DL, Moodie DS, Vacante M, et al. Marfan syndrome: natural history and long-term follow-up of cardiovascular involvement. J Am Coll Cardiol 1989;14:422.

29. Shores J, Berger KR, Murphy EA, Pyeritz RE. Progression of aortic dilatation and the benefit of long-term beta–adrenergic blockade in Marfan's syndrome. N Engl J Med 1994;330:1335.

30. McDonald GR, Schaff HV, Pyeritz RE, et al. Surgical management of patients with the Marfan's syndrome and dilatation of the ascending aorta. J Thorac Cardiovasc Surg 1981;81:180.

31. Gott VL, Pyeritz RE, Magovern GJ, et al. Surgical treatment of aneurysms of the ascending aorta in the Marfan syndrome: results of composite graft repair in 50 patients. N Engl J Med 1986;314:1070.

32. Smith JA, Fann JI, Miller DC, et al. Surgical management of aortic dissection in patients with the Marfan syndrome. Circulation 1994;90:235.

33. Crawford ES, Svensson LG, Coselli JS, et al. Aortic dissection and dissecting aortic aneurysms. Ann Surg 1988;208:254.

34. Pyeritz RE. Marfan's syndrome: current and future clinical and genetic management of cardiovascular manifestations. Semin Thorac Cardiovasc Surg 1993;5:11.

35. Amar D, Komer CA. Anesthetic implications of a ruptured aneurysm of the sinus of Valsalva. J Cardiothorac Vasc Anesth 1993;7:730.

36. Burakovsky VI, Podsolkov VP, Sabirow BOV, et al. Ruptured congenital aneurysm of the sinus of Valsalva: clinical manifestations, diagnosis and results of surgical corrections. J Thorac Cardiovasc Surg 1988;95:836.

37. Anderson CB, Butcher HR, Ballinger WF. Mycotic aneurysms. Arch Surg 1974;109:712.

38. Austen WG, Blennerhassett MB. Giant cell aortitis causing an aneurysm of the ascending aorta and aortic regurgitation. N Engl J Med 1965;272:80.

39. Lande A. Takayasu's arteritis and congenital coarctation of the descending thoracic and abdominal aorta. A critical review. AJR Am J Roentgenol 1976;127:227.

40. Cipriano PR, Silverman JF, Perlroth MG, et al. Coronary arterial narrowing in Takayasu's aortitis. Am J Cardiol 1977;39:744.

41. Davidson P, Bagenstoss AH, Slocumb CH, Daugherty GW. Cardiac and aortic lesions in rheumatoid spondylitis. Proc Mayo Clin 1963;36:427.

42. Zuaifler NJ, Weintraub AM. Aortitis and aortic insufficiency in chronic rheumatic disorders. A reappraisal. Arthritis Rheum 1963;6:241.

43. Pearson CM, Kroening R, Verity MA, Getzen JH. Aortic insufficiency and aortic aneurysm in relapsing polychondritis. Trans Assoc Am Phys 1967;80:71.

44. Paulus HE, Pearson CM, Pitts W. Aortic insufficiency in five patients with Reiter's syndrome. A detailed clinical and pathologic study. Am J Med 1972;53:464.

45. Muna WF, Roller DH, Craft J, et al. Psoriatic arthritis and aortic regurgitation. JAMA 1980;244:363.

46. Little AG, Zarins CK. Abdominal aortic aneurysm and Behçet's disease. Surgery 1982;91:359.

47. Sorenson HR, Olsen H. Ruptured and dissecting aneurysms of the aorta: incidence and prospects of surgery. Acta Chir Scand 1964;128:644.

48. Miller DC. Acute dissection of the aorta—continuing need for earlier diagnosis and treatment. Modern Concepts Cardiovascular Disease 1985;54:51.

49. Lillienfeld DE, Gunderson PD, Sprafka JM, Vargas C. Epidemiology of aortic aneurysms: I. Mortality trends in the United States, 1951–1981. Arteriosclerosis 1987;7:637.

50. Hirst AE Jr, Johns VJ Jr, Kime SW. Dissecting aneurysm of the aorta: a review of 505 cases. Medicine 1958;37:217.

51. Massumi A, Mathur VS. Clinical recognition of aortic dissection. Texas Heart Institute Journal 1990;17:254.

52. Hanley WB, Jones BN. Familial dissecting aortic aneurysm. A report of three cases within two generations. Br Heart J 1967;29:852.

53. Roberts WC, Honig HS. The spectrum of cardiovascular disease in the Marfan's syndrome: a clinico–morphologic study of 18 necropsy patients and comparison to 151 previously reported necropsy patients. Am Heart J 1982;104:115.

54. Hirst A, Gore I. The Etiology and Pathology of Aortic Dissection. In RM Doroghazi, EE Slater (eds), Aortic Dissection. New York: McGraw-Hill, 1983;13.

55. Fukuda T, Tadavarthy SM, Edwards JE. Dissecting aneurysm of aorta complicating aortic valvular stenosis. Circulation 1976;53:169.

56. Pedowitz P, Perell A. Aneurysm complicated by pregnancy. Am J Obstet Gynecol 1957;73:720.

57. Kitchen DH. Dissecting aneurysm of the aorta in pregnancy. Journal Obstetrical Gynecol–British Commonwealth 1974;81:410.

58. DeBakey ME, Henly WS, Cooley DA, Crawford ES. Surgical treatment of dissecting aneurysm of the aorta. Analysis of seventy-two cases. Circulation 1961;24:290.

59. DeBakey ME, Henly WS, Cooley DA, et al. Surgical management of dissecting aneurysms of the aorta. J Thorac Cardiovasc Surg 1965;49:130.

60. Crawford ES. Marfan's syndrome: broad spectral surgical treatment of cardiovascular manifestations. Ann Surg 1983;198:487.

61. Daily PO, Trueblood HW, Stinson EB, et al. Management of acute aortic dissection. Ann Thorac Surg 1970;10:237.

62. Wheat MW Jr. Pathogenesis of Aortic Dissection. In RM Doroghazi, EE Slater (eds), Aortic Dissection. New York: McGraw-Hill, 1983;55.

63. Carlson RG, Lillehei CW, Edwards JE. Cystic medial necrosis of the ascending aorta in relation to age and hypertension. Am J Cardiol 1970;25:411.

64. Schlatmann TJM, Becker AE. Pathogenesis of dissecting aneurysm of aorta: comparative histopathologic study of significance of medial changes. Am J Cardiol 1977;39:21.

65. Antani J, Srinivas HV. Ehlers-Danlos syndrome and cardiovascular abnormalities. Chest 1973;63:214.

66. Prokop EK, Palmer RD, Wheat MW. Hydrodynamic forces in dissecting aneurysm: in vitro studies in a tygon model and in dog aortas. Circ Res 1970;27:121.

67. Wheat MW Jr, Palmer RF. Dissecting aneurysms of the aorta—present status of drug versus surgical therapy. Prog Cardiovascular Dis 1968;11:198.

68. McFarland J, Willerson JT, Dinsmore RE, et al. The medical treatment of dissecting aortic aneurysms. N Engl J Med 1972;286:115.

69. Slater EE. Aortic Dissection: Presentation and Diagnosis. In RM Doroghazi, EE Slater (eds), Aortic Dissection. New York: McGraw-Hill, 1983;61.

70. Rose EA, McNicholas KW, Bethea MC, et al. Renovascular hypertension following surgical repair of dissecting aneurysm of the thoracic aorta. Surgery 1978;83:235.

71. Slater EE, DeSanctis RW. The clinical recognition of dissecting aortic aneurysm. Am J Med 1976;60:625.

72. DeSanctis RW, Doroghazi RM, Austen G, Buckley MJ. Aortic dissection. N Engl J Med 1987;317:1060.

73. Weisman AD, Adams RD. Neurological complications of dissecting aortic aneurysms. Brain 1944;67:69.

74. Moersch FP, Sayre GP. Neurologic manifestations associated with dissecting aneurysms of the aorta. JAMA 1950;144:1141.

75. Riley DJ, Liv RT, Saxanoff S. Aortic dissection: a rare cause of the superior vena cava syndrome. J Med Soc NJ 1981;78:187.

76. Buja ML, Ali N, Roberts WC. Stenosis of the right pulmonary artery: a complication of acute dissecting aneurysm of the ascending aorta. Am Heart J 1972;83:89.

77. McCarthy C, Dickson CH, Besterman EM, et al. Aortic dissection with rupture through ductus arteriosus into pulmonary artery. Br Heart J 1972;34:284.

78. Roth JA, Parekh MA. Dissecting aneurysms perforating the esophagus. N Engl J Med 1978;299:776.

79. Neustein SM, Narang J, Gribetz A, Krellenstein DJ. Spontaneous hemothorax due to subacute aortic dissection. J Cardiothorac Vasc Anesth 1993;7:79.

80. Thiene G, Rossi L, Becker AE. The atrioventricular conduction system in dissecting aneurysms of the aorta. Am Heart J 1979;98:447.

81. Tencate JW, Timmers H, Becker AE. Coagulopathy in ruptured or dissecting aortic aneurysms. Am J Med 1975;59:171.

82. Yacoub MH, Schottenfeld M, Kittle CF. Hematoma of the interatrial septum with heart block secondary to dissecting aneurysm of the aorta: a clinicopathologic entity. Circulation 1972;46:537.

83. Millward DJ, Robinson NJ, Craige E. Dissecting aortic aneurysm diagnosed echocardiographically in a patient with rupture of the aneurysm into the right atrium. Am J Cardiol 1972;30:407.

84. Victor MF, Mintz GS, Kotler MN, et al. Two dimensional echocardiographic diagnosis of aortic dissection. Am J Cardiol 1981;48:1155.

85. Heiberg E, Wolverson M, Sundarm M, et al. CT findings in thoracic aortic dissection. AJR Am J Roentgenol 1981;136:13.

86. Singh H, Fitzgerald E, Puttley MS. Computed tomography: the investigation of choice for aortic dissection. Br Heart J 1986;56:171.

87. Earnest F, Muhan Jr, Sheedy PF. Roentgenographic findings in thoracic aortic dissection. Mayo Clin Proc 1979;54:43.

88. Dinsmore RE, Willerson JT, Buckley MJ. Dissecting aneurysm of the aorta. Aortographic features affecting prognosis. Radiology 1972;105:567.

89. Borner N, Erbel R, Braun B, et al. Diagnosis of aortic dissection by transesophageal echocardiography. Am J Cardiol 1984;54:1157.

90. Nienaber CA, Spielmann RP, Kodolitsch YV, et al. Diagnosis of thoracic aortic dissection: magnetic resonance imaging versus transesophageal echocardiography. Circulation 1992;85:434.

91. Jamieson WRE, Munro AI, Miyagishima RT, et al. Aortic dissection: early diagnosis and surgical management are the keys to survival. Can J Surg 1982;25:145.

92. Nienaber CA, Kodolitsch YV, Nicolas V, et al. The diagnosis of thoracic aortic dissection by noninvasive imaging procedures. N Engl J Med 1993;328:1.

93. Fisher MR. Application of MRI in Vascular Surgery. In JJ Bergan, JS Yao (eds), Arterial Surgery—New Diagnostic and Operative Techniques. Orlando, FL: Grune & Stratton, 1988.

94. Kimbris D, Dreifus LS, Adam A, et al. Dissection and rupture of the ascending aorta. Chest 1975;68:313.

95. Litchford B, Okies JE, Sugimura S, Starr A. Acute aortic dissection from cross-clamp injury. J Thorac Cardiovasc Surg 1976;72:709.

96. Boruchow IB, Iyengar R, Jude JR. Injury to ascending aorta by partial-occlusion clamp during aorto-coronary bypass. J Thorac Cardiovasc Surg 1977;73:303.

97. Williams CD, Survansirikul S, Engelman RM. Thoracic aortic dissection following cannulation for perfusion. Ann Thorac Surg 1974;18:300.

98. Nicholson WS, Crawley IS, Cogue RB, et al. Aortic root dissection complicating coronary bypass surgery. Am J Cardiol 1978;41:103.

99. Benedict JS, Buhl TL, Henney RP. Acute aortic dissection during cardiopulmonary bypass. Arch Surg 1974;108:810.

100. Murphy DA, Craver JM, Jones EL, et al. Recognition and management of ascending aortic dissection complicating cardiac surgical operation. J Thorac Cardiovasc Surg 1983;85:247.

101. Troianos CA, Savino Jr, Weiss RL. Transesophageal echocardiographic diagnosis of aortic dissection during cardiac surgery. Anesthesiology 1991;75:149.

102. Bjerke RJ. Intraoperative diagnosis of aortic dissection using transesophageal echocardiography. J Cardiothorac Vasc Anesth 1992;6:720.

103. Smuckler AL, Nomeir AM, Watts LE, Hackshaw BT. Echocardiographic diagnosis of aortic root dissection by M-mode and two dimensional techniques. Am Heart J 1982;103:897.

104. Robbins RC, McManus RP, Mitchell RS, et al. Management of patients with intramural hematoma of the thoracic aorta. Circulation 1993;88:1.

105. Crawford ES. The diagnosis and management of aortic dissection. JAMA 1990;264:2537.

106. Wheat MW Jr. Intensive Drug Therapy. In RM Doroghazi, EE Slater (eds), Aortic Dissection. New York: McGraw-Hill, 1983;165.

107. Mori M, Chuma R, Kiichi Y, et al. The anesthetic management of a patient with a thoracic aortic aneurysm that caused compression of the left mainstem bronchus and the right pulmonary artery. J Cardiothorac Vasc Anesth 1993;7:579.

108. Jansen V, Milne B, Salerno T. Femoral–femoral cardiopulmonary bypass prior to induction of anaesthesia in the management of upper airway obstruction. Can Anaesth Soc J 1983;30:270.

109. Norman PH, Mycyk T. Dissection of ascending thoracic aorta complicated by cardiac tamponade. Can J Anaesth 1989;36:470.

110. Mayer JR Jr, Lindsay WG, Wang Y, et al. Composite replacement of the aortic valve and ascending aorta. J Thorac Cardiovasc Surg 1978;76:816.

111. Kouchoukos NT, Karp RB, Blackstone EH, et al. Replacement of the ascending aorta and aortic valve with a composite graft. Results in 86 patients. Ann Surg 1980;192:403.

112. Maurer W, Ablasser A, Tschada R, et al. Myocardial catecholamine metabolism in patients with chronic aortic regurgitation. Circulation 1982;66(Suppl):139.

113. Cooley DA, DeBakey ME. Resection of entire ascending aorta in fusiform aneurysm using cardiac bypass. JAMA 1956;162:1158.

114. Gibbon JH Jr. Application of mechanical heart and lung apparatus to cardiac surgery. Minn Med 1954;37:171.

115. Kay EB, Head LR, Nogueira C. Direct coronary artery perfusion for aortic valve surgery. JAMA 1958;168:1767.

116. Hufnagel CA, Conrad PW. Direct approach for correction of aortic insufficiency. JAMA 1961;178:275.

117. Wheat MW Jr, Wilson JR, Bartley TD. Successful replacement of the entire ascending aorta and aortic valve. JAMA 1964;188:717.

118. Bentall H, DeBono A. A technique for complete replacement of the ascending aorta. Thorax 1968;23:338.

119. Asano K, Ando T, Hanada S, Maruyama Y. Control of bleeding during the Bentall operation. J Cardiovasc Surg 1983;24:13.

120. McCready RA, Pluth JR. Surgical treatment of ascending aortic aneurysm associated with aortic valve insufficiency. Ann Thorac Surg 1979;28:307.

121. Cabrol C, Gandjbakhch I, Cham B. Aneurismes de l'aorte ascendante. Remplacement total avec reimplantation des artères coronaires. Nouv Presse Med 1978;7:363.

122. Cabrol C, Pavie A, Gandjbakhch I, et al. Complete replacement of the ascending aorta with reimplantation of the coronary arteries. New surgical approach. J Thorac Cardiovasc Surg 1981;81:309.

123. Cooley DA. Experience with hypothermic circulatory arrest and the treatment of aneurysms of the ascending aorta. Semin Thorac Cardiovasc Surg 1991;3:166.

124. Livesay JJ, Cooley DA, Duncan JM, et al. Open aortic anastomosis. Improved results in the treatment of aneurysms of the aortic arch. Circulation 1982;66(Suppl):122.

125. Kouchoukos NT, Davila-Roman VG, Spray TL, et al. Replacement of the aortic root with a pulmonary autograft in children and young adults with aortic-valve disease. N Engl J Med 1994;330:1.

126. Ross DN. Replacement of aortic and mitral valves with a pulmonary autograft. Lancet 1967;2:956.

127. Ross DN, Jackson M, Davies J. The pulmonary autograft—a permanent aortic valve. Eur J Cardiothorac Surg 1992;6:113.

128. Elkins RC, Santangelo K, Randolph JD, et al. Pulmonary autograft replacement in children: the ideal solution? Ann Surg 1992;216:363.

129. Gerosa G, McKay R, Davies J, Ross DN. Comparison of the aortic homograft and the pulmonary autograft for aortic valve or root replacement in children. J Thorac Cardiovasc Surg 1991;102:51.

130. Carpentier A. "Glue aortoplasty" as an alternative to resection and grafting for the treatment of aortic dissection. Semin Thorac Cardiovasc Surg 1991;3:213.

131. Guilmet D, Cachet J, Goudot B, et al. Use of biological glue in acute aortic dissections. A new surgical technique—preliminary results. J Thorac Cardiovasc Surg 1979;77:516.

132. Fabiani JN, Jebara VA, Deloche A, et al. Use of surgical glue without replacement in the treatment of type A aortic dissection. Circulation 1989;80(Suppl I):264.

Chapter 7

Anesthesia for Aortic Arch Aneurysm Surgery

Pierre A. Casthely and Mark Badach

In spite of advances in modern surgical techniques, aortic arch replacement remains a relatively infrequent procedure, demanding complex anesthetic management and surgical techniques.[1–3] It requires myocardial and brain protection, as well as individualization of both operative planning and perfusion techniques. Despite an improvement in surgical technique, mortality remains high at 10–25%. The following discussion is a review of aortic arch aneurysm surgery with special emphasis on anesthetic management, brain protection, and associated complications. Since the initial successful report by Griepp and coworkers in 1975,[4] there have been two traditional surgical options for the treatment of aneurysms involving the aortic arch. These options are selective perfusion of the arch vessels nourishing the brain and profound hypothermic circulatory arrest. In the early 1990s, retrograde cerebral perfusion emerged as yet another modality.

Pathology

The causes of aneurysms of the aortic arch are diverse. Three distinct patterns of proximal aortic atherosclerosis have been identified by Mills and Everson: (1) the so-called porcelain aorta, characterized by circumferential medial calcification; (2) the ragged, friable ulcerated type of disease; and (3) a pattern that is described as liquid, toothpaste-like cholesterol debris[5] (see Chapter 1).

All three patterns of atherosclerosis are dangerous and can be missed on both preoperative angiography and on initial surgical assessment of the aorta. Intraoperative transesophageal or epiaortic echocardiography has been used to scan the thoracic aorta to identify patients at risk.[6,7] The multiplane probe, with views obtained in the longitudinal plane in particular, has been useful for viewing the ascending aorta and the aortic arch.

An important pathologic distinction, made initially by Crawford and Snyder,[8] is the location and extent of the aneurysm. Aneurysms that are limited to the distal arch (usually on the concave surface of the aorta) are generally atherosclerotic in nature, characterized by considerable intimal debris. These distal aneurysms are frequently sacciform, involving less than 50% of the aortic circumference, lending themselves to patch repair. On the other hand, aneurysms involving the proximal or entire arch are usually degenerative in origin, characterized by medial degeneration with resultant circumferential aneurysmal dilation. Intimal debris, though often present, is not as impressive as in the more distally occurring aneurysms.

Aside from medial degeneration and atherosclerosis, the other major cause of aortic arch pathology is aortic dissection. Predisposing conditions to aortic dissections are included in Table 7-1. Additionally, aortic dissections have been classified by both Debakey and Daily (Figure 7-1). Mortality from aortic dissection remains high and requires prompt diagnosis and treatment. Acutely, dissection may originate in the arch with an intimal tear (<5% of dissections). More commonly, the intimal tear occurs proximally with the dissection propagating

Table 7-1. Predisposing Conditions to Aortic Dissections

History of hypertension	Present in 90% of patients
Advanced age	> 60 years
Sex	Male preponderance under age 60
Arachnodactyly (Marfan's syndrome)	Also other connective tissue disease
Congenital heart disease	Coarctation of aorta, biscuspid aortic valve
Pregnancy	Uncommon
Other causes	Toxins and diet

through the arch. Occasionally, dissections originating in the descending aorta may extend retrograde to involve the arch. Patients who survive the acute dissection may go on to form chronic, large dissecting aneurysms of the aortic arch.

Patients with Marfan's syndrome may present with diverse aortic pathology. The cystic medial necrosis characteristic of this syndrome leads to aneurysmal dilatation of any part or all of the aorta and additionally can be a precursor of dissection (see Chapter 1).

In the patient with aortic arch dissection, careful evaluation of neurologic, renal, and gastrointestinal function is important. The neurologic examination should be followed closely to detect signs of any change in neurologic status, as deterioration in function is an indication for immediate surgical intervention. Renal function should be followed closely after insertion of a urinary catheter. If aortic dissection has been diagnosed, the development of anuria or oliguria in the setting of euvolemia is an indication for immediate surgical intervention. Additionally, serial abdominal examinations should be performed. Arterial blood gas analysis should be done routinely to assess changes in acid–base status, as ischemic bowel can produce significant acidosis.

Anesthetic Management

The goals for anesthetic management of the patient for aortic arch surgery may be dictated by the urgency of the procedure, whether the patient has a full stomach, and other coexisting problems. In the patient with isolated arch aneurysm or dissection, the primary goals are the avoidance of hypertension and increased contractility. Hypertension can cause rupture of an aneurysm, especially in an aneurysm that is leaking. Increased contractility can lead to

increased shearing forces in the aorta and potentially to an extension of the dissection. Occasionally, a patient with arch dissection may present in extremis with pericardial tamponade secondary to retrograde propagation of the dissection.

In addition to these considerations, the usual considerations of ventricular function and coexisting vascular or coronary pathology affect the choices of anesthetic agents. Drugs that do not depress hemodynamics, such as narcotics, benzodiazepines, and etomidate, are usually chosen for induction and maintenance.

In addition to the monitoring techniques usually employed for aortic surgery (see Chapter 4), brain temperature is monitored via either the nasopharyngeal or tympanic membrane, core temperature is monitored via the rectum or bladder, and venous and arterial blood temperatures are monitored via temperature probes inserted in their respective oxygenator ports.

Arch Surgery and Brain Protection

To operate on the aortic arch, blood flow to the brain is interrupted. To prevent ischemic injury to the brain, several techniques have been used. These techniques include (1) hypothermic circulatory arrest, (2) selective cannulation and perfusion of the cerebral vessels, (3) retrograde cerebral perfusion, and (4) pharmacologic brain protection. More frequently, several of these techniques have been combined to allow for surgical repair of the arch.

Hypothermia

Hypothermia exerts numerous effects on all body organs. The relationship between metabolic rate and temperature is neither a linear nor an exponential

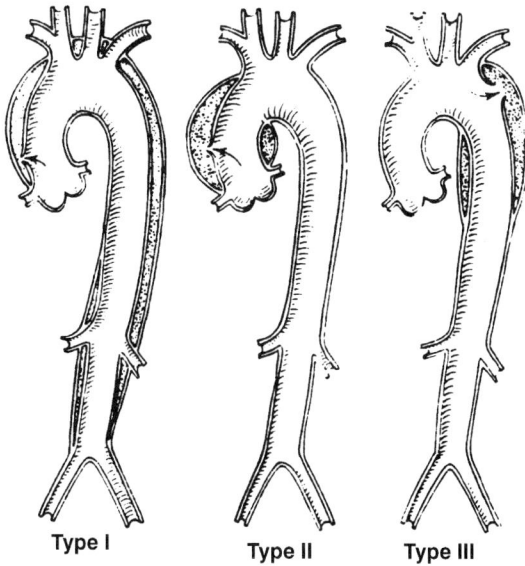

Type A (proximal)   Type B (distal)

Figure 7-1. DeBakey classification of dissections. This classification comprises three different types, depending on where the intimal tear is located and which section of the aorta is involved. Type I: The intimal tear is located in the ascending portion, but the dissection involves all portions (ascending, arch, and descending) of the thoracic aorta. Type II: The intimal tear is in the ascending aorta, but the dissection involves only the ascending aorta, stopping before the takeoff of the innominate artery. Type III: The intimal tear is located in the descending segment, and the dissection almost always involves the descending portion of the thoracic aorta only, starting just distal to the origin of the left subclavian artery. By definition, type III dissections can propagate proximally into the arch, but this is rare. (Reprinted with permission from EW Larson, WD Edwards. Risk factors for aortic dissection: a necropsy study of 161 cases. Am J Cardiol 1984;53:849. Excerpta Medica, Inc.)

function. However, the relationship between oxygen consumption and temperature is roughly exponential. In mammals, the decrease in oxygen consumption as the temperature is lowered can be transposed into a reduction of approximately 7% per degree.

The best approach for protecting the brain from temporary ischemia due to complete circulatory arrest is to reduce its demand for oxygen (or the cerebral metabolic rate of oxygen consumption [$CMRO_2$]). Hypothermia is the most effective means of reducing $CMRO_2$ during cardiopulmonary bypass (CPB).[9] Cooling the brain causes a slowing of biochemical processes, thus both the energy needed to maintain

cellular integrity (40–50% of the total $CMRO_2$) and the energy needed to maintain electrical activity (50–60% of the total $CMRO_2$) are decreased. The decrease in energy used is expressed as the Q10, which is the ratio of $CMRO_2$s after a cooling of 10°C has occurred. When electrical activity is present in the brain, the Q10 between 28°C and 18°C is about 15.[10] But when cerebral electrical activity has been suppressed prior to inducing hypothermia, as with barbiturates, the Q10 ranges from 2.1–2.4.

Hypothermia reduces cerebral blood flow and metabolism and confers protection in the face of ischemic and hypoxemic insults. Recent animal work shows even mild hypothermia (33–35°C) to be highly effective in ameliorating the effect of temporary cerebral ischemia. This protective effect is present despite tissue acidosis and depletion of energy sources equivalent to that occurring at normothermia.[11,12] More profound hypothermia may be effective in decreasing the damage of permanent lesions.[13] In addition to metabolic suppression, hypothermia modifies the postinjury response to ischemia, which may be an additional mechanism of protection. Mechanisms of this type of protection include (1) inhibition of excitatory neurotransmitters, (2) inhibition of postischemic edema and leukotriene formation, and (3) reduction of abnormal ion fluxes. Brain regions appear to be affected differently by hypothermia, some showing marked protection (hippocampus), and others less (thalamic nuclei).

Induction of Hypothermia

Profound hypothermia can be achieved by surface cooling, core cooling, or both.[14] Surface cooling is induced by placing the patient on a cooling blanket unit set at 27°C. The entire body including the head and neck is packed with small plastic bags filled with ice chips. The genital organs, nose, ears, eyes, toes, and fingers are protected with gauze pads to avoid thermal injuries. Ice packs are placed around the neck and head area to aid in reducing brain temperature, and they are not removed until after circulatory arrest is completed and the rewarming phase begins. Arterial blood gases are measured every 15 minutes during surface cooling. When the esophageal temperature reaches 30°C the ice is removed, the patient draped, and a median sternotomy performed. Ventricular fibrillation does not occur during surface

Table 7.2. Example of Hemodynamic Changes in a Patient During Hypothermia

Hemodynamic Parameters	35°C	33°C	30°C	28°C
Cardiac index L-min^{-1}-m^{-2}	2.85	2.69	2.1	1.75
Heart rate (beats/minute)	98	80	70	60
Mean arterial pressure (mm Hg)	98	85	75	70
Pulmonary artery pressure (mm Hg)	12	14	16	19
Pulmonary vascular resistance (dyne-sec-cm^{-5})	112	170	312	457
Systemic vascular resistance (dyne-sec-cm^{-5})	1,639	1,712	1,850	2,057

cooling if the core temperature is more than 28°C. Nevertheless, arrhythmias can occur, including premature ventricular contractions, atrial premature contractions, atrial fibrillation, and heart block.

Surface cooling prior to skin incision is no longer practiced in most institutions. The reasons for this are twofold. First, the temperature drop is hard to predict and control. The patient may cool faster than anticipated and ventricular fibrillation may occur. If hypothermia-induced ventricular fibrillation occurs and the chest is still closed, resuscitation is difficult, and the usual maneuvers such as direct current cardioversion may not work (as long as the hypothermia still exists). Additionally, if aortic insufficiency is present (as it frequently is with ascending dissection and aneurysm), then ventricular fibrillation will quickly lead to ventricular distention. Second, the surface-induced hypothermia can cause a coagulopathy, making initial surgical exposure more difficult. Therefore, most centers currently use CPB to achieve deep hypothermia. CPB with cooling is begun at a flow rate averaging 3.0–3.5 liters per minute using a disposable membrane oxygenator and an auxiliary heat exchanger. The cooling is continued until an esophageal temperature of 12–14°C is reached. At this point circulatory arrest can be performed. During circulatory arrest, care must be taken to avoid environment-induced rewarming. This can be accomplished by keeping the operating room temperature as low as possible and maintaining cooling with the hypothermia blanket.

Cardiac and Respiratory Function

Hypothermia produces prolonged systole and prolonged PR and QT intervals. Heart rate decreases during cooling and is accompanied by a progressive widening of the QRS complex.[14] Ventricular fibrillation may occur between 28 and 26°C. Myocardial

Table 7-3. Example of Arterial Blood Gases in a Patient During Hypothermia

Temperature	pH	PaCO$_2$	PaO$_2$
35°C	7.54	30.5	361
33°C	7.49	28.0	300
30°C	7.39	25.5	298
28°C	7.35	25.0	285

contractility and oxygen demand decrease. There is a progressive decrease of cardiac index during cooling. This is accompanied by a progressive decrease in mean arterial pressure and an increase in systemic and pulmonary vascular resistance (Table 7-2). There is also a progressive decrease in PaCO$_2$, PaO$_2$, and pH during cooling (Table 7-3).

Other Effects of Hypothermia

Glucose metabolism is depressed because of the diminished release of insulin. Therefore, the blood glucose level should be monitored during hypothermia when glucose utilization is diminished and glycogen stores are depleted. Renal function exhibits increased tolerance to ischemia, depression of tubular function, and diminished urinary output.

The oxyhemoglobin dissociation curve is also affected by hypothermia. Hypothermia shifts the curve to the left, with increased affinity of hemoglobin for oxygen and decreased oxygen availability to the tissues. There is also increased solubility of oxygen in plasma.

Because of the decreased metabolism seen during profound hypothermia, carbon dioxide production decreases. It has been recommended that CO$_2$ be added to the inspiratory mixture to increase the PaCO$_2$, and therefore correct the hypothermia-induced shift to the left of the oxygen hemoglobin dissociation curve. However, hypercarbia may increase the risk of arrhythmias.[15]

The effects of hypothermia on the electroencephalogram (EEG) include a decrease in amplitude of major frequency, burst suppression, and possible complete loss of major frequency. At 25°C zero waves are present. At 22–19°C the EEG becomes isoelectric.

Monitoring the Brain During Deep Hypothermia

The significance of EEG monitoring during CPB remains a hotly debated topic. Despite improvement in intraoperative EEG technology, recent data show no correlation between EEG abnormalities and neuropsychological outcome.[16] This lack of correlation between EEG findings and neurologic or neuropsychological outcome may be associated with the mechanism of injury. Small emboli may cause infarcts involving areas too small to have significant impact on the larger area monitored by surface EEG electrodes. This argument, although reasonable in nature, is contradicted by data from a study by Edmonds and colleagues that showed that an increase in relative low frequency power occurring over 5 minutes during rewarming was a significant predictor of cerebral cortical dysfunction (disorientation).[17]

EEG is a recording of localized spontaneous electrical activity of the brain limited to detection of events occurring within a small area surrounding a recording electrode (see Chapter 4). Adjacent cortex overshadows distant cortical activity, requiring that multiple recording electrodes be used to ensure EEG monitoring of all areas of the cortex. Leakage currents from electrical devices, ground loop interference, and electrocautery in the operating room can make recording and interpreting EEG data difficult or impossible unless the impedance of the electrodes is kept low (<5 kΩ).

Wave forms obtained on EEG records are described in terms of frequency, amplitude, distribution, regularity, and, most recently, phase interaction. The conventional EEG recording is the simplest example of time domain analysis, since it is in actuality a graph of signal amplitude (microvolts) as a function of time (seconds). Although widely employed in electrodiagnosis, this technique is generally impractical for routine intraoperative monitoring because it generates an enormous volume of data

and requires continuous assessment by a highly skilled medical or paramedical specialist. Power spectral analysis converts information from a time domain (frequency versus time) to a frequency domain (plot of power against frequency) for a given segment of the EEG. The compressed spectral array displays serial power spectra plotted one above the other to give a "mountain and valley" representation of EEG pattern. Computers using fast Fourier transformation can simultaneously plot power spectra for several channels. Reliability in predicting neurologic or neuropsychological outcome with neurologic monitoring may depend on newer forms of cerebral oxygen monitoring (see Chapter 4).

Spectroscopy

Advanced applications of the near infrared technology can detect oxyhemoglobin, cytochrome a,a3 redox status, and cerebral blood volume.[18,19] This method allows evaluation of brain oxygenation in children after deep hypothermic CPB and delineates a significant decrease in the oxidative state of cytochrome a,a3 in patients subjected to circulatory arrest versus low flow CPB.[20] This advanced technology has progressed slowly due to difficulties with spectral overlap occurring in the range of cytochrome a,a3. Multiple wavelength analysis continues to improve the accuracy of this promising monitor, but correlation with neurologic or neuropsychological outcome remains necessary to determine its future for monitoring in aortic arch surgery.

Acid–Base Management During Hypothermia

Hypothermia decreases plasma pH owing to the increased solubility of CO_2 in plasma. It also decreases the protein anion concentration and produces a change in the pH of bicarbonate buffer, leading to a net increase in pH of 0.005 units per 10°C decrease in temperature.

Acid–base management during hypothermic CPB remains controversial. Two specific forms of management may be used, pH-stat and alpha-stat. With pH-stat management, the clinical objective is to maintain a pH of 7.4 at the patient's core temperature. This requires the addition of exogenous CO_2 to the pump oxygenator to maintain a temperature corrected $PaCO_2$ at 35–40 mm Hg. Until recently, pH-stat was the most common method of management. Using the alpha-stat approach, $PaCO_2$ and pH are measured at 37°C and maintained at 40 mm Hg and a pH of 7.4, respectively, without regard to patient temperature. Blood gases are not temperature-corrected; therefore, the actual pH varies with body temperature. Using this technique, macromolecular structure and function are believed to be better preserved during hypothermia compared with pH-stat. pH-stat management produces relative hypercarbia and intracellular acidemia as compared with alpha-stat management. Because the CBF response to changing $PaCO_2$ is preserved during hypothermic bypass, pH-stat management leads to greater CBF than alpha-stat management, and cerebral vasodilation of pH-stat management can interfere with cerebral autoregulation.[21,22] Furthermore, autoregulation[23,24] and cerebral flow/metabolism coupling[21] preserve a more physiologic cerebral milieu, avoiding excessive cerebral blood flow with alpha-stat management. Nevertheless, Bashein and coworkers found no difference in neuropsychological outcome between patients randomized to alpha-stat or pH-stat management.[25] Additionally, animal studies indicate blood gas management has little to no effect on cerebral metabolism at 27°C, although at colder temperatures an effect may be present.[26] Additional animal works suggest brain acidosis may be less severe and recovery of brain oxygenation more effective following hypothermic circulatory arrest when alpha-stat management is used during cooling.[21]

The effects of acid–base management on myocardial function have also been studied. McConnell and associates[27] evaluated function in the canine heart during CPB at 28°C and made comparisons at a pH of 7.4 and 7.7. Under the alpha-stat regime (pH 7.7 corrected) they reported significant elevations in coronary blood flow, left ventricular oxygen consumption, and lactate use when compared with the pH-stat regimen (pH 7.4 corrected). Swan et al.[28] also reported a maintenance of left ventricular function after CPB with alpha-stat regimen as opposed to pH-stat. Poole-Wilson and Langer evaluated the performance of hypothermic perfused papillary muscle and found that a pH of perfusate on the alkaline side of pH 7.4 resulted in preservation of greater contractility. They later observed that acidosis, induced by increasing perfusate $PaCO_2$, was associated with a rapid decrease in myocardial tension development as well as alteration in calcium transport.[29]

Swain et al.[30] reported the effect of acid–base regulation on cardiac electrophysiology and noted that during hypothermia, electrical stability of the heart was increased using alpha-stat. Conversely, Gillen and colleagues reported a decrease in ventricular fibrillatory threshold in dogs using the pH-stat regimen.[31]

In conclusion, the alpha-stat method of acid-base management during profound hypothermia has theoretical advantages over pH-stat. However, recent evidence suggests no difference in neuropsychiatric outcome between patients randomized to receive either alpha-stat or pH-stat management.[32]

Glucose and Cerebral Ischemia

When cerebral oxygen delivery is inadequate (e.g., during hypoperfusion or embolism) anaerobic glucose oxidation becomes the main source of adenosine triphosphate (ATP) production, resulting in intracellular lactic acidosis. Hyperglycemia, by providing more glucose, increases the severity of intracellular acidosis, which correlates with the severity of subsequent injury in numerous animal studies. In a study of cardiac arrest patients, neurologic outcomes correlated negatively with elevated plasma glucose levels. Mild insulin-induced hypoglycemia has also been shown to improve neurologic function in cerebral ischemia.[33,34]

Although hyperglycemia in the presence of both global and focal cerebral ischemia is generally accepted as deleterious and euglycemia during bypass has been recommended, some human studies challenge these conclusions.[35] Metz and Keats reported no neurologic injury in 54 patients undergoing coronary artery bypass graft managed with glucose-containing fluids (serum glucose 700 mg/dl during bypass), as compared with one stroke and one case of encephalopathy in 53 patients in whom glucose was avoided during coronary artery bypass graft (glucose, 200 mg/dl).[36]

A more detailed study of neuropsychological performance found no correlation between serum glucose level during bypass (ranging from 103–379 mg/dl) and subsequent neuropsychological deterioration.[37] Presently, avoidance of hyperglycemia during periods of potential neurologic injury (circulatory arrest and bypass) appears prudent, although neurologic benefit is unproven.

Pharmacologic Brain Protection During Hypothermic Arrest

Proposed mechanisms by which drugs may exert protective effects include decreasing cerebral metabolic rate (CMRO$_2$), providing lysosomal membrane stabilization, allowing a decrease in the uptake of free extracellular calcium, and avoiding lipid peroxidation.[38,39]

Corticosteroids

A large dose of corticosteroids is often used before circulatory arrest, although experimental evidence for cerebral protection is equivocal. Corticosteroids may stabilize the microcirculation during hypothermia. Stabilization of cell membranes and prevention of lysosomal breakdown have also been suggested.[40,41]

Diuretics

Mannitol (0.5 g/kg) is often given as an osmotic diuretic to protect renal function and to attenuate increased intracranial pressure due to cerebral edema that may be seen in the perioperative period.[42,43] Mannitol may also function as a free radical scavenger. Furosemide can be administered to decrease the brain volume by systemic diuresis. It also causes decreased cerebrospinal fluid production, reduced astroglial cellular fluid transport, and capacitance relaxation.[44]

Barbiturates

The use of barbiturates to protect the brain during open heart surgery is controversial. Barbiturates are most effective in ameliorating injury in response to temporary focal insults, although protection from permanent focal lesions has been demonstrated with prolonged therapy (96 hours). In a study of 182 patients undergoing normothermic open cardiac procedures, Nussmeier et al. reported that maintenance of EEG burst-suppression with thiopental before and during bypass decreased postoperative neurologic abnormalities compared with nonbarbiturate controls.[45] In contrast, Zaidan and coworkers found no evidence of neurologic benefit with thiopental in 312 patients undergoing coronary artery bypass graft, although inotropic use and time to extubation were markedly greater in the thiopental group.[46] Of note, Nussmeier later published the results of neuropsychological testing not reported in the original paper, showing no benefit in the barbiturate group.

Barbiturates may be of benefit in ameliorating the effects of temporary focal lesions (gas emboli from bypass pump or open cardiac chamber) if metabolic suppression is not being achieved by hypothermia. But under usual conditions (i.e., membrane oxygenator, arterial filter, hypothermia, or any combination of these) these insults are either not created or are fairly well tolerated. In such a setting, short-term barbiturate therapy is probably not helpful and does not protect patients from permanent lesions (e.g., plaque, valve fragments).[47] Thus, the effectiveness of thiopental in reducing neurologic and neuropsychological sequelae of cardiac surgery must be seriously questioned and its use balanced against its significant cardiodepressant properties.

In experimental studies, normothermic deep pentobarbital anesthesia was associated with a 30% decrease in CMRO$_2$ and cerebral metabolic rate of glucose utilization (CMRG), as compared with lightly anesthetized controls. However, similar values were achieved with hypothermia (30°C) alone. The addition of hypothermia to pentobarbital anesthesia decreased CMRO$_2$ by 70% and decreased cerebral metabolic rate of glucose by 70%. Nevertheless, a moderate dose of thiopental (3–10 mg/kg) 3 minutes prior to circulatory arrest should decrease cerebral metabolism and may provide an added degree of protection.[48]

Calcium Channel Blockers

Recently, there has been renewed interest in the use of calcium channel blockers for cerebral protection. During ischemia there is a breakdown of membrane ion pumps, leading to a rapid increase in extracellular potassium, paradoxically stimulating neuron metabolism while further impeding substrate delivery by causing glial swelling and intracellular accumulation of sodium and calcium. Ischemic mitochondria and the endoplasmic reticulum cause further release of calcium. Under normal conditions, several defense mechanisms are available to counteract the intracellular calcium increase. They include a Na$^+$/Ca^{2+} exchange at the membrane level driven by the transmembrane sodium concentration gradient created by Na$^+$/K$^+$ ATPase; a membrane ATP-dependent calcium pump; an ATP-dependent sequestration of calcium by intracellular organelles; and a Ca^{2+}/H^+ exchange at the mitochondrial level occurring at the expense of oxidative phosphorylation. The increase in intracellular free calcium reinforces the initial insult and stimulates biochemical reactions, leading to further cell injury by encouraging uncoupling of oxidative phosphorylation at the mitochondrial level. Additionally, calcium affects the vasculature by direct vasconstriction. This may contribute to postischemic vasospasm and can result in sludging of red cells in the microvasculature.

Verapamil and diltiazem are almost ineffective due to their poor blood–brain barrier penetration. Nimodipine, which crosses the blood–brain barrier, has been shown to be effective when given after an ischemic insult in a primate model, but it has not been shown to improve surgical outcome after cardiopulmonary arrest in humans. Further use of these compounds may hold some promise in the future.[49,50]

Other calcium entry blockers have been found to be effective cerebral vasodilators. Nifedipine causes a dose-related relaxation of spasm induced in canine cerebral arteries by potassium or prostaglandin.[51] However, the doses required may produce complete heart block especially when used in patients undergoing aortic arch aneurysm resection under profound hypothermia and circulatory arrest.

Other Drugs

Two drugs, lidocaine and phenytoin, have been the subject of many studies. Lidocaine appears to have an effect on $CMRO_2$ even if the EEG is flat. Phenytoin and lidocaine both slow the release of potassium from ischemic neurons.[52,53] However, the large doses required experimentally to produce this effect make their use unpopular since clinical relevance has not been proven. The protective values of etomidate and flunarizine during surgery have also been studied, although their usefulness during complete circulatory arrest has not been reported.[54,55]

Retrograde Cerebral Perfusion

In 1980, Mills and Ochsner reported that retrograde perfusion via the superior vena cava with hypother-

mia at 20°C was effective in the management of massive air embolism during CPB.[56] Retrograde perfusion to expel air in the aortic arch and its branches after profound hypothermic circulatory arrest without cross clamping of any branches has been successfully applied by Ueda et al.[57]

Retrograde cerebral perfusion can be beneficial via two mechanisms: (1) It provides blood flow to the brain, thereby decreasing cerebral ischemia and prolonging the safe period of deep hypothermic circulatory arrest, and (2) it expels air and particulate emboli from the cerebral circulation.[56,58]

The method studied by Takamoto and colleagues of retrograde cerebral perfusion by elevating central venous pressure under profound hypothermia is simple and similar to the conventional pump technique.[59] The oxygen saturation of blood perfusing the lower half of the body under profound hypothermia (while an occlusion balloon is in the descending aorta) is high when it returns to the right atrium owing to the low oxygen consumption. High central venous pressure (15 mm Hg) in Trendelenburg's position with the aortic arch open during aortic arch surgery allows the oxygen-saturated venous blood to perfuse the brain tissue in retrograde fashion from the right atrium. During this retrograde cerebral perfusion, oxygen consumption occurs in brain tissue, causing darkening of the retrograde perfused blood returning through the carotid artery. Thus, significant oxygen consumption occurs in the brain even during profound hypothermia. This brain protection has lasted for as long as 93 minutes of circulatory arrest at 15°C.[59]

More recently, several authors have recommended selective cannulation of the superior vena cava with continuous direct perfusion at 100–500 ml per minute. Ueda et al. have demonstrated that moderate venous pressures seen with retrograde perfusion will not disrupt the blood–brain barrier and will not cause cerebral edema.[57] Okamoto and colleagues recommend direct jugular cannulation to avoid the problem of superior vena cava–jugular valves present in some patients.[60] In a recent study by Safi et al., 11 patients underwent retrograde cerebral perfusion with only one stroke reported.[61]

Further investigation is needed into the local cerebral circulation and metabolism during retrograde cerebral perfusion and into refinement of the retrograde perfusion technique (Figures 7-2 and 7-3).

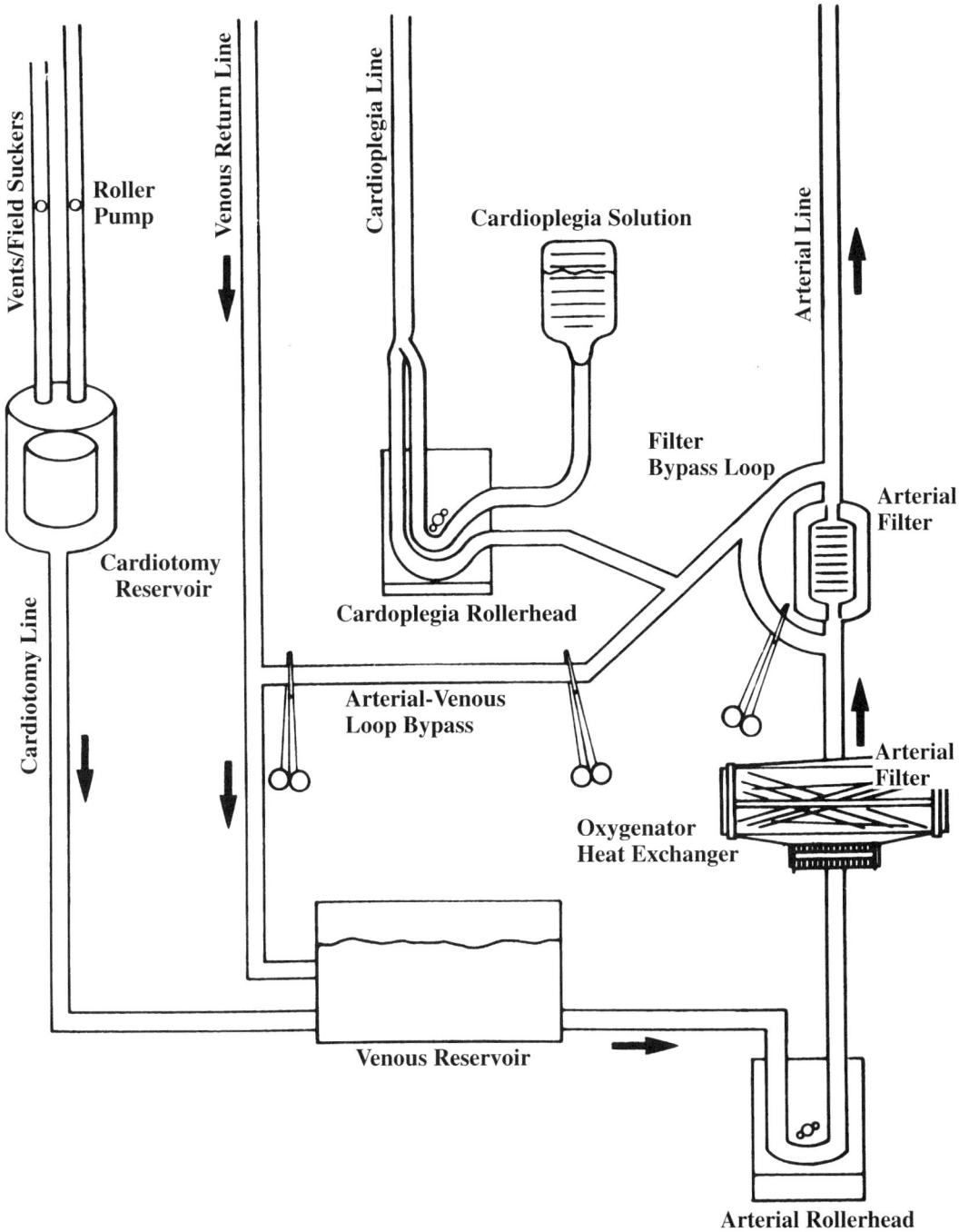

Figure 7-2. Diagram of cardiopulmonary bypass circuit used before and after systemic circulatory arrest. Clamps positioned as shown. Arrows indicate direction of perfusate flow. (Reprinted with permission from TM McLoughlin, WR Carter, CD King. Continuous retrograde cerebral perfusion as an adjunct to brain protection during deep hypothermic systemic circulatory arrest. J Cardiothorac Vasc Anesth 1995;9:205.)

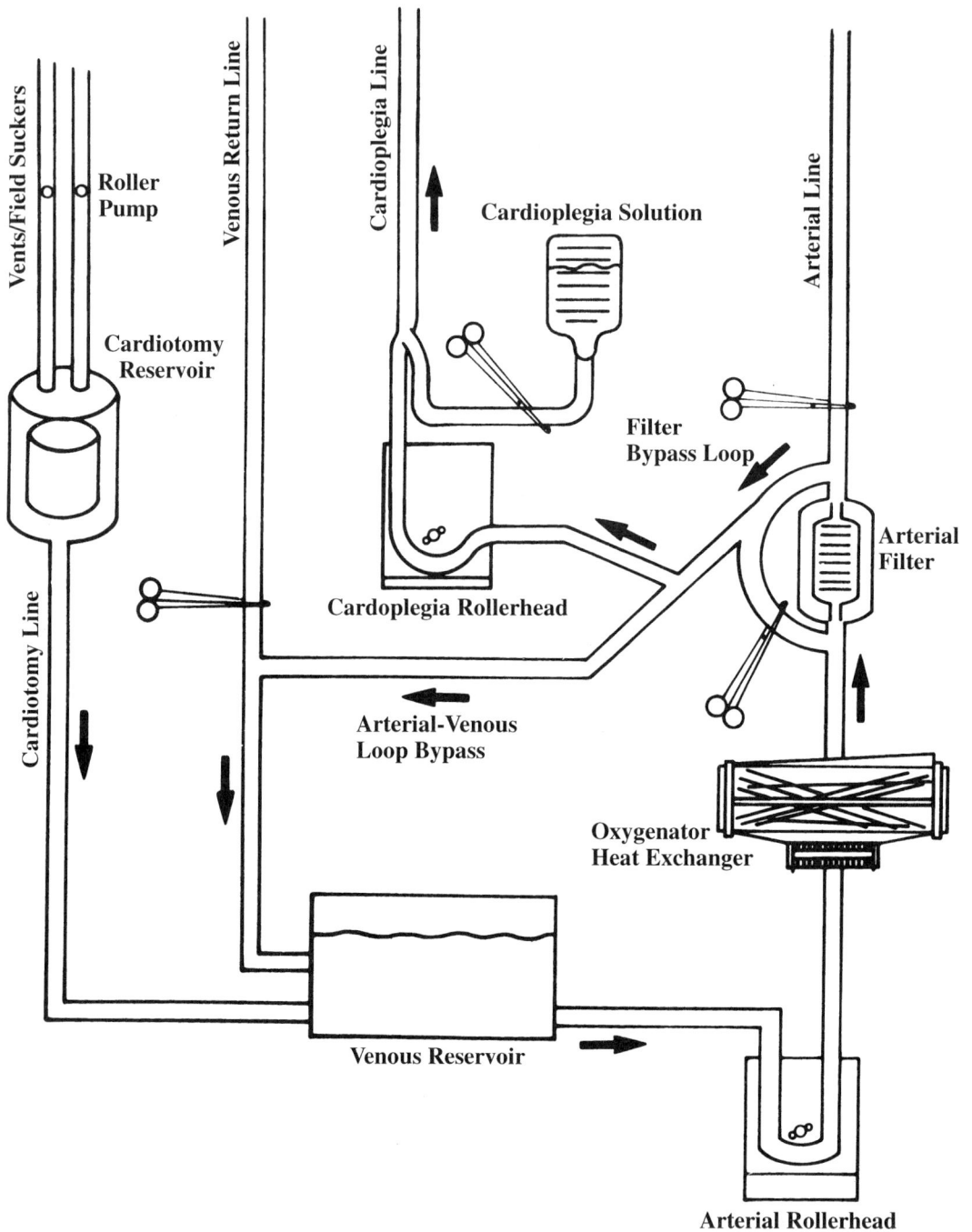

Figure 7-3. Diagram of cardiopulmonary bypass circuit used during continuous retrograde cerebral perfusion. Clamps positioned as shown. Arrows indicate direction of perfusate flow within arterial-venous loop bypass and from the "cardioplegia" line to the cannula positioned within the right internal jugular vein. (Reprinted with permission from TM McLoughlin, WR Carter, CD King. Continuous retrograde cerebral perfusion as an adjunct to brain protection during deep hypothermic systemic circulatory arrest. J Cardiothorac Vasc Anesth 1995;9:205.)

Neurologic Complications

The incidence of neurologic complications associated with surgery for aortic arch repair is low if the period of total circulatory arrest is of short duration and the peripheral circulation is maintained during cooling and rewarming. However, transient and permanent impairment of cerebral function after hypothermic circulatory arrest has been reported.[62,63] The incidence of neurologic disorders increases with the duration of total circulatory arrest. Intellectual development of children subjected to prolonged circulatory arrest during hypothermic open heart surgery in infancy was found to be the same as the normal population.[64] However, Wright and colleagues found more developmental abnormalities in infants treated under hypothermic arrest.[65] Morphologic alterations of the brain in seemingly normal patients following hypothermic circulatory arrest as well as following standard extracorporeal circulation have been documented by computerized tomography.[66] The incidence of neurologic complications ranges from 1–3%. Neurologic damage may result from the inadequacy of perfusion during cooling and rewarming rather than circulatory arrest.[67] However, the most important factor in avoiding neurologic complications is length of time of total circulatory arrest.[67]

In a recent retrospective study, multivariate predictors of postoperative neurologic injury included a history of cerebrovascular disease, previous descending aortic surgery, and circulatory arrest time. The occurrence of stroke was observed to increase after 40 minutes of circulatory arrest and mortality increased markedly after 65 minutes of arrest.[68] Even though hypothermia decreases $CMRO_2$, it is difficult to predict a safe time limit for circulatory arrest in humans.

The optimal level of hypothermia for cerebral protection in adults has been explored by several authors. Griepp et al.[4] and O'Connor et al.[69] showed good cerebral protection for 1 hour during circulatory arrest in the dog at 15°C, and for periods from 15–59 minutes at temperatures ranging from 11 to 18°C (surface and core cooling) in humans (Table 7-4). Crawford and Snyder used only core cooling, ranging between 12 and 20°C and found it to be protective in adults during periods of brachiocephalic artery clamping ranging from 19–75 minutes.[8] Cooling times in eight patients ranged from 31–59 minutes. Most temperatures were below 15°C, but higher temperatures were used in patients with simple operations requiring only brief periods of occlusion. Some have recommended low flow instead of total circulatory arrest during profound hypothermia.[70,71] Kirklin has pointed out the need to avoid total circulatory arrest for any protracted period and suggests trying to maintain a low flow (0.05 liters/m²/minute) because of the possibility of introducing air into the arterial system.[72] This approach seems prudent, because it also provides some blood flow to the brain and other vital organs.

Table 7-4. Safe Duration of Circulatory Arrest

Temperature (Degrees Celsius)	Oxygen Consumption (Percentage)	Circulatory Arrest Time (Minutes)
37	100	4–5
29	50	8–10
22	25	16–20
16	12	32–40
10	6	64–80

Hematologic Dysfunction

The coagulation system is profoundly affected by the foreign surfaces of the extracorporeal circuit, hemodilution, and hypothermia (see Chapter 5). Alteration in platelet function and number are the most common causes of hematologic dysfunction seen during CPB. Normally, platelets adhere to both foreign surfaces and to each other by the process of aggregation. Aggregation is activated by chemical substances including adenosine diphosphate, serotonin, arachidonic acid, and thromboxane A_2. Once activated, platelets undergo both structural and biochemical change and release thromboxane A_2 as well as additional serotonin and adenosine diphosphate. Thromboxane A_2, which is a powerful vasoconstrictor and platelet activator, promotes further platelet aggregation. Hypothermia is also associated with platelet dysfunction. In vitro platelet aggregation is abolished below 33°C,[73] while sequestration of platelets occurs below 25°C, primarily to the liver with return into the circulation during rewarming.[74] Platelet count also decreases during CPB due to dilution by the priming solution, blood loss, adhesion to the circuit, as well as fragmentation and destruc-

Table 7-5. Postoperative Hematologic Parameters Associated with Increased Risk of Hemorrhage

Test	Result
Prothrombin time	>19 seconds
Partial thromboplastin time	>45 seconds
Fibrinogen	<225 mg/dl
Platelets	<40,000/µl

tion. The platelet count usually decreases by 25–60% from baseline values. In addition, the cardiotomy suction exposes platelets to blood–air and blood–tissue interfaces, where activation, injury, and destruction occur. Other possible causes of thrombocytopenia or platelet dysfunction following CPB are platelet aggregation induced by pulmonary artery catheters, heparin, protamine, heparin-protamine complexes, and adenosine diphosphate released from hemolyzed red blood cells. The intravenous injection of protamine after CPB reduced platelet counts by one-third within minutes.[75] This effect is transient, lasting less than 1 hour, and may result from temporary sequestration of platelets in the liver.

Formed elements of the blood are affected, with blood viscosity increasing as a result of loss of plasma to the tissues or sequestration in small vessels, and reversible leukopenia and thrombocytopenia result.[76] With profound hypothermia there is also a reduction of coagulation factors, fibrinogen, and plasminogen. The reduction in coagulation factors is usually great enough to result in bleeding diathesis. Excessive red blood cell transfusion frequently seen in arch surgery coupled with hemodilution may further reduce these factors.[77] Hypofibrinogenemia and occasional elevated fibrin split products seen during profound hypothermia and massive transfusion may complicate the clinical picture.

Management of Patients Who Bleed

The management of patients with excessive hemorrhage after aortic arch surgery can be difficult because of the many variables involved, both surgical and nonsurgical (see Chapter 5). As many surgeons have found, reexploration of these patients is frustrating because often only generalized oozing is found (Table 7-5). Our approach to the patient with

a bleeding aortic arch is based on clinical evaluation in conjunction with a battery of simple laboratory tests that can be rapidly performed; namely prothrombin time (PT), partial thromboplastin time (PTT), fibrinogen, platelet count, and hematocrit. Bleeding is assessed by measuring chest tube drainage from tubes that have been regularly stripped, and also by inspecting the surgical wound.

Evaluation of Bleeding

A complete laboratory coagulation profile should be performed for excessive post-CPB bleeding (Table 7-6). Tests include PT, activated PTT, complete blood count with platelet count, examination of the peripheral smear, fibrinogen and fibrin split products, thrombin or reptilase time, and plasminogen levels.

Adequate protamine reversal of heparin can be assessed by measuring heparin concentration. An increased thrombin time is also seen with residual heparin. Platelet count and peripheral smear will reveal thrombocytopenia. Prolonged PT or activated PTT may indicate a deficiency in the coagulation factors. The clot from reptilase or thrombin time is observed for 5 minutes for evidence of lysis, which along with fibrinogen level and fibrinogen degradation products may give information about primary or secondary fibrinolysis. Euglobin lysis time is a measure of clot lysis in the euglobin fraction of plasma that contains fibrinogen, plasminogen, and plasminogen activator. Increase in plasminogen activator levels will shorten euglobin lysis time (normal, <80 minutes). Template bleeding time (normal, 1–8 minutes) is technically difficult to perform intraoperatively and is probably underused postoperatively. The bleeding time is more predictive of postoperative bleeding than platelet count. However, the test is subject to wide variations and lacks correlation with clinically significant bleeding. The

Table 7-6. Laboratory Evaluation of Postcardiopulmonary Bypass Hemorrhage

Complete blood and platelet count
Blood smear evaluation
Prothrombin time
Activated partial thromboplastin time
Heparin assay (synthetic substrate)
Thrombin time (observe for lysis)
Plasminogen and plasmin assay

utility of tests for platelet aggregation and function is limited by the time required for results.

Laboratory tests of coagulation measure specific coagulation parameters. With hemostatic alterations from CPB, hypothermia, and platelet dysfunction, the test results may be difficult to interpret. An abnormal laboratory test result in patients with adequate hemostasis is not an indication for therapy. Despite limitations of laboratory coagulation tests post-CPB, they may serve as a guide to therapy.

Thromboelastography, first introduced in 1948,[78] has gained interest as an intraoperative coagulation monitor for liver transplantation[79] and cardiac surgery.[80] Thromboelastography is a qualitative viscoelastic measure of clot formation from initial procoagulant activation and fibrin formation through fibrin cross linking and clot retraction to eventual clot lysis. Thromboelastography offers a number of important advantages over routine coagulation tests. It (1) is economical, using a simple reusable machine; (2) is easy to use; (3) is available in the operating room, allowing intraoperative monitoring of coagulation; (4) is highly predictive of postsurgical bleeding; (5) is able to assess heparinization and platelet-protein interaction; (6) is able to easily diagnose fibrinolysis, disseminated intravascular coagulation, and hypercoagulable states; and (7) allows assessment of coagulation factor, fibrinogen, and platelet activity, as well as clot maturation and lysis, all from a single blood sample.

The main disadvantage of thromboelastography is the time required to obtain a complete analysis. Initial evaluation of fibrin formation is available within 12–25 minutes. Platelet function may be assessed from the amplitude of the tracing in another 20 minutes. Evaluation of clot lysis for fibrinolysis requires a variable amount of time.

Thromboelastography, however, has been shown to loosely correlate with various coagulation tests. This lack of significant correlation may exist because coagulation tests examine isolated coagulation factors, whereas thromboelastography examines whole blood coagulation, interaction of the protein coagulation cascade, fibrinogen, and platelet surface.

The sonoclot is a device that uses changes in impedance to assess coagulation.[81,82] A typical tracing consists of the clotting, clot retraction, and clot lysis phases. The tracing is dependent on the number and function of platelets. While the sonoclot tracing is used primarily to assess functional integrity of

platelets, it also may be used to aid in the diagnosis of other coagulation deficits.

Activated Clotting Time. While an elevated activated clotting time (ACT) may indicate inadequate heparin reversal, a normal ACT does not ensure complete heparin neutralization.[83] Although the ACT may be affected by many factors, including severe depletion of intrinsic coagulation factors and severe thrombocytopenia due to insufficient platelet factor III, platelet dysfunction will not elevate the ACT. The ACT is also relatively insensitive to low heparin levels.

If the ACT remains elevated after initial protamine administration, an additional incremental dose of protamine is given. If there is no improvement in the ACT following additional administration of protamine, then the possibilities of excess protamine, fibrinolysis, or coagulation factor deficiency, must be addressed.

Fresh Whole Blood

Fresh whole blood administration is gaining popularity for decreasing blood loss post-CPB. Mohr and colleagues[84] compared the hemostatic effects of transfusion of 1 unit of fresh whole blood and 10 units of platelets. The whole blood group showed an increase in the platelet count equal to 4 units of platelets with normalization of bleeding time. Furthermore, postoperative platelet aggregation to collagen and epinephrine improved after whole blood, but not with platelet concentrates. The 24-hour blood loss was lower in the whole blood group. A recent study in children undergoing open heart surgery showed a significant decrease in postoperative blood loss in patients receiving fresh whole blood.[85] The benefit appears greatest for children less than 2 years of age who have had complex surgery. The difference in blood loss is probably due to better platelet function in fresh whole blood.

Heparin Rebound

Heparin rebound is the reappearance of free heparin after complete protamine neutralization. Proposed etiologies include the longer elimination time of heparin compared with protamine, greater body stores of heparin, incomplete rewarming with delayed heparin release from the tissues, exogenous heparin (heparin flush solutions and pump blood), and reentry of free heparin into the circulation via the lymphatic system.[86]

Heparin rebound is reported to occur in patients post-CPB.[87] Most cases of heparin rebound have been reported to occur within 8–9 hours after initial heparin neutralization, but delayed heparin rebound has been reported as late as 18 hours postoperatively.[88] Ellison et al.[87] demonstrated heparin rebound in all patients who received lower doses (0.56 mg of protamine per 1.00 mg of total heparin administered) of protamine. Others have reported a much lower incidence of heparin rebound (4.5%) without clinical significance.[89]

Whatever its cause, incidence, or clinical significance, heparin rebound is easily treated with additional protamine. Indeed, any diagnostic work-up of post-CPB bleeding should only be undertaken after eliminating heparin rebound.

References

1. Ergin MA, O'Connor J, Guinto R, Griepp R. Experience with hypothermia and circulatory arrest in the treatment of aneurysms of the aortic arch. J Thorac Cardiovasc Surg 1982;84:649.
2. Bailey LL, Takeuchi Y, Williams WG, et al. Surgical management of congenital cardiovascular anomalies with the use of profound hypothermia and circulatory arrest. Analysis of 180 consecutive cases. J Thorac Cardiovasc Surg 1976;71:485.
3. Ergin MA, Griepp RB. Progress in treatment of aneurysms of aortic arch. World J Surg 1980;4:535.
4. Griepp RB, Stenson EB, Hollingsworth JF, Buehler D. Prosthetic replacement of the aortic arch. J Thorac Cardiovasc Surg 1975;70:1051.
5. Mills NL, Everson CT. Atherosclerosis of the ascending aorta and coronary artery bypass: pathology, clinical correlates, and operative management. J Thorac Cardiovasc Surg 1991;102:546.
6. Wareing TH, Davila-Roman VG, Barzilai B, et al. Management of the severely atherosclerotic ascending aorta during cardiac operations: a strategy for detection and treatment. J Thorac Cardiovasc Surg 1992;103:453.
7. Ribakove GH, Katz ES, Galloway AC, et al. Surgical implications of transesophageal echocardiography to grade the atheromatous aortic arch. Ann Thorac Surg 1992;53:758.
8. Crawford ES, Snyder DM. Treatment of aneurysms of the aortic arch. J Thorac Cardiovasc Surg 1983;85:237.
9. Hickey RF, Hoar PF. Whole body oxygen consumption during low-flow hypothermic cardiopulmonary bypass. J Thorac Cardiovasc Surg 1983;86:903.
10. Fox LS, Blackstone MD, Kirklin JW, et al. The relationship of whole body oxygen consumption to perfusion flow rate during hypothermic cardiopulmonary bypass. J Thorac Cardiovasc Surg 1982;83:239.
11. Chopp M, Welch KM, Tidwell CD. Metabolic effect of mild hypothermia on global cerebral ischemia and recirculation in the cat: comparison to normothermia and hypothermia. J Cereb Blood Flow Metab 1989;9:141.
12. Busto R, Dietrich WD, Globus MY, et al. Small differences in intra ischemic brain temperature critically determine the extent of ischemic neuronal injury. J Cereb Blood Flow Metab 1987;7:729.
13. Onesti ST, Baker CJ, Sun PP, Solomon RA. Transient hypothermia reduces focal ischemia brain injury in the rat. Neurosurgery 1991;29:369.
14. Casthely PA, Griepp R, Ergin MA. Anaesthesia for aortic arch aneurysm: our experience with 17 patients. Canadian Anaesthetist's Society Journal 1985;32:73.
15. Minamisawa H, Nordstrom CH, Smith ML. The influence of mild body and brain hypothermia on ischemic brain damage. J Cereb Blood Flow Metab 1990;10:365.
16. Bashein G, Nessly ML, Bledsoe SW, et al. Electroencephalography during surgery with cardiopulmonary bypass and hypothermia. Anesthesiology 1992;76:878.
17. Edmonds HL, Griffiths LK, Van der Laken J, et al. Quantitative electroencephalographic monitoring during myocardial revascularization predicts postoperative disorientation and improves outcome. J Thorac Cardiovasc Surg 1992;103:555.
18. Jobsis FF, Piantadosi CA, Sylvia AL, et al. Near infrared monitoring of cerebral oxygen sufficiency. I. Spectra of cytochrome oxidase. Neurol Res 1988;10:7.
19. Hampson NB, Camporesi EM, Stolp BW, et al. Cerebral oxygen availability by NIR spectroscopy during transient hypoxia in man. J Appl Physiol 1990;69:907.
20. Greeley WJ, Bracey VA, Ungerleider RM, et al. Recovery of cerebral metabolism and mitochondrial oxidation state is delayed after hypothermic circulation arrest. Circulation 1991;84:400.
21. Murkin JM, Farrar JK, Tweed WA. Cerebral autoregulation and flow/metabolism coupling during cardiopulmonary bypass: the influence of $PaCO_2$. Anesth Analg 1987;66:825.
22. Rogers AT, Stump DA, Gravlee GP, et al. Response of cerebral blood flow to phenylephrine infusion during hypothermic cardiopulmonary bypass: influence of $PaCO_2$ management. Anesthesiology 1988;69:547.
23. Brusino FG, Reves JG, Smith LR, et al. The effect of age on cerebral blood flow during hypothermic cardiopulmonary bypass. J Thorac Cardiovasc Surg 1989;97:541.
24. Johnsson P, Messeter K, Ryding E. Cerebral blood flow and autoregulation during hypothermia cardiopulmonary bypass. Ann Thorac Surg 1987;43:386.

25. Bashein G, Toulnes BD, Nessly ML, et al. A randomized study of carbon dioxide management during hypothermia cardiopulmonary bypass. Anesthesiology 1990;72:7.

26. Javid H, Tufo HM, Najafi H, et al. Neurological abnormalities following open-heart surgery. J Thorac Cardiovasc Surg 1968;58:502.

27. McConnell DH, White FN, Nelson RL, et al. Importance of alkalosis in maintenance of "ideal" blood pH during hypothermia. Surg Forum 1975;26:263

28. Swan H. The importance of acid-base management for cardiac and cerebral preservation during open heart operations. Surg Gynecol Obstet 1984;158:391.

29. Poole-Wilson PA, Langer GA. Effect of pH on ionic exchange in rat and rabbit myocardium. Am J Physiol 1975;229:570.

30. Swain JA, White FN, Peter RM. The effect of pH on hypothermic ventricular fibrillation thresholds. J Thorac Cardiovasc Surg 1984;87:445.

31. Gillen JP, Vogel MFX, Holterman RK, et al. Ventricular fibrillation during orotracheal intubation of hypothermic dogs. Ann Emerg Med 1986;15:412.

32. Steen PA, Newberg LA, Milde JH. Cerebral blood flow and neurologic outcome when nimodipine is given after complete cerebral ischemia in the dog. J Cereb Blood Flow Metab 1984;4:82.

33. Lanier WL. Post-ischemic neurologic recovery and cerebral blood flow using a compression model of complete bloodless cerebral ischemia in dogs. Resuscitation 1988;16:271.

34. Lemay ER. Insulin administration protects neurologic function in cerebral ischemia in rats. Stroke 1988;19:411.

35. Lanier WL. Glucose management during cardiopulmonary bypass: cardiovascular and neurologic implications. Anesth Analg 1991;72:423.

36. Metz S, Keats AS. Benefits of a plasma containing solution for cardiopulmonary bypass. Anesth Analg 1991;72:428.

37. Frasco P, Croughwell N, Blumenthal J, et al. Association between blood glucose level during cardiopulmonary bypass and neuropsychiatric outcome. Anesthesiology 1991;75(Suppl):55.

38. Messick J, Milde L. Brain protection. Advances in Anesthesiology 1987;4:47.

39. Krisch JR, Dean JM, Rogers MC. Current concepts in brain resuscitation. Arch Intern Med 1986;146:1413.

40. Altman DI, Young RSK, Yagel SK. Effects of dexamethasone in hypoxic ischemic brain injury in the neonatal rat. Biol Neonate 1984;46:149.

41. Bass E. Cardiopulmonary arrest: pathophysiology and neurologic complications. Ann Intern Med 1985;103:920.

42. Yosiumoto T, Sakamoto T, Watanabe T, et al. Experimental cerebral infarction, part 3: protective effect of mannitol in thalamic infarction in dogs. Stroke 1978;9:217.

43. Yutani C, Imakita M, Ishibashi-Ueda H, et al. Cerebrospinal infarction caused by atheromatous emboli. Acta Pathol Jpn 1985;35:789.

44. Cottrell JE, Robustelli A, Post K, et al. Furosemide and mannitol induced changes in intracranial pressure and serum osmolarity and electrolytes. Anesthesiology 1977;47:28.

45. Nussmeier NA, Arlung C, Slogoff S. Neuropsychological dysfunction after cardiopulmonary bypass: cerebral protection by a barbiturate. J Cardiothorac Vasc Anesth 1991;5:584.

46. Zaidan JR, Klochany A, Martin WA, et al. Effects of thiopental on neurological outcome following coronary artery bypass grafting. Anesthesiology 1991;74:406.

47. Topol EJ, Humphrey LS, Borkon AM, et al. Value of intraoperative left ventricular microbubbles detected by transesophageal two dimensional echocardiography in predicting outcome after cardiac operations. Am J Cardiology 1985;56:773.

48. Baldy MM. Cerebral protection by drugs. Agressologie 1982;23:3.

49. Steen PA, Gisvold SE, Milde JH, et al. Nimodipine improves outcome when given after complete cerebral ischemia in primates. Anesthesiology 1985;62:406.

50. Wauquier A, Ashton D, Clincke G, et al. Calcium entry blockers as cerebral protecting agents comparative activity in tests of hypoxia and hyperexcitability. Jpn J Pharmacol 1985;38:1.

51. Allen GS, Bahr AL. Cerebral arterial spasm: reversal of acute and chronic spasm in dogs with orally administered nifedipine. J Neurosurg 1979;4:43.

52. Cullen JP, Aldrete JA, Jankousky L. Protective action of phenytoin in cerebral ischemia. Anesth Analg 1979;58:165.

53. Astrup J, Moller-Sorensen P, Rahbek-Sorensen H. Inhibition of cerebral oxygen and glucose consumption in the dog by hypothermia, pentobarbital and lidocaine. Anesthesiology 1981;55:263.

54. Wauquier A. Brain protective properties of etomidate and flunarizine. J Cereb Blood Flow Metab 1982;2:53.

55. Tulleken CAF, van Dieren A, Johnkan J, Kalenda Z. Clinical and experimental experience with etomidate as a brain protective agent. J Cereb Blood Flow Metab 1982;2:92.

56. Mills NL, Ochsner JL. Massive air embolism during cardiopulmonary bypass. J Thorac Cardiovasc Surg 1980;80:708.

57. Ueda Y, Miki S, Kusuhara K, et al. Surgical treatment of aneurysm or dissection involving the ascending aorta and aortic arch, utilizing circulatory arrest and retrograde cerebral perfusion. J Cardiovasc Surg 1990;31:553.

58. Kouchoukos N. Adjuncts to reduce the incidence of embolic brain injury during operations on the aortic arch. Ann Thorac Surg 1994;57:243.

59. Takamoto S, Matsuda T, Harada M, et al. Simple hypothermic retrograde cerebral perfusion during aortic arch surgery. J Cardiovasc Surg 1992;33:560.

60. Okamoto H, Sato K, Matsuura A, et al. Selective jugular cannulation for safer retrograde cerebral perfusion. Ann Thorac Surg 1993;55:538.

61. Safi HJ, Brien HW, Winter JN, et al. Brain protection via cerebral retrograde perfusion during aortic arch aneurysm repair. Ann Thorac Surg 1992;53:47.

62. Subramanian S, Wagner H. Correction of transposition of the great vessels in infants under surface induced deep hypothermia. Ann Thorac Surg 1973;16:391.

63. Subramanian S, Wagner H, Vlad P, Lambert E. Surface induced deep hypothermia in cardiac surgery J Pediat Surg 1971;6:612.

64. Stevenson JG, Steone EF, Dillard DH, Morgan BC. Intellectual development of children subjected to prolonged circulatory arrest during hypothermic open heart surgery in infancy. Circulation 1974;49:11.

65. Wright JH, Hicks RG, Newman DC. Deep hypothermic arrest: observations on later development in children. J Thorac Cardiovasc Surg 1979;77:466.

66. Muraoka R, Shirotani H. Open heart surgery in infants and small children utilizing profound hypothermia and limited cardiopulmonary bypass. J Jap Surg Soc 1977;78:1009.

67. Kawashima N. Central nervous system consequences in children from cardiac surgery using simple deep hypothermia and circulatory arrest. Proceedings of the Tenth Anniversary Meeting of Japan Society for Hypothermia 1979;62:64.

68. Svensson LG, Crawford ES, Hess KR, et al. Deep hypothermia with circulatory arrest. Determinants of stroke and early mortality in 656 patients. J Thorac Cardiovasc Surg 1993;106:19.

69. O'Connor JV, Wilding T, Farmer C, et al. The protective effect of profound hypothermia on the canine central nervous system during one hour of circulatory arrest. Ann Thorac Surg 1986;41:255.

70. Rubeyka IM, Coles JG, Wilson GJ, et al. The effect of low-flow cardiopulmonary bypass on cerebral function: an experimental and clinical study. Ann Thorac Surg 1987;43:391.

71. Thompson IR. The Influence of Cardiopulmonary Bypass on Cerebral Physiology and Function. In JH Tinker (ed), Cardiopulmonary Bypass: Current Concepts and Controversies. Philadelphia: Saunders, 1989;21.

72. Kirklin JW, Barratt-Boyes BG. Hypothermia, Circulatory Arrest and Cardiopulmonary Bypass. In JW Kirklin, BG Barratt-Boyes (eds), Cardiac Surgery. New York: Churchill Livingstone, 1988;35.

73. Holmson H, Karpatkin S. Metabolism of Platelets. In WJ Williams, E Beutler, AJ Erslev, et al (eds), Hematology (3rd ed). New York: McGraw-Hill 1983;1157.

74. Aster RH. Thrombocytopenia Due to Sequestration of Platelets. In WJ Williams, E Beutler, AJ Erslev, et al (eds), Hematology (3rd ed). New York: McGraw-Hill 1983;1338.

75. Heyns A. Kinetics and in vivo redistribution of 111 indium-labeled human platelets after intravenous protamine sulfate. Thromb Haemost 1980;44:605.

76. Shenaq S, Childres W. Management of aortic aneurysms. Semin Anesth 1991;10:108.

77. Thomas R, Hessel EA, Harker LA, et al. Platelet function during and after deep surface hypothermia. J Surg Res 1981;31:314.

78. Tuman KJ, Speiss BD, McCarthy RJ, et al. Comparison of viscoelastic measures of coagulation after CPB. Anesth Analg 1989;69:69.

79. Kang YG, Martin DJ, Marquez J, et al. Intraoperative changes in blood coagulation and thromboelastographic monitoring in liver transplantation. Anesth Analg 1985;64:888.

80. Speiss BD, Tuman KJ, McCarthy RJ, et al. Thromboelastography as an indicator of post-cardiopulmonary coagulopathies. J Clin Monit 1987;3:25.

81. vonKaulla KN, Ostendorf P, Von Kaulla E. The impedance machine: a new bedside coagulation recording device. J Med 1975;6:73.

82. Saleem A, Blifeld C, Saleh SA, et al. Viscoelastic measurement of clot formation: a new test of platelet function. Ann Clin Lab Sci 1983;13:115.

83. Gravelee G, Goldsmith J, Low J, et al. Heparin sensitivity comparison of the ACT, SCT, and aPTT. Anesthesiology 1989;71:4.

84. Mohr R, Martinowitz U, Lavee J, et al. The hemostatic effect of transfusion fresh whole blood versus platelet concentrates after cardiac operations. J Thorac Cardiovasc Surg 1988;96:530.

85. Lavee J, Martinowitz U, Mohr R, et al. The effects of transfusion of fresh whole blood versus platelet concentrates after cardiac operations. A scanning microscope study of platelet aggregation on extracellular matrix. J Thorac Cardiovasc Surg 1989;97:204.

86. Schreiner R. Discussion of our experience in regional heparinization by Naskamoto S, Holmes JH. Trans Am Soc Artif Organs 1958;4:36.

87. Ellison N, Beatty CP, Blake DR, et al. Heparin rebound, studies in patients and volunteers. J Thorac Cardiovasc Surg 1974;67:723.

88. Estas JW. Kinetics of the anticoagulant effect of heparin. J Am Med Assoc 1970;212:1492.

89. Esposito RA, Culliford AT, Colvin SB, et al. The role of activated clotting time in heparin administration and neutralization for cardiopulmonary bypass. J Thorac Cardiovasc Surg 1983;85:174.

Chapter 8

Anesthesia for Descending Thoracic Aortic Surgery

Joseph I. Simpson

Mortality following repair of thoracic aortic aneurysms remains at approximately 10%. Morbidity, including spinal cord injury, is significantly higher. Complications associated with descending thoracic aortic surgery include paraplegia, renal ischemia and postoperative renal failure, ischemia and infarction of other end organs (i.e., the bowel), massive blood loss, and death. Anesthetic management of descending thoracic aortic surgery requires a level of expertise and skill above that usually required for management of nonvascular thoracic surgery. In addition to the usual modalities of one-lung ventilation and invasive and noninvasive hemodynamic monitoring, one must be familiar with the indications and uses of temporary shunting, management of partial bypass, management of left-heart bypass, and protection from end-organ damage (most notably protection of the spinal cord in avoiding permanent ischemic injury).

Pathology

Descending thoracic aortic surgery may be indicated for a variety of lesions. Most commonly, descending thoracic surgery is performed for repair of aneurysmal dilatation of the descending thoracic aorta. Causes of the aneurysmal dilatation of the descending thoracic aorta include artherosclerotic disease, connective tissue disease, and aortitis. Aortitis may be secondary to inflammatory origins, infective origins, or both.[1]

Aside from aneurysmal disease of the aorta, two other types of disease present for surgical correction. The first is acute or chronic aortic dissection. The etiology of aortic dissection most commonly is involvement of the aorta in a generalized connective tissue disease. Marfan's syndrome is frequently associated with descending thoracic dissection.[2] Aortic dissection may also occur as a result of traumatic injury to the aorta. The "deceleration type injury" frequently seen at the aortic isthmus can lead to aortic disruption including transection and dissection of the descending thoracic aorta. Acute transection or disruption of the descending thoracic aorta secondary to deceleration-type injury is an indication for emergency repair of the descending thoracic aorta. A more complete discussion of aortic pathology and classification of aortic dissection is presented in Chapter 1 (Figure 8-1).

Thoracic aortic disease may also extend into the abdominal aorta, and thoracoabdominal disease is not uncommon (Figure 8-2). The implications of thoracoabdominal aortic surgery depend somewhat on the location of the disease process. The higher the lesion in the thoracic aorta, the more such surgery is likely to follow the pattern of thoracic aortic surgery. The lower the lesion, the more likely such surgery is to follow the pattern of abdominal aortic surgery (see Figure 8-2). In either case the issues of spinal cord ischemia, renal ischemia, bowel ischemia, and hemodynamic consequences of cross clamping apply.

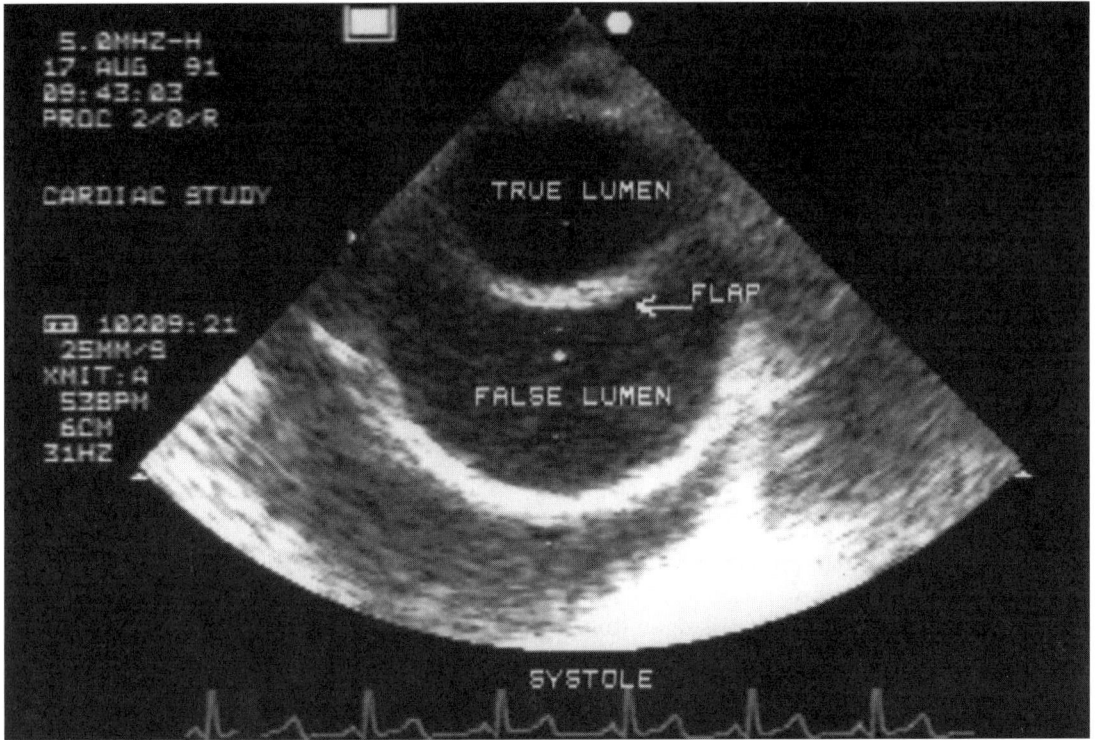

A

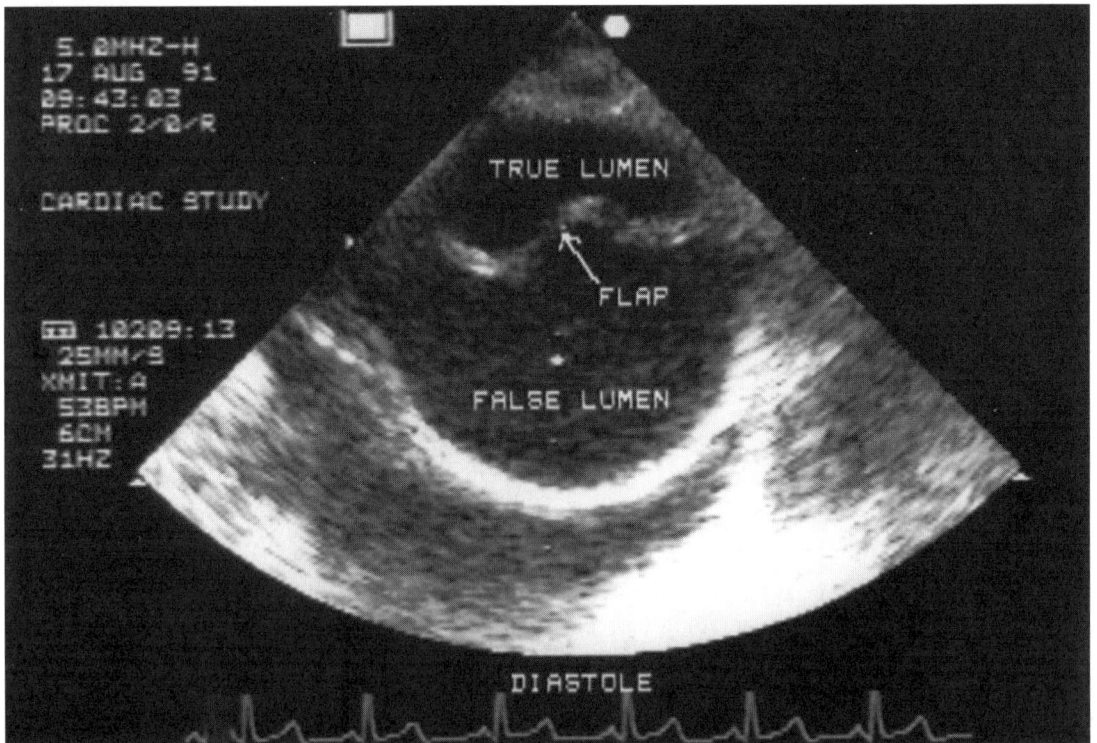

B

Figure 8-1. Transesophageal echocardiographic image of a dissecting aortic aneurysm in the descending thoracic aorta. A. Systole. B. Diastole. C. M-mode showing the movement of the intimal flap.

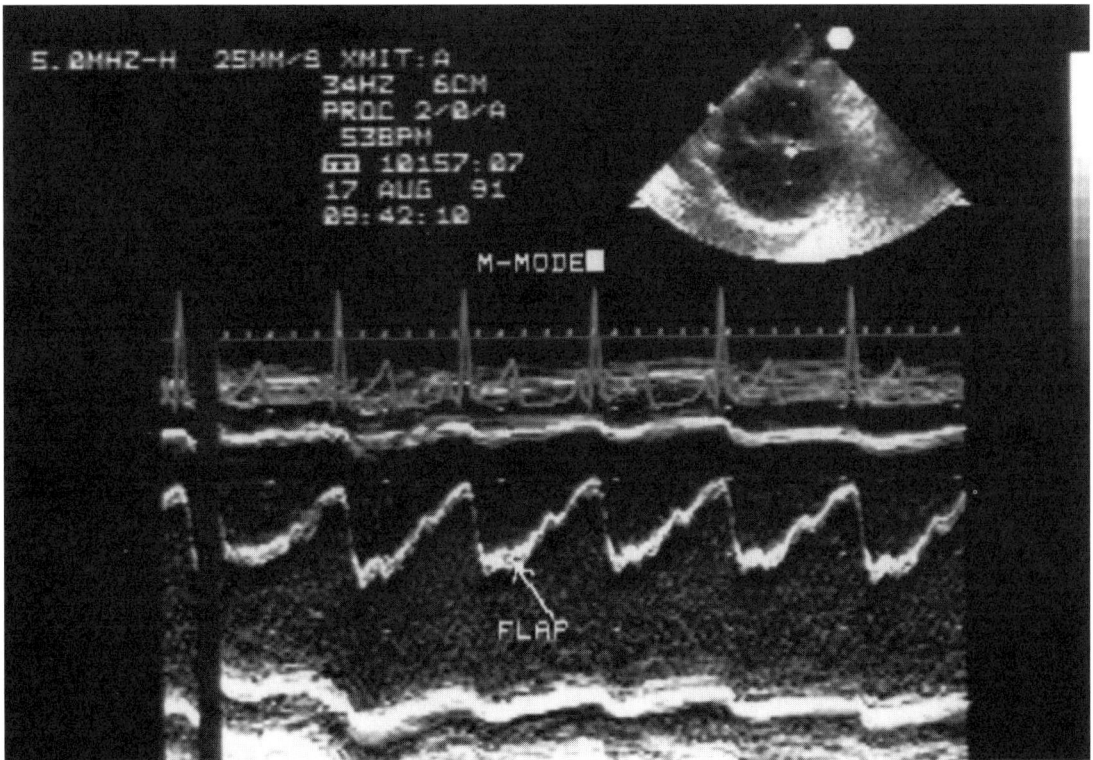

C

Consequences of Cross Clamping the Descending Thoracic Aorta

The most striking response to cross clamping the descending thoracic aorta is an acute increase in systemic vascular resistance or afterload.[3–5] The most commonly explained reason for this increase in systemic vascular resistance is the increase in impedance to aortic blood flow. In addition, filling pressures usually increase. Blood flow to the area the body supplied above the cross clamp will increase. However, this increase occurs in greater proportion than the effect of decreasing the flow distal to the cross clamp.[6] This is a result of the redistribution of blood flow. The mechanism involved in this redistribution is not entirely clear; however, it may involve differences in blood volume present in the splanchnic circulation. This effective volume redistribution is not present during infraceliac aortic cross clamping. This apparently occurs because of the greater shift of blood volume into the splanchnic circulation during infraceliac cross clamping.

Therefore, the effect on venous return to the heart and preload depends on the level of the aortic cross clamp. During high aortic cross clamping (i.e., supraceliac cross clamping) the more common effect is an increase in preload. Again, the most likely mechanism for this increase in preload is volume redistribution to areas of the body supplied proximal to the cross clamp. However, with low aortic cross clamping (i.e., infraceliac cross clamping) this redistribution occurs in the splanchnic circulation and does not involve an increase in left ventricular preload.[7] Blood flow distal to the aortic cross clamp clearly decreases. This involves a decrease in perfusion to all organs that receive their blood supply from parts of the aorta that are distal to the cross clamp (Figure 8-3).

Cardiac output usually decreases in response to aortic cross clamping.[5,8,9] However, this decrease in cardiac output may be attenuated by the use of an intravenous vasodilator[9,10] (Figure 8-4 and Table 8-1).

Management of this increased afterload and proximal blood pressure (BP) remains controver-

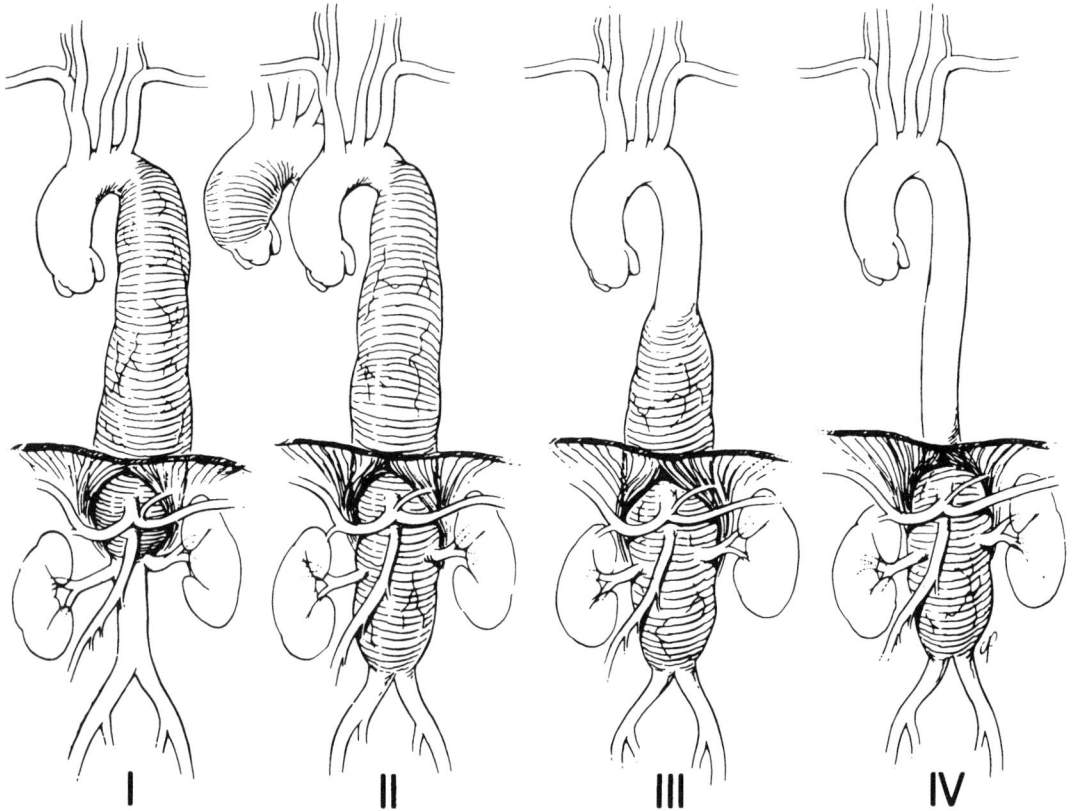

Figure 8-2. Crawford classification of thoracoabdominal aortic aneurysms. Type I extends from the proximal descending thoracic aorta to the upper abdominal aorta, but terminates before the renal arteries. Type II extends below the renal arteries. Type III begins in the distal half of the descending thoracic aorta and extends for a variable length into the abdomen. Type IV involves most of or the entire abdominal aorta. (Reprinted with permission from LG Svensson, ES Crawford. Aortic dissection and aortic aneurysm surgery: clinical observations, experimental investigations and statistical analyses. Part II. Curr Probl Surg 1992;29:923.)

sial. Many suggest the use of vasodilators such as nitroglycerin, nitroprusside, or trimethaphan. However, the use of vasodilators has been implicated in the potential increased incidence in the development of spinal cord ischemia (see the section on prevention of spinal cord ischemia). Others recommended the use of various shunts or partial bypass. The idea is to remove blood from areas proximal to the aortic cross clamp and shunt them to areas distal to the aortic cross clamp. This not only improves the increased afterload seen with aortic cross clamping, it also provides blood flow and tissue oxygenation to areas distal to the aortic cross clamp, thus helping prevent ischemia to major organ systems that are supplied distal to the aortic cross clamp. This

is discussed more fully in the section on spinal cord ischemia.

The increased preload and afterload seen with high aortic cross clamping requires an increase in myocardial contractility. In patients who are unable to mount this increased contractility, aortic cross clamping may be associated with hemodynamic decompensation. Coronary blood flow increases with high aortic cross clamping.[11,12] This can be further increased by the use of nitroglycerin.[11] However, in the presence of coronary disease, this increased coronary blood flow may not be enough to make up for the increased myocardial oxygen demand. Because coronary perfusion pressure is inversely related to left ventricular preload, coronary perfusion may decrease because of

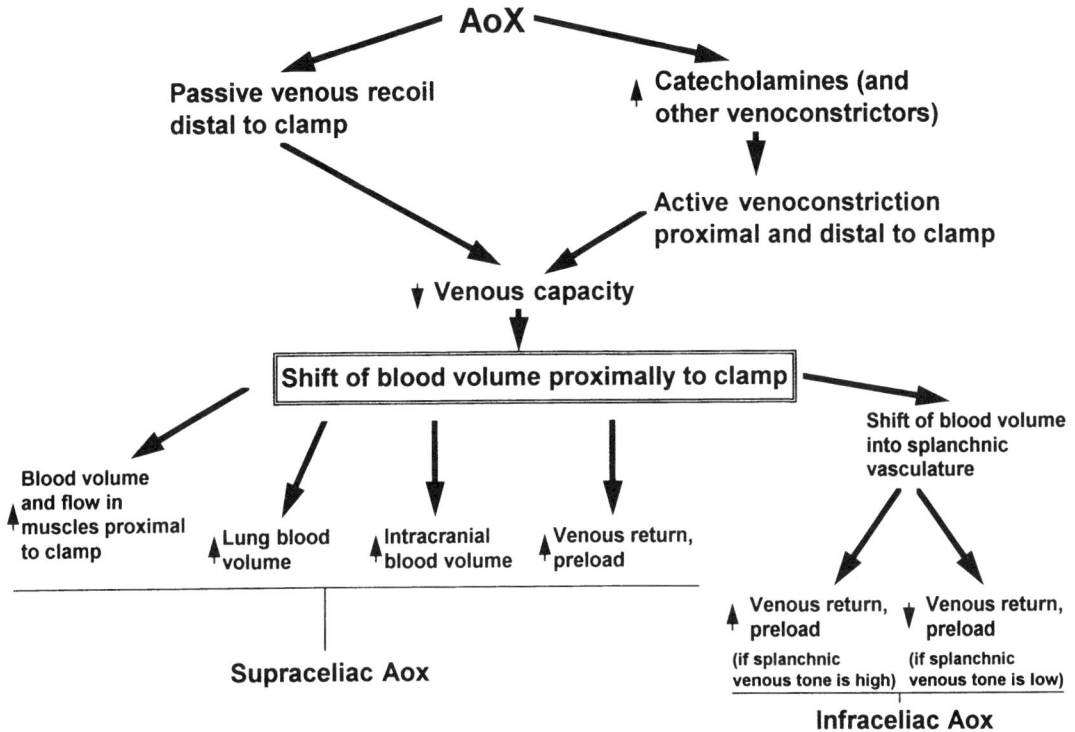

Figure 8-3. Blood volume redistribution during aortic cross clamping. This scheme depicts the reason for the decrease in venous capacity, which results in blood volume redistribution from the vasculature distal to the aortic cross clamp to the vasculature proximal to the aortic cross clamp. If the aorta is clamped above the splanchnic system, the blood volume travels to the heart, increasing preload and blood volume in all organs and tissues proximal to the clamp. However, if the aorta is clamped below the splanchnic system, blood volume may shift into the splanchnic system or into the vasculature of other tissues proximal to the clamp. The distribution of this blood volume between the splanchnic and nonsplanchnic vasculature determines changes in preload. (AoX = aortic cross clamping; ↑ and ↓ = increase and decrease, respectively.) (Reprinted with permission from S Gelman. Aortic cross-clamping and unclamping. Anesthesiology 1995;82:1026.)

the increase in preload seen with high thoracic aortic cross clamping. The use of vasodilators has been shown to improve myocardial function in patients undergoing high aortic cross clamping. This may be secondary to decreased afterload, decreased preload, and improved coronary blood flow caused by these vasodilators[4,10]

Longer duration of aortic cross clamping results in a further increase in systemic vascular resistance and a further decrease in cardiac output.[4,13] Using transesophageal echocardiography (TEE), Roizen et al. demonstrated that supraceliac cross clamping produced substantial increases in left ventricular, systolic, and diastolic areas with decreased ejection fractions. This occurred despite the administration of vasodilators. A high incidence of regional wall motion abnormalities was observed, suggesting the possibility of for myocardial ischemia. This was in contrast to infrarenal aortic cross clamping (see Figure 8-4).[8]

Management of Aortic Cross Clamping

Use of Vasodilators

Perhaps the most commonly used vasodilator to control proximal hypertension seen with thoracic aortic cross clamping is sodium nitroprusside. Sodium nitroprusside functions as a direct arterial dilator and reduces the increased afterload seen with thoracic aortic cross clamping. Sodium nitroprusside also decreases the preload increases that are seen with high thoracic aortic cross clamping.

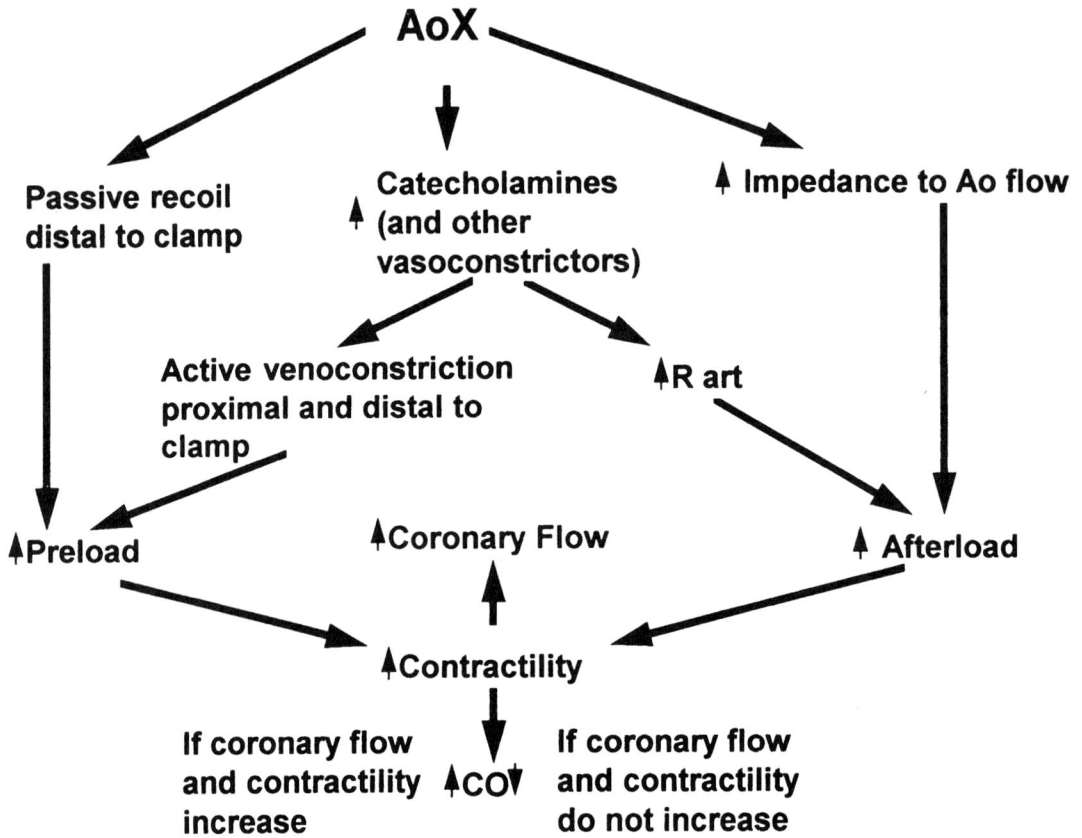

Figure 8-4. Systemic hemodynamic response to aortic cross clamping. Preload does not necessarily increase. If during infrarenal aortic cross clamping, blood volume shifts into the splanchnic vasculature, preload does not increase. (AoX = aortic cross clamping; Ao = aortic; R art = arterial resistance; $\uparrow$ and $\downarrow$ = increase and decrease, respectively; CO = cardiac output.) (Reprinted with permission from S Gelman. Aortic cross clamping and unclamping. Anesthesiology 1995;82:1026.)

Small doses of beta-adrenergic blocking agents, such as esmolol or labetalol, can be used to control heart rate and lower the dose requirement of nitroprusside. However, the use of sodium nitroprusside has been implicated in causing an increased incidence of paraplegia and spinal cord ischemia (see the section on prevention of spinal cord ischemia). Sodium nitroprusside, in addition to decreasing systemic vascular resistance, also causes vasodilatation in the cerebral vasculature. This increases cerebrospinal fluid (CSF) pressure. Sodium nitroprusside will also further decrease BP distal to the aortic cross clamp. The combination of these two mechanisms may further decrease the perfusion of the spinal cord.

Isoflurane has been used as a vasodilator to control the proximal hypertension seen with thoracic aortic cross clamping. Although isoflurane can be an effective vasodilator in this setting, the negative inotropic properties of the large doses of isoflurane that are needed may not be tolerated in patients who have preexisting coronary disease, myocardial dysfunction, or both. Additionally, this negative inotropy may not allow the ventricle to adequately compensate for the increased afterload seen with the aortic cross clamp. Isoflurane may add another potential beneficial effect in that it can help protect the spinal cord from spinal cord ischemia.[14]

Nitroglycerin has been used to decrease the afterload in patients undergoing thoracic aortic cross clamping. In addition to decreasing afterload, nitroglycerin decreases preload, which may improve coronary perfusion pressure and decrease the incidence of myocardial ischemia during tho-

Table 8-1. Hemodynamic Changes During Thoracic Aortic Cross Clamping in Animals

Author	Date	Species	Proximal Mean Arterial Pressure	Distal Mean Arterial Pressure	Left Ventricular End-Diastolic Pressure	Cardiac Output/Left Ventricular Contractility	Superior Vena Cava Flow	Inferior Vena Cava Flow
Stokland	1980	Dogs	↑↑	↓↓	↑	NC	↑	↓
Gelman	1988	Pigs	↑↑	↓↓	—	↑/NC	↑	↓
Gregoretti	1990	Dogs	↑↑	—	—	NC	↑	↓
Brusoni	1978	Dogs	↑↑	—	—	NC	—	—
Symbas	1983	Dogs	↑↑	↓↓	—	NC	—	—
Kien	1987	Dogs	↑↑	↓↓	↑	NC	—	—
Shine	1990	Dogs	↑↑	↓↓	—	NC	—	—
Katsamouris	1988	Dogs	↑↑	↓↓	NC	NC	—	—
Roberts	1983	Dogs	↑↑	—	↑	↓	—	—
Gelman	1983	Dogs	↑↑	↓↓	—	↓	—	—

↑ = increased; ↓ = decreased; ↑↑ = increased greatly; ↓↓ = decreased greatly; NC = no change; — = not assessed.
Source: Modified from KJ Tuman. Anesthetic considerations for descending thoracic aortic surgery: part II. J Cardiothorac Vasc Anesth 1995;9:734.

racic aortic cross clamping. However, nitroglycerin itself may not be adequate to treat the huge increase in proximal BP seen with thoracic aortic cross clamping. Additionally, nitroglycerin may further worsen spinal cord perfusion pressure and the incidence of paraplegia.[15]

Perfusing the Aorta Distal to the Cross Clamp

Maintaining perfusion distal to the cross clamp has two advantages. The first advantage is that it decreases the proximal hypertension and its attendant effects on the cardiovascular system during thoracic aortic cross clamping. The second advantage is an increase in perfusion below the cross clamp, potentially avoiding ischemia to various organ systems that are perfused distal to the aortic cross clamp. Perfusion distal to the cross clamp has traditionally been provided by one of the following three means (Figure 8-5 and Table 8-2):

1. The first technique is to insert a fixed shunt between the aorta proximal to the cross clamp and the aorta distal to the cross clamp. The most common shunt used is the Gott shunt. When using the Gott shunt, the proximal end of the shunt can be placed in the ascending aorta, aortic arch, left subclavian artery, or proximal descending aorta. However, if the proximal end of the shunt is put into the left subclavian artery, a subclavian steal phenome-

non may occur, causing flow reversal in the vertebral arteries. This may further decrease flow to the anterior spinal artery, because much of the upper part of anterior spinal artery blood flow is derived from the vertebral arteries. Therefore, the left subclavian artery is the least advisable place to position the proximal end of the Gott shunt.

2. The second most common method of providing perfusion to the aorta distal to the aortic cross clamp is the use of femoral venous-to-femoral arterial bypass. Blood is drained from the femoral vein, passed through an extracorporeal oxygenator, and pumped back into the femoral artery. This provides a continuous oxygenated blood supply to the area of the body distal to the aortic cross clamp. Additionally, this provides decreased preload, thus controlling the hypertensive response to aortic cross clamping. An added advantage of this technique is the ability to control the rate of flow (i.e., the rate of blood removal from the femoral venous system), thus allowing for decreases in circulating blood volume secondary to bleeding during repair of the thoracic aorta. Additionally, there is the ability to use the pump suction so that most of the shed blood can be returned to the cardiopulmonary bypass circuit and reinfused into the femoral artery. A major disadvantage of this method is the need for systemic heparinization and anticoagulation. This increases bleeding and may increase transfusion requirements. Additionally, all of the effects of cardiopul-

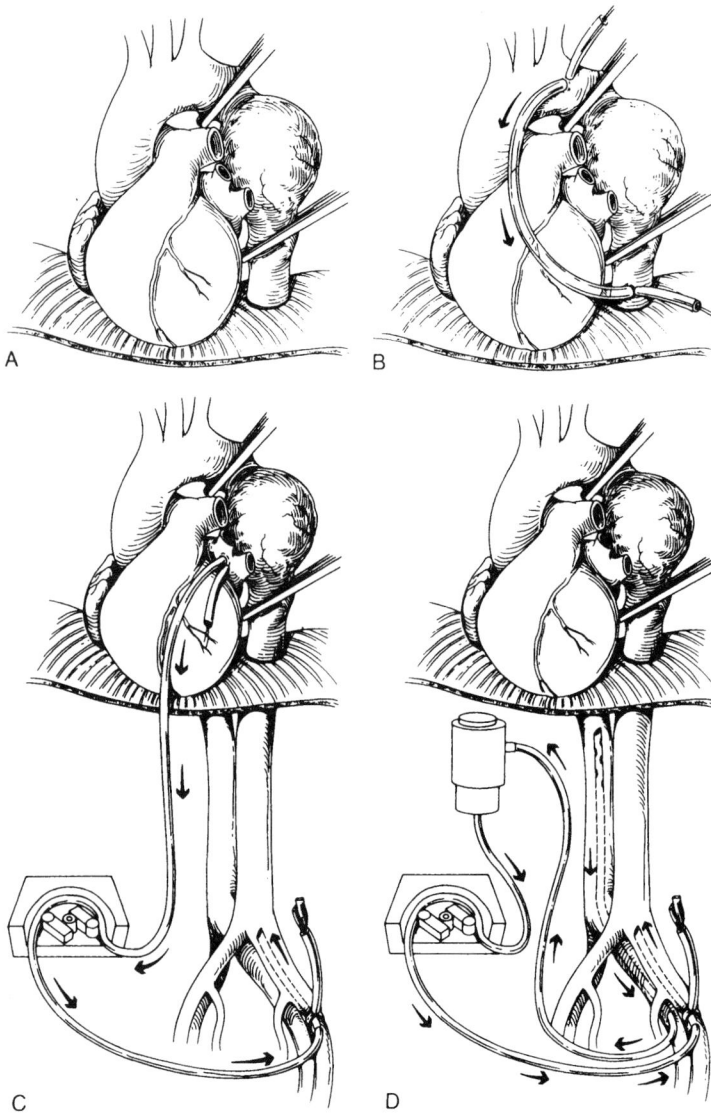

Figure 8-5. A. Simple cross clamping of the descending thoracic aorta. B. Aneurysm exclusion with a passive Gott shunt from the aortic arch to the distal descending thoracic aorta. C. Left atriofemoral by-pass with pump. D. Femoral-femoral bypass using a pump oxygenator. (Reprinted with permission from J Ochsnor, N Ancalmo. Descending thoracic aortic aneurysms. Chest Surg Clin North Am 1992;2:291.)

monary bypass on the coagulation system are present (see Chapter 5).

3. The third way of providing distal perfusion is via a left atrial–to–femoral artery pump. This is a closed system that does not use an oxygenator or reservoir. Blood is withdrawn from the left atrium and reinfused into the femoral artery. As with partial femoral-femoral bypass, the rate of blood flow to the femoral artery can be controlled. That is, in periods of increased blood loss and decreased blood volume, the amount of blood shunted from the left atrium to the femoral artery can be decreased;

whereas in periods of relative hypervolemia, the amount of blood shunted from the left atrium to the femoral artery can be increased. The proximal hypertension is controlled by the amount of blood withdrawn from the left atrium. This system does not require systemic heparinization. Instead, the system uses heparin-bonded tubing. Additionally, blood is not exposed to a reservoir bag and oxygenator, thus the effect of the extracorporeal system on platelets and other formed elements in the blood is greatly minimized. A potential disadvantage of this system is the need for continuous low-level

Table 8-2. Advantages and Disadvantages of Distal Perfusion Techniques

Advantages
    Control of proximal hypertension
    Reduction of visceral and renal ischemia
    Prevention of acidosis and declamping shock
    Ability to rapidly warm patients
    Access for rapid volume infusion
    Reduced incidence of paraplegia?
Disadvantages
    Air emboli or embolic stroke
    Increased operative time
    Potential for excess hemorrhage with anticoagulation
    Shunt dislodgement

Source: Modified from KJ Tuman. Anesthetic considerations for descending thoracic aortic surgery: part II. J Cardiothorac Vasc Anesth 1995;9:734.

pumping even in times of relative hypovolemia. This is necessary to prevent blood clotting in the tubing since systemic heparinization is not used.

Unclamping the Thoracic Aorta

Unclamping the thoracic aorta is associated with hypotension, decreased systemic vascular resistance, decreased cardiac output, and decreased preload.[3,12,16,17] These changes are much more profound in patients who did not have a shunting procedure to shunt blood to the distal aorta during the period of aortic cross clamping. The severity of these changes varies with the duration of aortic cross clamping, the level of the cross clamp, and the residual influence of vasodilators, beta-adrenergic antagonists, and inhaled anesthetics. Arterial pH usually decreases and pulmonary vascular resistance and pulmonary artery pressures usually increase. Causes for these hemodynamic effects are multifactorial.

Reactive hyperremia plays a large role in the hypotensive response seen with aortic unclamping. This reactive hyperremia is present secondary to maximal vasodilatation below the clamp during the period of relative ischemia.[18] In addition to reactive hyperremia, the influence of ischemic metabolites released from the underperfused tissues on myocardial contraction can play an important role.[18] Acidosis released from the ischemic bed causes further decreases in myocardial contractility and may increase systemic vasodilatation seen following tho-

racic aortic cross-clamp removal. Visceral ischemia may create increased permeability in the interstitium of the intestine. This may allow for release of bacterial endotoxins into the portal circulation and may in part account for some of the vasodilatation seen during aortic unclamping (Figure 8-6).[19]

Management of Aortic Unclamping

Volume loading prior to unclamping the thoracic aorta has been shown to decrease the hypotensive response to aortic unclamping. Maintaining a pulmonary capillary wedge pressure of 16–18 mm Hg before unclamping has been shown to obviate the decrease in preload seen with unclamping. One must be careful to discontinue vasodilator infusions and inhalational anesthetics several minutes before unclamping the thoracic aorta. However, turning off the inhalational anesthetic prior to declamping may cause an unwanted lightening of anesthesia with hypertension and tachycardia. Additionally, removal of the inhalational agent takes time and may be difficult to titrate during the period of aortic declamping. Acidosis immediately after unclamping should be treated with sodium bicarbonate. If acidosis is present before unclamping, it should be treated with sodium bicarbonate because additional acidosis will surely develop after the aortic cross clamp is removed.

In spite of volume loading and decreasing the vasodilator infusions prior to unclamping, hypotension will usually occur. This hypotension, however, may not be as severe as it would have been had the previously mentioned maneuvers not been taken. This hypotension should be treated carefully with vasopressors. One must be careful not to overshoot and cause even momentary episodes of hypertension, as this may compromise vascular anastamosis on the aorta. The physician must also be cognizant of the fact that suture line bleeding may necessitate the reapplication of the aortic cross clamp shortly after its release. If hypotension is treated too vigorously, severe hypertension may occur on reapplication of the aortic cross clamp.

The effects of declamping the thoracic aorta are significantly decreased when one uses partial bypass or shunting during the cross clamp period. This may be secondary to the fact that reactive hyperremia does not develop during shunting or may de-

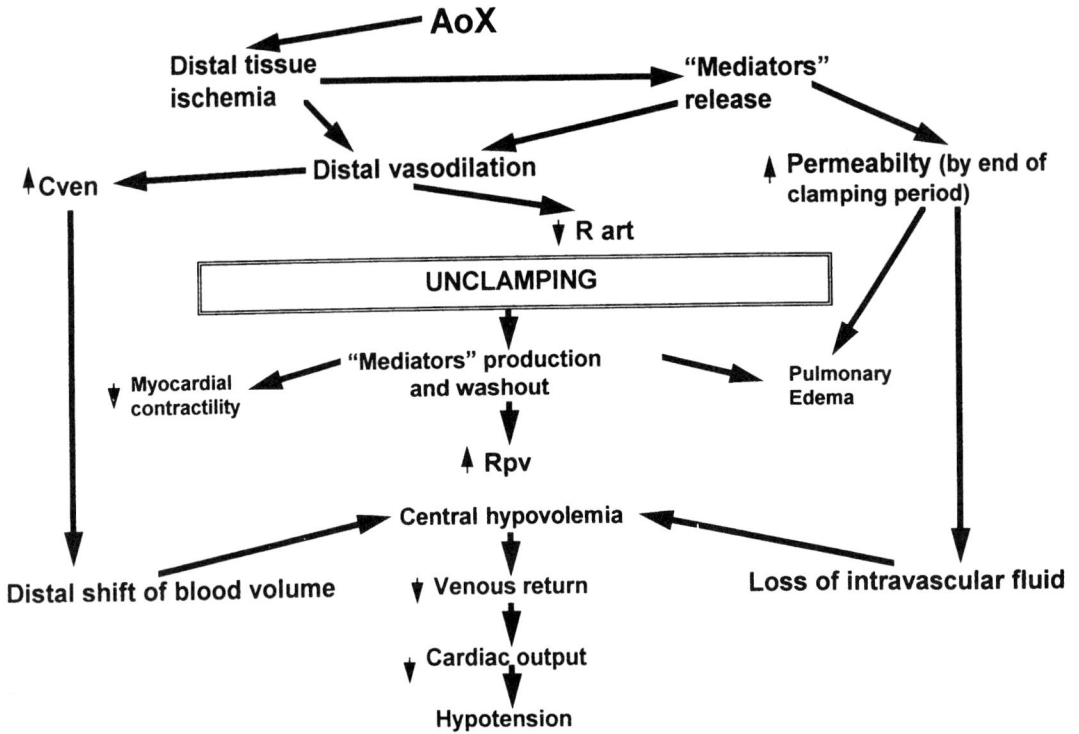

Figure 8-6. Systemic hemodynamic response to aortic unclamping. (AoX = aortic cross clamping; Cven = venous capacitance; R art = arterial resistance; Rpv = pulmonary vascular resistance; ↑ and ↓ = increase and decrease, respectively.) (Reprinted with permission from S Gelman. Aortic cross-clamping and unclamping. Anesthesiology 1995;82:1026.)

velop to a much smaller degree. Additionally, washout of ischemic factors may not occur as the area below the clamp remains perfused during most of the cross clamp period. Nevertheless, in spite of all of these factors, some degree of hypotension is present following cross clamp removal, even when partial shunting or partial bypass is used during cross clamp application.

Anesthetic Management for Descending Thoracic Aortic Surgery

Monitoring

Basic monitoring for descending thoracic aortic surgery should include an arterial line. As discussed previously, BP control during the period of thoracic aortic cross clamping and declamping necessitates minute-to-minute and beat-to-beat

availability of BP measurement. Additionally, one must always remember the possibility of acute rapid blood loss in a setting of descending thoracic aortic surgery, again making the presence of an arterial line mandatory. Ideally, the arterial cannulae should be placed in the right radial artery. This is true because, during cross clamping of the descending thoracic aorta, especially if the cross clamp is placed high, blood flow to the left radial artery may be compromised by the cross clamp. In addition to the radial artery catheter, many prefer to use a femoral artery catheter as well. This is mandatory in cases in which shunting is used. This is so because during the shunting procedure, whether shunting with a Gott shunt, a left atrial-to-femoral artery pump, or partial femoral-femoral bypass, there is no way to assess the distal perfusion pressure without the femoral artery catheter (or another distal source of continuous pressure measurement).

Pulmonary artery catheter monitoring is an important adjunct during this type of surgery. As discussed previously, significant hemodynamic changes occur on both cross clamp application and cross clamp removal. Additionally, myocardial dysfunction, including myocardial failure and myocardial ischemia, may occur during this period of time. The need to use vasoactive drugs, both vasodilators and vasopressors, during this procedure will be easier with the presence of a pulmonary artery catheter. However, since this surgery is usually performed through a left thoracotomy with one-lung anesthesia and collapse of the left lung, it is important to make sure that the tip of the pulmonary artery catheter is in the right main pulmonary artery.

Recently, TEE has been used during descending thoracic aortic surgery. TEE can be helpful in the estimation of left ventricular preload as well as in diagnosing ischemia by the onset of new regional wall motion abnormalities. TEE may also be helpful in managing postclamp hypotension. TEE may be useful in the initial diagnosis of the extent of a thoracic aortic dissection (see Figure 8-1). Confirmation of preoperative diagnosis and identification of true and false lumen can all be aided by the use of TEE.

CSF pressure monitoring by the use of a spinal catheter may be useful in an attempt to prevent paraplegia by maintaining an increased level of spinal cord perfusion pressure (see the section on prevention of spinal cord ischemia).

Temperature monitoring is critically important in descending thoracic aortic surgery. Massive volume shifts and blood loss with large transfusion requirements frequently cause hypothermia. While this hypothermia may have some benefit during the period of aortic cross clamping vis-à-vis spinal cord and renal ischemia (see the section on prevention of spinal cord ischemia), post–cross clamp release hypothermia can be a considerable problem vis-à-vis coagulation (see Chapter 5).

Induction of Anesthesia

The major hemodynamic goals during induction of anesthesia for descending thoracic aortic surgery are the avoidance of tachycardia, hypertension, and increased dp/dt. This is important in attempting to avoid aneurysm rupture or propagation of an existing dissection. Frequently, patients with descending thoracic aortic pathology also have coronary and cerebral vascular pathology; therefore, hypotension needs to be avoided as well. A high-dose opioid technique, with its lack of cardiovascular depression, seems best suited for these procedures. As is the case with surgery on the ascending and aortic arch, choice of anesthetic medications is primarily related to the presence of coexisting disease and myocardial function. However, enflurane should probably be avoided because it is known to cause increased CSF production and may further aggravate spinal cord ischemia during the period of aortic cross clamping.[20]

One-Lung Anesthesia

Surgery on the descending thoracic aorta is usually performed through the left chest. Consequently, one-lung anesthesia is frequently required. A double-lumen endotracheal tube is usually inserted on induction. One must remember that this tube needs to be changed at the end of the procedure to a single-lumen tube if the patient is to remain intubated. If a difficult intubation is anticipated, the single-lumen Univent (Fuji Systems, Japan) tube with the built-in bronchial blocker may be useful. Use of the Univent tube obviates the need for endotracheal tube change at the end of the procedure. A potential difficulty may occur during placement of the left-sided endobronchial tube. This may be because the left main stem bronchus can be displaced by a large descending thoracic aortic aneurysm. When placement of the left endobronchial tube is difficult, the fiberoptic bronchoscope may be helpful. There have been rare case reports of massive fatal hemorrhage occurring during placement of a left-sided endobronchial tube secondary to aneurysm erosion into the left main stem bronchus.

Prevention of Spinal Cord Ischemia

The most devastating complication following surgery on the descending thoracic and thoracoabdominal aorta is paraplegia. The reported incidence of this complication continues to be high and ranges from 1–40%.[21–23] Cross clamp time has been shown to be related to the incidence of paraplegia, with the incidence markedly increasing with cross clamp times greater than 30 minutes (Figure 8-7).[24] The incidence

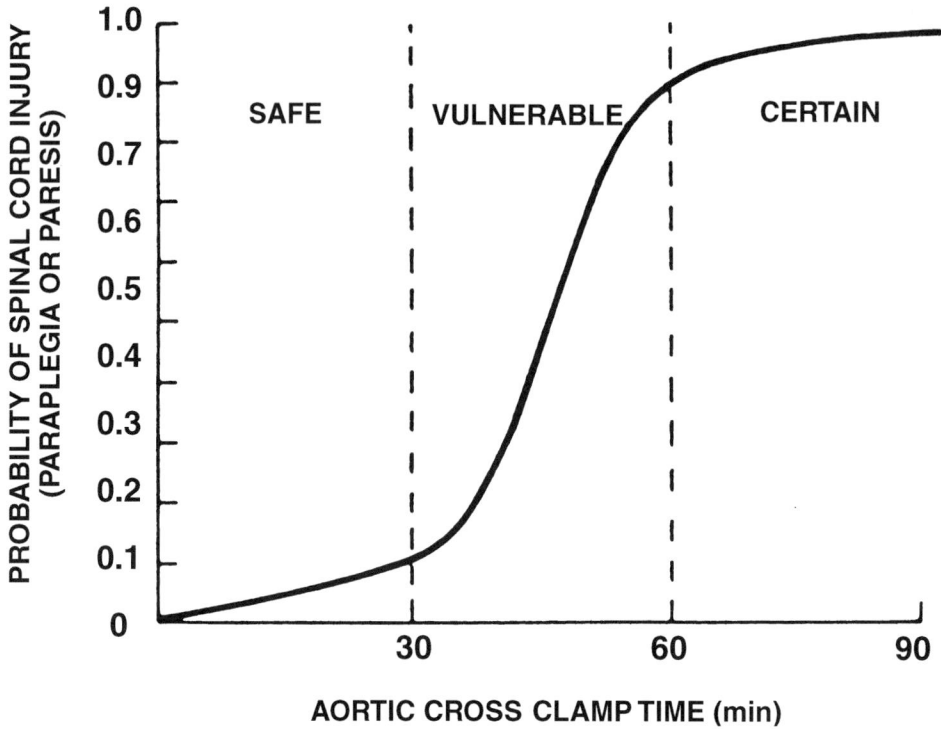

Figure 8-7. Relationships of duration of aortic cross clamping in high-risk patients to probability of spinal cord injury. (Reprinted with permission from LG Svensson, FD Loop. Prevention of Spinal Cord Ischemia in Aortic Surgery. In JJ Bergan, JST Yao [eds], Arterial Surgery: New Diagnostic and Operative Techniques. New York: Grune & Stratton, 1988;273.)

of paraplegia is also higher in patients greater than 70 years old, during emergency surgery, and in those patients with large dissecting aneurysms.[24] Clinically, the injury that occurs is similar to that seen in anterior spinal artery syndrome, after occlusion of the arteria radicularis magna anterior (the artery of Adamkiewicz). Motor function and pin-prick sensation are lost while vibratory sensation and position sensation are maintained.

Blood Supply to the Spinal Cord

The spinal cord is supplied by two posterior spinal arteries and one anterior spinal artery. The anterior spinal artery supplies at least 75% of the cord, leaving only 25% or less to be supplied by the posterior spinal arteries. The cervical part of the anterior spinal artery is primarily supplied by branches of the vertebral arteries (Figure 8-8). This part of the ante-

rior spinal artery circulation is usually well preserved and protected during thoracic aortic cross clamping. The lumbosacral part of the anterior spinal artery is supplied by branches from the internal iliac arteries. The remainder of the anterior spinal artery blood flow is supplied by six to eight radicular arteries, which are branches of the intercostal arteries. The largest radicular artery supplying the anterior spinal artery is the artery of Adamkiewicz. The posterior spinal artery is supplied by 10–20 radicular arteries.

The origin of the artery of Adamkiewicz is variable. This artery can originate from any level between T5 and L3. In 15% of patients, the artery arises between T5 and T8. In 60% of patients, the artery arises between T9 and T12; and in 14% of patients, the artery arises at L1 with the remainder arising between L2 and L3.

During clamping of the descending thoracic aorta, blood supply to the anterior spinal artery can

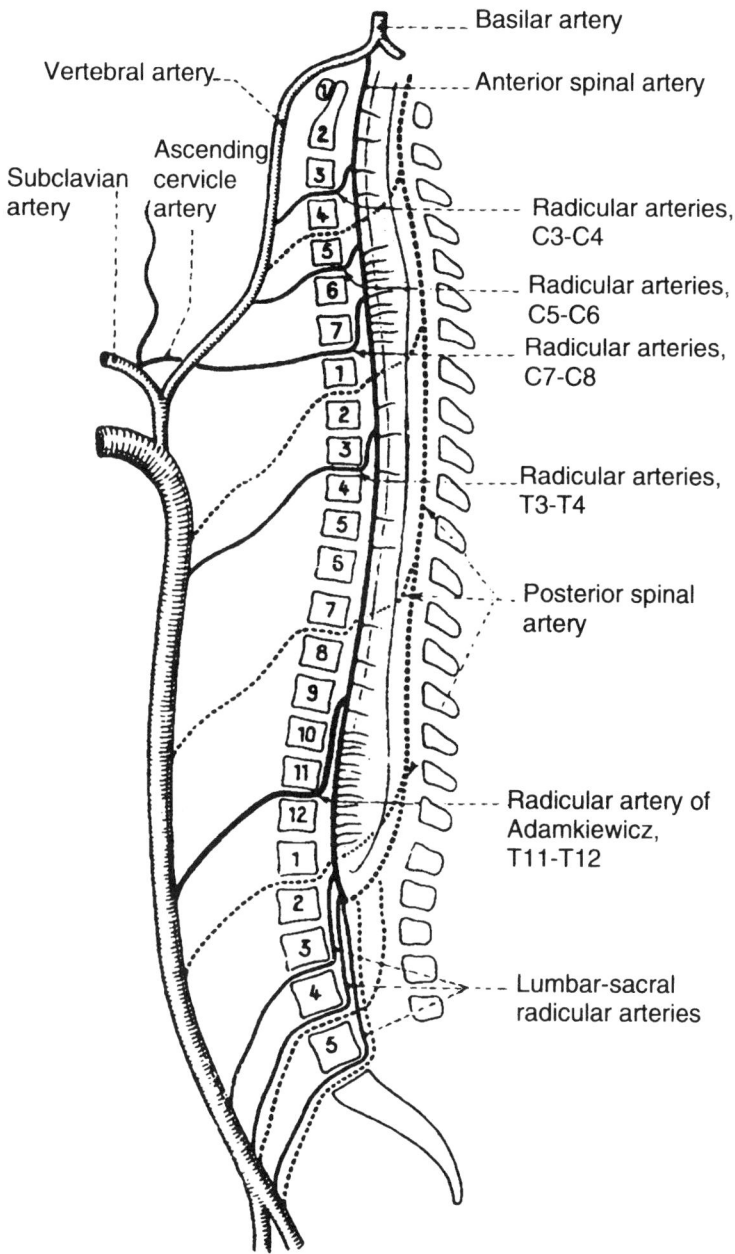

Figure 8-8. Diagram of the blood supply of the spinal cord showing the anterior and posterior radiculomedullary branches seen in a lateral view. (Modified from R Djindjian. Arteriography of the spinal cord. AJR Am J Roentgenol 1969;107:461.)

be significantly decreased. If the artery of Adamkiewicz branches off the part of the aorta that is being replaced, or if the origin of the artery of Adamkiewicz lies distal to the proximal aortic cross clamp, then blood supply to the anterior spinal artery will significantly decrease. Collateral blood supply to the spinal cord at this level is ex-

tremely poor. Ischemia can occur either from permanent exclusion of the artery of Adamkiewicz from the graft or from temporary exclusion of the artery of Adamkiewicz (during the cross clamp period) from the circulation. Late ischemia can occur in patients who have had the artery of Adamkiewicz or its origin resected and who have

Table 8-3. Incidence of Paraplegia and Renal Failure Related to Cross Clamp Time

Time (Minutes)	Paraplegia (Percentage)	Renal Failure (Percentage)
0–15	0	0
16–30	3.5	4.2
31–45	10.0	7.8
46–60	12.5	6.3
>60	25.0	0

Source: Modified from JJ Livesay, DA Cooley, RA Ventemiglia, et al. Surgical experience in descending thoracic aneurysmectomy with and without adjuncts to avoid ischemia. Ann Thorac Surg 1984;39:37.

marginal, pressure-dependent collateral circulation. This can occur during periods of hypotension in the postoperative period (Table 8-3).

Monitoring for the Onset of Spinal Cord Ischemia

Somatosensory Evoked Potential

Laschinger et al. demonstrated that the use of somatosensory evoked potentials (SSEPs) can accurately predict injury to the spinal cord.[25,26] The idea is that if a change is seen on the SSEP, a search can be made for the artery of Adamkiewicz or another radicular artery supplying the anterior spinal artery at that level and those radicular arteries can be re-anastomosed to the graft. Alternatively, a distal shunt or partial bypass procedure can be used to supply blood flow distal to the aortic cross clamp. This use of SSEP monitoring is also advocated by other authors.[27,28]

The use of SSEP monitoring does, however, have its drawbacks. First, SSEPs measure conduction primarily through the posterior spinal cord. Most of the posterior part of the spinal cord is supplied by the posterior spinal arteries. The posterior part of the cord is not the most likely to become ischemic during cross clamping of the descending thoracic aorta. The use of SSEP monitoring in this setting relies on ischemia produced in the most lateral portions of the posterior columns that are supplied by the "watershed" area between the posterior and anterior spinal artery

circulations. Second, SSEPs can be affected by external factors such as general inhalational anesthetics, as well as temperature and other drugs given to the patient (see Chapter 4). Not surprisingly there have been several case reports of the development of paraplegia following thoracic aortic cross clamping in spite of maintaining normal SSEPs.[29,30] Crawford et al.[31] demonstrated that SSEP monitoring had no significant impact on prevention of neurologic deficits.

Motor evoked potentials monitor the anterior segment of the cord and the area of the cord supplied by the anterior spinal artery. Laschinger et al.[32] demonstrated that motor evoked potentials in dogs are an accurate predictor of ischemic injury to the anterior part of the spinal cord. Svensson et al. demonstrated motor evoked potentials to be an accurate predictor in identifying segmental arteries supplying the anterior spinal artery.[33] However, Reuter et al. showed that motor evoked potentials may be too sensitive a monitor, in that they may demonstrate abnormal motor evoked potentials in spite of a normal clinical result in a dog model.[34] Unfortunately, the use of motor evoked potentials at present remains cumbersome and difficult in the operating room setting.

Spinal Cord Perfusion Pressure

Perfusion pressure to the anterior part of the spinal cord is the arterial pressure in the anterior spinal artery minus the venous pressure in the spinal venous plexus. From a practical point of view, these measurements are impossible to obtain. Therefore, spinal cord perfusion pressure can be estimated as the distal aortic pressure, which is the pressure distal to the aortic cross clamp, minus the CSF pressure. The arterial pressure distal to the aortic cross clamp is the pressure available to the arteries feeding the anterior spinal artery in the area below the clamp, and thus should approximate anterior spinal artery pressure supplying that area of the cord. CSF pressure should approximate the venous plexus pressure of the spinal cord. On application of the thoracic aortic cross clamp, the distal aortic pressure, which is the pressure distal to the aortic cross clamp, drops markedly, and the CSF pressure increases.[35]

Several authors have shown in various animal models that the level of spinal cord perfusion pressure, calculated as the distal mean arterial pressure minus the CSF pressure, correlates with the incidence of paraplegia following thoracic aortic cross clamping. Grubbs et al.,[36] in a canine model, demonstrated that the minimum level of spinal cord perfusion pressure needed to prevent paraplegia is 11 mm Hg. In a human study, Maeda et al.[37] demonstrated that 40 mm Hg is the minimum spinal cord perfusion pressure necessary to prevent paraplegia. Similarly, Berendes et al.[38] demonstrated a low spinal cord perfusion pressure to be related to a higher incidence of paraplegia. Dasmahapatra et al.[39] demonstrated a direct relationship between spinal cord perfusion pressure and paraplegia as well.

Prevention of Spinal Cord Injury

Distal Perfusion

Improving spinal cord perfusion pressure by increasing perfusion pressure in the aorta distal to the aortic cross clamp has been advocated by many as a method to prevent paraplegia (Table 8-4). The mechanics of increasing the distal perfusion are less important than the fact that distal perfusion allows for maintenance of a much higher distal aortic BP. As discussed earlier, this distal perfusion may come from the Gott shunt, partial bypass, or left atrial-to-femoral artery pump flow.[40,41] The advantages and disadvantages of the various methods of perfusion were discussed in the section on management of aortic cross clamping. However, one must remember that distal shunting alone may not be enough to protect the spinal cord. This may be because the blood supply to the anterior spinal artery may be present between the aortic cross clamps, i.e., between the proximal and distal aortic clamp. Increasing BP distal to the distal clamp will not affect blood flow in between the clamps. Additionally, if the major collateral circulation to the anterior spinal artery is in the area of the aorta that is being replaced and no reimplantation of collateral circulation occurs, then spinal cord ischemia can occur regardless of the spinal cord perfusion pressure during the procedure.

Weimann et al. and others have demonstrated successful completion of thoracic aortic aneurysm

Table 8-4. Prevention of Paraplegia During Descending Thoracic Aneurysm Repair

Blood flow enhancement
Shunts and bypasses
Cerebrospinal fluid drainage
Improvement in spinal cord perfusion pressure
Monitoring spinal cord ischemia
Somatosensory evoked potentials
Motor evoked potentials
Hypothermia
Systemic
Local (to spinal cord)
Drugs
Sodium thiopental
Naloxone
Corticosteroids
Oxygen radical scavengers
Localization of the blood supply of the spinal cord
Angiographic
Hydrogen-induced current impulse
Intrathecal drugs?

Source: Modified from S Shenaq, L Svensson. Paraplegia following aortic surgery. J Cardiothorac Vasc Anesth 1993;7:81.

surgery without the occurrence of paraplegia in patients who were not shunted at all.[42] Others have recommended progressive movement of the clamp with intermittent partial surgical repair of the aortic aneurysm for maximal segmental aortic perfusion throughout the procedure.[43]

Reimplantation of Intercostal Arteries

Radiographic identification of the spinal cord blood supply is possible prior to aortic surgery. Identification of the artery of Adamkiewicz by radiologic means in the preoperative period would aid the surgeon in knowing which radicular artery to reimplant into the graft, thus decreasing the incidence of paraplegia.[44] Unfortunately, the radiologic procedure itself may be complicated by paraplegia as a result of injury to the intercostal supply of the anterior spinal artery. There is, however, evidence that reimplantation of large collateral intercostal vessels to the new aortic graft does decrease the incidence of paraplegia.[35,45] Recently, a new method was developed for intraoperative identification of the intercostal arteries that contribute to the anterior spinal cord blood flow. This involves injecting hydrogen-saturated saline into the ostia of the intercostal arteries within the aneurysm. An intrathecal platinum electrode can then detect a current that is applied to the intercostal artery, thus better identifying the intercostal arteries that have the greatest impact on blood flow to the anterior spinal artery.[35,45] However, Lowell et al., in an animal model, showed that selective shunting through intercostal arteries did not prevent spinal cord ischemia during thoracic aortic cross clamping.[46]

Cerebrospinal Fluid Drainage

As discussed earlier, thoracic aortic cross clamping causes a large increase in CSF pressure. The mechanism for this increase in CSF pressure is not entirely understood, but is probably due in part to the increased blood flow to areas of the central nervous system that are supplied from the aorta proximal to the proximal aortic cross clamp. This increase in CSF pressure has a negative impact on spinal cord perfusion pressure. Several authors have recommended CSF drainage to attenuate this increase in CSF pressure and improve spinal cord perfusion pressure. Nevertheless, the use of CSF drainage remains controversial.[47,48] In a dog study, Bower and coworkers demonstrated that CSF drainage during thoracic aortic occlusion maintained spinal cord perfusion above critical levels, diminished reperfusion hyperemia, and improved neurologic outcome.[49] Similarly, Woloszyn et al.[50] demonstrated that CSF drainage in combination with steroids provided protection during thoracic aortic cross clamping, whereas steroids without CSF drainage did not. McCullough and coworkers[51] also demonstrated CSF drainage to be useful in preventing paraplegia in a dog model. However, in a prospective study on humans, Crawford et al. were not able to demonstrate any benefit of CSF drainage in preventing paraplegia.[52] Similarly, Murray and colleagues[53] were unable to demonstrate improved outcome with the use of CSF drainage.

CSF drainage may not be protective because the calculation of spinal cord perfusion pressure is only an estimation. It does not take into account local regional factors such as regional vascular resistance, as well as the possibility of other collateral flow. Additionally, decreasing CSF pressure alone may not change venous pressure in the cord. Risks of CSF drainage include those related to the

placement of the catheter, including nerve injury and epidural hematoma, and the possibility of herniation when large amounts of CSF are rapidly removed. However, there have been no reports in the literature of these complications occurring in patients who are having CSF drainage for thoracic aortic surgery.

Use of Sodium Nitroprusside

Sodium nitroprusside has been used to decrease the proximal arterial hypertension that is present during thoracic aortic cross clamping. However, the use of sodium nitroprusside in this setting has been associated with an increase in CSF pressure and a decrease in distal aortic BP, with consequent worsening of spinal cord perfusion pressure. Several studies have shown that the use of sodium nitroprusside leads to an increased incidence of paraplegia. Marini and colleagues[54] and, more recently, Cernaianu and colleagues[55] have shown in the dog model that sodium nitroprusside increases CSF pressure, decreases spinal cord perfusion pressure, and increases the incidence of ischemia. Ryan et al.[56] have shown that sodium nitroprusside, when used to control proximal hypertension, produced a worse neurologic outcome as compared with when esmolol was used to control hypertension in a dog model. Similarly, Clark and coworkers have shown that when nitroprusside is combined with isoflurane for the control of hypertension, there are significant increases in CSF pressure and consequent decreases in spinal cord perfusion pressure.[57] Woloszyn et al.[58] have shown that the increase in the incidence of neurologic injury seen with sodium nitroprusside is not reversible with the use of CSF drainage.

Berendes and colleagues have reported a case of a patient undergoing coarctation repair with a large increase in CSF pressure occurring on administration of nitroprusside.[59] This patient was paraplegic after the surgery, in spite of the fact that coarctation repair rarely leads to paraplegia.

Pharmacologic Intervention

Free radical scavenging or the decrease in production of free radicals can theoretically prevent some of the injury seen in ischemic neural tissue that occurs during reperfusion. Agee and colleagues[60] have shown in a rabbit model that the use of superoxide dismutase increases the tolerance of the spinal cord to ischemia. Similarly, Kirshner et al.[61] have shown that superoxide dismutase when used in combination with barbiturates and hypothermia significantly improves neurologic outcome following thoracic aortic cross clamping in an animal model. Qayumi and colleagues have shown in a swine model of thoracic aortic cross clamping, where the spinal cords were exposed to 30 minutes of ischemia, that superoxide dismutase significantly improved neurologic outcome.[62] Francel et al. showed that the use of 21-aminosteroid (a free radical scavenger)[63] decreased CSF pressure during thoracic aortic cross clamping and improved neurologic outcome. It was not clear whether the effect on neurologic outcome was primarily due to the lower CSF pressure or to the free radical scavenging properties of the drug.

Intrathecal papaverine has been shown in an animal model to protect against paraplegia seen with thoracic aortic cross clamping. Svensson et al.[64] looked at 11 patients undergoing descending thoracic or thoracoabdominal aortic surgery where intrathecal papaverine resulted in a low incidence of paraplegia.

CSF levels of beta-endorphin increase during spinal cord ischemia. Intrathecal opioids have been shown to decrease spinal blood flow and depress firing of neurons.[65] Naloxone has been shown to improve neurologic recovery from spinal cord ischemia. Following trauma, naloxone has been shown to improve spinal cord blood flow.[66] When CSF drainage and naloxone are combined, the incidence of neurologic outcome following thoracic aortic cross clamping decreases.[67]

Barbiturates are known to protect the central nervous system from focal ischemia.[68] Barbiturates may protect the spinal cord by decreasing spinal cord metabolism during the period of spinal cord ischemia. However, once again, barbiturates would not be expected to be of any assistance if blood flow to the spinal cord remains diminished after aneurysm repair owing to exclusion of the spinal cord collateral circulation from the graft. Barbiturates have been shown to protect the spinal cord in a dog model.[69] However, when barbiturates were compared with isoflurane in a dog model, no benefit of the use of barbiturates was found.[70]

Spinal cord ischemia can result in the release of excitatory amino acid neurotransmitters.[71,72] Glutamate and aspartate are two of these excitatory amino

neurotransmitters. They bind to various amino acid receptors including N-methyl-D-aspartate receptors (NMDA), which are abundant in the spinal cord. When these receptors are stimulated by excitatory amino acid neurotransmitters, calcium and sodium channels are opened and calcium and sodium enter the cell.[73] Blocking these NMDA receptors has been shown to decrease central nervous system ischemic injury. MK-801, an NMDA receptor antagonist, has been shown to prevent the hypersensitivity induced by spinal cord ischemia in the rat[74] and rabbit.[75] Propentofylline, a drug that is known to inhibit glutamate release, has been shown to improve the incidence of paraplegia in a rabbit model of spinal cord ischemia. However, when given before ischemia, the drug did not improve the incidence of paraplegia. When given after ischemia, the drug had a significant effect on the incidence of paraplegia. This suggests that perhaps the neuroprotective effect of this drug is not related to decreased glutamate release, but rather some unknown mechanism.[76] Simpson et al. have shown that intrathecal magnesium prevents spinal cord ischemia in a canine model. The mechanism for this protection is unclear, but may involve modulation of the NMDA receptor. The NMDA receptor is known to have a magnesium gate on it, and increasing intrathecal magnesium levels may decrease the amount of calcium flow through the NMDA receptor.[77]

The use of steroids for spinal cord protection remains controversial. Laschinger and coworkers[78] have shown that the use of steroids is protective in a canine model of spinal cord ischemia. It is thought that the protective effect of steroids may be related to their ability to scavenge free radicals and stabilize membranes, particularly lysosomal membranes. This is further supported by the recent finding that the use of steroids in traumatic spinal cord injury improves patient outcome.

Choice of Anesthetic Agents and Their Influence on Spinal Cord Ischemia

Enflurane has been shown to increase CSF production and decrease the rate of removal of CSF in the central nervous system.[79] Enflurane should therefore be avoided in these cases. The use of isoflurane, on the other hand, may be beneficial. Isoflurane is known to provide cerebral protection during hypoxia. Additionally, in an animal model of thoracic aortic cross clamping, the use of isoflurane was shown to decrease the incidence of spinal cord ischemia.[14]

Ketamine has weak NMDA antagonist effects. Therefore, its use may seem beneficial from the point of view of spinal cord ischemia. However, the use of ketamine, and its attendant cardiovascular effects in the setting of thoracic aneurysm or dissection, can be problematic. The hypertension and tachycardia frequently seen with the use of intravenous ketamine can prove deleterious to the aneurysm and dissection.

Use of Other Vasodilators

As discussed previously, the use of sodium nitroprusside for the control of proximal hypertension during thoracic aortic cross clamping has been shown to be associated with an increased incidence of spinal cord ischemia and paraplegia. In a canine model of thoracic aortic cross clamping, Simpson et al. have shown that nitroglycerin similarly increases CSF pressure and decreases spinal cord perfusion pressure. The incidence of paraplegia was no different between the nitroglycerin group and a sodium nitroprusside group.[15] On the other hand, the use of trimethaphan has been shown by Simpson et al. not to be associated with decreased spinal cord perfusion pressure; and, in fact, when trimethephan was compared with sodium nitroprusside, the incidence of spinal cord ischemia was significantly decreased.[80]

Hypothermia

Hypothermia is known to protect central nervous system tissue from ischemic injury. In an animal study of whole body hypothermia, Naslund et al. demonstrated significant protection of the spinal cord from ischemia during aortic clamping by the use of whole body hypothermia to 30°C.[81] Vacanti reported that a reduction in temperature of 3°C doubled the duration of tolerance to spinal cord ischemia in a rabbit model.[82] If partial bypass is used for shunting blood from the proximal to the distal aorta (see previous section on Management of Aortic Cross Clamping), then a heater/cooler could be added to the pump circuit so that systemic blood going to the lower half of the body can be cooled. Alternatively, the patient's temperature may be allowed to drift down several degrees. This will

occur if the ambient temperature in the operating room is cooled and no attempt is made to actively warm the patient. Conversely, if inadvertent heating (i.e., overaggressive attempt at maintaining patient temperature) results in an actual increase in patient temperature, then increased spinal cord metabolism may occur with an attendant increased incidence in paraplegia. Crawford and Sade[83] reported three cases of children whose temperature was allowed to rise to 39°C during aortic coarctation repair who all suffered paraplegia, paraplegia being an extremely uncommon complication of aortic coarctation repair.

Hypothermia does, however, have its negative aspects. Even mild hypothermia to 34°C has been shown to affect the coagulation system. This may be especially deleterious in the setting of thoracic aortic surgery where massive bleeding and transfusion are common. Additionally, if cardiopulmonary bypass is not used, cooling is often difficult to control and the temperature may rapidly drift down to levels at which it is difficult to warm the patient. This may result in prolongation of anesthetic effect as well as prolongation of muscle relaxant effect. If the patient is allowed to become too cold (i.e., below 30°C), the danger of ventricular arrythmias will arise.

As an alternative to whole body cooling, several authors have attempted selective cooling of the spinal cord during thoracic aortic surgery. Wisselink et al.[84] have shown that circulating normal saline at a temperature of 2°C through the CSF of a dog produced a significant improvement in the incidence of paraplegia. Vanicky et al.[85] have shown that in rabbits, the use of epidural cooling solutions (5°C isotonic saline) caused significant cooling of the spinal cord, and there was a significant protective effect vis-à-vis spinal cord ischemia. This was again confirmed by Berguer et al.[86] in a dog model with subarachnoid infusion of cold saline. More recently, Davidson and colleagues infused ice saline into the epidural space of eight patients undergoing resection of thoracoabdominal aneurysms. None of the patients developed postoperative neurologic injury. Ice saline solution at 4°C in the epidural space produced CSF temperatures of 25°C.[87] One of the potential downsides of such a technique is the potential for increased CSF pressure secondary to the cold solution being infused either into the epidural or subarachnoid space.

Table 8-5. Glucose Loading Versus Paraplegia

Infusion (5% Dextrose in Water) Over 90 Minutes (17 ml/kg/hour)	
Serum glucose	
Control	137 ± 13
Experiment	177 ± 38
Paraplegia	
Control	3:10
Experiment	9:10

Source: Modified from JC Drummond, SS Moore. The influence of dextrose administration on neurologic outcome after temporary spinal cord ischemia in the rabbit. Anesthesiology 1989;70:64.

Alternative Nutrition Sources for the Spinal Cord

Recently, Maughan et al.[88] demonstrated that intrathecal perfusion of an oxgenated perfluorocarbon emuslion prevented paraplegia during aortic cross clamping in a dog model. While this has not yet been done in humans, this represents an exciting area of further study (see Table 8-4).

Hyperglycemia

Several studies have addressed the issue of increased blood glucose levels in cerebral ischemia.[89] In a rabbit model of spinal cord ischemia, Drummond et al. demonstrated that intravenous glucose infusion worsened the incidence of paraplegia.[90] Therefore, glucose levels should be vigorously controlled during thoracic aortic cross clamping and serum glucose should be below 150 mg per dl prior to aortic cross clamp application. Hemmila et al. also demonstrated that glucose given after an ischemic injury to the spinal cord worsens neurologic outcome.[91] Thus, it would seem prudent for strict and tight glucose control to continue after aortic cross clamp removal. This may be particularly difficult given the fact that following cross-clamp removal the patient may be receiving infusions of various inotropic and catecholamine-like drugs, which are all known to increase serum glucose. Therefore, serum glucose needs to be followed closely and treated with insulin as necessary (Table 8-5).

Renal Protection

Prolonged aortic cross clamping may lead to ischemia-induced renal failure following descending thoracic aortic surgery. The incidence of renal failure after thoracic aortic surgery is between 3% and 14%.[92] The incidence of renal injury is directly related to the cross clamp time. Where the cross clamp time is greater than 30 minutes, the incidence of renal injury significantly increases (see Table 8-3). The use of a shunting procedure, partial bypass, or left atrial femoral artery bypass has been shown to decrease the incidence of renal failure following thoracic aortic surgery.[43] As is the case with spinal cord perfusion pressure, the use of sodium nitroprusside has been shown to decrease renal perfusion pressure in the setting of thoracic aortic cross clamping.[93] Cross clamping of the thoracic aorta causes a decreased renal blood flow, decreased glomerular filtration rate, and decreased urine output.[94] Unclamping the thoracic aorta is associated with a prolonged continued decrease in both renal blood flow and glomerular filtration rate.[94,95] This may occur because of activation of the renin-angiotensin system causing renal vasoconstriction during thoracic aortic cross clamping. Pretreatment with an angiotensin-converting enzyme inhibitor prevents the decreases in glomerular filtration rate and renal blood flow that are seen after cross clamp release.[95] Aside from activation of the renin-angiotensin system, the sympathetic nervous system is activated during thoracic aortic cross clamping. Activation of the sympathetic nervous system can further decrease blood flow to the kidney.

The use of mannitol and loop diuretics has been recommended by some in an attempt to decrease the incidence of renal failure after thoracic aortic cross clamping. Mannitol causes an osmotic diuresis and may help in preserving renal blood flow. Mannitol also causes decreased blood viscosity, which may cause diminished renin release and therefore diminished renal vasoconstriction.[60,96]

Some authors have recommended the use of low-dose dopamine (i.e., 3 µg/kg/minute) in addition to diuretic therapy to further promote renal vasodilitation and increase renal blood flow.[97]

The most important maneuver that can be done to avoid renal failure following thoracic aortic cross clamping is the adequate maintenance of intravascular volume, particularly before and after aortic

Table 8-6. Methods of Renal Protection During Descending Thoracic Aortic Surgery

Maintenance of intravascular volume
Minimization of aortic cross-clamp time
Avoidance of distal hypotension during aortic clamping
Atriofemoral bypass
"Low-dose" dopamine
Mannitol
Furosemide
Superoxide dismutase

Source: Modified from KJ Tuman. Anesthetic considerations for descending thoracic aortic surgery: part II. J Cardiothorac Vasc Anesth 1995;9:734.

cross clamp release. Maintenance of adequate intravascular volume has been shown to increase renal blood flow. Renal failure in a setting of thoracic aortic surgery carries a mortality of up to 40%. Therefore, preservation of renal function is an important aspect of the anesthetic management of these patients (Table 8-6).

Pulmonary Injury Following Thoracic Aortic Surgery

Postoperative respiratory failure in the setting of thoracic aortic aneurysm repair can be a life-threatening complication. Svensson et al. demonstrated an 8% incidence of pulmonary complications requiring prolonged respiratory support and tracheotomy following thoracic aortic surgery.[98] Fifty percent of these patients died in the hospital.

During thoracic aortic cross clamping, pulmonary vascular resistance is increased. This increase in pulmonary vascular resistance remains even after clamp removal.[99] The mechanism for the increased pulmonary vascular resistance during thoracic aortic cross clamping is probably secondary at least in part to the increased blood flow to the pulmonary circulation. The mechanism for increased pulmonary vascular resistance following thoracic aortic cross unclamping is not clear. Tissue ischemia generates thromboxane, which has been shown to increase pulmonary artery pressure. In contrast, infusion of prostaglandin E_1 has been shown to decrease pulmonary vascular resistance in the period of time following thoracic unclamping. Furthermore, the prevention of thromboxane for-

mation led to a low level of pulmonary hypertension and prevention of sequestration of leukocytes in the lung.

An additional mechanism that may be responsible for this pulmonary injury is the generation of oxygen free radicals by ischemic tissue. In an animal model, superoxide dismutase caused a decreased level of pulmonary vascular resistance increase after unclamping of the thoracic aorta.[100] Aside from the increase in pulmonary vascular resistance seen after unclamping of the thoracic aorta, there is an increase in pulmonary vascular permeability. This may lead to pulmonary edema in the face of low left ventricular filling pressures.

The use of mannitol has been advocated by some because it interferes with the effect of thromboxane on platelets and neutrophils. Additionally, mannitol has some weak activity in terms of oxygen free radicals.

Blood Loss and Transfusion During Thoracic Aortic Surgery

Surgery on the thoracic aorta is frequently accompanied by massive blood loss. Although the aorta is cross clamped above and below, opening the aneurysm sac exposes several intercostal arterial bleeders that are often difficult to control. Frequently bleeding is so massive that is difficult to keep up with the blood loss. It is difficult for the surgeon to clamp these vessels and they frequently need to be oversewn, which increases the incidence of spinal cord ischemia, as discussed previously. In preparation for this massive blood loss, the patient should have several large-bore intravenous lines placed prior to the procedure. Additionally, a cell saver should be available with rapid processing capabilities, so that shed blood can be reinfused as rapidly as possible. Frequently, 8–12 units of packed red blood cells as well as fresh frozen plasma and platelets are required. Rapid infusion systems, such as the Level One Auto Transfuser (Level One Technologies, Rockland, MA) should be available. Care must taken to avoid significant hypothermia (i.e., below 30°C), which can occur with massive and rapid transfusion. While some hypothermia may be beneficial in terms of renal and spinal cord protection (see above), profound hypothermia or hypothermia below 30°C can be associated with ventricular irritability as well as significant coagulation abnormalities in the setting of vascular bleeding.

Coagulopathy may develop in the setting of descending thoracic aortic surgery. This may be occur secondary to massive blood loss and transfusion. This may also occur secondary to hypothermia. Rarely, fibrinolysis and disseminated intravascular coagulation may develop secondary to the cycle of massive transfusion, hypothermia, and hypotension. Some of the problems associated with massive rapid transfusion in this setting may include metabolic acidosis, hyperkalemia, and citrate-induced hypocalcemia. See Chapter 5 for a more complete discussion of these issues.

References

1. Svensson LG, Crawford ES. Aortic dissection and aortic aneurysm surgery: clinical observations, experimental investigations and statistical analyses, part III. Curr Probl Surg 1993;10:163.
2. Svensson LG, Crawford ES. Aortic dissection and aortic aneurysm surgery: clinical observations, experimental investigations and statistical analyses, part II. Curr Probl Surg 1992;12:913.
3. Robert AJ, Nova JD, Hughes WA, et al. Cardiac and renal responses to cross clamping of the descending thoracic aorta. J Thorac Cardiovasc Surg 1983;86:732.
4. Carroll RM, Laravisco RB, Schauble JF. Left ventricular function during aortic surgery. Arch Surg 1976;111:740.
5. Meloche R, Pottecher T, Audet J, et al. Hemodynamic changes due to clamping of the abdominal aorta. Can Anaesth Soc J 1977;24:20.
6. Gelman S, Khazaeli MB, Orr R, Henderson T. Blood volume redistribution during cross-clamping of the descending aorta. Anesth Analg 1994;78:219.
7. Van Der Linden P, Gilbart E, Engleman E, et al. Determination of right ventricular volumes during aortic operations. J Cardiothoracic Anesth 1989;3:280.
8. Roizen MF, Beaupre PN, Alpert RA, et al. Monitoring with two-dimensional transesophageal echocardiography: comparison of myocardial function in patients undergoing supraceliac, suprarenal-infraceliac or infrarenal aortic occlusion. J Vasc Surg 1984;1:300.
9. Gelman S, McDowell H, Varner PD, et al. The reason for cardiac output reduction following aortic cross clamping. Am J Surg 1988;155:578.
10. Zaidan JR, Guffin AV, Perdue G, et al. Hemodynamics of intravenous nitroglycerin during aortic cross clamping. Arch Surg 1982;117:1285.
11. Hummel BW, Raess DH, Gewertz BL, et al. Effect of nitroglycerin and aortic occlusion on myocardial blood flow. Surgery 1982;92:159.
12. Brunsoni B, Colombo A, Merlo L, et al. Hemodynamic and metabolic changes induced by temporary clamping of the thoracic aorta. Eur Surg Res 1978;10:206.
13. Farrand EA, Horvath SM. Cardiovascular and hemodynamic functions in dogs subject to prolonged aortic occlusion. Arch Surg 1958;76:951.
14. Simpson JI, Eide TR, Schiff GA, et al. Isoflurane vs. sodium nitroprusside for the control of proximal hypertension during thoracic aortic cross clamping: effects on spinal cord ischemia. J Cardiothoracic Vasc Anesth 1995;9:491.
15. Simpson JI, Eide TR, Schiff GA, et al. Effect of nitroglycerin on spinal cord ischemia after thoracic aortic cross clamping. Ann Thorac Surg 1996;61:113.
16. Symbas PN, Pfaender LM, Drucker MH, et al. Cross-clamping of the descending aorta. J Thorac Cardiovasc Surg 1983;85:300.
17. Brant B, Armstrong R, Vetto RM. Vasodepressor factor in declamp shock production. Surgery 1970;67:650.
18. Lee Y, Jihayel A. Thoracic Aortic Aneurysm Repair. Hemodynamic Changes and Complications. In P Casthely, D Bergman (eds), Cardiopulmonary Bypass: Physiology, Related Complications and Pharmacology. New York: Futura, 1991;489.
19. Cohen JR, Sardardi F, Paul J, et al. Increased intestinal permeability: implications for thoracoabdominal aneurysm repair. Ann Vasc Surg 1992;6:433.
20. Artru AA. Relationship between cerebral blood volume and CSF pressure during anesthesia with halothane or enflurane in dogs. Anesthesiology 1983;58:533.
21. Crawford ES, Fenstermocker JM, Richardson W, et al. Reappraisal of adjuncts to avoid ischemia in the treatment of thoracic aneurysms. Surgery 1970;67:182.
22. Najafi H, Javid H, Hunter J, et al. Descending aortic aneurysmectomy without adjuncts to avoid ischemia. Ann Thorac Surg 1980;30:326.
23. Crawford ES, Crawford JL, Safi HJ, et al. Thoracoabdominal aortic aneurysms: preoperative and intraoperative factors determining immediate and long term results of operations in 605 patients. J Vasc Surg 1986;3:389.
24. Livesay JJ, Cooley DA, Venemiglia RA, et al. Surgical experience in descending thoracic aneurysmectomy with and without adjuncts to avoid ischemia. Ann Thorac Surg 1985;39:37.
25. Laschinger JC, Cunningham JN, Isom OW, et al. Definition of the safe lower limits of aortic resection during surgical procedures on the thoracoabdominal aorta: use of somatosensory evoked potential. J Am Coll Cardiol 1983;2:959.
26. Laschinger JC, Cunningham JN, Baumann FG, et al. Monitoring of somatosensory evoked potentials during surgical procedures on the thoracoabdominal aorta. II. Use of somatosensory evoked potentials to assess adequacy of distal aortic bypass and perfusion after thoracic aortic cross clamping. J Thorac Cardiovasc Surg 1987;94:266.

27. Mizrahi EM, Crawford ES. Somatosensory evoked potentials during reversible spinal cord ischemia in man. Electroencephalogr Clin Neurophysiol 1984;58:120.

28. Coles JG, Wilson GJ, Sima AF. Intraoperative detection of spinal cord ischemia using somatosensory evoked potentials during thoracic occlusion. Ann Thorac Surg 1980;34:299.

29. Ginsburg HH, Shetter AG, Raudzens PA. Postoperative paraplegia with preserved intraoperative somatosensory evoked potentials. J Neurosurg 1985;63:296.

30. Takaki O, Okumura F. Application and limitation of somatosensory evoked potential monitoring during thoracic aortic aneurysm surgery: a case report. Anesthesiology 1985;63:700.

31. Crawford ES, Mizrahi EM, Hess KR, et al. The impact of distal aortic perfusion and somatosensory evoked potential monitoring on prevention of paraplegia after aortic aneurysm. J Thorac Cardiovasc Surg 1988;95:357.

32. Laschinger JC, Owen J, Rosenbloom M, et al. Directed noninvasive monitoring of spinal cord motor function during thoracic aortic occlusion. Use of motor evoked potentials. J Vasc Surg 1988;7:161.

33. Svensson LG, Patel V, Robinson MF, et al. The influence of preservation or perfusion of intraoperatively identified spinal cord blood supply on spinal motor evoked potentials and paraplegia after aortic surgery. J Vasc Surg 1991;13:355.

34. Reuter DG, Tacker WA, Badylak SF, et al. Correlation of motor-evoked potential response to ischemic spinal cord damage. J Thorac Cardiovasc Surg 1992;104:262.

35. D'Ambra MN, Dewhirst W, Jacobs M, et al. Cross clamping the thoracic aorta: effect on intracranial pressure. Circulation 1988;78(Suppl 3):198.

36. Grubbs PE, Marini C, Toporoff B, et al. Somatosensory evoked potentials and spinal cord perfusion are significant predictors of postoperative neurologic dysfunction. Surgery 1988;104:216.

37. Maeda S, Miyamoto T, Murata H, Yamashita K. Prevention of spinal cord ischemia by monitoring spinal cord perfusion pressure and somatosensory evoked potentials. J Cardiovasc Surg 1989;30:565.

38. Berendes JN, Bredee JJ, Schipperheyn JJ, Mashhour YAS. Mechanisms of spinal cord injury after cross clamping of the descending thoracic aorta. Circulation 1982;66(Suppl 1):112.

39. Dasmahapatra HK, Coles JG, Wilson GJ, et al. Relationship between cerebrospinal fluid dynamics and reversible spinal cord ischemia during experimental thoracic aortic occlusion. J Thorac Cardiovasc Surg 1988;95:920.

40. Verdant A. Descending thoracic aortic aneurysms: surgical treatment with the Gott shunt. Can J Surg 1992;35:493.

41. Svensson LG, Crawford ES, Hess KR, et al. Variables predictive of outcome in 832 patients undergoing repairs of the descending thoracic aorta. Chest 1993;104:1248.

42. Weimann S, Balogh D, Furtwangler W, et al. Graft replacement of post-traumatic thoracic aortic aneurysm: results without bypass or shunting. Eur J Vasc Surg 1992;6:381.

43. Wadouh F, Wadouh R, Hartmann M, Crisp-Lindgren N. Prevention of paraplegia during aortic operations. Ann Thorac Surg 1990;50:543.

44. Doppman JL, Dichiro G, Morton DL. Arteriographic identification of spinal cord blood supply prior to aortic surgery. JAMA 1978;204:172.

45. Svensson LG, Patel V, Coselli JS, Crawford ES. Preliminary report of localization of spinal cord blood supply by hydrogen during aortic operations. Ann Thorac Surg 1990;49:528.

46. Lowell RC, Gloviczki P, Bergman RT, et al. Failure of selective shunting to intercostal arteries to prevent spinal cord ischemia during experimental thoracoabdominal aortic occlusion. Int Angiol 1992;2:281.

47. Wynands JEA. Pro and con: pro: cerebrospinal fluid drainage prevents paraplegia. J Cardiothoracic Vasc Anesth 1992;6:366.

48. Shenaq SA, Svensson LG. Con: cerebrospinal fluid drainage does not afford spinal cord protection during resection of thoracic aneurysm. J Cardiothorac Vasc Anesth 1992;6:369.

49. Bower TC, Murray MJ, Gloviczki P, et al. Effects of thoracic aortic occlusion and cerebrospinal fluid drainage on regional spinal cord blood flow in dogs: correlation with neurologic outcome. J Vasc Surg 1988;9:135.

50. Woloszyn TT, Corrado PM, Coons MS, et al. Cerebrospinal fluid drainage and steroids provide better spinal cord protection during aortic cross clamping than does either treatment alone. Ann Thorac Surg 1990;49:78.

51. McCullough JL, Hollier L, Nugent M. Paraplegia after thoracic aortic occlusion: influence of cerebrospinal fluid drainage. J Vasc Surg 1988;7:153.

52. Crawford ES, Svensson LG, Hess KR, et al. A prospective randomized study of cerebrospinal fluid drainage to prevent paraplegia after high-risk surgery on the thoracoabdominal aorta. J Vasc Surg 1990;13:36.

53. Murray MJ, Bower TC, Oliver WC, et al. Effects of cerebrospinal fluid drainage in patients undergoing thoracic and thoracoabdominal aortic surgery. J Cardiothoracic Vasc Surg 1993;7:266.

54. Marini CP, Grubbs PE, Toporoff B, et al. Effect of sodium nitroprusside on spinal cord perfusion and paraplegia during aortic cross clamping. Ann Thorac Surg 1989;47:379.

55. Cernaianu AC, Olah A, Cilley JH, et al. Effect of sodium nitroprusside on paraplegia during cross clamping of the thoracic aorta. Ann Thorac Surg 1993;56:1035.

56. Ryan T, Mannion D, O'Brien W, et al. Spinal cord perfusion pressure in dogs after control of proximal aortic hypertension during thoracic aortic cross clamping with esmolol or sodium nitroprusside. Anesthesiology 1993;8:317.

57. Clark FJS, Mutch WAC, Sutton R, et al. Treatment of proximal aortic hypertension after thoracic aortic cross clamping in dogs. Anesthesiology 1992;77:357.

58. Woloszyn TT, Marini CP, Coons MS, et al. Cerebrospinal fluid drainage does not counteract the negative effect of sodium nitroprusside on spinal cord perfusion and paraplegia during aortic cross clamping. Ann Thorac Surg 1989;47:379.

59. Berendes JN, Bredee JJ, Schipperheyn JJ. Mechanisms of spinal cord injury after cross-clamping of the descending thoracic aorta. Circulation 1982;66(Suppl):112.

60. Agee JM, Flanagan T, Blackbourne LH, et al. Reducing postischemic paraplegia using conjugated superoxide dismutase. Ann Thorac Surg 1995;51:911.

61. Kirshner DL, Kirshner RL, Heggeness LM, DeWeese JA. Spinal cord ischemia: an evaluation of pharmacologic agents in minimizing paraplegia after aortic occlusion. J Vasc Surg 1989;9:305.

62. Qayumi AK, Janusz MT, Jamieson RE, Lyster DM. Pharmacologic interventions for prevention of spinal cord injury caused by aortic cross clamping. J Thorac Cardiovasc Surg 1992;104:256.

63. Francel PC, Long BA, Malik JM, et al. Limiting ischemic spinal cord injury using a free radical scavenger 21-aminosteroid and/or cerebrospinal fluid drainage. J Neurosurg 1993;79:742.

64. Svensson LG, Cosgrove DM, Bevens EG, et al. Intrathecal papaverine for the prevention of paraplegia after operation on the thoracic or thoracoabdominal aorta. J Thorac Cardiovasc Surg 1988;96:823.

65. De Riu PL, Petruzzi V, Palmieri G, et al. β-endorphin in experimental canine spinal ischemia. Stroke 1989;20:253.

66. Baskin DS, Hosobuchi T. Naloxone reversal of ischemic neurological deficits in man. Lancet 1981;2:272.

67. Archer CW, Wynn MM, Hoch JR, et al. Combined use of cerebrospinal fluid and naloxone reduces the risk of paraplegia in thoracoabdominal aneurysm repair. J Vasc Surg 1994;19:236.

68. Robertson S, Foltz R, Grossman RG, et al. Protection against experimental ischemic injury. J Neurosurg 1986;64:633.

69. Nylander WA, Plunkett RJ, Hummon JW, et al. Thiopental modification of ischemic spinal cord injury in the dog. Ann Thorac Surg 1982;33:64.

70. Mutch WAC, Graham MR, Halliday WC, et al. Paraplegia following thoracic aortic cross clamping in dogs: no difference in neurological outcome with a barbiturate vs. isoflurane. Stroke 1993;24:1554.

71. Benveniste H, Drejer J, Schousboe A, Diemer NH. Elevation of the extracellular concentrations of glutamate and aspartate in rat hippocampus during transient cerebral ischemia monitored by intracerebral microdialysis. J Neurochem 1984;43:1369.

72. Simpson RK Jr, Robertson CS, Goodman JC. Spinal cord ischemia-induced elevation of amino acids: extracellular measurement with microdialysis. Neurochem Res 1990;15:635.

73. Choi DW. Ionic dependence of glutamate neurotoxicity. J Neurosci 1987;7:369.

74. Hao JX, Xu XJ, Aldskogius H, et al. The excitatory amino acid receptor antagonist MK-801 prevents the hypersensitivity induced by spinal cord ischemia in the rat. Exp Neurol 1991;113:182.

75. Martinez-Arizala A, Rigamonti DD, Long JB, et al. Effects of NMDA receptor antagonists following spinal ischemia in the rabbit. Exp Neurol 1990;108:232.

76. Danielisova V, Chavko M. Amelioration of ischemic spinal cord damage by postischemic treatment with propentofylline (HWA 285). Brain Res 1992;590:321.

77. Simpson JI, Eide TR, Schiff GA, et al. Intrathecal magnesium sulfate protects the spinal cord from ischemic injury during thoracic aortic cross clamping. Anesthesiology 1994;81:1493.

78. Laschinger JC, Cunningham JN, Cooper MM, et al. Prevention of ischemic spinal cord injury following aortic cross clamping: use of corticosteroids. Ann Thorac Surg 1984;38:500.

79. Artru AA, Nugent M, Michenfeld JD. Enflurane causes a prolonged and reversible increase in the rate of CSF production in the dog. Anesthesiology 1982;57:255.

80. Simpson JI, Eide TR, Newman SB, et al. Trimethephan vs. sodium nitroprusside for the control of proximal hypertension during thoracic aortic cross clamping: the effects on spinal cord ischemia. Anesth Analg 1996;82:68.

81. Naslund TC, Hollier LH, Money SR, et al. Protecting the ischemic spinal cord during aortic clamping: the influence of anesthetics and hypothermia. Ann Surg 1992;215:409.

82. Vacanti FX, Ames A III. Mild hypothermia and MG protect against irreversible damage during CNS ischemia. Stroke 1984;15:695.

83. Crawford FA Jr, Sade RM. Spinal cord injury associated with hyperthermia during aortic coarctation repair. J Thorac Cardiovasc Surg 1984;87:616.

84. Wisselink W, Becker MO, Nguyen JH, et al. Protecting the ischemic spinal cord during aortic clamping: the influence of selective hypothermia and spinal cord perfusion pressure. J Vasc Surg 1994;19:788.

85. Vanicky I, Marsala M, Galik J, Marsala J. Epidural perfusion cooling protection against protracted spinal cord ischemia in rabbits. J Neurosurg 1993;79:736.

86. Berguer R, Porto J, Fedoronko B, Dragovic L. Selective deep hypothermia of the spinal cord prevents paraplegia after aortic cross clamping in the dog model. J Vasc Surg 1992;15:62.

87. Davison JK, Cambria RP, Vierra DJ, et al. Epidural cooling for regional spinal cord hypothermia during thoracoabdominal aneurysm repair. J Vasc Surg 1994;20:304.

88. Maughan RE, Mohan C, Nathan IM, et al. Intrathecal perfusion of an oxygenated perfluorocarbon prevents paraplegia after aortic occlusion. Ann Thorac Surg 1992;54:818.

89. Lanier WL, Strangland KJ, Scheithauer BW, et al. The effects of dextrose infusion and head position on neurologic

outcome after complete cerebral ischemia in primates: examination of a model. Anesthesiology 1987;66:39.

90. Drummond JC, Moore SS. The influence of dextrose administration on neurologic outcome after temporary spinal cord ischemia in the rabbit. Anesthesiology 1989;70:64.

91. Hemmila MR, Zelenock GB, D'Alecy LG. Post-ischemic hyperglycemia worsens neurologic outcome after spinal cord ischemia. J Vasc Surg 1993;17:661.

92. Crawford ES, Walker HSJ, Saleh SA, et al. Graft replacement of the aneurysm in descending thoracic aorta: results without bypass or shunting. Surgery 1981;89:73.

93. Gelman S, Reves JG, Fowler K, et al. Regional blood flow during cross clamping of the thoracic aorta and infusion of sodium nitroprusside. J Thorac Cardiovasc Surg 1983;85:287.

94. Oyama M, McNamara J, Suehiro A, Sue-Ako K. The effects of thoracic aortic cross-clamping and declamping of visceral organ blood flow. Ann Surg 1983;197:459.

95. Joob AW, Dunn C, Miller E, et al. Effect of left atrial to left femoral artery bypass and renin-angiotensin system blockade on renal blood flow and function during and after thoracic aortic occlusion. J Vasc Surg 1987;5:329.

96. Goldberg AH, Lilienfeld LS. Effects of hypertonic mannitol and renal vascular resistance. Proc Soc Exp Biol Med 1965;119:635.

97. Goldberg LI. Cardiovascular and renal actions of dopamine: potential clinical applications. Pharmacol Rev 1972;24:1.

98. Svensson LG, Hess KR, Coselli JS, et al. A prospective study of respiratory failure after high-risk surgery of the thoracoabdominal aorta. J Vasc Surg 1991;14:271.

99. Shenaq SA, Chelly JE, Karlberg H, et al. Use of nitroprusside during surgery for thoracoabdominal aortic aneurysm. Circulation 1984;70(Suppl 1):1.

100. Casthely PA, Dluzneski J, Jones R, et al. Superoxide dismutase and hemodynamic changes following aortic cross clamp release. J Cardiothorac Anesth 1988;2:450.

Chapter 9

Anesthesia for Surgery to Repair Aortic Coarctation

Kevin Whitrock

Coarctation of the aorta consists anatomically of a narrowing of the aortic lumen. The term *coarctation* is derived from the Latin word *coarctatio,* which means "a drawing together to make tight."[1] Coarctation is often associated with other important cardiovascular abnormalities that can affect the age of clinical presentation and timing and choice of medical or surgical interventions, as well as the overall morbidity and mortality. While this vascular lesion was first described by Meckel in 1760, the first successful surgical repair of this lesion was not reported until 1945 by Gross and by Crafoord and Nylin.[2–5] Before the introduction of surgical therapy, this lesion was associated with a high morbidity and mortality by the third decade of life. Advances in both surgical intervention and long-term medical care have significantly improved the quality of life of patients with aortic coarctation, and advances in anesthetic techniques have improved perioperative outcome.[6–8]

To successfully care for these patients, the anesthesiologist must (1) have an understanding of the anatomy of the aortic coarctation and any associated abnormalities, (2) be able to evaluate the severity of the pathophysiologic effects of the lesion and the effectiveness of medical interventions, and (3) be familiar with the various surgical repairs and their perioperative implications. By having a clear understanding of these important points, the anesthesiologist can best formulate an anesthetic plan that will benefit the patient during the perioperative period.

Epidemiology

As an isolated lesion, aortic coarctation is the fifth or sixth most common congenital cardiovascular defect.[9] In one large survey, it ranked fourth in frequency (7.5% of cases) among lesions requiring surgery or cardiac catheterization during the first year of life.[10] Its discovery rate is 2 in 10,000 live births. The true incidence is actually higher, at about 1 in 1,200 live births, since many individuals remain undiagnosed during the first year of life.[2]

Coarctation affects men and boys more than women and girls. The relative incidence of coarctation in male subjects is 1.27 to 1.00 in infancy and 1.74 to 1.00 in older patients.[10–12] It usually occurs sporadically, although there has been a report of 27 families with coarctation occurring in more than one family member and of one family with an autosomal dominant pattern of inheritance.[13] There is an unusually high prevalence (35%) of aortic coarctation among patients with Turner's syndrome (XO karyotype), where it is the most common cardiovascular abnormality.[2,14] Associated coarctation of the abdominal aorta has been reported in 2% of cases and may result in severe hypertension if the renal arteries are involved.[3]

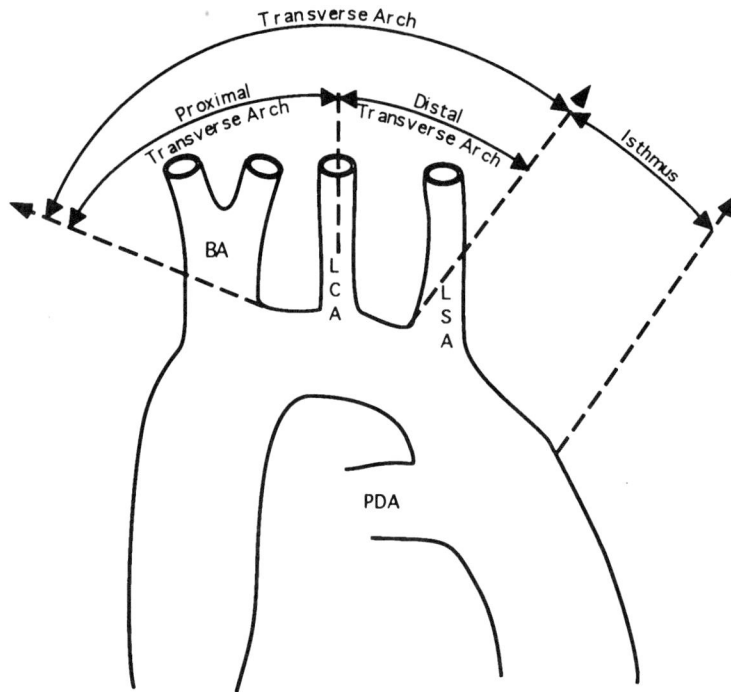

Figure 9-1. Neonatal aortic arch. The relationship of the brachiocephalic artery (BA), left carotid artery (LCA), left subclavian artery (LSA), and patent ductus arteriosus (PDA) to the aortic arch is depicted. The aortic isthmus, which lies between the left subclavian artery and the ductus arteriosus, is a common site for preductal coarctation and associated aortic tubular hypoplasia. (Modified with permission from F Lacour-Gayet, J Bruniaux, A Serraf, et al. Hypoplastic transverse arch and coarctation in neonates. J Thorac Cardiovasc Surg 1990;100:808.)

Pathology and Pathophysiology

Anatomy and Classification

Classically, this lesion has been described as a discrete lesion, but may be associated with a variety of cardiovascular lesions that can affect the diagnostic features and clinical course. It is commonly found as an abrupt constriction in the aortic isthmus located between the origin of the left subclavian artery proximally and the junction of the ductus arteriosus and the aorta distally (Figures 9-1 and 9-2).[15] Although the lesion is commonly located in the aortic isthmus, it occurs rarely as an isolated discrete lesion in other locations, including the aortic arch, descending aorta, or abdominal aorta with renal artery involvement.[16] Histologic studies of aortic coarctation have demonstrated an abnormality of the aortic media giving rise to a ridge-like infolding of the aortic wall that narrows the lumen eccentrically, often in the posterior wall immediately opposite the junction of the ductus arteriosus.[17] This abnormality of the aortic media has been referred to as a *posterior shelf* or *curtain lesion*.[18]

Another lesion that produces restriction to flow in this region is preductal tubular hypoplasia, which is a zone of diffuse narrowing of the distal aortic arch or isthmus that may or may not be associated with a curtain lesion.[1] Tubular hypoplasia has a higher association with aortic coarctation when severe intracardiac anomalies are present.[19] In the most severe form, tubular hypoplasia may be associated with an interrupted aortic arch or aortic atresia and a patent ductus arteriosus, which provides blood flow to the distal aorta.

The presence of aortic narrowing above the ductus arteriosus has been termed *preductal* or *infantile type*, since this is the anatomic location of 80% of coarctations diagnosed during infancy. The presence of the narrowed aortic segment below the ductus arteriosus has been termed *postductal* or *adult type*, since 77% of coarctations identified after infancy are in this location (see Figure 9-2).[20] Even though most of the preductal lesions occur in infants, they do occur in adults, and postductal coarctation can occur in infants. Since the imprecise age-related terms have caused confusion regarding the classification and description of aortic coarctation over the years, the site-related terms *preductal* and *postductal* are preferable. The term *juxtaductal* refers to the location of the coarctation opposite the entry of the ductus arteriosus, patent or ligamentous

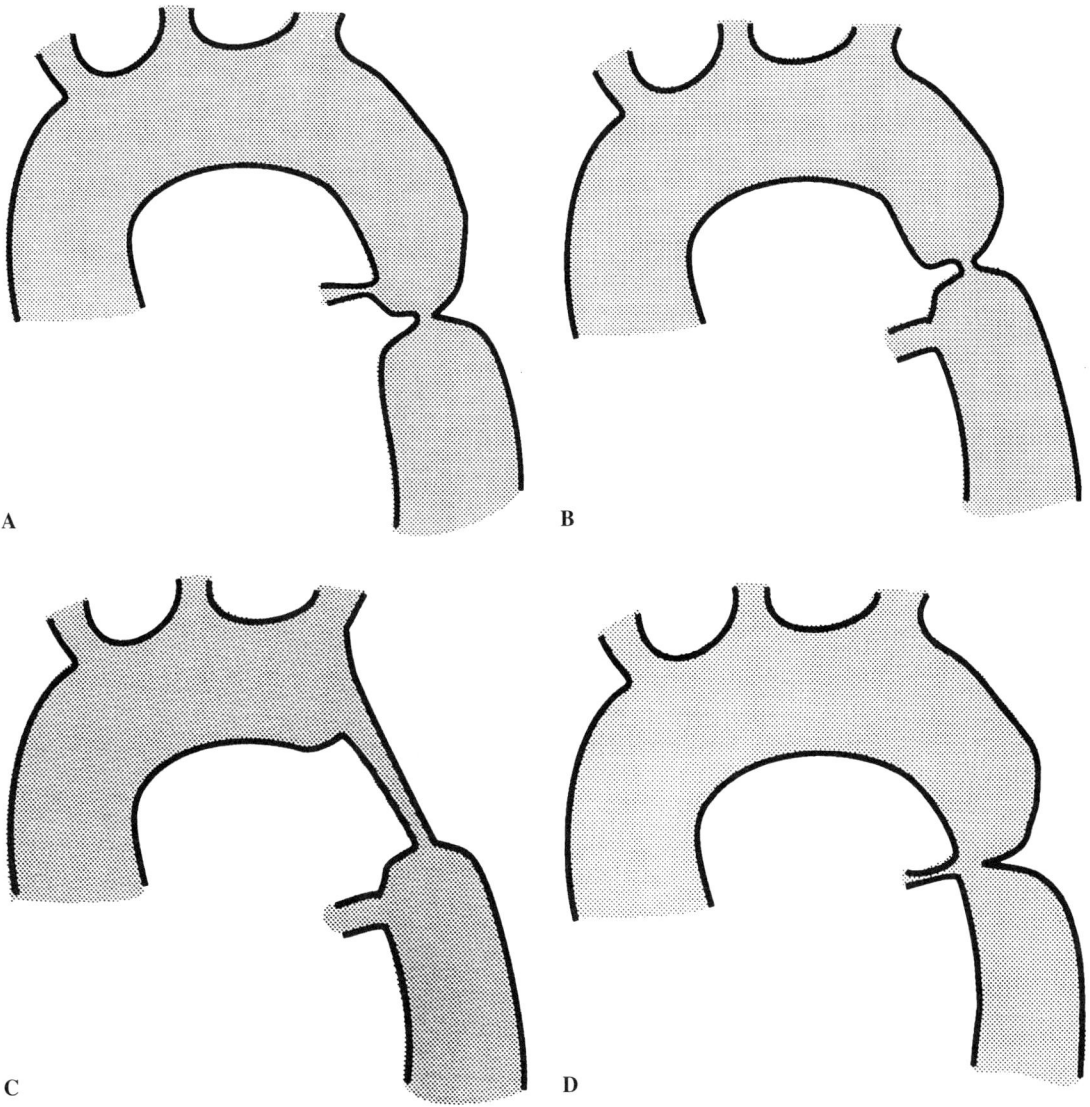

Figure 9-2. Types of aortic coarctation. A. Postductal coarctation. B. Preductal coarctation. C. Preductal coarctation with isthmal hypoplasia. D. Juxtaductal coarctation.

(see Figure 9-2).[2,18,21] The majority of aortic coarctation lesions are actually best described by this term, since the most marked degree of infolding of the coarctation lesion usually occurs at this site.[22]

The terms *simple* and *complex* describe isolated coarctation and coarctation associated with significant intracardiac abnormalities, respectively. Associated cardiac abnormalities are present in 40% of preductal coarctations and 14% of postductal lesions.

In symptomatic infants, coarctation is often complex. Two-thirds of symptomatic infants have a patent ductus arteriosus.[23] A ventricular septal defect will be present in 35% of symptomatic infants; and it is this group that will most often require urgent surgery.[14] Mitral abnormalities are common, but severe dysfunction is noted in only 10% of symptomatic infants.[9] The mitral valve may become incompetent in the presence of severe aortic coarctation, while mitral stenosis may result from dysplasia of leaflets and short-fused chordae tendineae.[24] Shone syndrome comprises the constellation of aortic coarctation and subaortic valvular and mitral stenosis.[25]

The cardiovascular malformation most frequently associated with aortic coarctation is a bicuspid aortic valve, which in one series has been reported to have an associated prevalence as high as 85% in patients with a bicuspid aortic valve.[17,26,27] Cystic medial necrosis is also commonly identified in patients with aortic coarctation, as well as in patients with bicuspid aortic valves.[28,29] This intrinsic weakness of the arterial wall may explain why these patients are commonly predisposed to develop single or multiple aneurysms of the aorta and other vessels, as well as dissecting lesions both proximal and distal to the site of coarctation.[30] Likewise, an inherent weakness in the aortic media may explain why these individuals may have aortic rupture after successful repair of coarctation, even in patients without evidence of hypertension.[31–34] The existence of so many associated arterial abnormalities with coarctation of the aorta strongly suggests that a generalized arterial disease may be a possible etiology in many individuals.[35]

Other abnormalities associated with coarctation include cerebral aneurysms, which may predispose a patient to a cerebrovascular hemorrhage in hypertensive patients and aberrant origin of the right subclavian artery distal to the coarctation.[36] Very rarely, both right and left subclavian arteries are aberrant and arise below the coarctation segment.[22] Associated noncardiovascular malformations have been reported to occur in 7–25% of patients and include hypospadias, club foot deformity, and ocular defects.[11,37]

Pathogenesis

Various theories have been postulated to explain the pathogenesis of aortic coarctation that probably occurs during the first 6–8 weeks of gestation. In utero, the left fourth primitive aortic arch gives rise to the aortic arch proximal to the site of insertion of the ductus arteriosus, the dorsal aorta gives rise to the descending thoracic aorta, and the sixth primitive aortic arch forms the ductus arteriosus. Coarctation arises from the anomalous development of the aorta from these primitive structures (Figure 9-3) (see Chapter 1).[1,14]

A hemodynamic theory can best explain the development of the large variation of anatomic abnormalities observed, which range from discrete aortic coarctation to severe segmental narrowing of the aortic isthmus and, finally, to complete interruption of the aortic arch.[14,38] This theory has been based on observations in fetal lambs and postmortem human fetal studies.[18] The hemodynamic theory requires the presence of a cardiac abnormality early during embryologic development, which decreases the normal antegrade flow from the left ventricle to the aorta, along with a compensatory increase in flow through the pulmonary artery and patent ductus arteriosus into the aorta. While the normal fetus has approximately 25% of the combined ventricular output flowing through the aortic isthmus, it has been postulated that diminished left ventricular output in utero may be inadequate to promote normal development of the aortic arch. The result would be aortic coarctation or tubular hypoplasia above the level of the ductus arteriosus. An example of such a cardiac abnormality would be a malaligned ventricular septal defect that has a narrowed and posteriorly displaced aortic orifice that, beginning in utero, would limit left ventricular outflow and favor flow through the pulmonary artery and ductus arteriosus.[14] Normally, individuals with preductal coarctation have adequate lower body perfusion via the patent ductus arteriosus and, therefore, do not develop extensive collateral circulation in utero. The drawback to this theory is that it does not explain the pathogenesis of isolated simple aortic coarctation in individuals who had normal left ventricular outflow in utero.

In individuals with simple isolated aortic coarctation, the lesion is often juxtaductal or postductal. This observation has lead to the theory that the aortic coarctation segment is composed of aberrrant or ectopic tissue from the ductus arteriosus that has extended into the wall of the aorta at the site of entry of the ductus arteriosus (see Figure 9-3). This theory proposes that the ectopic ductal tissue constricts in response to the same factors that initiate closure of the ductus arteriosus (i.e., increasing oxygen partial pressure) shortly after birth. Support for this theory is based on histologic studies. In normal subjects, histologic examination of the ductus arteriosus reveals a structure different from the adjoining great arteries. Examination of specimens of aortic coarctation, on the other hand, demonstrates that ductal tissue extends into the aortic wall and

A

B

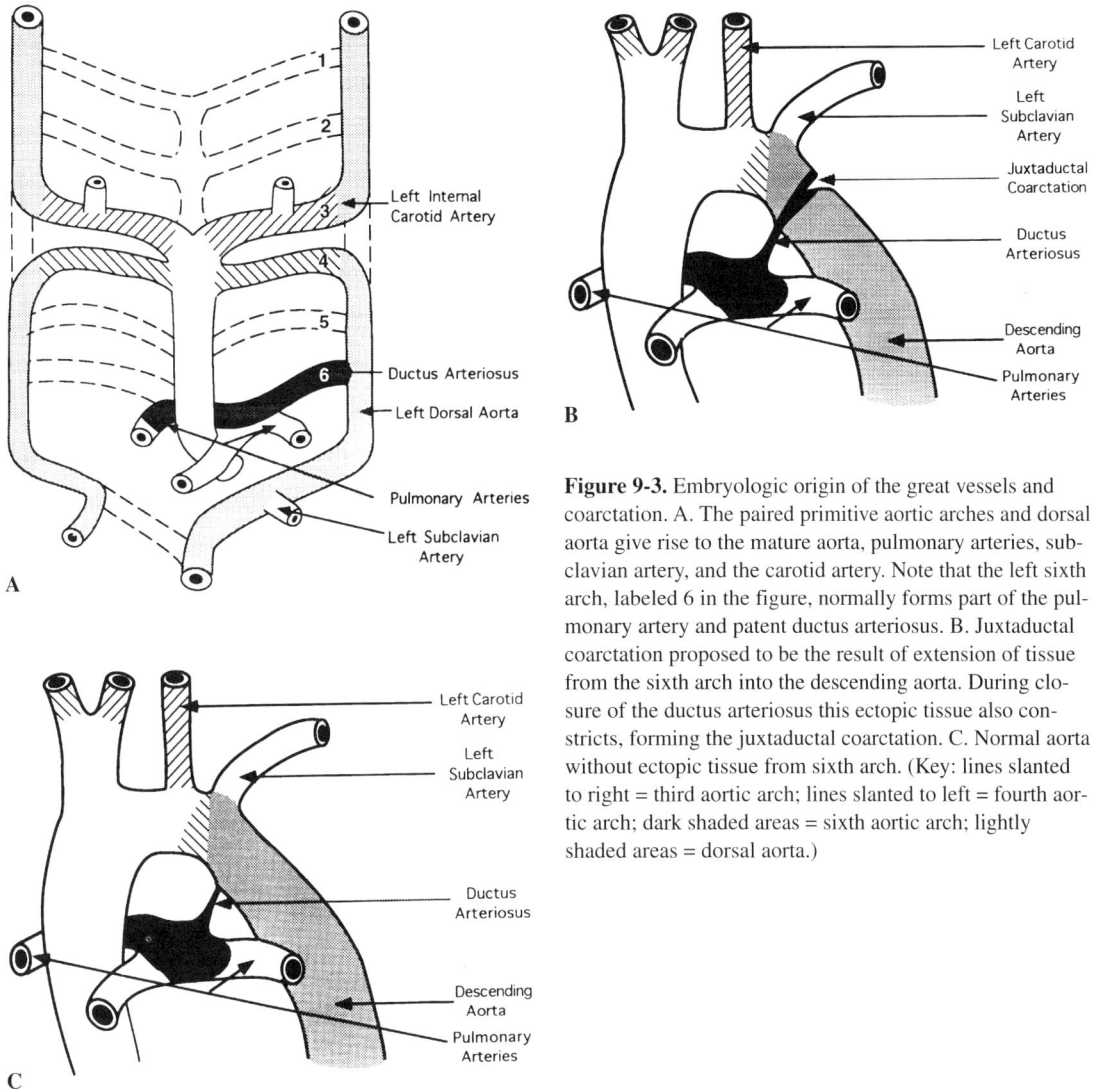

Figure 9-3. Embryologic origin of the great vessels and coarctation. A. The paired primitive aortic arches and dorsal aorta give rise to the mature aorta, pulmonary arteries, subclavian artery, and the carotid artery. Note that the left sixth arch, labeled 6 in the figure, normally forms part of the pulmonary artery and patent ductus arteriosus. B. Juxtaductal coarctation proposed to be the result of extension of tissue from the sixth arch into the descending aorta. During closure of the ductus arteriosus this ectopic tissue also constricts, forming the juxtaductal coarctation. C. Normal aorta without ectopic tissue from sixth arch. (Key: lines slanted to right = third aortic arch; lines slanted to left = fourth aortic arch; dark shaded areas = sixth aortic arch; lightly shaded areas = dorsal aorta.)

C

encircles the aorta like a diaphragm.[1] This histologic finding also supports the theory proposed by Rosenberg that the sixth left aortic arch in utero forms not only the ductus arteriosus, but also may give rise to a segment of the descending aorta adjacent to the ductus arteriosus.[39] The possible role of anomalous fibroductal tissue arising from the ductus arteriosus in the pathogenesis of aortic coarctation is debated, since it does not satisfactorily account for those cases in which aortic coarctation exists in the presence of a patent ductus arteriosus.[2,39,40]

Pathophysiology

The primary cardiovascular disturbance associated with aortic coarctation is increased impedance to left ventricular ejection. Mechanisms that potentially may compensate for this increased impedance include (1) myocardial hypertrophy, (2) activation of the sympathetic nervous system, and (3) the Frank-Starling mechanism (i.e., preload reserve).[41] Unfortunately, the neonatal myocardium is often incapable of fully using these mechanisms because the immature neonatal myocardium is less compliant, has limited preload reserve, and has sympathetic innervation that is incomplete.[42] If impedance to left ventricular ejection rapidly develops in the young infant, there may be inadequate time for development of arterial collateral circulation, and congestive heart failure may develop due to pressure overload.

Patients with complex coarctation lesions may develop cardiac decompensation due to hemodynamic disturbances other than left ventricular pressure overload. Lesions such as large ventricular septal defects or endocardial cushion defects may contribute to left-to-right intracardiac shunting. This intracardiac shunt increases the volume load on an already pressure-overloaded ventricle, which may lead to mitral regurgitation, pulmonary hypertension, and congestive heart failure.[2]

The other potentially serious hemodynamic disturbance is inadequate systemic perfusion distal to the aortic coarctation lesion. Systemic perfusion distal to the coarctation may be maintained by (1) increased systolic pressure proximal to the coarctation, (2) development of arterial collateral circulation, or (3) a patent ductus arteriosus. Individuals with a large patent ductus arteriosus and a large ventricular septal defect may have descending aortic blood flow that is well-oxygenated and at systemic levels of pressure.[2] For patients dependent on the presence of a patent ductus arteriosus, acute ductal closure or left ventricular failure can cause systemic hypoperfusion resulting in mesenteric and renal ischemia leading to metabolic acidosis, further myocardial depression, necrotizing enterocolitis, and renal failure.

The coarctation lesion usually becomes more obstructive as the individual grows.[22] This gradually increasing obstruction caused by intimal proliferation is usually balanced by recruitment of collateral arterial vessels. Arterial collateral circulation may develop in infancy and is comprised of a posterior and anterior system. The posterior collateral system allows arterial blood from branches of the thyrocervical trunk to flow in a retrograde fashion into the descending aorta via the posterior intercostal arteries. These dilated, tortuous intercostal arteries erode the inferior rib margins in older children and produce the characteristic "rib notching" seen on chest radiography. The anterior spinal artery may also become dilated and tortuous due to collateral flow through branches from the proximal and distal aorta. The anterior collateral system allows arterial blood

from internal thoracic arteries to pass to the external iliac arteries in a retrograde fashion via the superior and inferior epigastric arteries.[2] In the presence of an isolated aortic coarctation lesion, this collateral system may be well developed, even in infants.[43]

Natural History

Approximately one-fifth of infants admitted with heart failure during the first few weeks of life have simple coarctation without significant associated cardiovascular defects.[44] The majority of these patients respond to medical management and can mature to an age of at least 2–3 years before undergoing surgical repair. Those infants treated medically generally improve as the upper extremity hypertension present in the first few months of life diminishes and the collateral arterial system develops.[44]

The location of the aortic coarctation and the severity of coexisting cardiovascular abnormalities determine the clinical presentation. The timing of closure of the ductus arteriosus often plays a decisive role in the onset and progression of symptoms in most patients with preductal and juxtaductal coarctation.[2,13] In some neonates with preductal aortic coarctation, the ductus arteriosus remains patent and may result in shunting of systemic venous blood from the pulmonary artery to the descending aorta. This persistent patency of the ductus arteriosus may provide differential cyanosis and only a small blood pressure gradient between the upper and lower extremities. Hypoperfusion and ventricular failure develop usually during the first few weeks of life when the ductus arteriosus begins to constrict.

Likewise, an isolated juxtaductal aortic coarctation may initially be of little hemodynamic consequence in the presence of a patent ductus arteriosus in some children. For this group of patients, it is the unconstricted ampulla of the ductus arteriosus that often provides an adequate channel for antegrade blood flow in the descending aorta. Therefore, these children may remain asymptomatic even after the ductus arteriosus begins its normal constriction from the pulmonary end to the aortic end in response to elevated arterial oxygen partial pressure after birth.[18] If the aortic ampulla of the ductus closes rapidly, aortic blood flow to the descending aorta is impeded and left ventricular afterload increases suddenly. Left ventricular failure, systemic hypoperfusion, elevation of left atrial pressure, left-to-right shunting across the foramen ovale, and pulmonary hypertension can result. Since the constriction of the aortic ampulla may be delayed, these infants may not present with isolated juxtaductal aortic coarctation until 3 weeks of age. Often the anatomic closure of the pulmonary end of the ductus arteriosus may be complete at the time of clinical presentation and can explain why these patients are more refractory to infusion of prostaglandin E_1 (PGE$_1$) than patients with preductal coarctations. On the other hand, if closure of the aortic ampulla is delayed for many weeks or months and aortic flow is obstructed gradually, cardiac failure may not occur during early infancy. The progressive development of left ventricular hypertrophy and collateral circulation may allow these infants to compensate for the developing coarctation.[45]

The hemodynamics of a postductal aortic coarctation are different. First, in utero a collateral circulation has to be present for the fetus to survive if the coarctation is severe. Second, closure of the ductus arteriosus does not compromise lower body perfusion. Therefore, the infant with postductal coarctation and a well-developed collateral circulation is often able to adapt to postnatal life and is usually diagnosed as an asymptomatic older child, adolescent, or adult, when hypertension, a blood pressure gradient, diminished pulses, or murmur is noted on a routine examination.[22] For these patients, the median age of diagnosis is 10 years old.[14] The majority of these patients presenting in childhood will not have a patent ductus arteriosus. The arterial collateral circulation is usually well developed and concentric left ventricular hypertrophy is common.[46] Symptoms sometimes noted in older children or adults include headache, epistaxis, or leg claudication.[14,47] Systolic hypertension in an upper extremity, murmur, or endocarditis involving a bicuspid aortic valve or dilated poststenotic segment of the aorta are common findings in older children.[46] The suspicion of coarctation usually arises when repeated measurements of systolic blood pressure are higher in the arm than in the leg. Repeated differences of 20 mm Hg or greater represent significant obstruction, since the systolic blood pressure in the femoral artery is usually as much as 20 mm Hg higher than in the arm in normal individuals.[22]

The morbidity and mortality in patients with uncorrected coarctation is significant, since associated cardiovascular disease progresses with age. The estimated first-year mortality for untreated symptomatic coarctation in infancy is 84%. For those individuals who are not identified during infancy and remain untreated, the mean age of survival is 34 years (Figure 9-4).[12] The most common causes of death in unrepaired aortic coarctation are congestive heart failure (25%), bacterial endocarditis (18%), aortic rupture (21%), and cerebrovascular hemorrhage from circle of Willis aneurysm rupture (11%).[12] Aortic rupture occurs most often in the third decade of life.[12,48] Patients who develop endocarditis usually have involvement of a bicuspid aortic valve, but may present with endarteritis at the site of coarctation instead.[44,49] Therefore, these individuals require appropriate antibiotic prophylaxis throughout their lives.

For children, the long-term postoperative prognosis is determined by the severity of coexisting cardiovascular anomalies.[50] For older individuals, the incidence of late postoperative cardiovascular complications (e.g., residual hypertension, aneurysm rupture, aortic dissection, and premature cardiovascular death) increases with the age at which the repair is performed.[2] A study of patients 20 years after surgical repair during adolescence revealed that late cardiovascular complications developed in the majority of individuals. Rebound hypertension following surgical repair is particularly common in these patients, especially if moderate-to-severe hypertension was present preoperatively.[51] Therefore, all patients require follow-up cardiovascular evaluation for the remainder of their lives.

Preoperative Evaluation

Physical Examination

The physical examination of a symptomatic infant will vary depending on the presence and severity of coexisting defects. The moribund infant may appear pale, diaphoretic, tachycardic, and tachypneic. The lungs are usually clear, but rales may be present in severe heart failure. Congestive heart failure may present with hepatomegaly, extremity edema, and diminished arterial pulses throughout. Hypertension may be absent in the upper extremities.[2]

Well-compensated infants, i.e., those without significant ventricular dysfunction, and those with mild heart failure usually have normal or bounding pulses

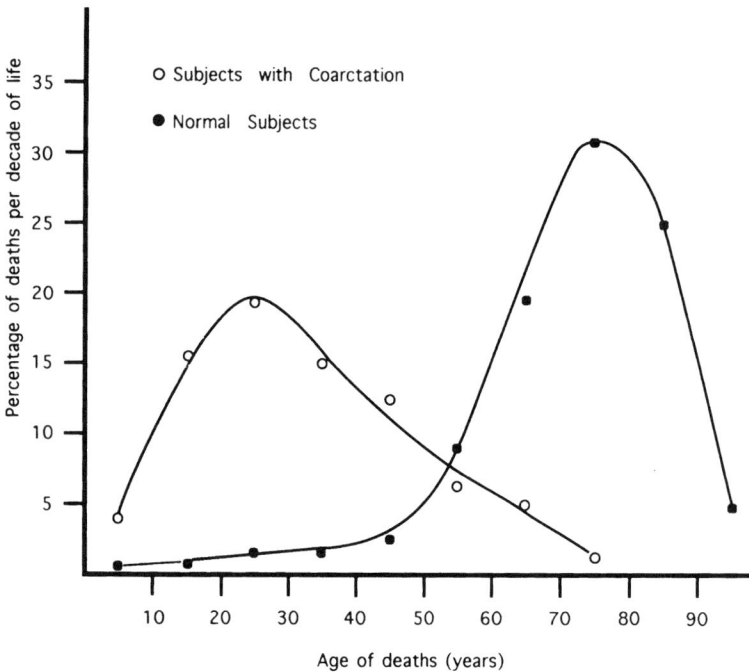

Figure 9-4. The distribution of deaths per decade of life for normal subjects and patients with uncorrected aortic coarctation. The coarctation curve is derived from 304 subjects who survived past 1 year of age and were noted to have aortic coarctation during autopsy. The curve for normal subjects is derived from 1,000 subjects who survived past the first year of life. Note that there is significant mortality by the third decade of life for individuals with uncorrected aortic coarctation. (Modified with permission from M Campbell. Natural history of aortic coarctation. Br Heart J 1970;32:633.)

in the right arm and diminished or absent pulses in the legs. Systolic pressure is higher in the right arm than in the legs, with gradients ranging between 20 and 140 mm Hg.[14] Blood pressure values in the right arm that are less than the left arm, but equal to the lower extremities, are suggestive of an anomalous right subclavian artery originating below the coarctation.[2] The presence of a large patent ductus arteriosus or well-developed collateral circulation may result in minimal differences in the pressures measured between upper and lower extremities, while cyanosis of the lower body is often present with a patent ductus arteriosus unless a ventricular septal defect promotes left-to-right intracardiac shunting.

The cardiac examination commonly includes a heaving left precordium and a medium-pitched systolic blowing murmur originating from the coarctation that is best heard posteriorly in the interscapular area (usually with radiation to the left axilla, apex, and anterior precordium). Well-developed arterial collateral circulation produces a low-pitched, continuous murmur, which is best heard over the posterior chest wall, particularly in the subscapular area. A ventricular septal defect produces a harsh pansystolic murmur along the left lower sternal border. Patients with mild congestive heart failure may have a S_3 gallop, while patients in severe heart failure may

have no audible murmurs until aggressive therapy compensates for the low cardiac output.[14,44]

Diagnostic Studies

The electrocardiogram (ECG) is usually abnormal, especially if there are coexisting cardiac anomalies. The ECG of a young infant normally shows right axis deviation and right ventricular hypertrophy due to the increased right ventricular afterload in utero. Older infants and children normally have evidence of left ventricular hypertrophy. The presence of severe left ventricular hypertrophy and inverted T waves in the left precordial leads of an infant suggests severe aortic stenosis, coarctation, or endocardial fibroelastosis.[2]

Chest radiography in the symptomatic infant may show cardiac enlargement, pulmonary venous congestion, and possibly increased pulmonary arterial markings if a large left-to-right shunt is present. The older asymptomatic child may only show a heart size that is the upper limit of normal. Older children and adults with a discrete thoracic coarctation may have a figure of 3 sign on the left margin of the aorta at the level of the coarctation on an overpenetrated frontal chest radiograph. This radiographic finding is produced by the contour of the dilated aorta just above the coarctation, the central indentation of the coarctation, and the poststenotic dilation below the coarctation.[52] The reverse 3 sign or E sign may be noted on the left anterior oblique projection of radiologic barium swallow studies from indentation by the same structures on the esophagus.[2] Due to the risk of aspiration in critically ill patients and availability of safer diagnostic approaches, barium studies are rarely performed. Notching of the inferior border of the posterior fourth to ninth ribs is commonly not observed until after 8 years of age.[2]

Echocardiography can be used to noninvasively assess simple and complex aortic coarctation. Two-dimensional long-axis views from the suprasternal notch permit visualization of isthmic hypoplasia.[44,53,54] Since this portion of the aorta may be difficult to image, associated findings of poststenotic dilation and diminished pulsation of the descending aorta are sought. A characteristic finding in simple coarctation is indentation of the posterior and lateral aspects of the aorta by a wedged-shaped shelf of tissue. Because there is often associated hypoplasia of the aortic arch, the transverse arch should be imaged and measured using a parasternal notch view.[22] Intracardiac anomalies and left ventricular function can be assessed by various two-dimensional views. Doppler echocardiography is used to detect ventricular septal defects, mitral insufficiency, shunting through a ductus arteriosus, and estimate gradients across obstructive lesions.[55] Color Doppler echocardiography has been shown to correlate well with angiographic evaluation of aortic coarctation.[56]

Sine magnetic resonance imaging has been used to noninvasively evaluate flow through the ductus arteriosus and the coarctation in patients with chest deformities or a lung disease that would limit the usefulness of echocardiography.[57] It provides an excellent alternative method to visualize the aortic isthmus and proximal descending aorta, particularly in older individuals. This method of evaluation requires the patient to lie perfectly still, which may limit its usefulness in some patients.

The decision to perform a cardiac catheterization prior to surgical correction varies among cardiologists, since invasive diagnostic procedures have significant risks in small children and noninvasive diagnostic studies are often sufficient. In the infant with multiple cardiovascular abnormalities, cardiac catheterization is often essential to determine whether repair of the aortic coarctation alone will be of sufficient hemodynamic benefit to warrant a delay in the surgical repair of the other correctable lesions.[14] The majority of older children diagnosed with aortic coarctation never require cardiac catheterization, since complex intracardiac defects are rare in this group. Noninvasive echocardiography is often sufficient for evaluation. On the other hand, angiography may be necessary to delineate the anatomy of severe long segment coarctation or the presence of collateral circulation. This information may be invaluable for assessing the need for left heart bypass or the optimal placement of aortic cross clamps intraoperatively.

Preoperative Management

The approach to each patient must be individualized and guided by the patient's response to medical therapy, associated lesions, and the practitioner's experience. In general, asymptomatic infants without hypertension who are diagnosed during routine examination may wait until 3–5 years of age to undergo elective repair of aortic coarctation. Infants with severe hypertension without heart failure, but who have cardiomegaly or significant left ventricular hypertrophy on echocardiography, often do not respond to antihypertensive therapy and require early surgical intervention.[2]

The treatment of infants with aortic coarctation who present with heart failure varies depending on the presence of coexisting cardiovascular anomalies. These infants require rapid stabilization with diuretics and digoxin. Only after aggressive treatment of coexisting problems, such as acidosis, anemia, hypoglycemia, or hypothermia, will cardiac catheterization be considered to establish a diagnosis and plan therapy.[2]

The critically ill neonate may require intubation, mechanical ventilation, inotropic support, diuresis, and bicarbonate infusion. Newborns who develop severe congestive heart failure due to closure of the ductus arteriosus may improve dramatically with infusion of PGE_1, which may reopen the ductus arteriosus. The use of PGE_1 infusion, starting at 0.05 µg per kg per minute, to open or maintain the patency of a ductus arteriosus may result in dramatic clinical improvement and stabilization. These infants need to be monitored for potential serious side effects of PGE_1 therapy such as hypotension, bradycardia, apnea, and hyperthermia.[45,58,59] In infants with severe heart failure and serious defects, who fail to improve with PGE_1, surgical intervention is the only chance for survival. Improved perioperative care and the use of PGE_1 has also decreased the early postoperative death rate for simple and complex coarctation.[6]

Treatment has been controversial for infants who present with congestive heart failure and simple aortic coarctation. Both medical management and early surgical repair have been advocated for this group of patients.[6,60,61] Proponents of medical management are influenced by concerns that there may be inadequate growth of the aortic anastomotic site, which would increase the likelihood of residual or recurrent stenosis if surgical repair is performed during infancy. They recommend delaying surgery until 2–4 years of age if the infant responds to management with digitalis and diuretics and there is no major intracardiac defect or ductal flow to the descending aorta. This age range has been recommended for two reasons: (1) avoiding early surgical repair decreases the likelihood of recoarctation, which has a high incidence during infancy; and (2) the incidence of persistent postoperative hypertension is lower in older children.[48]

On the other hand, proponents of early surgical repair in this group of patients base their decision on several factors. Most importantly, improvements in anesthetic techniques, operative procedures, and postoperative care have shifted the risk-benefit ratio toward performing the repair at an earlier age.[7,8,14] For example, Beekman reports no 1-month postoperative deaths in infants with simple coarctation and heart failure who received 2 days of stabilization preoperatively in his institution since 1977.[2] Although most infants in this group improve with medical therapy, some develop recurrent heart failure and some die acutely of left ventricular failure.[61] Therefore, proponents of early surgical repair argue that even though early operative intervention has risks (e.g., an increased risk of restenosis), early surgical repair should ensure survival of most infants in this group.

The management of infants with aortic coarctation and complex cardiac lesions is determined by the severity of the coexisting cardiovascular anomalies. In the majority of patients, the aortic coarctation lesion produces the major hemodynamic burden and is responsible for cardiac decompensation. For example, infants with aortic coarctation and an associated ventricular septal defect often improve dramatically with coarctation repair alone.[62] Combined repair of the ventricular septal defect and the coarctation during infancy is rarely required in this group. Pulmonary artery banding is advocated by some cardiologists if the pulmonary artery pressures remain elevated after completion of the coarctation repair.[63] Others recommend avoiding pulmonary artery banding in infants with membranous ventricular septal defects, because the distortion of the pulmonary arteries caused by the banding is an unnecessary complication not always completely amendable to later procedures.[64] Only if the patient fails medical management because of severe left-to-right shunting is the ventricular septal defect repaired.[62,65] Banding of the pulmonary artery along with repair of the coarctation is often performed in infants with large apical muscular septal defects or single ventricle or other complex lesions.[14]

Likewise, for most infants with coexisting aortic valvular stenosis or mitral valve abnormalities, only repair of the coarctation lesion during infancy is usually required. Repair of aortic valvular stenosis can often wait until later in childhood, and mitral valve function often improves over time following repair of coarctation.[14,66,67]

Preoperative Anesthetic Preparation

The anesthesiologist should obtain a detailed history, perform a thorough physical examination, and review all pertinent laboratory and investigational studies. A thorough discussion of the case with the cardiologist and cardiac surgeon preoperatively can be invaluable, because the clinical presentation can vary from a sick acidotic newborn dependent on a patent ductus arteriosus to an asymptomatic child with minimal hypertension.

Patients with Turner's syndrome should be evaluated for potentially difficult laryngoscopy and tracheal intubation. Associated congenital abnormalities should be evaluated. The site and type of aortic coarctation should be noted as well as the presence and significance of coexisting cardiovascular lesions (e.g., ventricular septal defects and valvular disease). The range of blood pressures recorded preoperatively from a site proximal to the coarctation should be noted since it provides a guide for the range of acceptable blood pressures during surgery and induced hypotension. The presence of an aberrant right subclavian artery may limit the usefulness of the right extremity for measurement of the proximal aortic blood pressure during aortic cross clamping. The presence and adequacy of collateral circulation can often be assessed by review of angiograms and evaluation of peripheral pulses, as well as identification of rib notching and subscapular bruits in older patients.

Patients with congestive heart failure should be optimized preoperatively. They may require treatment with diuretics, digoxin, and occasionally infusions of inotropic agents and sodium bicarbonate. Likewise, patients who are dependent on a patent ductus arteriosus should be identified, optimized with an infusion of PGE_1, and observed for the side effects of this therapy. Since resting hypertension is common in older individuals, it should be controlled medically prior to elective surgery, and antihypertensive therapy should be continued until the day of surgery.[3,47]

Individuals prone to develop anxiety should be well sedated to minimize hypertension preoperatively.[46] The patient's age, physical status, and level of anxiety are important factors when choosing a sedative for premedication. Premedication should rarely be necessary for patients under 1 year of age. Often anxiety can be allayed by having a parent accompany the child. Asymptomatic children may be premedicated with oral midazolam (0.5 mg/kg) 30 minutes before surgery or with intramuscular scopolamine (0.004 mg/kg) and morphine (0.15 mg/kg) 60 minutes prior to anesthetic induction if an intravenous line is unavailable preoperatively. Patients with limited cardiac reserves or other concerns should have the premedication dosage decreased by 30–50% or withheld until the patient arrives in the operating room suite. This will allow the anesthesiologist to administer additional sedative agents under direct supervision. Older children and adults may require no premedication if they are not anxious or hypertensive.

Operative Procedures

Surgical procedures to repair aortic coarctation include subclavian patch angioplasty, synthetic patch angioplasty, and end-to-end anastomosis after resection of the coarctation segment.[68–70] In addition, conduit insertion between the ascending and descending aorta can be used in selected cases for long segment obstruction in older individuals.[71] The procedure of choice during infancy varies from institution to institution and is a matter of current debate.[72,68]

The surgical technique chosen depends on the patient's age, the position and length of the coarctation segment, the presence of coexisting cardiovascular lesions, procedure success and complication rates, as well as the surgeon's experience. For all procedures, the ductus arteriosus is always divided. The surgical approach is usually via a left thoracotomy, unless there is a complex lesion such as coexisting aortic arch hypoplasia requiring median sternotomy.

The first surgical procedure to successfully correct aortic coarctation in an infant was resection of the coarctation segment with end-to-end anastamosis by Kirklin in 1952 (Figure 9-5).[73,74] Direct end-to-end anastomosis is easiest when it requires excision of a discrete narrow coarctation segment, although increased elasticity of the aorta in neonates may allow mobilization and excision of several centimeters of tubular aortic hypoplasia. The surgical approach is usually via the third or fourth intercostal space. The aorta is mobilized upward to the aortic arch and downward distal to the anastomotic site. The coarctation site can often be identified visually as a discrete narrowed segment that is excised after placement of proximal and distal aortic clamps. An anastomosis is then performed between the proximal and distal ends of the aorta by running a continuous suture line posteriorly and an interrupted suture line anteriorly.[75] Modifications of this repair may include insertion of a tubular vascular prosthesis to bridge an aortic segment in cases in which the coarctation is long, the aortic isthmus is hypoplastic, or there is an associated aneurysmal dilation.[44]

As experience with end-to-end anastomosis in infants and young children increased, it became apparent that this group of patients had a high incidence of residual or recurrent coarctation following this procedure. Inadequate growth of a circular suture line at the site of the anastomosis was thought to be the cause. This problem led to the development of other procedures.[76] End-to-end anastomosis is still commonly used in older children and adults in whom the incidence of restenosis is lower. Proponents of the use of this technique during infancy claim that restenosis occurs less frequently now that newer suture techniques are being used.[75] In addi-

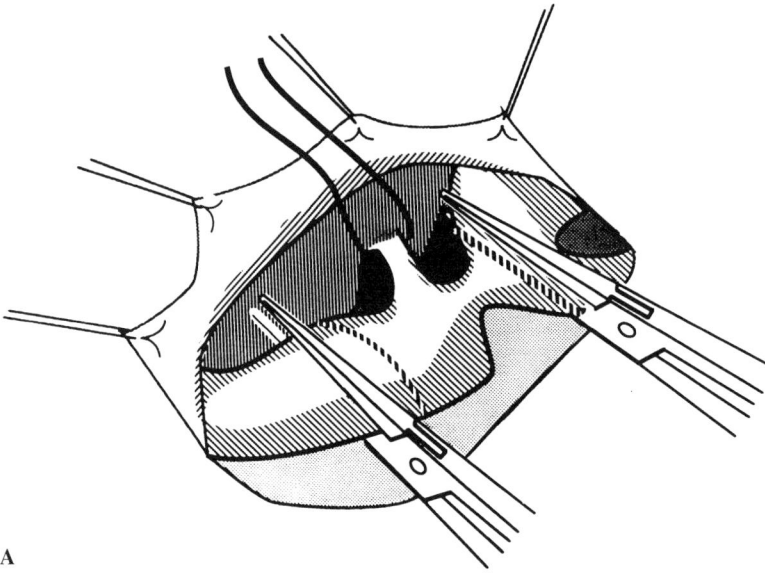

A

Figure 9-5. Resection and end-to-end anastomosis of aortic coarctation. A. Vascular clamps placed above and below the coarctation. B. Coarctation segment is excised. Anastomosis begun posteriorly with continuous suture. C. Anastomosis completed anteriorly with interrupted sutures. (Modified with permission from AG Coran, DM Behrendt, WH Weintraub. Surgery of the Neonate. Boston: Little, Brown, 1978;93.)

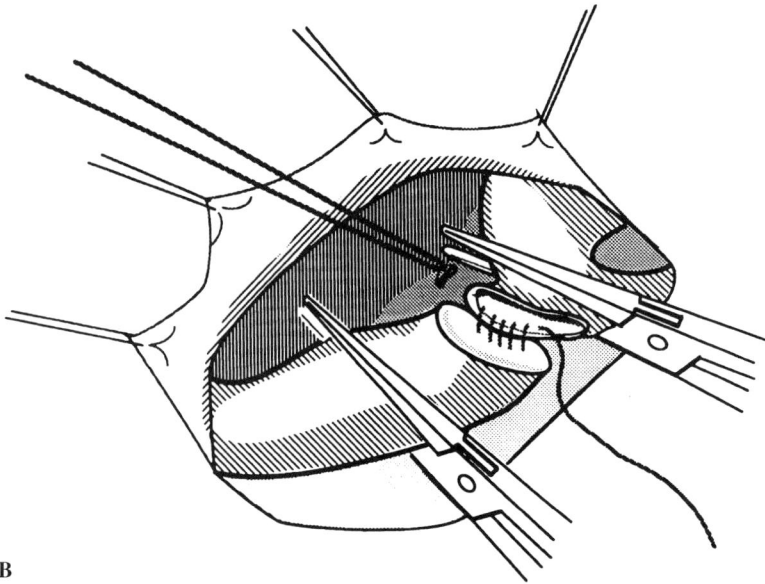

B

tion, extreme elasticity of the aorta in young patients allows full resection of even long coarctation segments, while avoiding the possible hazards arising from the division of major vessels required by the subclavian flap procedure.[77]

In 1966, Waldhausen and Nahrwold introduced the subclavian flap procedure, which is now widely used for coarctation repair during infancy (Figure 9-6).[78] This procedure is performed via a left thoracotomy. The surgeon dissects and mobilizes the ductus arteriosus, distal aortic arch, left subclavian artery, and the aorta distal to the coarctation segment. Extension of the dissection distal to the site of coarctation may involve intercostal arteries responsible for collateral blood flow. The left vertebral artery is often ligated to prevent the development of a vertebral steal syndrome from the cerebral circulation to the left

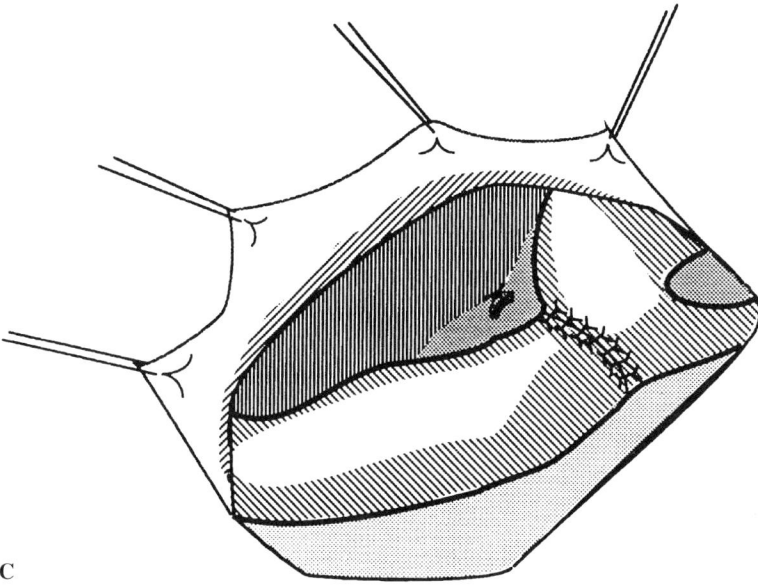

C

arm later in life.[7,79] A longitudinal incision is made from the proximal left subclavian artery into the descending aorta across the coarctation. The posterior shelf lesion is excised, and the subclavian artery is used anteriorly as a patch graft that is sutured with continuous sutures.[7,75] Since this procedure avoids a circumferential scar, uses living tissue for the patch, and uses absorbable sutures, the potential for growth at the repair site is thought to be maximized.[80–82] Although collateral arterial circulation of the left arm usually develops, there is a potential for decreased arm growth, reduced perfusion, and brachial plexus injury.[79] Repair of aortic coarctation by subclavian flap procedure probably offers the greatest likelihood of a surgical cure during the first year of life, although there is considerable debate concerning which procedure is best for this age group.[72,83]

In the patch aortoplasty procedure, the aorta is opened longitudinally across the segment of aortic coarctation. In an older individual with a postductal coarctation, this would require an aortomy from the inferior portion of the left subclavian to the largest portion of the descending aorta. The fibrous shelf contributing to aortic luminal narrowing is excised and an elliptical woven Dacron patch is sutured in place to augment the diameter of the aortic segment.[14] Patch aortoplasty is no longer used for the primary repair in children because in the long-term there is an unacceptably high incidence (24%) of aortic aneurysm formation in young individuals.[84]

Experience with balloon angioplasty of aortic coarctation has yielded mixed results.[85] Successful attempts at balloon angioplasty succeed by tearing the vascular intima and part or all of the media.[86] While unrepaired aortic coarctation lesions may be dilated with good initial relief of the gradient and minimal short-term complications, the decrease in the pressure gradient is usually less than that obtained surgically.[87,88] Early restenosis is common following this procedure in neonates. Balloon angioplasty of lesions, such as preductal coarctation with associated isthmal hypoplasia, may lead to aortic dissection or the development of aneurysms in children.[89] In the patient with restenosis following surgical repair, balloon angioplasty is safer and more successful because of the coexisting scarring around the repaired coarctation segment. The indications for balloon angioplasty, therefore, are limited mainly to treatment of recoarctation in children following subclavian flap repair or end-to-end anastomotic repair during infancy. It is not indicated for the routine management of unrepaired coarctation, but may be useful in the selected sick infant or child

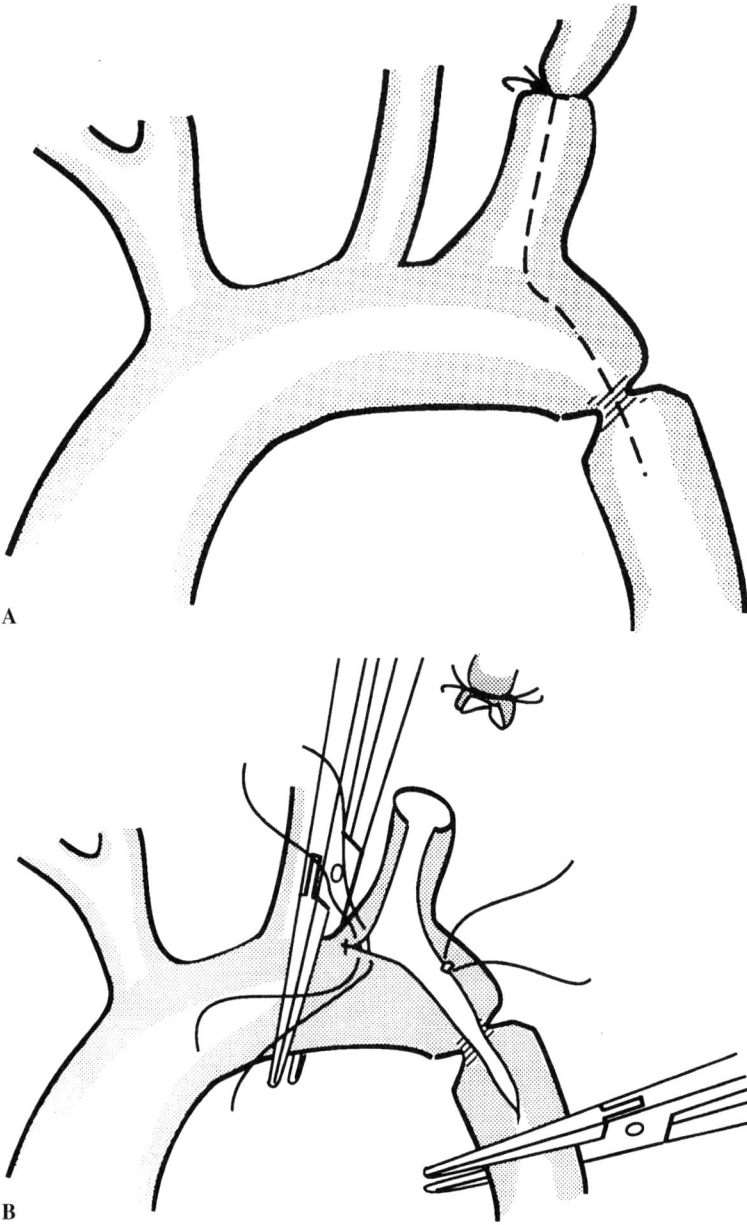

Figure 9-6. Left subclavian artery flap angioplasty repair of aortic coarctation. A. Subclavian artery is ligated and divided. A longitudinal incision is made from the left subclavian and extended across the coarctation to the descending aorta. B. After excision of the intraluminal coarctation shelf, the subclavian artery flap is folded down and sutured over the incised aorta. C. The completed subclavian flap allows aortic growth. (Modified with permission from AG Coran, DM Behrendt, WH Weintraub. Surgery of the Neonate. Boston: Little, Brown, 1978;93.)

with associated complex anomalies who is judged to be at high risk with surgical intervention.[90–92]

Perioperative Complications

Surgical Complications

Complications of surgical repair of aortic coarctation include hemorrhage, chylothorax, mesenteric arteri-tis, paraplegia, and recurrent laryngeal, phrenic, and vagus nerve injury.[45,46] Operative mortality and morbidity depend on age, overall physical condition, emergency status, surgical experience, as well as the presence and severity of coexisting cardiovascular lesions.[14] Over the past few decades the operative mortality has progressively decreased for repair of simple aortic coarctation, while the operative and long-term follow-up mortality remains high for complex coarctation. The operative and postoperative mortality for

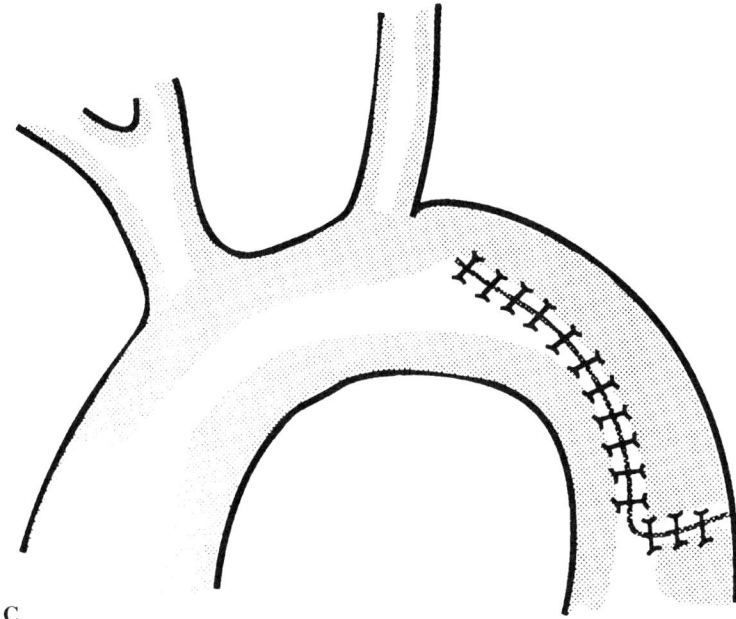

C

infants with simple coarctatation has been reported as low as 0–4%, whereas the overall mortality of infants with complex coarctation who undergo surgical repair is 38–50%.[6,93] Causes of intraoperative death include ventricular fibrillation, asystole, and hemorrhage.[20] Hemorrhage usually occurs in individuals with associated aneurysmal disease or those patients undergoing repeat coarctation repair. The primary cause of postoperative death is low cardiac output syndrome, which is almost always present preoperatively and has a higher incidence in individuals with complex cardiovascular lesions.[20]

The long-term prognosis for a child who had a coarctation repair during infancy depends on residual or recurrent coarctation, persistent hypertension, and residual cardiovascular lesions.[2] The major long-term problem encountered in infants and children who survive surgery is recoarctation. The reported incidence of restenosis varies and is higher in younger age groups. While the type of surgical repair appears to influence the incidence of residual stenosis and recoarctation, there remains considerable debate over which technique offers the best protection. Recurrent stenosis following resection with end-to-end anastomotic repair during infancy has a reported incidence of 25–60%.[75,76,94–96] The reported incidence of clinically significant restenosis following subclavian flap repair has been

reported to be as low as 0–13%.[7,8,97] However, restenosis requiring reoperation has been reported as high as 25% in patients undergoing the subclavian flap repair before 3 months of age.[75] While the initial reports of lower restenosis rates following subclavian flap repair appear promising, this procedure has a shorter history of long-term follow-up compared with the end-to-end anastomotic repair.[72]

For patients undergoing reoperation for recurrent coarctation, the risk for mortality has been reported to be 7–33%.[98] The majority of these patients have dense adhesions in the area of the coarctation, which increases the risk of hemorrhage and complicates attempts at end-to-end anastomotic repairs. To minimize hemorrhage, graft insertion has been recommended by some.[99,100] In a review of 21 cases of reoperation by Beekman, 9 of 21 patients required left-sided heart bypass, and the lowest operative morbidity was noted with synthetic patch aortoplasty.[76]

Early Hypertension

Most patients undergoing repair during early childhood have arterial blood pressures decrease toward normal levels immediately following surgery. Occasionally, paradoxical postoperative hypertension can become a serious complication. It requires spe-

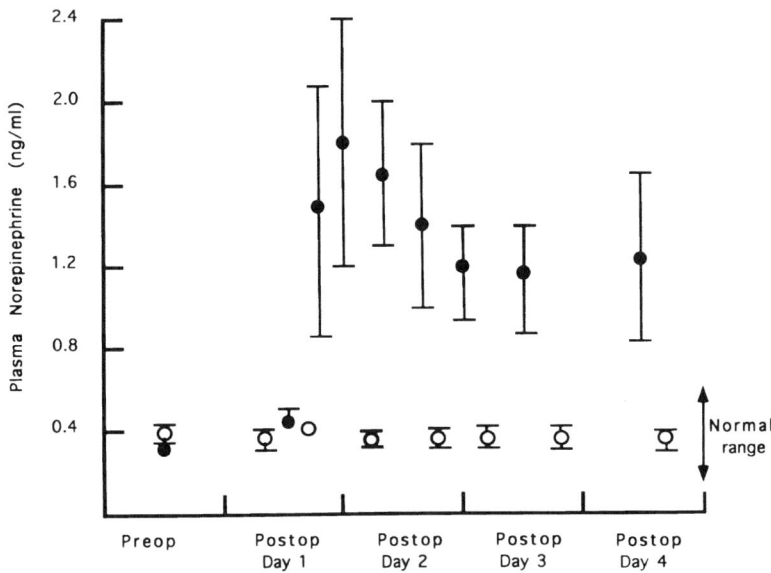

Figure 9-7. Postoperative plasma norepinephrine concentrations. The postoperative plasma norepinephrine concentrations (mean + standard error of the mean) remain elevated in the group of patients following repair of aortic coarctation (●) in comparison with a control group following major surgery (O). (Modified with permission from A Fischer, CR Benedict. Adult coarctation of of the aorta: anesthesia and postoperative management. Anaesthesia 1977;32:533.)

cialized care during the immediate postoperative period to minimize problems such as mesenteric arteritis, intracranial hemorrhage, tearing of the suture line, or rupture of aortic segments with residual aneurysmal dilation, which can result if postoperative hypertension is inadequately controlled.[47,51] The exact etiology of paradoxical postoperative hypertension is unclear, and there appear to be multiple contributing factors. The hypertension may be diastolic and systolic in nature and may present in two phases.[101] The early phase presents during the first 12–24 hours after surgery. It has been proposed that this early increase in blood pressure is reflexive in nature. The carotid baroreceptors proximal to the coarctation are adapted to a greater degree of stretch due to the chronic preexisting proximal hypertension.[47] These baroceptors react to decreased stretch following surgical repair with increased sympathetic activity.[102] This theory is supported by measurement of plasma norepinephrine levels in the postoperative period. The degree of elevation of plasma norepinephrine levels at 12 hours after surgery correlates positively with the preoperative peak pressure gradient across the coarctation.[46] As early as 12 hours following coarctation repair, plasma norepinephrine levels have been elevated by as much as as 750% above preoperative levels compared with only a 40% increase following major surgery in patients who served as a control group.[103] While patients in the control group have normal

levels of norepinephrine by the end of the third day, norepinephrine levels remain elevated in the coarctation repair group and may remain elevated for as long as 6 months (Figure 9-7).[46] This initial phase of hypertension usually subsides with treatment.

The second phase of paradoxical postoperative hypertension generally begins 2–3 days after surgery. It has been postulated that in addition to the reflexive baroceptor mechanism and increased sympathetic activity, hormonal effects moderated by renin and angiotensin may play a role in the etiology of hypertension in this second phase.[104–107] Perioperative administration of saralasin acetate, a specific antagonist of angiotensin II, to patients undergoing coarctation repair results in lower blood pressure and is strong evidence that the renin-angiotensin system plays an important role in postoperative hypertension.[108,109]

Agents that have been used to control hypertension in the postoperative period include chlorpromazine, reserpine, hydralazine, phentolamine, methyldopa, diuretics, ganglionic blockers, nitroprusside, and nitroglycerin. Nitroglycerin is often ineffective and nitroprusside may be effective only at high infusion rates. Therefore, beta-blockers and angiotension inhibitors are commonly used. Nonselective beta-blockers (e.g., propranolol) provide blood pressure control via negative chronotropic and inotropic mechanisms, as well as inhibiting renin release by blocking sympathetic activity at the juxtaglomerular complex.[47] The therapeutic response to angiotensin-converting enzyme inhibitors, arterial smooth muscle dilators, and beta-blockers has proved useful in controlling the blood pressure of these patients.[110–114] When a patient can resume oral intake, antihypertensive therapy, which may be required for several days or weeks after surgical repair, can usually be converted to oral medication.

Late Hypertension

Residual hypertension that is unrelated to residual aortic coarctation and requires prolonged medical therapy occurs in 10–60% of older individuals.[2,47,115,116] After 10 years of age, the increase of incidence of residual hypertension correlates with an increase in the age of the patient at the time of the repair.[117] The exact etiology of residual hypertension is unclear but is probably related to the factors that contribute to hypertension in the postoperative period.[118,119] There is a subset of patients without restenosis who are normotensive at rest, but may develop upper extremity hypertension and a significant arm-leg gradient during dynamic exercise after coarctation repair.[120,121] It has been proposed that increased cardiac output, residual coarctation stenosis, diminished compliance of the repair site, and altered vascular reactivity are possible contributing factors in this exercise-induced hypertension. Since exercise-induced hypertension is associated with accelerated progression of cardiovascular disease and early mortality, it is important for patients to be evaluated for the remainder of their lives following surgery. In an effort to minimize rapid progression of cardiovascular disease in this group of patients, long-term antihypertensive therapy may be required.[122]

Mesenteric Arteritis

Postcoarctectomy syndrome, also known as mesenteric arteritis, is a complication that was first reported in 1951.[123] This syndrome results from severe vasoconstriction of the mesenteric arteries leading to ischemia of the abdominal viscera. It is most likely a result of elevated sympathetic activity. In its most severe form, it is characterized by hypertension, abdominal pain, pyrexia, intestinal bleeding or obstruction, and vomiting. It typically presents 1–5 days postoperatively.[46] While postcoarctectomy syndrome complicated approximately 10% of surgical repairs at one time and had a 10% mortality,[124] it is now less prevalent due in part to improved postoperative blood pressure control. Additionally, restriction of postoperative oral fluids, nasogastric decompression, and aggressive treatment of postoperative hypertension has significantly reduced this postoperative complication.[14] The hypertension associated with this syndrome responds well to the administration of beta-blockers, arterial smooth muscle dilators, and angiotensin-converting enzyme inhibitors.[114]

Spinal Cord Ischemia

A devastating complication of surgical repair of aortic coarctation is spinal cord ischemia and paresis, which has a reported incidence of 0.14–0.41%.[125–127] Possible mechanisms include (1) direct compromise of the intercostal arterial supply to the anterior spinal artery that may occur from cross clamping and mobilization of the aorta, (2) inadequate distal aortic blood flow via collateral circulation during aortic cross clamping, and (3) increased cerebrospinal fluid (CSF) pressure.[128,129] Interestingly, paralysis has been reported to occur spontaneously without surgery in eight older individuals (10–57 years old) with aortic coarctation. Paralysis resulted from rupture of an intercostal artery aneurysm or from compression of the spinal cord by an intercostal artery aneurysm.[125]

To best understand the pathogenesis of spinal cord ischemia and the proposed measures to minimize its occurrence, it is important to understand the anatomy of the blood supply to the spinal cord. There are many variations of the blood supply of the anterior spinal artery, which originates from the vertebral arteries at the base of the skull and extends to the lumbar region.[125,130] The anterior spinal artery is not a continuous vessel in most individuals. Instead, it is divided into end arteries with the lower divisions supplied by segmental intercostal arteries. Normally, there is little arterial continuity between the divisions, and collateral arterial supply between divisions of the anterior spinal arteries is often limited or nonexistent. Therefore, the spinal cord is at risk of ischemia whenever the intercostal arterial supply to anterior spinal end arteries is compromised. This may occur if there is interruption of a critical segmental supply to the anterior spinal artery, such as when the intercostal arteries are divided by the surgeon or when distal aortic blood flow decreases during aortic cross clamping.[131] A dangerous situation arises when the anterior spinal artery is interrupted at the level of an aortic coarctation and the entire blood supply for the lower spinal cord originates from an intercostal vessel at or near the T9 level. Even in patients with coarctation and well-developed thoracoabdominal collateral circulation, the blood supply to the lower spinal cord may be inadequate during surgical repair (see Chapters 1 and 8).[125]

Brewer and coworkers conducted the largest retrospective review of over 12,000 cases of surgical coarctation repair and found the incidence of paraplegia to be 0.41%.[125] This study revealed that paraplegia was more prevalent among older individuals. The average age for this complication was 21, while the youngest patient was 3 years of age. There appeared to be no critical number of intercostal arteries that was unsafe to divide, and the author recommended dividing as many intercostal arteries as deemed necessary to expedite the procedure. Risk factors associated with paraplegia include hyperthermia, poor collateral circulation to the descending aorta, cross clamp time greater than 30 minutes, low blood pressure proximal and distal to the cross clamp, and elevated CSF pressure during aortic cross clamping (see Chapter 8).[125,132,133]

Management of Aortic Cross Clamping During Coarctation Repair

Cross clamping of the aorta increases both aortic blood pressure proximal to the cross clamp and the CSF pressure, while decreasing distal aortic pressure.[134–136] It is postulated that arterial hypertension of the cerebral circulation during aortic cross clamping results in increased cerebral blood flow and an elevation of CSF pressure. Efforts to normalize proximal aortic blood pressure with vasodilators (e.g., nitroprusside) to prevent left ventricular dysfunction and the deleterious effects of hypertension may further increase CSF pressure and decrease distal aortic pressure. The result of vasodilator therapy in conjunction with aortic cross clamping may therefore lead to further reductions in spinal cord perfusion resulting in ischemic injury (see Chapter 8 for a detailed discussion of this issue).

Despite these concerns, controlled hypotension may be beneficial during surgical repair of aortic coarctation for various reasons. Control of arterial blood pressure may shorten the operative time by providing a drier operative field. Induced hypotension provides a lax aorta during the repair that may facilitate suturing, clamping, and creation of the anastomosis.[137] In addition, induced hypotension can not only minimize blood loss in patients requiring extensive mobilization of long aortic segments, but also decrease the risk of aortic rupture in patients with associated aortic aneurysms.[46,138,139] In patients with a well-developed collateral circulation, blood pressure control has been advocated from the beginning of the surgical procedure in order to minimize blood loss from tortuous blood vessels.[139,140]

In patients who have limited collateral circulation but adequate aortic lumen diameter, blood pressure control is required to reduce the incidence of hemodynamic complications of aortic cross clamping (e.g., dysrhythmias, left ventricular failure, cerebrovascular hemorrhage, or cardiac arrest).[46,137,140,141] Therefore, a period of testing aortic cross clamping should be used in most patients to evaluate the adequacy of collateral circulation, the need for blood pressure control, and the possible need for circulatory support.[47] An increase in blood pressure of more than 25–30 mm Hg proximal to the aortic cross clamp suggests inadequate collaterals and is an indication for blood pressure control.[142] The clamp should be removed and after adequate control of blood pressure is attained, the cross clamp can be reapplied.

Vasodilators have traditionally been effective in controlling proximal blood pressure during aortic cross clamping even though a major portion of the vasculature is excluded.[45,139,143,144] Children may be more resistant to these agents and may benefit from the use of more than one agent.[145–147] The addition of beta-blocking agents may minimize tachycardia, as well as reduce the infusion rate of vasodilators during controlled hypotension. Doses of propranolol up to 0.06 mg/kg that are administered slowly and divided doses have been used successfully in children.[147] Likewise, labetalol (1.0 mg/kg) in divided doses has provided satisfactory blood pressure and heart rate control during coarctation repair in nine children (1–14 years old) anesthetized with halothane.[141] The mean arterial pressure decreased an average of 30% and heart rate decreased 8% from preoperative values. Hypertension was not

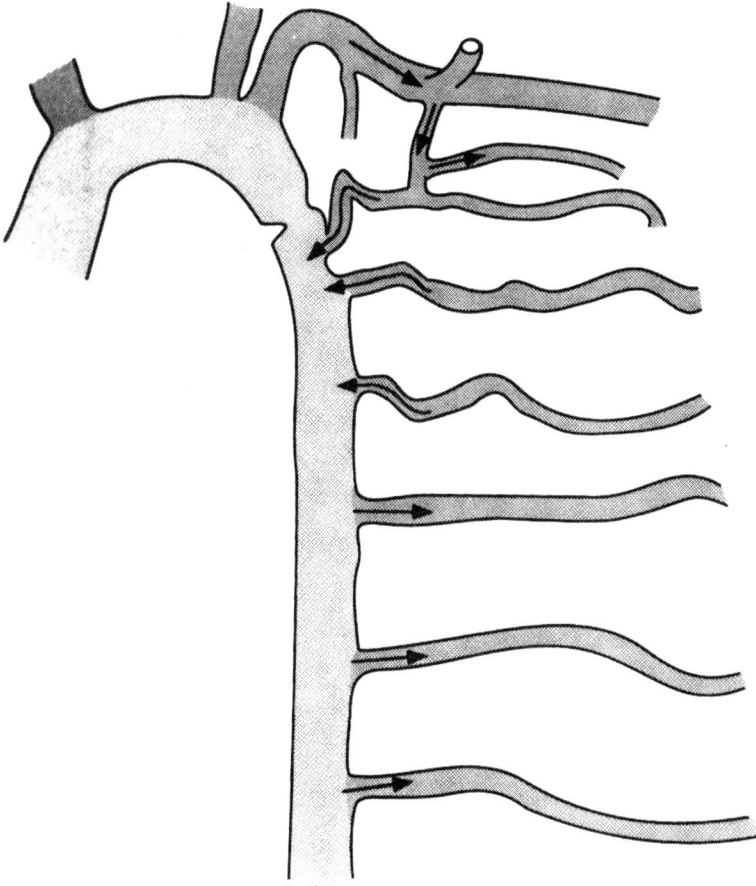

Figure 9-8. Intercostal arterial collateral flow in coarctation of the aorta. Collateral flow to the distal aorta may occur via reverse blood through the intercostal arteries from vessels originating from the subclavian arteries. The extent of reverse collateral flow varies among individuals. It commonly involves the second intercostal artery and in some cases involves the second through the seventh intercostal arteries. (Modified with permission from RW Barnes, EA Rittenhouse, C Kontahworn, et al. Reversed intercostal arterial flow in coarctation of the aorta. Intraoperative assessment with the Doppler ultrasonic velocity detector. Ann Thorac Surg 1975;19:27. The Society of Thoracic Surgeons.)

observed with aortic cross clamping. Release of the aortic cross clamp produced an average decrease in blood presure of 25% that was followed by rapid recovery. It is important for the anesthesiologist to understand that beta-blocking agents decrease blood pressure primarily by reducing cardiac output and may prevent restoration of cardiac output in the event of sudden severe blood loss.[148] The use of esmolol, which has a short plasma half-life, may prove to be more advantageous.

It is important to avoid profound hypotension, which may increase the risk of hypoperfusion. Usually, maintenance of normotension or a slight reduction in blood pressure is all that is required for optimal surgical exposure. While control of the blood pressure proximal to the aortic cross clamp may facilitate surgery, maintenance of blood pressure below the coarctation is important since blood

flow is often dependent on collateral flow arising from branches of subclavian arteries.[46] One of the major sources of collateral blood flow is via reverse blood flow in the second to sixth intercostal arteries (Figure 9-8).[149] The adequacy of collateral flow can be tested most accurately by measuring the intraaortic pressure above and below the aortic cross clamps.[150] Measurement of the distal aortic pressure is especially important when a cross clamp must be placed above the subclavian artery.[125] A mean arterial pressure of 50 mm Hg in the distal aortic segment is regarded by some as the critical pressure below which perfusion becomes inadequate and circulatory support is necessary.[46,151]

The effects of anesthetic agents, antihypertensive drugs, and cross clamp repositioning on distal aortic pressure during aortic cross clamping in coarctation repair has been investigated.[129] Watterson and colleagues studied 133 patients undergoing coarctation repair and determined that the critical level for arterial pressure in the leg during aortic cross clamping is 45 mm Hg in children over 1 year of age.[129] Often, the distal arterial pressure increased slightly during the first 10 minutes of aortic cross clamping from a mean pressure of 53–59 mm Hg. Based on this study, Watterson et al. recommend that if distal aortic pressure is less than 45 mm Hg, an effort should be made to readjust the proximal and distal cross clamps to allow maximal collateral blood flow. If distal perfusion pressure remains low, then reduction of agents that affect blood pressure should be tried. The author found that the use of halothane, enflurane, nitroprusside, or labetalol to lower proximal aortic systolic pressure to 150 mm Hg or less contributed to unacceptably low levels of distal aortic pressure in some patients.[129] Acceptance of proximal aortic systolic pressures as high as 180 mm Hg allowed for less vasodilator use and higher distal aortic pressures. However, the potential for increased risk of cerebral hemorrhage or acute left ventricular failure remains unknown especially in younger children.[129] In the young infant there is no evidence that allowing proximal systolic pressures to increase greater than 80–90 mm Hg offers any benefit. Therefore, excessive increases in systolic pressure above preoperative levels should be treated in infants to avoid ventricular failure or cerebral injury.

If the initial maneuvers fail to maintain adequate distal aortic pressure, placement of a temporary shunt from the distal aortic arch to the descending aorta or use of left heart bypass is recommended by many authors.[129,152–155] The requirement of a vascular shunt is rare in most patients, especially in older patients who tend to have well-developed collateral circulation.[156]

Additional measures that may minimize spinal cord injury should be used. Hyperthermia should definitely be avoided. Mild hypothermia (32–35°C) may allow longer aortic occlusion time.[45,156] Greater degrees of hypothermia increase the risk of ventricular fibrillation. Arterial PCO_2 should be monitored and maintained in the normal range, since respiratory alkalosis could potentially contribute to further decreases in CNS blood flow (see Chapter 8).[129,157]

Somatosensory evoked potential (SSEP) monitoring has been used by a few investigators to evaluate the adequacy of spinal cord perfusion during coarctation repair, although few studies have included patients with well-developed collateral circulation.[157,158] Krieger and Spence used SSEP to assess cord ischemia in five patients undergoing coarctation repair.[133] The distal aortic pressure was maintained over 60 mm Hg during aortic cross clamping. The evoked potential remained unchanged and no patients developed paraplegia. Dasmahapatra and coworkers demonstrated reversible spinal cord ischemia by the loss or diminution of SSEP in 38 patients undergoing repair of aortic coarctation.[157] In 31 patients, the distal aortic pressure was measured and the mean pressure was 32 mm Hg during aortic cross clamping. A low distal aortic pressure was associated with reversible spinal cord ischemia. Factors identified to be associated with reduced distal aortic pressure included use of vasodilators and low arterial CO_2 partial pressure.[129] However, it must be remembered that SSEP monitors only the posterior spinal cord, which has a separate blood supply from the anterior spinal cord. Therefore, patients may develop anterior spinal cord ischemia and postoperative paraplegia while displaying normal evoked potentials during intraoperative SSEP monitoring (see Chapters 4 and 8).[159–161]

Anesthetic Management

The most important factor in determining the anesthetic plan should be the overall physical condition of the patient. All patients require antibiotic prophylaxis preoperatively and postoperatively.[3] The choice of anesthetic agents and techniques should be guided by such factors as personal experience, type and severity of the coarctation lesion, presence and severity of associated cardiovascular anomalies, adequacy of ventricular function and reserve, presence and adequacy of collateral circulation, patient age, possible use of SSEP monitoring, and planned surgical repair. The goal for a safe anesthetic should be to maintain normal heart rate, contractility, and preload.[162] Patients who have limited ventricular function and reserve, such as neonates or individuals with severe cardiac anomalies, may not tolerate myocardial depressant agents or increases in left ventricular afterload.

While all patients undergoing surgical repair of aortic coarctation are at risk of developing any of the complications discussed earlier in this chapter, anesthesiologists must be aware that certain anatomic lesions have higher associated surgical risks. Dalal et al. were the first to emphasize that special considerations should be made when formulating the anesthetic plan based on the presence of the following anatomic features.[139] Patients with good collateral circulation and without severe stenosis of the aortic coarctation usually tolerate aortic cross clamping with minimal cardiovascular instability (e.g., severe hypertension and acute left ventricular dysfunction) as long as the adequacy of collateral flow is not compromised. The greatest problem encountered may be blood loss primarily from collateral vessels in the chest wall. This may be best minimized by using induced hypotension at the start of surgery. It is imperative that the anesthesiologist have adequate vascular access, hemodynamic monitoring, vasoactive infusions, and blood products available from the start of the case. Patients with good collateral circulation and severe narrowing of the aortic lumen usually tolerate aortic cross clamping, but may have even greater blood losses during surgical exposure.

Patients with minimal aortic narrowing and poorly developed collateral circulation are at an increased risk of acute cardiovascular instability at the time of aortic cross clamping (i.e., acute left ventricular failure, reflex cardiac arrest, or cerebrovascular hemorrhage), life-threatening rupture of a tense aorta during mobilization, and hypoperfusion distal to the aortic cross clamp. The anesthesiologist should be prepared to rapidly titrate vasoactive agents to minimze proximal hypertension while avoiding distal hypotension. In addition to pharmacologic manipulations, surgical interventions with trial aortic cross clamping, cross clamp repositioning, shunt insertion, or left heart bypass may be required to proceed safely.

Patients with severe narrowing of the aorta and poor collateral circulation have the greatest risk of developing spinal cord injury.[139] This risk is greatest when mobilization of the aorta is extensive, replacement of blood loss is inadequate, distal hypotension is prolonged, and spinal cord protection is inadequate (see Chapter 8).

Monitoring

During surgical repair, the blood pressure above and below the level of coarctation should be monitored to prevent severe hypertension, hypotension, and organ damage. Unless there is an anomalous right subclavian artery, the right arm should be used for blood pressure readings. Since these patients are usually in the right lateral decubitus position, to obtain reliable readings compression of the blood pressure cuff should be avoided by a properly positioned axillary roll. The use of an arterial line to measure the proximal aortic pressure is essential. Placement of an indwelling arterial line distal to the site of aortic coarctation may prove difficult in small infants and individuals with inadequate distal perfusion due to limited collateral circulation. These individuals may require placement of a needle in the descending aorta by the surgeon in order to monitor distal aortic pressure.[46] In older individuals, placement of a blood pressure cuff on a lower extremity may provide a measure of distal aortic pressure if the collateral circulation is well developed.[158] Likewise, a lower extremity blood pressure cuff may provide a measure of the pressure gradient before and after the repair. With placement of the aortic cross clamps, ligation of intercostal arteries, and possible infusion of vasoactive drugs, the accuracy of a lower extremity blood pressure cuff may be limited compared with a distal indwelling arterial line (i.e., femoral artery, dorsalis pedis, or posterior tibial arterial lines).

Adequate intravenous access is required for volume replacement and possible resuscitation due to bleeding from dilated intercostal arteries during thoracotomy incision, the mobilization and dissection of the thoracic aorta, or rupture of coexisting aneurysms. For the older child and adult, at least two 14-gauge intravenous catheters are recommended.[163] Patients who have cardiovascular lesions that may allow potential right-to-left or left-to-right shunting should have all intravenous lines meticulously purged of air bubbles.

A urinary catheter should be present intraoperatively and the urine output should be noted before, during, and after the period of aortic cross clamping. Urinary output provides one measure of the adequacy of organ perfusion distal to the site of aortic coarctation. This is particularly important in patients who require inotropes perioperatively, have prolonged cross clamp times, or require volume resuscitation due to extensive bleeding.

The use of central venous pressure (CVP) catheters intraoperatively is advocated by most anesthesiologists. A CVP catheter may be invaluable when (1) managing individuals with complex or severe lesions who required inotropic support preoperatively, (2) monitoring the effects of induced hypotension, and (3) evaluating the response to fluid resuscitation. The CVP catheter should be positioned so as not to enter an anomalous left superior vena cava that is found in some individuals. This vessel, which runs medially across the junction of the coarctation and ductus arteriosus, may need to be ligated for surgical access.[139] Insertion of a CVP catheter via the subclavian approach should be avoided in individuals with associated major arterial malformations that may distort the normal subclavicular anatomy.[46]

The placement of two separate pulse oximeter probes above and below the site of surgery, which are connected to oximeters that display plethysmyographic tracings, can be useful. In individuals with complex congenital heart disease and a patent ductus arteriosus, a sudden change in the direction and magnitude of the shunting of blood may be detected by changes in the arterial saturation of blood perfusing above and below the level of the coarctation. Likewise, a change in the character and amplitude of the oximeter plethysmyographic tracings may provide a measure of the adequacy of perfusion, especially when correlation is made with the mean arterial blood pressures.

Other important monitors include the ECG, temperature probe, and capnography, which are used for other pediatric cardiovascular procedures. An esophageal stethoscope is also essential because it may provide important and early warning of changes in heart tones and ventilation.

Anticoagulation

Anticoagulation should be attained with heparin in the vast majority of patients before placement of the aortic cross clamp. However, in some patients with extensive arterial collateral circulation, the aortic cross clamp can be applied without prior heparinization if there is sufficient perfusion distal to the aortic cross clamp to minimize the occurrence of thrombosis during brief periods of aortic cross clamping.[156,164] When anticoagulation is desired, at least 1 mg/kg of heparin should be administered through a well-secured intravenous catheter or CVP. The adequacy of anticoagulation should be evaluated using the acti-

vated coagulation time before initiating cross clamping to avoid thrombosis. Likewise, after reversal of anticoagulation with protamine the activated coagulation time should be checked (see Chapter 5).[164,165]

Cross Clamp Release

Regardless of the patient's age, there is a risk of hypotension associated with the release of the aortic cross clamp. This can be minimized by (1) the appropriate replacement of operative blood loss, (2) cautious administration of intravenous fluids to achieve a slightly hypervolemic state in individuals with adequate ventricular reserve, (3) reduction in inspired inhalational agent concentration, (4) slow release of the cross clamp, and (5) discontinuation of the vasodilator infusion 5–10 minutes before the anticipated release of the aortic cross clamp.[139] It is not uncommon for mild hypotension to occur for several minutes after the release of the cross clamp despite these efforts. Cautious volume infusion and further decreases in inhalational agent concentration usually is sufficent to correct hypotension. While a vasopressor should always be available, it should not be used routinely as a first-line intervention. If it is required, it should be titrated cautiously to avoid hypertension and disruption of the surgical repair. It is always important to inspect the surgical field after release of the aortic cross clamp, because hypotension associated with significant surgical bleeding requires repeat cross clamping of the aorta and immediate volume replacement.

Acidosis associated with aortic cross clamping is always a potential cause of hypotension, although the degree of acidosis observed and the need to treat it varies. For many individuals with simple coarctation, the surgical repair can be accomplished quickly, and the degree of acidosis that develops is minimal and resolves with adequate reperfusion. Administration of sodium bicarbonate is usually unnecessary and often the only short-term intervention that may be required is an increase in minute ventilation to produce mild respiratory alkalosis in order to compensate for a mild metabolic acidosis. Acidosis may develop more rapidly in individuals with low cardiac output states preoperatively (e.g., individuals with complex coarctation and individuals requiring inotropes), inadequate collateral circulation, and prolonged aortic cross-clamp times. These individuals may require frequent arterial blood gas analysis to guide sodium bicarbonate infusion, inotropic support, adjustments in ventilation, and fluid administration.

Anesthetic Management of Neonates and Infants

Neonates and young infants require special consideration. They normally have immature and poorly compliant ventricles, as well as incomplete development of sympathetic innervation to the heart. When these individuals present for aortic coarctation surgery, they often have poor collateral arterial circulation and are dependent on a patent ductus arteriosus for lower body perfusion. The group of infants that can be particularly challenging to manage are those who develop rapid closure of the ductus arteriosus that is refractory to infusion to PGE_1. An acute increase in left ventricular afterload usually follows, resulting in acute left ventricular distention and reduced cardiac output. Placement of the aortic cross clamp during the repair in these infants may cause even greater increases in left ventricular afterload.

Due to these concerns, these individuals are not candidates for inhalational agents, which cause myocardial depression. Otherwise, inhalational agents may be carefully titrated and supplemented with a narcotic (e.g., fentanyl at 10–25 µg/kg) in hemodynamically stable patients.[45,47,156] Ketamine, which may increase systemic vascular resistance, should likewise be avoided. For the very sick neonate, an anesthetic technique that primarily uses a narcotic (e.g., fentanyl at 25–50 µg/kg) supplemented with a muscle relaxant is probably the safest, since myocardial depression is avoided and acute increases in systemic vascular resistance caused by surgical stress is minimized.[45,156,162] Nitrous oxide offers little advantage as an adjunct to other agents. It may produce myocardial depression in patients with impaired ventricular function and increases the size of air bubbles that may be accidentally entrained intravenously.

Since the cardiac output of neonates and infants is heart rate dependent, the anticholinergic and sympathomimetic effects of pancuronium may be beneficial in offsetting the vagotonic effects of higher doses of narcotics such as fentanyl. If early extubation is a goal, then shorter-acting nondepolarizing muscle relaxants and an anticholinergic (e.g., at-ropine, 0.01 mg/kg) may be used. Atropine should always be available for immediate injection, since bradycardia can occur particularly during airway and ductal manipulation. Inotropes are rarely needed in the postoperative period unless they were required during the preoperative period.

Special consideration is required for individuals with complex cardiac lesions who undergo pulmonary artery banding at the time of coarctation repair. Multiple factors can influence the direction and degree of intracardiac shunting. Neonates with large ventricular septal defects are at risk of developing increased left-to-right shunting, resulting in pulmonary congestion and ventricular overload during their anesthesia. One must be careful to avoid excessive increases in preload, systemic vascular resistance, respiratory alkalosis, hyperoxemia, as well as decreases in hematocrit or pulmonary vascular resistance.

Infants less than 46 weeks postconceptual age require careful administration of inspired oxygen in order to minimize retinopathy of prematurity. Measurement of the oxygen saturation must be made from a site supplied by the ascending aorta in individuals with a patent ductus arteriosus. The inspired oxygen concentration should be administered so as to maintain an oxygen saturation of 92–96%. Since the surgical repair is almost always via a left thoracotomy, arterial desaturation and decreased pulmonary compliance are not uncommon due to lung retraction by the surgeon. The capnogram should be closely monitored for changes that may indicate impaired ventilation or impaired pulmonary perfusion. Therefore, vigilant inspection of the surgical field and controlled ventilation by hand is recommended. Postoperative ventilation is usually required for young infants, especially if a high-dose narcotic technique was used, or if congestive heart failure or respiratory insufficiency was present preoperatively.

Anesthetic Management of Children

The approach to the older child, who is often asymptomatic at the time of the surgical repair, is different. Most of these individuals have proximal hypertension, and concentric hypertrophy of the left ventricle is often present due to the increased afterload imposed by the coarctation lesion. The arterial blood pressure should be monitored continuously at a site proximal to the planned site of the repair. Regardless of the anesthetic technique chosen, sudden and exaggerated hypertensive responses may occur, particularly in individuals with long-standing proximal hypertension.[162] Most children have adequate collateral arterial circulation and exhibit minimal blood pressure responses due to aortic cross clamping and unclamping.[156]

Careful titration of intravenous or inhalational agents is well tolerated. Halothane has been reported to provide adequate maintenance of anesthesia and induced hypotension, but there have been reported cases in which the use of halothane failed to control hypertension intraoperatively.[110,148,166] Isoflurane, on the other hand, provides rapid control of arterial blood pressure and reduction of left ventricular afterload, which can be particularly advantageous in individuals with significant left-to-right shunting.[156] Therefore, when an inhalant is chosen, induction with halothane followed by maintenance of anesthesia with isoflurane is advantageous.

Most intravenous anesthetic agents, including potent synthetic narcotics, benzodiazepines, and barbiturates can be used for anesthetic induction and maintenance if carefully titrated. While ketamine has been used for anesthetic induction of individuals with limited cardiac reserve, it should be avoided for most patients with aortic coarctation because it can cause unwanted sympathetic stimulation and serious hypertension, particularly in individuals with preexisting hypertension.[156,162] In those individuals with limited ventricular function either etomidate (0.15–0.30 mg/kg) or high doses of a narcotic would be a good alternative. Likewise, agents with significant sympathomimetic or vagolytic effects, such as pancuronium and atropine, should be be used cautiously.

Patients with long-standing hypertension are prone to exaggerated hypertensive responses when stimulated. It is imperative that an adequate depth of anesthesia be achieved before initiating laryngoscopy and other potent stimuli, since serious life-threatening cardiovascular events can occur (e.g., arrhythmias, cardiac arrest, and cerebrovascular hemorrhage). The hypertensive responses can be attenuated by administering an increased concentration of inhalational agents, topical local anesthetics to the airway, and intravenous lidocaine (1.5 mg/kg), beta-blockers (e.g., esmolol), or narcotic before anticipated stimulation. Placement of an arterial catheter in a vessel arising proximal to the aortic coarctation (e.g., usually the right radial artery) should be done either before or shortly after induction of anesthesia in order to facilitate safe blood pressure control.

If the child was asymptomatic preoperatively, early extubation should be considered. Since these individuals are prone to hypertensive responses on emergence of anesthesia, adequate analgesia will be required. In addition to the use of intravenous narcotics, regional analgesic techniques may be used. Intercostal nerve block two ribs above and below the surgical site using 0.5% bupivacaine has been recommended by some, but should be used cautiously in individuals with dilated, tortuous intercostal vessels.[46,139] Thoracic epidural catheters may be used to provide segmental thoracic analgesia. Blockade below the level of T10 should be avoided since it may mask the abdominal symptoms associated with mesenteric arteritis.[46]

Anesthetic Management of Adolescents and Adults

Many of the same considerations for children will apply for adolescents and adults, although there are some additional considerations. For adolescents and adults, the placement of a double-lumen endotracheal tube can improve surgical exposure and thereby facilitate dissection and reduce the risk of hemorrhage.[46] Consideration should be given to provide adequate intravenous access for rapid volume resuscitation due to bleeding from arterial collateral sites or ruptured aneurysms.

Likewise, similiar considerations are required for the repair of recurrent aortic coarctation. These individuals may have significant fibrosis at the site of the coarctation that may result in excessive bleeding and prolonged aortic cross clamp times. The surgeon may therefore have to make a decision intraoperatively to place a temporary shunt or insert a bypass graft.

Conclusion

There has been significant improvement in the care of patients with aortic coarctation over the past few decades. Technical advances now allow a more detailed cardiovascular evaluation that helps guide the timing and choice of therapy.

Advances in surgical techniques and perioperative management have improved patient survival, particularly for infants without associated complex cardiovascular lesions. Further research continues to develop anesthetic and surgical techniques that will improve spinal cord protection during aortic cross clamping. To provide a safe anesthetic, it is essential for the anesthesiologist to have a clear understanding of the anatomy and pathophysiology of aortic coarctation and any coexisting anomalies, the nature of the planned surgical procedure, and the possible perioperative complications.

References

1. Ho SY, Anderson RH. Coarctation, tubular hypoplasia, and the ductus arteriosus: histological study of 35 specimens. Br Heart J 1979;41:268.

2. Beekman RH, Rocchini AP. Coarctation of the Aorta and Interruption of the Aortic Arch. In JH Moller, WA Neal (eds), Fetal, Neonatal, and Infant Cardiac Disease. Norwalk, CT: Appleton & Lange, 1990;497.

3. Hollinger IB. Diseases of the Cardiovascular System. In J Katz, DJ Steward (eds), Anesthesia and Uncommon Pediatric Diseases (2nd ed). Philadelphia: Saunders, 1993;176.

4. Gross RE. Surgical correction for coarctation of the aorta. Surgery 1945;18:673.

5. Crafoord C, Nylin G. Congenital coarctation of the aorta and its surgical treatment. J Thorac Surg 1945;14:347.

6. Hesslein PS, Gutgesell HP, McNamara DG. Prognosis of symptomatic coarctation of the aorta in infancy. Am J Cardiol 1983;51:299.

7. Thibault WN, Sperling DR, Gazzaniga AB. Subclavian artery patch angioplasty. Treatment of infants and young children with aortic coarctation. Arch Surg 1975;110:1095.

8. Pierce WS, Waldhausen JA, Berman W, Whitman V. Late results of the subclavian flap procedure in infants with coarctation of the thoracic aorta. Circulation 1978;58(Suppl 1):78.

9. Keith JD. Coarctation of the Aorta. In JD Keith, RD Rowe, P Vlad (eds), Heart Disease in Infancy and Childhood (3rd ed). New York: Macmillan, 1978;736.

10. Fyler DC, Buckley LP, Hellenbrand WE, Cohn HE. Report of the New England regional infant cardiac program. Pediatrics 1980;65:432.

11. Campbell M, Polani PE. The aetiology of coarctation of the aorta. Lancet 1961;1:463.

12. Campbell M. Natural history of coarctation of the aorta. Br Heart J 1970;32:633.

13. Beekman RH, Robinow M. Coarctation of the aorta inherited as an autosomal dominant trait. Am J Cardiol 1985;56:818.

14. Gersony W. Coarctation of the Aorta. In FH Adams, GC Emmanouilides (eds), Moss' Heart Disease in Infants, Children, and Adolescents (3rd ed). Baltimore: Williams & Wilkins, 1983;188.

15. Lacour-Gayet F, Bruniaux J, Serraf A, et al. Hypoplastic transverse arch and coarctation in neonates. J Thorac Cardiovasc Surg 1990;100:808.

16. Graham LM, Zelenock GB, Erlandson EE, et al. Abdominal aortic coarctation and segmental hypoplasia. Surgery 1979;86:519.

17. Edwards JE, Christensen NA, Clagett OT. Pathologic considerations in coarctation of the aorta. Mayo Clin Proc 1948;23:324.

18. Rudolph AM, Heymann MA, Spitznas U. Hemodynamic considerations in the development of narrowing of the aorta. Am J Cardiol 1972;30:514.

19. Moene RJ, Oppenheimer L, Decker A, Wenink AC. Relation between aortic arch hypoplasia of variable severity and central muscular ventricular septal defects: emphasis on associated left ventricular anomalies. Am J Cardiol 1981;48:111.

20. Chang JT, Burrington JD. Coarctation of the aorta in infants and children. J Pediatr Surg 1972;7:127.

21. Rudolph AM, Heymann MA. The circulation of the fetus in utero: methods for studying distribution of blood flow, cardiac output and organ flow. Circ Res 1967;21:163.

22. Fyler DC. Coarctation of the Aorta. In DC Fyler (ed), Nadas' Pediatric Cardiology. Philadelphia: Hanley & Belfus, 1992;535.

23. Fyler DC. Coarctation of the Aorta. In AS Nadas, DC Fyler (eds), Pediatric Cardiology (3rd ed). Philadelphia: Saunders, 1972;460.

24. Easthope RN, Tawes RL, Bonham-Carter S. Congenital mitral valve disease associated with coarctation of the aorta. Am Heart J 1969;77:743.

25. Shone JD, Sellers RD, Anderson RC. The developmental complex of "parachute mitral valve," supravalvar ring of left atrium, subaortic stenosis and coarctation of the aorta. Am J Cardiol 1963;11:714.

26. Tawes RL, Berr CL, Aberdeen E. Congenital biscupid aortic valves associated with coarctation of the aorta in children. Br Heart J 1969;31:127.

27. Isabel-Jones JB, Gyepes MT, Crudup C. Echocardiographic incidence of bicuspid aortic valve. Pediatric Digest 1977;19:13.

28. Lindsay J. Coarctation of the aorta, bicuspid aortic valve and abnormal ascending aortic wall. Am J Cardiol 1988;61:182.

29. Isner JM, Donaldson RF, Fulton D, et al. Cystic medial necrosis in coarctation of the aorta. Circulation 1987;75:689.

30. Skandalakis JE, Edwards BF, Gray SW, et al. Coarctation of the aorta with aneurysm. Surg Gynecol Obstet 1960;111:307.

31. Wilson SK, Hutchins GM. Aortic dissecting aneurysms: causative factors in 204 subjects. Arch Pathol Lab Med 1982;106:175.

32. Lindsay J, Rosenberg J, Ross JW, Garcia JM. Anuloaortic ectasia as a late complication following repair of coarctation of the aorta. Vasc Surg 1986;20:288.

33. White CW, Zoller RP. Left aortic dissection following repair of coarctation of the aorta. Chest 1973;63:573.

34. McCombs HL, Crocker DW. Dissecting aneurysm distal to coarctation of the aorta with long survival. Am Heart J 1967;74:675.

35. Mitchell IM, Pollock JCS. Coarctation of the aorta and post-stenotic aneurysm formation. Br Heart J 1990;65:332.

36. Becker AE, Becker MJ, Edwards JE. Anomalies associated with coarctation of the aorta: particular reference to infancy. Circulation 1970;41:1067.

37. Greenwood RD, Rosenthal A, Parisi L, et al. Extracardiac abnormalities in infants with congenital heart disease. Pediatrics 1975;55:485.

38. Hutchins GM. Coarctation of the aorta explained as a branch point of the ductus arteriosus. Am J Pathol 1971;63:203.

39. Rosenberg HS. Coarctation of the aorta: morphology and pathogenetic considerations. Perspectives in Pediatric Pathology 1973;1:339.

40. Wielenga G, Dankmeijer J. Coarctation of the aorta. J Pathol Bacteriol 1968;95:265.

41. Graham TP, Lewis BW, Jarmakani MM, et al. Left heart volume and mass quantification in children with left ventricular pressure overload. Circulation 1970;41:203.

42. Friedman WF. The Intrinsic Physiologic Properties of the Developing Heart. In WF Friedman, M Lesch, EH Sonnenblick (eds), Neonatal Heart Disease. New York: Grune & Stratton, 1973;21.

43. Mathew R, Simon G, Joseph M. Collateral circulation in coarctation of the aorta in infancy and childhood. Arch Dis Child 1972;47:950.

44. Schlant RC. The Pathology, Pathophysiology, Recognition, and Treatment of Congenital Heart Disease. In RC Schlant, RW Alexander (eds), The Heart, Arteries, and Veins (8th ed). New York: McGraw-Hill, 1990;1785.

45. Davis PJ, Cook DR. Anesthesia for Pediatric Vascular Lesions. In JA Kaplan (ed), Vascular Anesthesia. New York: Churchill Livingstone, 1991;491.

46. Fischer A, Benedict CR. Adult coarctation of the aorta: anesthesia and postoperative management. Anaesthesia 1977;32:533.

47. Salem MR, Hall SC, Motoyama ES. Anesthesia for Thoracic and Cardiovascular Surgery. In EK Motoyama, PJ Davis (eds), Anesthesia for Infants and Children (5th ed). St. Louis: Mosby, 1990;501.

48. Liberthson RR, Pennington DG, Jacobs ML, Dagget WM. Coarctation of the aorta. Review of 234 patients and clarification of management problems. Am J Cardiol 1979;43:835.

49. Campbell M, Baylis JH. Course and prognosis of coarctation of the aorta. Br Heart J 1956;18:475.

50. Morriss JH, McNamara DG. Residua, Sequelae and Complications of Surgery for Congenital Heart Disease. In A Rosenthal, E Sonnenblock, M Lesch (eds), Postoperative Congenital Heart Disease. New York: Grune & Stratton, 1975;3.

51. Maron BJ, Humphries JO, Rowe RD, Mellitis ED. Prognosis of surgically corrected coarctation of the aorta. A 20 year postoperative appraisal. Circulation 1973;47:119.

52. Garman JE, Hinson RE, Eyler WR. Coarctation of the aorta in infancy. Detection on chest radiographs. Radiology 1965;85:418.

53. Sahn DJ, Allen HD, McDonald G, Goldberg SJ. Real-time cross-sectional echocardiographic diagnosis of coarctation of the aorta. A prospective study of echocardiographic-angiographic correlations. Circulation 1977;56:762.

54. Huhta JC, Gutgesell HP, Latson LA. Two-dimensional echocardiographic assessment of the aorta in infants and children with congenital heart disease. Circulation 1984;70:417.

55. Marx GR, Allen HD. Accuracy and pitfalls of Doppler evaluation of the pressure gradient in aortic coarctation. J Am Coll Cardiol 1986;7:1379.

56. Carvalho JS, Redington AN, Shinebourne EA. Continuous wave Doppler echocardiography and coarctation of the aorta. Gradients and flow patterns in the assessment of severity. Br Heart J 1990;64:133.

57. Simpson IA, Soho DJ, Valdez-Cruz LM. Color Doppler flow mapping in patients with coarctation of the aorta. New observations and improved evaluation with color flow diameter and proximal acceleration as predictors of severity. Circulation 1988;77:736.

58. Heymann MA. Pharmacologic use of prostaglandin E1 in infants with congenital heart disease. Am Heart J 1981;101:837.

59. Lewis AB, Freed MA, Heymann MA, Roehl SL, et al. Side effects of therapy with prostaglandin E1 in infants with critical congenital heart disease. Circulation 1981;64:893.

60. Connors JP, Hartman AF, Weldon CS. Considerations in the surgical management of infantile coarctation of the aorta. Am J Cardiol 1975;36:489.

61. Waldhausen JA, Whitman V, Werner JC. Surgical intervention in infants with coarctation of the aorta. J Thorac Cardiovasc Surg 1981;81:323.

62. Neches WH, Park SC, Lenox CC, et al. Coarctation of the aorta with ventricular septal defect. Circulation 1977;55:189.

63. Litwin SB, Bernhard WF, Rosenthal A, Gross RE. Surgical resection of coarctation of the aorta in infancy. J Pediatr Surg 1971;6:307.

64. Kopf GS, Hellenbrand W, Kleinman C. Repair of aortic coarctation in the first three months of life: immediate and long term results. Ann Thorac Surg 1986;41:425.

65. Strattford MA, Hayes CJ, Griffiths SP, et al. Management of the infant with coarctation of the aorta and ventricular septal defect [abstract]. Am J Cardiol 1980;45:450.
66. Freed MD, Keane JF, Van Praagh R, et al. Coarctation of the aorta with congenital mitral regurgitation. Circulation 1974;48:1175.
67. Wood WC, Wood JC, Lower RR, et al. Associated coarctation of the aorta and mitral valve disease. J Pediatr 1975;87:87.
68. Zeimer G, Jonas RA, Perry SB. Surgery for coarctation in the neonate. Circulation 1986;74(Suppl 1):25.
69. Del Nido PJ, Williams WG, Wilson GJ. Synthetic patch angioplasty for repair of coarctation of the aorta: experience with aneurysm formation. Circulation 1986;74(Suppl 1):31.
70. Gross RE. Coarctation of the aorta. Surgical treatment of 100 cases. Circulation 1950;1:41.
71. Pennington DG, Liberthson RR, Jacobs M, et al. Critical review of experience with surgical repair of coarctation of the aorta. J Thorac Cardiovasc Surg 1979;77:217.
72. Beekman RH, Rocchini AP, Behrendt DM, et al. Long-term outcome after repair of coarctation in infancy: subclavian angioplasty does not reduce the need for re-operation. J Am Coll Cardiol 1986;8:1406.
73. Kirklin JW, Burchell HB, Pugh DG. Surgical treatment of coarctation of the aorta in a ten-week old infant. Report of a case. Circulation 1952;6:411.
74. Coran AG, Behrendt DM, Weintraub WH. Surgery of the Neonate. Boston: Little, Brown, 1978;93.
75. Cobanoglu A, Teply JF, Grunkemeier GL, et al. Coarctation of the aorta in patients younger than three months: a critique of the subclavian flap procedure. J Thorac Cardiovasc Surg 1985;89:128.
76. Beekman RH, Rocchini AP, Berendt DM. Reoperation for coarctation of the aorta. Am J Cardiol 1981;48:1108.
77. Todd PJ, Dangerfield PH, Hamilton DI, Wilkinson JL. Late effects on the left upper limb of subclavian flap aortoplasty. J Thorac Cardiovasc Surg 1983;85:678.
78. Waldhausen JA, Nahrwold DL. Repair of coarctation of the aorta with a subclavian flap. J Thorac Cardiovasc Surg 1966;51:532.
79. Van Son JAM, Van Asten W N, Van Lier HJJ, et al. A comparison of coarctation resection and subclavian flap angioplasty using ultrasonographically monitored postocclusive reactive hyperemia. J Thorac Cardiovasc Surg 1990;100:817.
80. Myers JL, Waldhausen JA. Management of Complications Following Repair of Coarctation of the Aorta, Patent Ductus Arteriosus, Interrupted Aortic Arch, and Vascular Rings. In JA Waldhausen, MB Orringer (eds), Complications in Cardiothoracic Surgery. St. Louis: Mosby-Year Book, 1991;135.
81. Reul GJ, Kabbani SS, Sandiford FM, et al. Repair of coarctation of the thoracic aorta by patch graft aortoplasty. J Thorac Cardiovasc Surg 1974;68:696.
82. Myers JL, Waldhausen JA, Pae WE, et al. Vascular anastomoses in growing vessels: the use of absorbable sutures. Ann Thorac Surg 1982;34:529.
83. Trinquet F, Vouhe PR, Vernant F, et al. Coarctation of the aorta in infants: which operation? Ann Thoracic Surg 1988;45:186.
84. Bromberg BI, Beekman RH, Rocchini AP, et al. Aortic aneurysm after patch aortoplasty repair of coarctation: a prospective analysis of prevalence, screening tests and risks. J Am Coll Cardiol 1989;14:734.
85. Cooper RS, Ritter SB, Rothe WB, et al. Angioplasty for coarctation of the aorta: long-term results. Circulation 1987;75:600.
86. Lock JE, Bass JL, Amplatz K. Balloon dilation angioplasty of coarctation in infants and children. Circulation 1983;68:109.
87. Beekman RH, Rocchini AP, Dick M. Percutaneous balloon angioplasty for native coarctation of the aorta. J Am Coll Cardiol 1987;10:1078.
88. Sperling DR, Dorsey TJ, Rowen M. Percutaneous transluminal angioplasty of congenital coarctation of the aorta. Am J Cardiol 1983;51:562.
89. Brandt B, Marvin WJ, Rose EF. Surgical treatment of coarctation of the aorta after balloon angioplasty. J Thorac Cardiovasc Surg 1987;94:715.
90. Rocchini AP, Beekman RH. Balloon angioplasty in the treatment of pulmonary valve stenosis and coarctation of the aorta. Texas Heart Institute Journal 1986;13:377.
91. Choy M, Rocchini AP, Beekman RH. No paradoxical hypertension after balloon angioplasty of coarctation of the aorta [abstract]. Circulation 1985;72(Suppl 3):260.
92. Reddington AN, Booth P, Shore DF, Rigby ML. Primary balloon dilation of coarctation of the aorta in neonates. Br Heart J 1990;64:277.
93. Williams WG, Shindo G, Trusler GA, et al. Results of repair of coarctation of the aorta during infancy. J Thorac Cardiovasc Surg 1980;79:603.
94. Patel R, Singh SP, Abrams L, Roberts KD. Coarctation of aorta with special reference to infants. Long-term results of operation in 126 cases. Br Heart J 1977;39:1246.
95. Eshaghpour E, Olley PM. Recoarctation of the aorta following coarctectomy in the first year of life. A follow-up study. J Pediatr 1972;80:809.
96. Hartmann AF, Goldring D, Hernandez A. Recurrent coarctation of the aorta after successful repair in infancy. Am J Cardiol 1970;25:405.
97. Hamilton DI, DiEusanio G, Sandrasagra FA, Donnelly RJ. Early and late results of aortoplasty with a left subclavian flap for coarctation of the aorta in infancy. J Thorac Cardiovasc Surg 1978;75:699.
98. Cerilli J, Lauridsen P. Reoperation for coarctation of the aorta. Acta Chir Scand 1965;129:391.
99. Weldon CS, Hartmann AF, Steinhoff NG, Morrissey JD. A simple, safe, and rapid technique for the management of recurrent coarctation of the aorta. Ann Thorac Surg 1973;15:510.

100. Eide RN, Janani J, Attai LA, Robinson G. Bypass grafts for recurrent or complex coarctations of the aorta. Ann Thorac Surg 1975;20:558.

101. Sealy WC. Coarctation of the aorta and hypertension. Ann Thorac Surg 1967;3:15.

102. Goodall M, Sealy WC. Increased sympathetic nerve activity following resection of coarctation of the thoracic aorta. Circulation 1969;39:345.

103. Benedict CR, Grahame-Smith DG, Fisher A. Changes in plasma catecholamines and dopamine beta-hydroxylase after corrective surgery for coarctation of the aorta. Circulation 1978;57:598.

104. Werning C, Schonbeck M, Weidman P. Plasma renin activity in patients with coarctation of the aorta. Circulation 1969;40:731.

105. Parker FB, Streeten DHP, Farrell A. Preoperative and postoperative renin levels in coarctation of the aorta. Circulation 1982;66:513.

106. Fox S, Pierce WS, Waldhausen JA. Pathogenesis of paradoxical hypertension after coarctation repair. Ann Thorac Surg 1980;29:135.

107. Beekman RH, Katz BP, Moorhead-Steffens C. Altered baroreceptor function in children with systolic hypertension after coarctation repair. Am J Cardiol 1983;52:112.

108. Ribeiro AB, Krakoff LR. Angiotensin blockade in coarctation of the aorta. N Engl J Med 1976;295:148.

109. Parker FB, Streeten DHP, Sondhenner HM, et al. Hypertensive mechanisms in coarctation of the aorta. J Thorac Cardiovasc Surg 1980;80:568.

110. Wilkinson C, Clark H. Refractory hypertension during coarctectomy. Anesthesiology 1982;57:540.

111. Rocchini AP, Rosenthal A, Barger AC, et al. Pathogenesis of paradoxical hypertension after coarctation resection. Circulation 1976;54:382.

112. Alpert BS, Bain HH, Balfe JW. Role of the renin-angiotensin-aldosterone system in hypertensive children with coarctation of the aorta. Am J Cardiol 1979;43:828.

113. Gidding SS, Rocchini AP, Beekman R, et al. Therapeutic effects of propranolol on paradoxical hypertension after repair of coarctation of the aorta. N Engl J Med 1985;312:1224.

114. Choy M, Rocchini AP, Beekman RH. Paradoxical hypertension after repair of coarctation of the aorta in children. Balloon angioplasty versus surgical repair. Circulation 1987;75:1186.

115. Sealy WC, Harris JS, Young WG, Callaway HA. Paradoxical hypertension following resection of coarctation of the aorta. Surgery 1957;42:135.

116. Malan JE, Benatar A, Levin SE. Long-term follow-up of coarctation of the aorta repaired by patch angioplasty. Int J Cardiol 1991;30:23.

117. Clarkson PM, Nicholson MR, Barrett-Boyes BG. Results after repair of coarctation of the aorta beyond infancy: a 10 to 28 year follow-up with particular reference to late systemic hypertension. Am J Cardiol 1983;51:1481.

118. Gidding SS, Rocchini AP, Moorehead C, Schork MA, et al. Increased forearm vascular reactivity in patients with hypertension after repair of coarctation. Circulation 1985;71:495.

119. Nanton MA, Olley WM. Residual hypertension after coarctectomy in children. Am J Cardiol 1976;37:769.

120. Markel H, Rocchini AP, Beekman RH. Exercise-induced hypertension after repair of coarctation of the aorta: arm versus leg exercise. J Am Coll Card 1986;8:165.

121. Freed MD, Rocchini A, Rosenthal A. Exercise-induced hypertension after surgical repair of coarctation of the aorta. Am J Cardiol 1979;43:253.

122. Kavey REW, Cotton JL, Blackman MS. Atenolol therapy for exercise-induced hypertension after aortic coarctation repair. Am J Cardiol 1990;66:1233.

123. Ring DM, Lewis FY. Abdominal pain following surgical correction of coarctation of the aorta: a syndrome. J Thorac Surg 1951;31:718.

124. Ho ECK, Moss AJ. The syndrome of mesenteric arteritis following surgical repair of aortic coarctation. Report of nine cases and review of the literature. Pediatrics 1972;49:40.

125. Brewer LA, Fosburg RG, Mulder GA, Verska JJ. Spinal cord complications following surgery for coarctation of the aorta. J Thorac Cardiovasc Surg 1972;64:368.

126. Keen G. Spinal cord damage and operations for coarctation of the aorta: aetiology, practice and prospects. Thorax 1987;42:11.

127. Crawford FA, Sade RM. Spinal cord injury associated with hyperthermia during aortic coarctation repair. J Thorac Cardiovasc Surg 1984;87:616.

128. Schuster AB, Gross RE. Surgery for coarctation of the aorta. A review of 500 cases. J Cardiovasc Surg 1962;43:54.

129. Watterson KG, Dhasmana JP, O'Higging JW, Wiseheart JD. Distal aortic pressure during coarctation operation. Ann Thorac Surg 1990;49:978.

130. Costello TG, Fisher A. Neurologic complications following aortic surgery. Case reports and review of the literature. Anaesthesia 1983;38:230.

131. Wadouh F, Arndt CF, Opperman E, et al. The mechanism of spinal cord injury after simple and double aortic clamping. J Thoarac Cardiovasc Surg 1986;92:121.

132. Symbas PN, Pfaender LM, Drucker MH. Cross clamping of the descending aorta. J Thorac Cardiovasc Surg 1983;85:300.

133. Krieger KH, Spence FC. Is paraplegia after repair of coarctation of the aorta due principally to distal hypoperfusion during aortic cross clamping? Surgery 1985;97:2.

134. Hantler CB, Knight PR. Intracranial hypertension following cross clamping of the thoracic aorta. Anesthesiology 1982;56:146.

135. D'Ambra MN, Dewhurst W, Jacobs M. Cross clamping the thoracic aorta. Effect on intracranial pressure. Circulation 1988;78(Suppl 3):198.

136. Nugent M, Kaye MP, McGoon DC. Effects of nitroprusside on aortic and intraspinal pressures during tho-

racic aortic crossclamping [abstract]. Anesthesiology 1984;61:68.

137. Salem MR, Toyama T, Wong AY, et al. Haemodynamic reponses to induced arterial hypotension in children. Br J Anaesth 1978;50:489.

138. Salem MR, El-Etr AA, Rattenborg CC. Deliberate hypotension for the management of threatening hemorrhage. Anesthesiology 1968;29:155.

139. Dalal FY, Bennett EJ, Salem MR, El-Etr AA. Anaesthesia for coarctation: a new classification for rational anaesthetic management. Anaesthesia 1974;29:704.

140. Bennett EJ, Dalal FY. Hypotensive anaesthesia for coarctation: a method of prevention of post-operative hypertension. Anaesthesia 1974;29:269.

141. Jones SEF. Coarctation in children: controlled hypotension using labetalol and halothane. Anaesthesia 1979;34:1052.

142. Bland JW, Reedy JC, Williams WH. Pediatric and Neonatal Thoracic Surgery. In JA Kaplan (ed), Thoracic Anesthesia. New York: Churchill Livingstone, 1983;505.

143. Salem MR. Therapeutic uses of ganglionic blocking drugs. Int Anesthesiol Clin 1978;16:171.

144. Kouchoukos NT, Lell WA, Karp RB, Samuelson PN. Hemodynamic effects of aortic clamping and decompression with a temporary shunt for resection of the descending thoracic aorta. Surgery 1979;85:25.

145. Anderson SM. Controlled hypotension with arfonad in pediatric surgery. BMJ 1955;2:103.

146. Larson AG. Deliberate hypotension. Anesthesiology 1964;25:682.

147. Salem MR, Wong AY, Bennett EJ, Mani M. Deliberate hypotension in infants and children. Anesth Analg 1974;53:975.

148. Adams AP. Techniques of vascular control for deliberate hypotension during anaesthesia. Br J Anaesth 1975;47:777.

149. Barnes RW, Rittenhouse EA, Kontahworn C, et al. Reversed intercostal arterial flow in coarctation of the aorta. Intraoperative assessment with the Doppler ultrasonic velocity detector. Ann Thorac Surg 1975;19:27.

150. Ross JK, Monro JL, Sbokos CG. Late complications of surgery for coarctation of the aorta. Thorax 1975;30:31.

151. Hughes RK, Reemtsma K. Correction of coarctation of the aorta. Manometric determination of safety during test occlusion. J Thorac Cardiovasc Surg 1971;62:31.

152. Moreno NN, deCampo T, Kaiser GA, Pallares VS. Technical and pharmacologic management of distal hypotension during repair of coarctation of the aorta. J Thorac Cardiovasc Surg 1980;80:182.

153. Pennington DG, Dennis HM, Swartz MT, et al. Repair of aortic coarctation in infants: experience with an intraluminal shunt. Ann Thorac Surg 1985;40:35.

154. Alexander JC. Maintenance of distal aortic perfusion by a heparin-bonded shunt during repair of coarctation of the aorta with minimal collateral circulation. Ann Thorac Surg 1981;32:304.

155. Lam CR, Arciniegas E. Surgical management of coarctation of the aorta with minimal collateral circulation. Ann Surg 1973;178:693.

156. Rosen DA, Rosen KR. Anomalies of the Aortic Arch and Valve. In CL Lake (ed), Pediatric Cardiac Anesthesia (2nd ed). Norwalk, CT: Appleton & Lange, 1993;356.

157. Dasmahapatra HK, Coles JG, Taylor MJ. Identification of risk factors for spinal cord ischemia by the use of monitoring of somatosensory evoked potentials during coarctation repair. Circulation 1987;76(Suppl 3):14.

158. Pollock JC, Jamieson MP, McWilliam R. Somatosensory evoked potentials in the detection of spinal cord ischemia in aortic coarctation repair. Ann Thoracic Surg 1985;41:251.

159. Lesser RP, Raudzens P, Luders R, et al. Postoperative neurologic deficits despite unchanged intraoperative somatosensory evoked potentials. Ann Neurol 1986;19:22.

160. Ginsburg HH, Shetter AG, Raudzens PA. Postoperative paraplegia with preserved intraoperative somatosensory evoked potentials. J Neurosurg 1985;63:296.

161. Coles JG, Wilson GJ, Sima AF, et al. Intraoperative detection of spinal cord ischemia using somatosensory cortical evoked potentials during thoracic aortic occlusion. Ann Thorac Surg 1982;34:299.

162. DiNardo JA. Anesthesia for Congenital Heart Disease. In JA DiNardo (ed), Anesthesia for Cardiac Surgery. Englewood Cliffs, NJ: Appleton & Lange, 1990;157.

163. Gilston A. Anaesthesia for coarctation. Anaesthesia 1975;30:242.

164. Walsh DB, McDaniel MD. Surgical Technique and Judgement: The Vascular Surgeon at Work. In MP Yeager, DD Glass (eds), Anesthesiology and Vascular Surgery. Englewood Cliffs, NJ: Appleton & Lange, 1990;31.

165. Effeney DJ, Goldstone J, Chin D. Intraoperative anticoagulation in cardiovascular surgery. Surgery 1981;90:1068.

166. Davis TB, Morrow DH, Herbert CL, Cooper T. An increased incidence of paradoxical hypertension following resection of aortic coarctation under halothane anesthesia. Anesthesiology 1961;22:132.

Chapter 10

Anesthesia for Surgery of the Abdominal and Distal Aorta

Ronald S. Levy and John Francis Clagnaz

Epidemiology

Aneurysms constitute approximately 10% or more of most active vascular surgeons' practices. The most common aneurysm, the arteriosclerotic abdominal aortic aneurysm (AAA), has been found in almost 2% of postmortem examinations.[1] AAA is found to occur in more than 5% of the United States population above the age of 60. A 30-year study, conducted from 1951 to 1980 by Bickerstaff et al.[2] at the Mayo Clinic, showed an increasing occurrence of AAA. The incidence increased from 7.5 per 100,000 person-years between 1951 and 1956 to 36.5 per 100,000 person-years between 1976 and 1980. The male to female ratio of age-adjusted incidence rose from 3.0 to 1 from 1951–1960 to 3.8 to 1 from 1971–1980. The mean age at the time of diagnosis was 69 for men and 78 for women. Clinically, approximately one-fifth of patients sought medical attention based on specific symptoms, while most were found to have aneurysms as an incidental finding during routine examination. Seventy-four percent of patients had small or medium-sized aneurysms, while approximately 20% had aneurysms 7 cm or greater. The overall rate of rupture was 20.3%.[1]

The major cause of morbidity and mortality in AAA is aneurysmal rupture. The chance of survival after aneurysmal rupture varies from 17–66%, with less than 10% survival for those presenting in shock with free intraperitoneal rupture.[3] The single most important factor that correlates with the risk of rupture is the aneurysm size. The 5-year risk of rupture for a 4-cm aneurysm is less than 15%, compared with an 8-cm aneurysm, which carries a 75% risk of rupture. When aneurysm size is plotted against 5-year risk of rupture, the slope increases most sharply as the aneurysm reaches 6 cm (Figure 10-1).

Pathogenesis and Pathophysiology

AAAs are always found in association with significant aortic atherosclerosis, and as such, the pathogenesis has been presumed to be related to atherosclerosis at weakened areas of the aorta, which then expand before they eventually rupture. Newer evidence, however, disputes this and implicates an alteration in systemic connective tissue metabolism.[4,5] Numerous studies[6–13] have linked aneurysmal pathogenesis to cellular, enzymatic, and genetic factors (see Chapter 1) (Figure 10-2).

From a genetic standpoint, there have been a number of reports of familial predisposition to AAA. In one study of 250 patients with AAA, 19% of patients had a relative with a known aneurysm as compared with less than 3% of controls.[14] Another report studied 34 families and found that in one-half of affected individuals at least one parent was affected and 20% of siblings were affected.[15] There was even one case report of three brothers, all of whom required emergency surgery for ruptured AAA.

There are many mechanisms by which genetic factors may predispose to the development of AAA. These include inherited defects in collagen and elastin, which may lead to an inherent weakness in

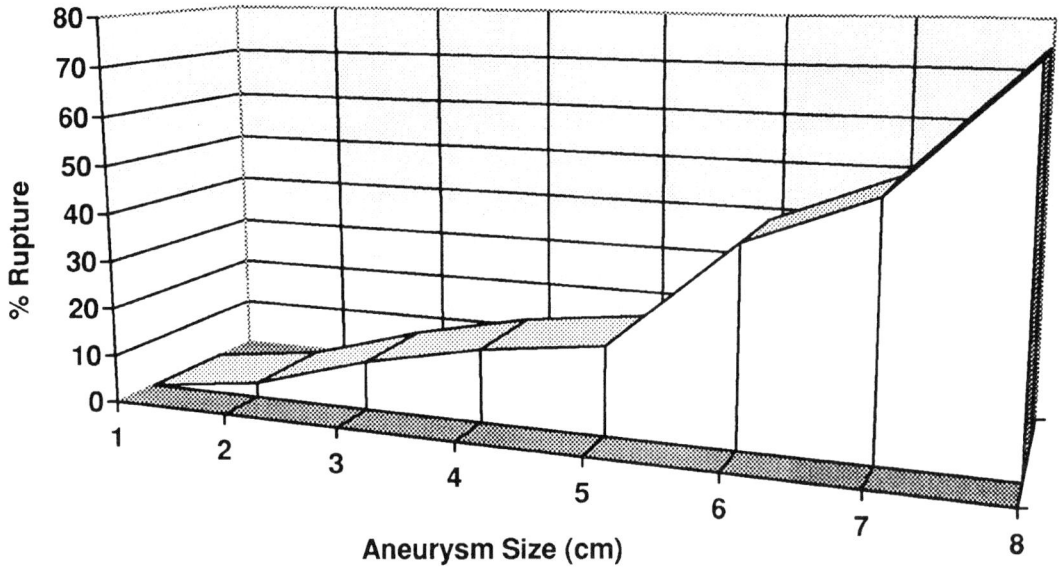

Figure 10-1. Five-year risk of abdominal aortic aneurysm rupture based on aneurysm size.

the aortic wall. Genetic factors may also cause an increase in enzymatic breakdown of structural components of the aortic wall (see Chapter 1).

Elastin metabolism was implicated in the pathogenesis of AAA as early as 1982, when elastase concentration was noted to be increased in the aortic wall of patients with AAA. Other implicated markers were serum antiprotease, alpha$_1$-antitrypsin inhibitor, and collagen metabolism. Elastase activity in the media of the aorta has been shown to be increased in aneurysm patients with respect to atherosclerotic and normal aortas.[14,16–18] Mature elastin is not synthesized in the adult abdominal aorta and appears to have a half-life of 70 years. This corresponds to the age of onset of aneurysmal disease and implies that elastin content is dependent on the degree of its destruction.[13] In a study on rat aortas, Anidjar and coworkers[19] showed that by injecting elastase intraarterially, elastin could be disrupted and aneurysmal dilatation of the aorta would form, but the degree of elastin degradation was independent of aneurysm diameter. One study by Powell and Greenhalgh[14] showed elastase activity to be 4.4 ± 1.1 U/ng DNA in the controls as compared with 8.3 ± 2.2 U/ng DNA for atherosclerotic patients and 17.8 ± 3.5 U/ng DNA for patients with aneurysmal disease. There

was a corresponding reciprocal decrease in medial elastin levels (as a percentage of dry weight) from 35% in controls, 23% in atherosclerosis, and 8% in aneurysms (Figure 10-3).[2]

Collagen type III has also been implicated in aneurysm formation.[20–22] It has been found in higher concentrations in aneurysmal aortas relative to the normal aorta.[20] Interestingly, decreased levels have also been shown in patients with ruptured intracerebral aneurysms.[21] Although increased collagenolytic activity has been shown in patients with aneurysmal disease, it has been difficult to show increased collagenase levels in nonruptured aneurysms.[20,23]

Smoking has long been associated with AAAs. A review of the Whitehall study[24] showed that there was a fourfold increase in the incidence of death from ruptured AAA in smokers than in nonsmokers. Furthermore, in smokers who hand-rolled their cigarettes, the incidence of death was 14 times more common. The specific toxic component of tobacco has yet to be identified. Cigarette smoking is a greater risk factor for aortic atherosclerosis than coronary atherosclerosis.[25]

Inflammatory changes in the wall of the aneurysm are seen in 2.5–10.0% of patients undergoing surgery for AAAs.[26,27] It is thought that this aneurysmal vari-

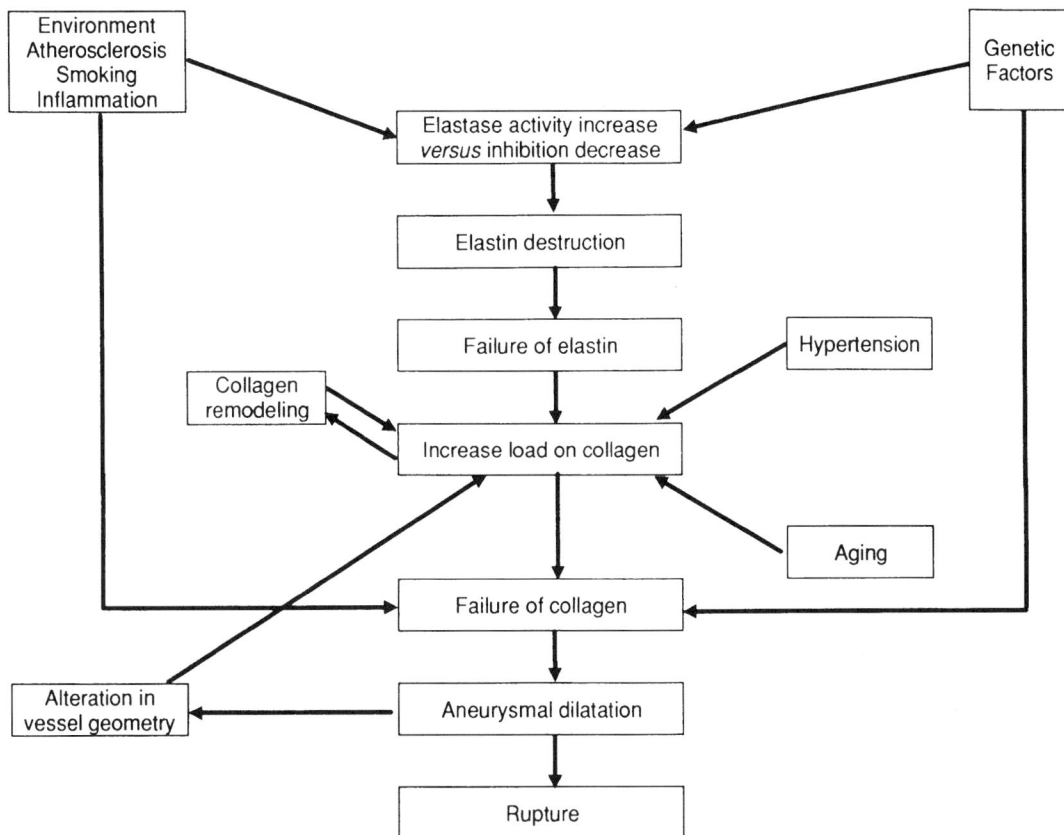

Figure 10-2. Pathogenesis of abdominal aortic aneurysm. (Reprinted with permission from STR MacSweeney, JT Powell, RM Greenhalgh. Pathogenesis of abdominal aortic aneurysm. Br J Surg 1994;81:935.)

ant is an autoimmune response to components of the aortic wall, specifically ceroid.[28] Several authors have suggested that the release of inflammatory mediators in response to the atherosclerotic process leads to weakening and destruction of the aortic media.[28–30]

AAA is primarily a disease of age. It is rare in patients under 50 years of age and increases in prevalence up to 85 and beyond. The aorta of a 20-year-old subject is approximately three times more elastic than that of a 70-year-old subject.[31,32]

Preoperative Assessment

Aortic surgery can be categorized as the repair of either aneurysmal or occlusive disease. AAA surgery can be further divided into elective and emergent repair. Patients undergoing aortic surgery for aneurys-

mal disease are twice as likely to die or have perioperative morbidity as are patients undergoing aortic surgery for occlusive disease. However, median survival time is lower in patients with occlusive disease (5.8 years as compared with 10.7 years).[33] Resection can be further subdivided into suprarenal and infrarenal AAA. The associated mortalities are 2–5% (infrarenal), greater than 30% (suprarenal),[34] and 17–66% (ruptured). This classification has clinical significance in regard to preoperative assessment and intraoperative management. Infrarenal AAAs are by far the most common (>90%) of all AAAs.

Elective Resection

Approximately 75% of AAAs are asymptomatic and found unexpectedly on routine physical examination or

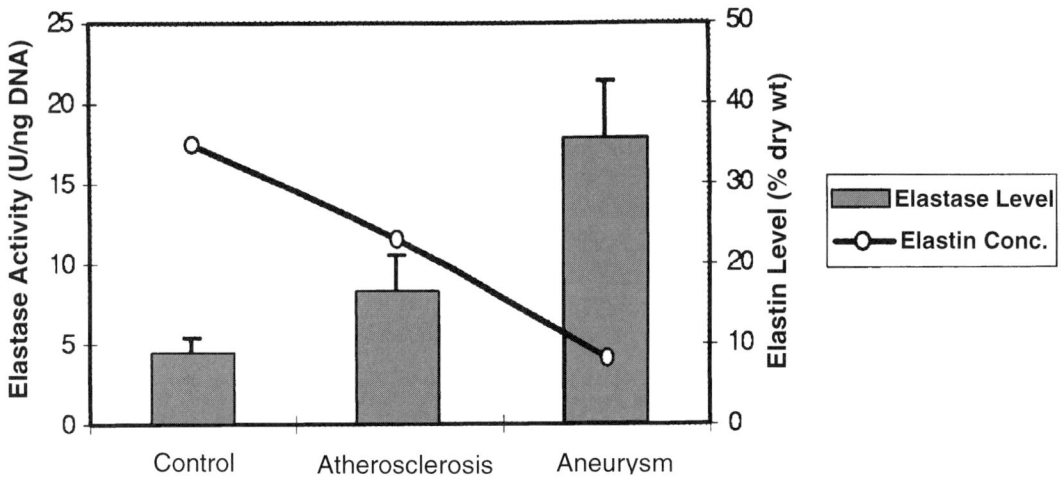

Figure 10-3. Elastin levels and elastase activity in patients with aneurysms versus patients with atherosclerosis and controls. Note the reciprocal relationship between elastase activity and elastin levels. (Modified from J Powell, R Greenhalgh. Cellular, enzymatic and genetic factors in the pathogenesis of abdominal aortic aneurysm. J Vasc Surg 1989;9:297.)

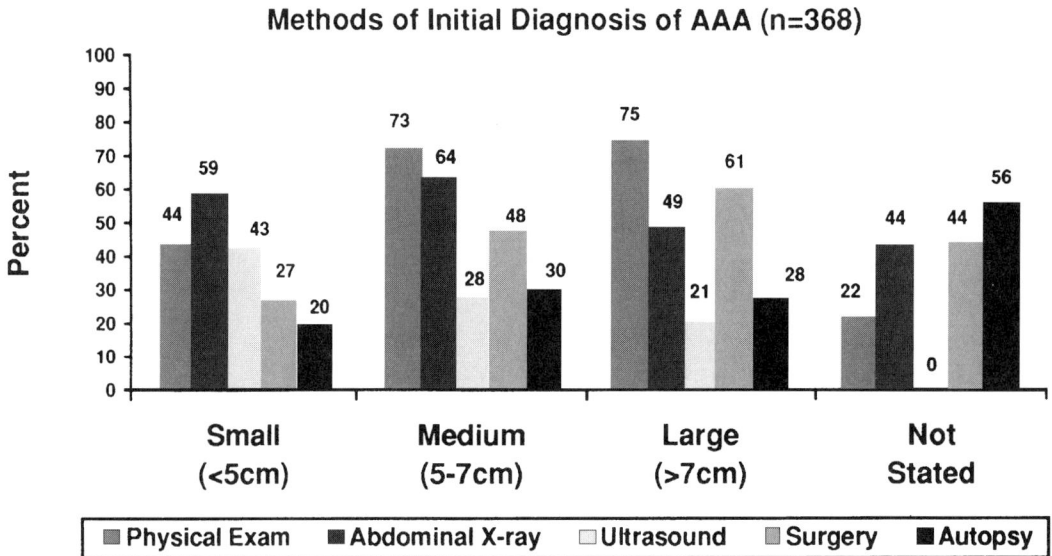

Figure 10-4. Relationship of aneurysm size to method of initial diagnosis in patients with newly diagnosed abdominal aortic aneurysms (AAA), 1951–1980 (n = 368; patients may be counted more than once). (Modified from LJ Melton, LK Bickerstaff. Changing incidence of abdominal aortic aneurysms: a population-based study. Am J Epidemiol 1984;120:379.)

during radiographic or operative procedures for unrelated reasons (Figures 10-4 and 10-5). It is beyond the scope of this chapter to describe the relative merits of the various methods used to determine the presence of an aneurysm. What is important to note is that aneurysm size is probably the most significant factor in determining the need for surgical intervention. As shown in Figure 10-1 and Table 10-1, as the aneurysm size increases above 6 cm, the 5-year risk of rupture increases from 15% for a 4-cm aneurysm to 75% for

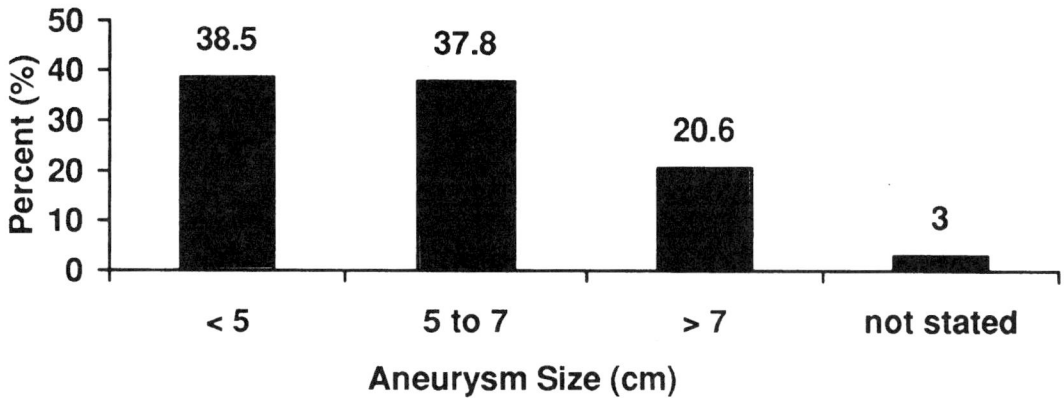

Figure 10-5. Aneurysm size at time of detection. (Modified from LK Bickerstaff, LH Hollier. Abdominal aortic aneurysms: the changing natural history. J Vasc Surg 1984;1:6.)

Table 10-1. Risk of Aneurysm Rupture Based on Size

Aneurysm Size (cm)	Five-Year Risk Rupture (Percentage)
4	15
5	20
6	30
7	50
8	75

an 8-cm aneurysm. Figure 10-6 shows the percent survival for aneurysms greater than 6 cm (large) as compared with aneurysms less than 6 cm (small), when treated both operatively and nonoperatively.

Coexisting Disease

There are a number of coexisting disease states associated with aortic disease (Table 10-2). Forty to fifty percent of patients have a history of a prior myocardial infarction, whereas 10–20% suffer from angina and 10–15% suffer from from congestive heart failure (see Chapter 2).

Preoperative studies should focus on identifying associated disease processes with the goal of correctly quantifying perioperative risk and optimizing a patient's associated diseases. This will always begin with the history and physical examination and indicated laboratory tests. The high correlation of atherosclerotic disease in the carotid and coronary vessels cannot be overstated. Noninvasive cardiac studies, such as adenosine or dipyridamole -hallium scintigraphy, may be used for identifying areas of myocardium at risk for ischemia. Additionally, coronary angiography may be required based on the results of the previously mentioned studies (see Chapter 2) (Figure 10-7).

With the introduction of magnetic resonance imaging and high-resolution helical computed tomography scanning, the need for aortography has greatly diminished and is now only recommended for specific indications. With aortography, aneurysm size can be falsely reported as small or normal because dye may only fill the central channel and thus not demonstrate the luminal clot that may make up a large portion of the aneurysm. Similarly, using aortography to delineate the upper and lower extent of the aneurysm can be misleading and is better demonstrated using computed tomography and Doppler ultrasound (see Chapter 3). Aortography, however, may be indicated to (1) rule out other suspected aneurysms (renal artery, splenic, popliteal, etc.), (2) evaluate associated renovascular hypertension, (3) rule out horseshoe kidney (as suggested by other studies), or (4) evaluate patients with intestinal angina.

Emergent Resection

In the case of emergent AAA resection, the physician does not have the luxury of an adequate pre-

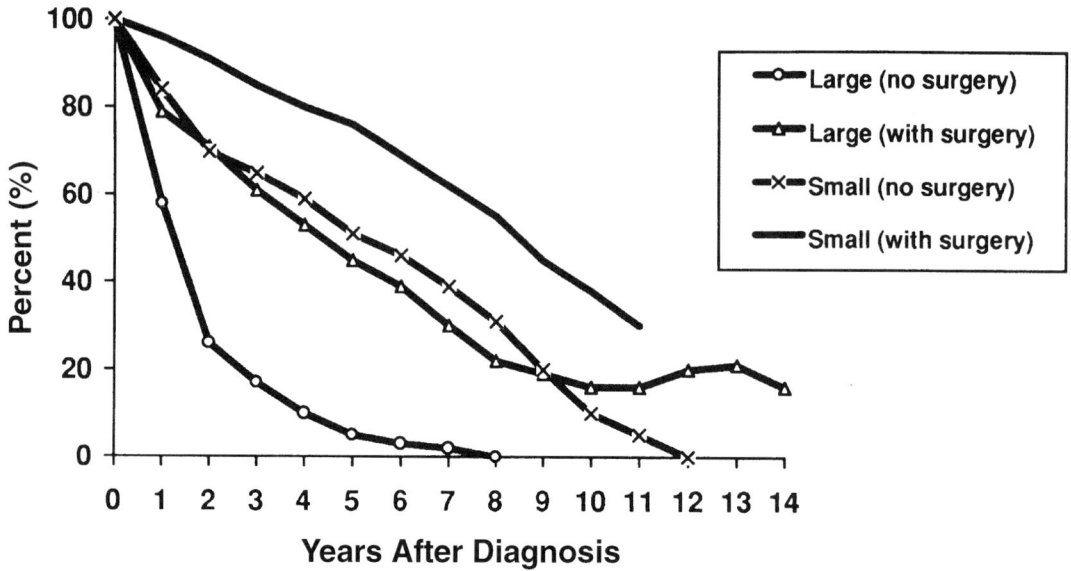

Figure 10-6. Survival curves for patients with small (<6 cm) and large (>6 cm) abdominal aortic aneurysms that received operative and nonoperative management. (Modified from DE Szilagyi, RF Smith. Contribution of abdominal aortic aneurysmectomy to prolongation of life. Ann Surg 1966;164:678.)

Table 10-2. Comorbid Diseases Associated with Abdominal Aortic Aneurysms

Comorbid Disease	Percentage
Heart disease	
Previous myocardial infarction	40–50
Angina	10–20
Congestive heart failure	10–15
Hypertension	50–60
Chronic obstructive pulmonary disease	25–50
Diabetes mellitus	9–12
Renal impairment	5–17

Source: Reprinted with permission from AS Cunningham. Anesthesia for abdominal aortic surgery—a review (Part I). Can J Anaesth 1989;36:426.

operative assessment. When a ruptured aneurysm is suspected, time is of utmost importance because the time from diagnosis to operation is highly correlated with survival. In these cases preoperative assessment may consist of no more than a rapid history and physical examination and basic laboratory, electrocardiographic, and radiologic examinations.

Monitoring

Myocardial Function and Ischemia Detection

All patients undergoing aortic surgery should have continuous intravascular monitoring of arterial pressure. The need for pulmonary artery catheters in patients undergoing aortic cross-clamp procedures has been debated. Some have recommended that pulmonary artery catheters be used in all cases,[35–37] whereas others use them based on the cross-clamp level and extent of comorbid disease.[38]

Increase in pulmonary artery diastolic pressure is a sensitive but nonspecific measure of myocardial ischemia. Pulmonary artery catheters offer the anesthesiologist the ability to monitor pulmonary artery pressures, pulmonary artery occlusion pressure, cardiac output, and mixed venous oxygen saturation. They additionally allow the clinician the ability to calculate a number of derived values including (1) systemic and pulmonary vascular resistance, (2) left ventricular stroke work index, and (3) arteriovenous oxygen difference.

The high incidence of coronary artery disease associated with both aortic aneurysm and aortoiliac

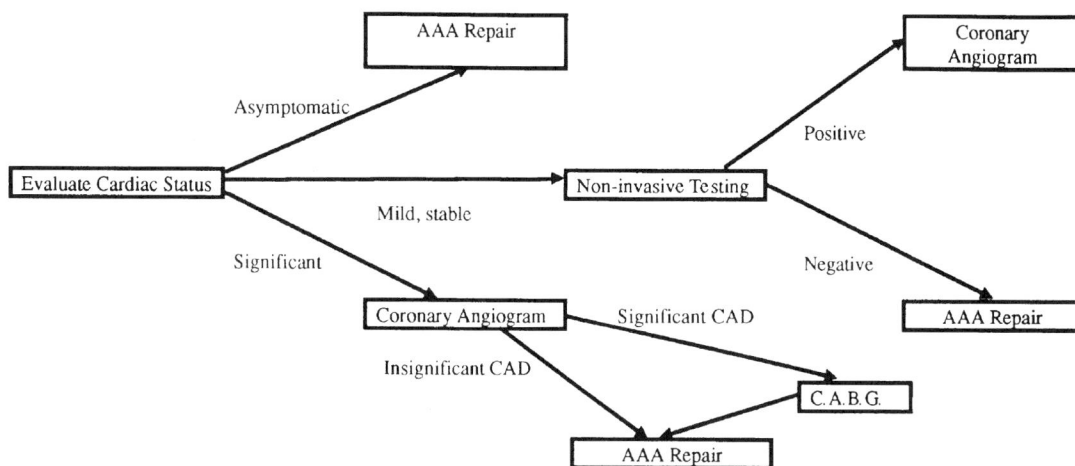

Figure 10-7. Algorithm to determine necessity of preoperative testing. (AAA = abdominal aortic aneurysm; CAD = coronary artery disease; CABG = coronary artery bypass graft.)

occlusive disease has been well documented. Two studies looking at angiographic evidence of significant coronary artery atherosclerosis showed that as many as 73% of patients with AAA disease and 40% of patients with aortoiliac disease demonstrated significant occlusion on coronary angiography.[39] Most significantly, 15–47% of clinically asymptomatic patients demonstrated angiographic evidence of significant coronary atherosclerosis.[39,40]

However, Isaacson et al.[41] compared pulmonary artery catheterization to central venous catheterization in a selected, randomized study. They selected out those patients with known severe or inoperable coronary artery disease (based on the concept that pulmonary artery catheterization would be mandatory in this population) and studied the rest of the patients. They found no significant difference in morbidity, mortality, length of stay in surgical intensive care unit or hospital, or cost of hospitalization. The only significant difference was in the professional fee charged by the anesthesiologist. They concluded that in the otherwise asymptomatic patient or in patients after coronary revascularization, the use of central venous catheterization was sufficient for abdominal aortic reconstruction (see Chapter 4).

Electrocardiography

The detection of ischemia using electrocardiography is most sensitive when leads II and V_5 or a modified

Table 10-3. Monitoring Criteria for Significant ST-Segment Changes

New ST depression ≥ 1 mm (0.1 mV) in a horizontal or downsloping ST segment measured 60 m after the J point
ST-segment depression ≥ 1.5 mm in a slowly upsloping ST segment
ST-segment elevation ≥ 1.5 mm from baseline in a non–Q-wave lead
ST-segment elevation ≥ 1.0 mm if associated with a simultaneous ST elevation of ≥ 1.5 mm of another electrocardiogram lead

Source: Modified from HC Gilbert, JS Vender. Cardiovascular Monitoring. In RR Kirby, N Gravenstein (eds), Clinical Anesthesia Practice. Philadelphia: Saunders, 1994;360.

chest lead are monitored (Table 10-3).[42] The majority of ST-segment changes that are detected on 12-lead electrocardiography will be found in lead V_5.[43] Changes in the ST segment and T wave are secondary to delayed repolarization of ischemic myocardial cells during periods of coronary insufficiency (Figure 10-8). ST-segment and T-wave changes also may result from conduction defects, left ventricular hypertrophy, electrolyte disorders, and drug effects.[42,44]

Transesophageal Echocardiography

Transesophageal echocardiography (TEE) has also been used with increasing frequency during repair of

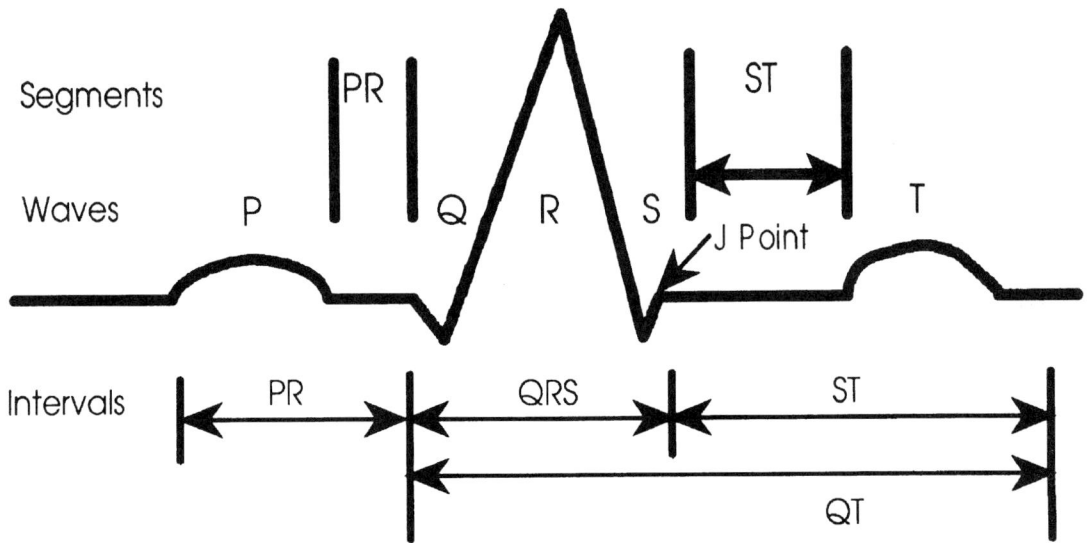

Figure 10-8. The electrocardiographic waves and intervals. (Reprinted with permission from DM Thys. The Normal ECG. In DM Thys, JA Kaplan (eds), The ECG in Anesthesia and Critical Care. New York: Churchill Livingstone, 1987;14.)

Table 10-4. Percent Change in Cardiovascular Variables on Initiation of Aortic Occlusion

	Percent Change After Aortic Occlusion		
Level of Occlusion	Supraceliac	Suprarenal–Infraceliac	Infrarenal
Mean arterial blood pressure	54	5*	2*
Pulmonary capillary wedge pressure	38	10*	0*
End-diastolic area	28	2*	9*
End-systolic area	69	10*	11*
Ejection fraction	−38	−10*	−3*
Patients with wall motion abnormalities	92	33	0
New myocardial infarctions	8	0	0

*Statistically different ($P < 0.05$) from group undergoing supraceliac aortic occlusion.
Source: Reprinted with permission from MF Roizen, PN Beaupre, RA Alpert. Monitoring with two-dimensional transesophageal echocardiography: comparison of myocardial function in patients undergoing supraceliac, suprarenal-infraceliac or infrarenal aortic occlusion. J Vasc Surg 1984;1:300.

AAAs. TEE is an effective and sensitive means of evaluating myocardial performance and detecting early myocardial ischemia. Roizen et al.[45] showed that cross clamp occlusion of the supraceliac aorta causes large increases in left ventricular end-systolic and end-diastolic areas, decreases in ejection fraction, and often results in wall motion abnormalities, which may be an early sign of myocardial ischemia. As shown in Table 10-4, after occlusion of the supraceliac aorta, significant increases in mean arterial pressure, pulmonary capillary occlusion pressure, and TEE-visualized wall motion abnormalities can be seen. Concomitantly, there is a significant decrease in ejection fraction. These changes were less for suprarenal-infraceliac occlusion and were essentially normal for infrarenal aortic occlusion (see Chapter 4).[46]

Electrocardiographic monitoring may be the most specific indicator of myocardial ischemia, but continuous monitoring of segmental wall motion abnormalities with the use of TEE is thought by many to be the most sensitive.[47] Segmental wall motion abnormalities may occur before, simultaneously, or in the absence of ST-segment changes.[46] In a study by Smith and colleagues[46] comparing ST-segment changes with segmental wall motion abnormalities, all the patients who suffered intraoperative myocardial infarctions had persistent intraoperative wall motion abnormalities, whereas only one of these patients had ST-segment changes. Ten patients in this study, who did not undergo cardiovascular surgery and had no history of cardiac disease, did not demonstrate ST-segment changes, wall motion abnormalities, or experience intraoperative myocardial infarction. TEE is also a valuable tool when used in patients with lung disease where pulmonary artery pressures may not accurately reflect left ventricular filling pressures.

TEE can also provide a real-time assessment of left ventricular volume status and the ventricle's response to fluid administration and inotropic agents. Its use also allows the anesthesiologist to observe changes in wall motion that may occur with aortic cross clamping so that appropriate interventions or therapy can be initiated (see Chapter 4 for a complete discussion of myocardial ischemia monitoring).[45]

Neurologic Monitoring

Where supraceliac aortic cross clamping is likely, the measurement of intraoperative spinal cord function has been advocated.[48] This is due to the higher incidence of paraplegia following aortic surgery with higher cross clamping. This incidence ranges from 0.11% to 0.90% in AAAs[49] and to 40% in thoracic aortic surgery.[48,50,51] Somatosensory evoked potentials have been used as a monitor for spinal cord ischemia; however, there is concern that since it only measures the posterior columns, it could theoretically fail to identify anterior motor tract ischemia (see Chapters 4 and 8).[52] The anterior spinal cord is at a higher risk for ischemia due to blood flow decreases that would occur initially in the distribution of the anterior spinal artery (artery of Adamkiewicz) (see Chapters 4 and 8). Spinal cord perfusion pressure (SCPP) can be estimated by the following equation:

$$SCPP = DAP - CSFP$$

where DAP = distal mean aortic pressure; and CSFP = cerebrospinal fluid pressure. Thoracic and high abdominal aortic cross clamping is associated with a decrease in distal aortic pressure and an increase in cerebrospinal fluid pressure (and a decrease in the compliance of the spinal fluid space), thus leading to decreased SCPP.[53] Many methods have been suggested to improve spinal cord perfusion pressure including phlebotomy,[54] cerebrospinal fluid drainage,[51,55,56] and the use of external shunts from the ascending thoracic aorta.[57] Use of sodium nitroprusside during aortic cross clamping has been shown to increase the incidence of neurologic deficit in dogs, although this has not been documented in humans and its use remains controversial.[58,59] Use of different anesthetic agents has been shown to reduce the incidence of paraplegia in animals. These include sodium thiopental alone and thiopental in combination with ketamine.[60] The mechanism of action in the former is probably related to the decrease in cerebral blood flow seen with barbiturates.

Renal Function

Surgery on the infrarenal aorta may be associated with a 5% incidence of renal failure necessitating hemodialysis while suprarenal aortic surgery has an incidence of renal failure approaching 17%.[61,62] Monitoring and maintenance of adequate volume status and urine output is of paramount importance in reducing the incidence of postoperative renal failure (see following discussions on acute renal failure and protection of renal function).

Anesthetic Considerations

Blood Loss

Although there has been a marked decrease in the chance of viral transmission during blood transfusion (Table 10-5),[63] other risks such as allergic reactions, transfusion of a septic unit, volume overload, and adult respiratory distress syndrome still exist. The use of autotransfusion systems has been shown to reduce the need for multiple donors in patients undergoing major vascular surgery. They also may be the only means of blood replacement in patients with rare blood types and in patients who, for religious reasons, will not accept homologous blood, yet will

Table 10-5. Infectious Rates of Viral Agents in Blood Transfusion

Viral Agent	Risk of Infection
Hepatitis C	1/3,000 units transfused
Hepatitis B	1/200,000 units transfused
Human immunodeficiency virus	1/255,000 units transfused
Human T-cell lymphotropic virus I or II	1/50,000 units transfused

Source: Reprinted with permission from JG Donahue, A Munoz, PM Ness. The declining risk of post-transfusion hepatitis C virus infection. N Engl J Med 1992;327:369.

allow use of these systems. One study showed a 25–57% reduction in the number of different donors when autotransfusion systems are used.[64] Anesthetic technique does play a role in the amount of hemorrhage incurred during surgery. Data from the orthopedic literature have shown that regional anesthesia, with its attendant sympathetic blockade, probably has a role in decreasing the venous tone and venous pressure, thus reducing blood loss.[65,66]

Regional anesthetic techniques have also been shown to reduce the risk of postoperative thromboembolism and vascular thrombosis when used for several days after surgery.[67]

Temperature Conservation

Hypothermia caused by exposure of abdominal contents, rapid transfusion of intravenous fluids and blood products, and the effects of anesthesia can be minimized by the use of intravenous fluid warmers, heated anesthesia circuits, heated operating room table pads, irrigation with warm fluids, and use of upper body warming blankets. Hypothermia is associated with vasoconstriction that can worsen hypertension at the end of surgery and can cause depression of myocardial contractility. Severe hypothermia (<30°C) can lead to intractable ventricular arrhythmia. Hypothermia causes a decrease in the rate of all enzymatic reactions. Because the coagulation cascade is a series of proteolytic enzymes, this is one of the earliest systems affected. Hypothermia is characterized by a marked increase in fibrinolytic activity, thrombocytopenia, and a decrease in collagen-induced platelet aggregation.[68] Selective hy-

pothermia of the spinal cord has been shown to prolong the safe ischemic time by reduction of metabolic rate and oxygen requirements.[69,70] The benefits of global hypothermia on spinal cord protection need to be weighed against the adverse effects of hypothermia on coagulation and hemodynamics.

Temperature monitoring can be done in a variety of ways, including use of an esophageal temperature probe rectally or using the pulmonary artery catheter's thermistor (see Chapter 4).

Effects of Aortic Cross Clamping

Hemodynamic Changes

A major goal of anesthetic management is to preserve vital organ function (myocardial, renal, central nervous system, pulmonary, and visceral) by maintaining oxygen delivery. The most significant physiologic changes occurring during abdominal aortic surgery are related to the application of the aortic cross clamp. Occluding the aorta results in hypertension in the proximal vasculature and hypotension in the distal vasculature. This increases the afterload on the heart, systemic vascular resistance, and myocardial oxygen consumption. These increases are all proportional to the level of occlusion. As can be seen in Table 10-4, cross clamping the supraceliac aorta causes significant increases in mean arterial pressure, pulmonary capillary occlusion pressure, and the incidence of wall motion abnormalities and decreases the ejection fraction. Myocardial performance, however, is minimally affected when the aorta is occluded infrarenally. It has been further shown by numerous studies[71–74] that vasodilators such as nitroglycerin can significantly reverse these changes. The mechanism for this action is presumably a decrease in peripheral vascular resistance and afterload, with subsequent increases in cardiac output and ejection fraction.

The hemodynamic changes during AAA surgery are influenced by the patient's preexisting coronary circulation and myocardial function, site of the aneurysm, volume status, and anesthetic technique. On clamping the aorta one might expect to see an increased afterload due to the increased impedance to ventricular ejection and a decreased preload secondary to decreased venous return, but this is not necessarily the case. Cross clamping results in an increase in blood pressure, an increase in systemic vascular resistance, a decrease in stroke volume, and a reduction in cardiac output.[75,76] However, the filling pressures may actually increase. This increase in filling pressures (i.e., central venous pressure, pulmonary artery occlusion pressure, and left ventricular end-diastolic pressure) is often seen with cross clamping of the thoracic aorta in animals as well as humans.[77,78] The degree of hemodynamic response seen after aortic cross clamping at different levels may result in part from different degrees and patterns of blood volume distribution.[79] During supraceliac aortic cross clamping, venous capacitance below the clamp decreases, which sends blood away from the splanchnic and nonsplanchnic beds toward the heart. There is a substantial increase in preload as manifested by elevated filling pressures and increases in the end-diastolic area of the left ventricle.[79] With infraceliac aortic cross clamping these findings may not be seen.[45,80,81] The more distal the cross clamp, the more arterial collateral flow will be present to minimize impedance changes. Preclamp blood flow is also determined by the degree of atherosclerotic disease in the aorta. In the patient with a significantly reduced aortic blood flow secondary to aortoiliac occlusive disease, the application of the aortic cross clamp may cause little or no change in hemodynamics.[82]

Myocardial Effects

Changes in myocardial function appear to be related to preexisting coronary disease. Aortic cross clamping is associated with substantial increases in preload and afterload, which lead to an increase in myocardial oxygen demand with a corresponding increase in coronary blood flow.[83] The data concerning nitroglycerin are conflicting. Nitroglycerin administration during infrarenal aortic cross clamping demonstrated a decrease in vascular resistance and an increase in cardiac output.[84] Cross clamping of the distal thoracic aorta led to a 33% decrease in coronary arteriovenous oxygen difference and a 10% decrease in oxygen extraction; while nitroglycerin infusion was associated with a greater decrease in coronary arteriovenous oxygen difference and myocardial oxygen extraction, despite a 12% increase in cardiac work.[79] The main beneficial effect of nitroglycerin may be related to a decrease in preload, resulting from an increase in

venous capacitance, allowing a more favorable stretch-contraction relationship.[79] Other mechanisms can be a decrease in afterload resulting from dilation of resistive vessels and dilation of the coronary vasculature with a subsequent increase in coronary blood flow. Anrep observed in 1912 that sudden aortic constriction resulted in left ventricular dilation followed by partial recovery, even when arterial blood pressure was maintained at a constant increased level. This results in decreases in left ventricular end-diastolic volume and pressure to control values, thereby exerting a positive inotropic effect termed the *Anrep effect*.[79]

Among the effects of aortic occlusion on myocardial function, the most important is increased ventricular wall stress. Elevated wall tension can contribute to decreased global ventricular function and possible myocardial ischemia secondary to increased myocardial oxygen consumption and reduced subendocardial perfusion.[85] Attia and coworkers[81] found that patients without preexisting coronary artery disease demonstrated a decrease in pulmonary artery pressure, pulmonary artery occlusion pressure, and central venous pressure when the aorta was clamped. Patients with clinical evidence of coronary artery disease responded to cross clamping with increased right- and left-sided filling pressures. Additionally, they found evidence of myocardial ischemia in three patients who exhibited a greater than 7 mm increase in pulmonary artery occlusion pressure.[81] Gooding et al.[86] confirmed these findings and showed that patients with coronary artery disease sustained a greater reduction in cardiac index as compared with patients without coronary disease. This suggests that patients with coronary artery disease and impaired myocardial contractility or increased left ventricular end-diastolic volumes may be unable to mobilize the Frank-Starling mechanism further and may proceed to develop myocardial ischemia and left ventricular failure following abrupt increases in afterload.[35]

There is also some evidence supporting the role of prostaglandin E in reducing aortic pressure and systemic vascular resistance and increasing cardiac output with cross clamping,[87] while prostaglandin F secretion is associated with unclamping the aorta.[88] Increased levels of prostacyclin (PGF_2), thromboxane A_2, and thromboxane X_2 have also been implicated in the reduction of cardiac output seen with aortic clamping.[89]

Pulmonary Effects

Pulmonary complications are often seen after abdominal and thoracic aortic surgery. One study by Golden et al.[90] showed a 26% incidence of postoperative respiratory failure following thoracoabdominal aortic aneurysm surgery. Patients undergoing thoracic aortic cross clamping have been shown to have an increase in pulmonary vascular resistance.[80,91] This may be due to an increased volume of blood in the lungs or to an increase in left ventricular end-diastolic pressure and volume. A similar increase in pulmonary vascular resistance is seen after unclamping of the aorta,[80,92] although the mechanism for this is unclear. Prostaglandins, specifically thromboxane, have been shown to play a role in the pulmonary circulatory complications seen with aortic cross clamping. Ischemia is known to generate thromboxane,[93] which, during reperfusion, can cause an increase in mean pulmonary artery pressure and increases in pulmonary microvascular permeability.[94] Other mediators implicated as possible causes for the increased pulmonary vascular resistance include oxygen free radicals,[95] complement activation,[96] and the renin-angiotensin system (see Chapter 11).

Renal Effects

The renin-angiotensin system plays an important role in the development of renal hemodynamic changes during aortic cross clamping. There is a large increase in sodium reabsorption and renal vascular resistance due to angiotensin II. This effect was effectively eliminated in patients receiving pretreatment with angiotensin-converting enzyme inhibitors.[97] It is interesting to note that during cross clamping, patients pretreated with angiotensin-converting enzyme inhibitors had lower values for renal blood flow than the controls but had higher values immediately after unclamping, suggesting that the protective effect of angiotensin-converting enzyme inhibitors functions after, but not during, aortic cross clamping.[79] A minor role is played by the activation of the sympathetic nervous system. However, epidural anesthesia, which significantly decreases sympathetic outflow to the kidneys, has little effect on the glomerular filtration rate.[98] (See the section on protection of renal function.)

Spinal Cord Ischemia

Spinal cord injuries after distal aortic surgery have been reported with an incidence far lower than in thoracic aortic surgery. In a study by Szilargyi et al.[99] there was a reported 0.25% incidence of spinal cord injury following abdominal aortic surgery, with a higher percentage (as much as ten times) of those occurring after emergency surgery. Spinal cord damage was not reported during surgery for aortoiliac disease.[99] The site of clamp placement and the ligation of critical lumbar and lower intercostal arteries were the predominant etiologies. The artery of Adamkiewicz, which arises most often at the T9–T12 level, is thought to be the major radicular arterial supply of the anterior spinal cord[100]; however, its location can vary. This artery can be interrupted when the cross clamp is placed either subdiaphragmatically or occasionally when placed just below the renal arteries. Hence, in the presence of inadequate collateral circulation, spinal cord ischemia can result. Somatosensory evoked potential measurements have been used in an attempt to detect cord ischemia; however, somatosensory evoked potentials principally assess dorsal column function and not the anterior cord, which is primarily at risk.[101,102] Anterior cord ischemia with motor loss during aortic cross clamping with complete preservation of somatosensory evoked potential has been demonstrated (see Chapters 4 and 8).[103]

Motor evoked potentials monitor anterior cord function[104–106] and are being studied. However, more studies are needed to evaluate their ability to improve outcome (see Chapter 4).

Effects of Abdominal Aortic Unclamping

Aortic unclamping is associated with a number of hemodynamic and physiologic responses. These responses are summarized in Figure 10-9.

Hemodynamic Changes

During cross clamping, tissues below the level of the cross clamp are perfused only by collateral vessels and may undergo ischemic metabolism. Lactic acid and other products of anaerobic metabolism accumulate during this period and are recirculated after unclamping.[107] Other substances,

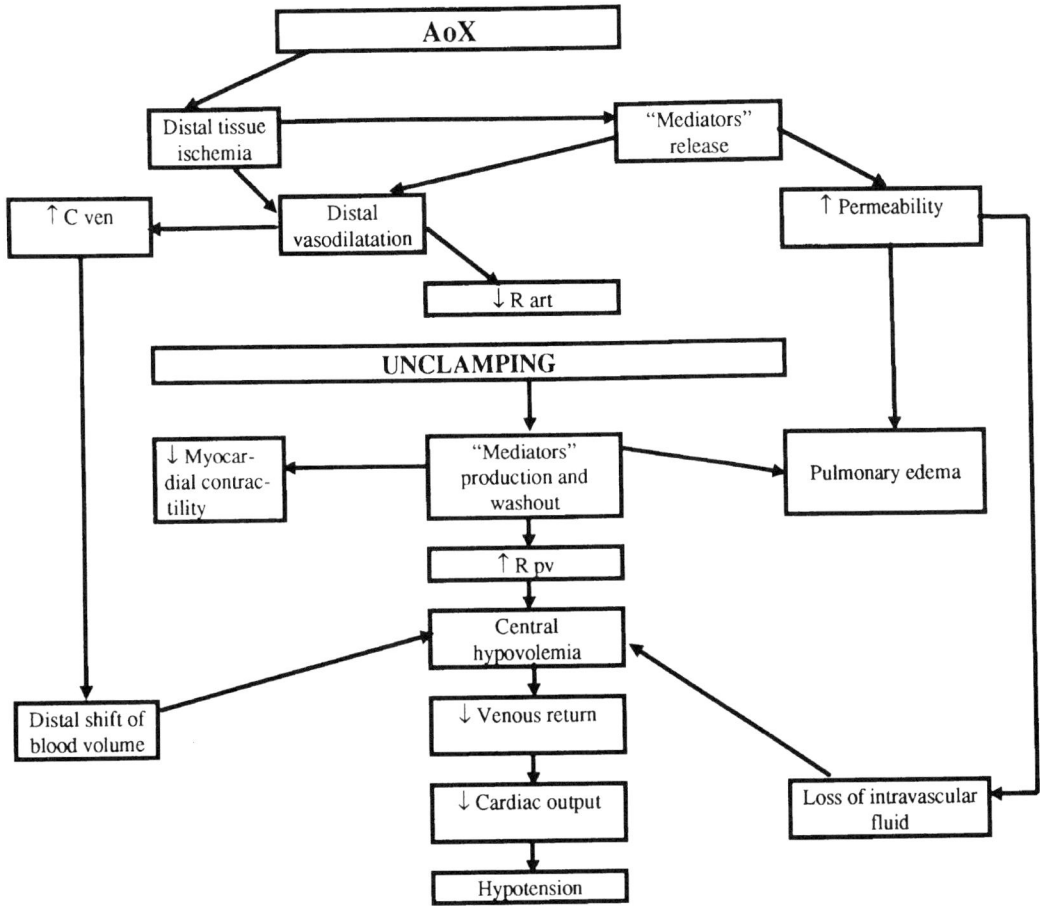

Figure 10-9. Systemic hemodynamic response to aortic unclamping. (AoX = aortic cross clamping; Cven = central venous capacitance; R art = arterial resistance; R pv = pulmonary vascular resistance; ↑ = increase; ↓ = decrease.) (Reprinted with permission from SG Gelman. The pathophysiology of aortic cross-clamping and unclamping. Anesthesiology 1995;82:1026.)

such as the myocardial depressant factor[108,109] and plasma levels of purine derivatives (i.e., xanthine, hypoxanthine, inosine, and adenosine),[110] have been shown to be increased after unclamping and may be implicated in causing the decreased cardiac output, vasodilatation, and hypotension often seen after unclamping.

The hemodynamic response to unclamping is variable. Cardiac output has been shown to decrease, increase, and remain the same.[79] The only consistent findings are a decrease in vascular resistance and arterial blood pressure, a decrease in left ventricular end-diastolic pressure, and an increase in myocardial blood flow.[79]

Vasoconstrictors, used systemically, may constrict the vasculature above the aortic clamp more than below the clamp, because the area above the clamp, which is nonischemic, would respond better to vasopressors than the area below the clamp, which is ischemic and acidotic. This may promote redistribution of blood volume from the upper to the lower part of the body, further reducing the flow above the aortic clamp.[79] Vasodilators given during cross clamp may paradoxically decrease cardiac output and increase filling pressures. This decrease in cardiac output may be caused by vasodilator promotion of washout of cardiodepressant substances as suggested by Grindlinger and colleagues.[111,112]

Metabolic acidosis from the release of substances from ischemic tissue distal to the cross clamp has been shown to occur during periods of aortic cross clamping.[113] The degree of acidosis is related in part to the underlying disease (i.e., aneurysm as opposed to occlusive disease). Presumably, patients with occlusive disease have developed better collateral circulation and thus better tissue perfusion distal to the clamp site. Metabolic acidosis may develop because of recirculation release of deoxygenated blood from ischemic legs; however, Baue et al.[114] showed that even after correcting the acidosis, there was no change in the arterial hypotension seen after unclamping. This leads to the conclusion that while the acidosis in the blood may be corrected, the tissue acidosis may not be.

Reactive hyperemia is one of the most important features of the response to aortic unclamping. There are several hypotheses to explain this phenomenon. The first person to describe this effect was Bayliss in 1902, who noted that after clamping an artery, the smooth muscle in the arterial wall relaxes, facilitating high flow after unclamping.[115] Another theory by Barcroft states that anoxia in the occluded artery causes the smooth muscle relaxation and the resulting increased flow after clamp removal.[116] A third theory involves the accumulation of vasodilating metabolites in the distal arterial segments.[117] The maximal hyperemic response was seen 15 minutes after aortic unclamping, suggesting a metabolic mediated response; however, an initial response was seen 10–60 seconds after clamp removal, which is consistent with a reflex phenomenon.[118]

Several objectives should be kept in mind during unclamping. Volume loading the patient prior to release of the cross clamp serves a dual role, both as a volume source and a diluent to dissipate the release of vasoactive and cardiodepressant mediators. Gradual release of the cross clamp has been advocated by some investigators to allow for a slower washout of these substances and may reduce the degree of abrupt reoxygenation to the ischemic limbs, thereby decreasing the production of oxygen free radicals.[119,120]

Acute Renal Failure

In addition to its cardiovascular effects, aortic clamping also has profound impact on the kidneys.

Gamulin and colleagues[121] studied ^{125}I hippuran clearance during infrarenal aortic cross clamping and found a 29% decrease in ^{125}I hippuran clearance and a 38% decrease in renal blood flow that persisted for 1 hour after the cross clamp was removed. There was also a 75% increase in renal vascular resistance. Gamulin et al.[121] stated that this decrease in ^{125}I hippuran clearance indicated a global diminution of renal perfusion with redistribution of the renal blood flow toward the cortical compartment. They believed that this phenomenon was beneficial and could prevent the development of acute tubular necrosis. Kountz et al.,[122] however, did not note any significant negative effect on blood flow or perfusion. Using microspheres, Cronenwett et al.[123] showed no change in distribution of renal blood flow when cardiac output and intravascular volume were maintained.

Acute renal failure following aortic cross clamping has been shown to have an incidence of up to 3% in patients following elective infrarenal cross clamping.[61] There are several predisposing factors that may contribute to this problem, including the residual presence of iodinated contrast dye,[124] preoperative hypovolemia seen after bowel preparation,[125] and age. The effect on renal outcome from the changes in renal perfusion and renal blood flow following infrarenal aortic cross clamping remains controversial. A number of authors[121,126] have shown a decrease in renal cortical blood flow during and after aortic cross clamping.

Diuretics and renal dose dopamine have been used to improve renal perfusion, but their role remains controversial. Several authors have reported a benefit from mannitol and the loop diuretics.[127,128] Mannitol reduces the degree of reduction in renal blood flow during periods of infrarenal cross clamping, but renal blood flow failed to return to baseline levels after unclamping.[128] This was also true for dopamine and the combination of dopamine and mannitol.[129,130] Nevertheless, these results are controversial because these studies consisted of few patients and the results could easily be explained by other confounding factors. The use of diuretics requires close monitoring of fluid balance. If replacement is insufficient, diuretic therapy may be more harmful than beneficial. Fluid replacement again is a key element in decreasing the incidence of renal complications[37] (see Chapter 8).

Management for Elective Abdominal Aortic Aneurysmectomy

Anesthetic Agents and Techniques

A variety of anesthetic agents and techniques has been used for patients undergoing surgery on the abdominal aorta. There have been few reports in the literature on the effect of anesthetic technique on cardiac and major organ performance during aortic vascular surgery. The choice of agents or technique used may be influenced by the anesthesiologist's personal bias, clinical experience, and familiarity with certain techniques, as well as the presence of coexisting disease. Although many anesthetic techniques and drugs have been used successfully for these patients, the diligence of the anesthesiologist in correcting hemodynamic alterations and maintaining organ perfusion (ensuring adequate oxygen delivery by maintaining adequate cardiac output and oxygen carrying capacity) during cross clamping may be the most important factor contributing to a positive outcome (Table 10-6). Nevertheless coexisting disease does play a role in anesthetic choice.

Attia and coworkers[81] showed that patients without coronary artery disease tolerate inhalational agents to a greater degree than those with severe coronary artery disease and also tolerate the hemodynamic effects of aortic cross clamping with less dependence on vasoactive agents. Patients with severe coronary artery disease usually require a narcotic-based anesthetic and have a greater reliance on vasoactive agents.

As mentioned earlier, it is important to continuously monitor myocardial performance in these patients. Any evidence of myocardial ischemia should be aggressively treated by attempting to improve the myocardial oxygen supply/demand ratio by using vasodilators such as nitroglycerin (0.5–1.0 µg/kg/minute initially and then titrated to effect), vasoconstrictors such as phenylephrine (used to improve coronary perfusion pressure), and beta-blockers. Transfusion to improve the hematocrit can also help.

Inhalational Agents

The halogenated hydrocarbons have all been used as either the principal anesthetic[131,132] or as part of a balanced technique.[113,133] Halothane and enflurane pro-

Table 10-6. Anesthetic Goals During Abdominal Aortic Surgery

Provide stable hemodynamics and preserve myocardial function
Preserve a favorable oxygen supply/demand ratio to the heart by decreasing oxygen consumption and increasing oxygen delivery
Increase oxygen-carrying capacity by maintaining intravascular volume and hematocrit
Protect the kidneys by maintaining adequate urine output with proper hydration and the use of dopamine, diuretics, or both when necessary
Preserve body temperature to prevent coagulopathy
Correct any derangements in electrolyte and acid–base status

duce dose-dependent reductions in cardiac output secondary to reduced myocardial contractility and reduced stroke volume. Isoflurane has a minimal effect on cardiac output because the decreased stroke volume is offset by increased heart rate. Isoflurane and enflurane are both potent vasodilators, with isoflurane having a greater effect. Halothane has less of an effect on peripheral vascular resistance. The vasodilating effects of enflurane and isoflurane may be beneficial by decreasing preload and afterload, especially during aortic cross clamping. These agents may also produce reductions in coronary vascular resistance.[134] Roizen and Hamilton showed that increases in pulmonary capillary wedge pressure and systemic blood pressure consequent to aortic cross clamping can be treated by titrating the dose of inhalational anesthetic to control hemodynamics.[134]

Increasing the depth of anesthesia reduces total peripheral vascular resistance secondary to dilation of vascular beds predominantly in skin and muscle, but also in the cerebral and perhaps coronary circulations.[134] A theoretical disadvantage is the possible need for increasing intravascular volume, which may lead to subsequent fluid overload and pulmonary edema as anesthetic depth is decreased and volume is shifted from the peripheral to the central compartment.

Nitrous oxide has several theoretical deleterious effects on hemodynamics that may limit its use during abdominal aortic surgery. It is a direct negative inotrope and may decrease cardiac output and increase afterload.[135] It also may decrease renal and splanchnic blood flow, which would contribute to ischemia during aortic cross clamping. Prolonged use of nitrous oxide may also lead to bowel distention, which may interfere with surgical exposure during prolonged cases.

Opioids

Benefiel and colleagues[136] randomly assigned 100 patients undergoing abdominal or thoracoabdominal reconstruction to receive isoflurane or sufentanil as their primary anesthetic. Intraoperative and postoperative measurements of systemic blood pressure, pulmonary capillary wedge pressure, and heart rate were kept within 20% of mean preoperative values. The authors found that although intraoperative fluid requirements did not differ between the two groups, fewer patients in the sufentanil group experienced severe postoperative complications. This included a lower incidence of congestive heart failure and renal insufficiency.[136] The results suggested a protective effect of a sufentanil-based anesthetic technique. The commonly used opioids have become increasingly popular as the primary and often sole anesthetic agent for patients undergoing aortic surgery because of their cardiovascular stability. This is extremely valuable in a population with a high incidence of underlying cardiovascular disease.[137,138] Other reasons cited include suppression of metabolic and humoral responses to anesthesia and surgery with prolonged postoperative analgesia.[138] However, Friesen et al.[139] and Thomson et al.[140] showed that high-dose fentanyl (100 μg/kg), oxygen, and a relaxant anesthetic can be associated with a higher incidence of hyperdynamic circulatory response to surgical stimuli before, during, and after aortic cross clamping.

Opioids in higher doses produce a mild decrease in cardiac output and blood pressure secondary to reduced sympathetic tone.[141] Significant doses of opioids, especially when administered concurrently with benzodiazepines can lead to significant decreases in systemic vascular resistance. A high-dose narcotic anesthetic technique has both advantages and disadvantages in these patients. In sufficient doses, narcotics minimally decrease myocardial contractility and blood pressure while providing analgesia and hypnosis. A major disadvantage may be the need for postoperative ventilatory support and prolonged tracheal intubation, which may increase the risk of pulmonary complications. Never-

theless, postoperative intubation and sedation have the advantage of allowing the patient to mobilize intraoperative fluids and allow for more gradual recovery from the stresses of major surgery (see Chapter 11).

Epidural Anesthesia

Epidural anesthesia has been used successfully alone and in combination with general anesthesia for surgery on the abdominal aorta.[80,142,143] A theoretical concern is the possibility of developing an epidural hematoma leading to neurologic deficit after the administration of heparin. Rao and El-Etr[142] looked at the incidence of neurologic complications after anticoagulation therapy following epidural or subarachnoid catheterizations in 3,164 and 847 patients, respectively. Twenty patients experienced minor neurologic complications or low back pain, which was self-limiting and resolved with time. None of the patients in the study developed peridural hematomas leading to spinal cord compression. Another retrospective study of 912 patients receiving continuous epidural analgesia undergoing vascular reconstruction of a lower extremity found no patients with a neurologic deficit that could be attributed to an epidural hematoma.[144]

Yeager et al.[143] performed a randomized clinical trial to evaluate the effect of epidural anesthesia and postoperative analgesia on postoperative morbidity in a group of high-risk patients. Urinary cortisol excretion was measured as a marker of stress response. They found a significantly decreased cortisol excretion during the first 24 hours after surgery in patients receiving epidural anesthesia and analgesia. Additionally, they found that patients who received epidural anesthesia and analgesia had a reduction in the overall postoperative rate of cardiovascular failure and major infectious complications. There was also a decrease in hospital costs in these patients. They concluded that epidural anesthesia and analgesia exerted a significant beneficial effect on operative outcome.[143] Epidural anesthesia may also decrease intraoperative blood loss and reduce postoperative pulmonary dysfunction.[145]

In their randomized study of 173 patients scheduled for abdominal aortic reconstruction, Baron and colleagues found results that conflicted with those of Yeager's group.[146] High-risk surgical patients re-

Table 10-7. Mortality and Major Postoperative Morbidity

Mortality and Morbidity	Group 1*	Group 2*	P Value
Mortality	4	3	0.93 (NS)
Cardiac complications	22	19	0.89 (NS)
Myocardial infarction	5	5	0.82 (NS)
Congestive heart failure	7	5	0.83 (NS)
Prolonged myocardial ischemia	16	16	1.00 (NS)
Ventricular tachyarrhythmia	0	1	0.98 (NS)
Respiratory complications	52	45	0.63 (NS)
Atelectasis minor	35	35	0.86 (NS)
Atelectasis major	2	5	0.39 (NS)
Pneumonia suspected	15	11	0.63 (NS)
Pneumonia confirmed	16	8	0.16 (NS)
Acute respiratory failure	8	4	0.42 (NS)
Renal failure	2	4	0.62 (NS)
Gastrointestinal bleeding	0	3	0.22 (NS)
General sepsis	4	2	0.73 (NS)
Major surgical complications	9	6	0.67 (NS)

Group 1 = general anesthesia; Group 2 = thoracic epidural anesthesia in combination with light general anesthesia; NS = non-significant.
*Number of patients who developed at least one complication.
Source: Reprinted with permission from J-F Baron, M Bertrand, E Bavre, et al. Combined epidural and general anesthesia versus general anesthesia for abdominal aortic surgery. Anesthesiology 1991;75:611.

ceived either a combination of thoracic epidural anesthesia with light general anesthesia or a standard technique of balanced general anesthesia. They found no benefit with intraoperative epidural anesthesia when comparing cardiovascular and respiratory morbidity and mortality (Table 10-7).[146]

In our practice, preoperative epidural placement is offered to all appropriate patients admitted for abdominal aortic surgery. After catheter placement in the operating room, the patients receive a general anesthetic that we believe will be best tolerated based on the patient's preoperative cardiovascular status. We do not administer local anesthetics through the catheter during surgery because of the increased volume loading necessary secondary to local anesthetic–induced sympathectomy. This excess perioperative fluid administration can lead to intravascular volume overloading and left ventricular dysfunction in patients with minimal myocardial reserve.[147] Patients remain intubated postoperatively as intraoperative fluids are mobilized and cardiovascular stability is maintained. Postoperatively, an epidural dose of morphine is given and the patient is started on a continuous epidural infusion of morphine and low dose local anesthetic (see Chap-

ter 13). The majority of patients are extubated within 8–12 hours with minimal discomfort.

Management of Aortic Cross Clamping

The hemodynamics and physiologic effects of aortic cross clamping are discussed earlier in this chapter in the section on effects of aortic cross clamping. The most important variables that determine the cardiovascular responses to aortic cross clamping are initial left ventricular function, level of cross clamp application, and the degree of collateral circulation. To attenuate the increase in afterload and systemic blood pressure associated with cross clamping, we recommend maintaining the patient at a normovolemic or slightly hypovolemic state prior to application of the clamp. It is also useful to increase anesthetic depth, as well as initiating vasodilator therapy at this time. The vasodilating effects of isoflurane make it a particularly useful agent before and during aortic cross clamping. Nitroglycerin or sodium nitroprusside can also be infused before cross clamping. During the time of aortic cross clamping, vasodilator infusion and deepening anesthetic depth allow for intravascular volume loading in preparation for cross clamp release. The main objective during the period of aortic cross clamping is to maintain intravascular volume and myocardial performance, which is achieved by the infusion of crystalloid, colloid, or blood products with the use of vasodilator and inotropic support when necessary. As mentioned earlier, one must be extremely vigilant in monitoring for myocardial ischemia during the cross clamp interval.

Preparing for Unclamping

Volume loading assisted with vasodilator therapy prepares for the hemodynamic changes that will follow unclamping of the aorta. Surgeons will commonly inform the anesthesiologists 5–10 minutes prior to release of the clamp. This gives the anesthesiologist time to decrease or discontinue vasodilator infusions and also decrease the anesthetic depth. As mentioned earlier, during cross clamping, tissues below the level of the clamp are perfused only by collateral vessels and may undergo ischemic metabolism with the accumulation of lactic acid and other products of anaerobic metabolism. These substances act as myocardial depressants, leading to decreased cardiac performance after clamp release. The release of the clamp also greatly decreases systemic vascular resistance; this, along with the released and recirculated vasodilating metabolites, leads to the hypotension commonly seen after release of the clamp. If the patient has been adequately volume loaded during clamping and myocardial function has been preserved, slow release of the clamp will cause minimal changes in blood pressure and cardiac output.[119,120] Larger changes in systemic blood pressure can be treated with small doses of phenylephrine (40–80 µg) and calcium chloride (300–400 mg). In patients with impaired left ventricular function (i.e., ejection fraction < 40%) or prolonged aortic cross clamp times, we start to infuse an inotropic agent (usually dopamine at 5–6 mg/kg/minute) before removal of the clamp. In these patients, ephedrine (5–10 mg) and calcium chloride (300–400 mg) are useful as both inotropes and vasoconstrictors to offset the myocardial depressant effects of acidic metabolites and the decreased systemic vascular resistance. We do not routinely administer sodium bicarbonate be-

fore or at the time of aortic unclamping as is common practice by some clinicians. Once perfusion is reestablished to the organs distal to the clamp site, lactate production diminishes and the transient acidosis is in most cases readily resolved. If on subsequent arterial blood gas analysis, acidosis persists, bicarbonate is administered and other causes for the acidosis are sought (e.g., low cardiac output and low blood pressure).

Patients are at high risk for myocardial ischemia during the period of time immediately after removal of the cross clamp due to the sudden decrease in blood pressure and systemic vascular resistance. Careful attention to the pulmonary artery catheter and the TEE is of paramount importance during this period. Early recognition and treatment with partial reapplication of the clamp or, for moderate decreases, small doses of phenylephrine (50–150 µg) may be critical in reducing the incidence of myocardial infarction.

Protection of Renal Function

Renal function during repair of AAA depends greatly on the level at which the aorta is cross clamped. Infrarenal cross clamping reduces renal blood flow by approximately 40% and increases renal vascular resistance by 75%, even in the absence of changes in cardiovascular and hemodynamic variables.[121] Clamping above the supraceliac vessels reduces renal blood flow by approximately 90%[59] and urine output frequently ceases with cross clamping at levels above the renal arteries. Renal failure following aortic surgery involving suprarenal cross clamping carries a mortality of greater than 30%.[34]

Preoperative volume loading and increased urine output are associated with a lower postoperative serum creatinine and other indices of preserved renal function. In a retrospective study, Bush and Huse found that the pulmonary capillary wedge pressure was more accurate than the central venous pressure as a measure of optimal volume replacement before and during AAA surgery. This volume replacement was associated with a lower incidence of postoperative renal insufficiency.[37,125] Episodes of hypovolemia and hypotension must be avoided because autoregulation of the renal vasculature is lost after periods of ischemic renal insult.[148]

Pharmacologic measures are also used in an attempt to preserve renal blood flow and protect

Table 10-8. Time Between Onset of Symptoms and Admission to Massachusetts General Hospital

Time	Survivors	Deaths	Total	Mortality (Percentage)
0–6 hrs	3	4	7	57
6–12 hrs	7	13	20	65
12–24 hrs	5	7	12	58
1–2 days	5	4	9	44
2–3 days	4	2	6	33
>3 days	5	19	24	67
Unknown	15	16	31	52

Source: Reprinted with permission from LW Ottinger. Ruptured arteriosclerotic aneurysms of the abdominal aorta. Reducing mortality. JAMA 1975;233:147. Copyright 1975, American Medical Association.

against renal injury. Administration of mannitol (0.50–0.75 g/kg) before aortic cross clamping causes an osmotic diuresis that has been shown to decrease renal tubular injury after periods of total renal ischemia.[149] Mannitol also increases renal cortical blood flow and may decrease reperfusion injury following release of the cross clamp secondary to its ability to scavenge free radicals.[34]

Low-dose dopamine (2–5 µg per kg per minute) acts as a renal vasodilator by increasing renal blood flow and inducing a diuresis. We prefer the use of low-dose dopamine since administration of mannitol will transiently increase intravascular volume and may lead to volume overload in patients with limited cardiovascular reserve. The use of mannitol, dopamine, or other diuretics (loop diuretics), although controversial as mentioned earlier, is most beneficial when the patient has been adequately hydrated preoperatively and optimal intravascular volume and hemodynamics are main-

tained throughout surgery and particularly during the period of renal ischemia.[37,125]

Management for Emergent Repair of Ruptured Abdominal Aortic Aneurysm

Preparation

The patient brought to the operating room emergently for repair of an unstable AAA represents one of the most challenging and labor-intensive cases seen in anesthetic practice. Patients may present with a wide spectrum of symptoms from abdominal, back, and lower extremity pain to cardiovascular collapse and shock. The successful care of these patients demands strict control of hemodynamics, acid–base status, maintenance of core temperature, and normal coagulation. These goals are similar to those presenting for elective repair, but in the emergent setting, survival depends on rapid volume resuscitation to treat hypovolemia and hypotension and improve tissue perfusion.

Abdominal aortic aneurysms usually rupture into the retroperitoneum. This provides a tamponade effect, decreasing acute blood loss. Free intraperitoneal rupture is associated with a greater degree of blood loss. Ottinger[150] found free intraperitoneal rupture to be one of the lethal factors influencing patient outcome, along with age, concomitant cardiac disease, preoperative hypotension, cardiac arrest, and anuria (Tables 10-8 and 10-9). Although rare, other presentations have been reported. Snow[151] reported a fatal hemopericardium resulting from a proximal dissection of an atherosclerotic AAA.

Other factors shown to influence operative mortality were duration of operation, blood loss, and the amount of fluid necessary for resuscitation. Wakefield

Table 10-9. Mortality in the Presence or Absence of Lethal Factors

Factor	Incidence of Death (Percentage)	
	With Factor	Without Factor
Preoperative episode of systolic pressure < 80 mm Hg	80	41
Preoperative cardiac arrest	82	55
Free intraperitoneal rupture	80	46
Preoperative anuria	93	41

Source: Reprinted with permission from LW Ottinger. Ruptured arteriosclerotic aneurysms of the abdominal aorta. Reducing mortality. JAMA 1975;233:147. Copyright 1975, American Medical Association.

Table 10-10. Factors That Differ Significantly Between Groups of Survivors and Nonsurvivors[a]

Factor	Survival	Death	Intraoperative Death	Postoperative Hospital Death
Preoperative				
Emergency room blood pressure	110/67	84/50[b]	76/43[b]	89/55[c]
White blood count (per cm^3)	13,000	15,500[b]	—	—
CO_2 (mm Hg)	24.8	22.2[b]	—	22[b]
Blood urea nitrogen (mg/dl)	19.3	28.6[c]	34.9[b]	25.1[b]
Creatinine (mg/dl)	1.5	2.2[b]	—	2.0[b]
Glucose (mg/dl)	180	260[b]	—	267[b]
Prothrombin time (seconds)	67.5	—	44.1[b]	—
Time from the emergency room to the operating room (minutes)	160	84[b]	—	81[b]
Intraoperative				
Operative time (minutes)	234	—	112[c]	300[c]
Lowest blood pressure (mm Hg)	69	30[c]	—	51[c]
Duration of hypotension (minutes)	22	64[c]	—	62[c]
Blood pressure at end of operation (mm Hg)	146	—	—	121[c]
Estimated blood loss (ml)	5,946	8,870[c]	—	10,013[c]
Blood transfusion (U)	12.5	18.2[c]	—	20.5[c]
Fluids administered (ml)	4,236	6,389[c]	—	7,309[c]

[a]Standard deviations and number not shown in table.
[b]$P <0.05$.
[c]$P <0.01$.
Source: Modified from TW Wakefield, WM Whitehouse Jr, SC Wu, et al. Abdominal aortic aneurysm rupture: statistical analysis of factors affecting outcome of surgical treatment. Surgery 1982;91:586.

et al.[152] studied 116 patients undergoing emergency surgery for repair of AAA. They found intraoperative and postoperative mortalities of 21% and 52%, respectively. Increased postoperative mortalities were associated with a duration of operation greater than 400 minutes (100%), hypotension lasting longer than 110 minutes (88%), estimated blood loss greater than 11 liters (75%), more than 17 units of blood transfused (68%), fluid administration in excess of 7 liters (70%), and a systolic blood pressure lower than 100 mm Hg at the conclusion of the operation (88%) (Table 10-10).[152]

Anesthetic Management

When preparing the operating room for the arrival of the patient with a leaking or ruptured AAA, multiple volume lines should be set up, each with the capability of warming and rapidly administering intravenous fluids. Maintaining normothermia is critical because hypothermia can lead to derangement in normal coagulation and myocardial function. A humidified breathing circuit is also used to minimize heat losses.

These patients may arrive from the emergency room with several large-bore intravenous lines in place. If they are not present, they are placed immediately as the patient enters the operating room so volume resuscitation can begin. A rapid-sequence induction with tracheal intubation is performed and the patient is ventilated with 100% oxygen. If the patient comes to the operating room conscious and fluid resuscitated, an arterial line is placed while the patient is being preoxygenated. No other invasive lines should be placed at this time. Induction should not be instituted until the patient is prepared and draped and the surgeon is ready to make an incision. This is because induction is likely to cause a decrease in the blood pressure and the time it takes to restore the pressure by cross clamping the aorta should be minimized. Induction of general anesthesia can be accomplished with minimal changes in blood pressure with succinylcholine and either etomidate (0.1–0.2 mg/kg) or ketamine (1–3 mg/kg). We prefer to use etomidate because of the potential of tachycardia, hypertension, further aneurysm leakage, and increased oxygen consumption that can occur with ketamine. Small doses of narcotics (fentanyl, 25–50 µg) or low-dose volatile agents can be titrated as blood pressure tolerates. Once the aorta is cross clamped, additional anesthesia may be titrated. If hemodynamics remain tenuous, small doses of scopolamine can at least provide amnesia at little hemodynamic cost.

TEE can be a valuable tool to follow changes in left ventricular wall motion and volume status. After the abdomen is opened and the aorta is cross clamped, volume resuscitation is continued and metabolic and acid–base derangements are corrected.

Maintaining normothermia is a difficult and critical task but must be accomplished to avoid problems with coagulopathy, myocardial depression, and arrhythmias. In contrast to the elective setting where the primary goal is the preservation of myocardial function by maintaining normal filling pressures and an adequate cardiac output, fluid resuscitation and the correction of hypotension are the primary goals in the emergent care of the patient with a ruptured AAA.

References

1. Melton LJ, Bickerstaff LK. Changing incidence of abdominal aortic aneurysms: a population-based study. Am J Epidemiol 1984;120:379.
2. Bickerstaff LK, Hollier LH. Abdominal aortic aneurysms: the changing natural history. J Vasc Surg 1984;1:6.
3. Fitzgerald JF, Stillman RM. A suggested classification and reappraisal of mortality statistics for ruptured atherosclerotic infrarenal aortic aneurysms. Surg Gynecol Obstet 1978;146:344.
4. Brown SL, Backstrom B, Busuttil RW. A new serum proteolytic enzyme in aneurysm pathogenesis. J Vasc Surg 1985;2:393.
5. Baxter BT, Davis VA, Minion DJ. Abdominal aortic aneurysms are associated with altered matrix proteins of the nonaneurysmal segments. J Vasc Surg 1994;18:797.
6. Powell JT, Greenhalgh RM. Multifactorial inheritance of abdominal aortic aneurysm. Eur J Vasc Surg 1987;1:29.
7. Busuttil RW, Rinderbreicht M. Elastase activity: the role of elastase in aortic aneurysm formation. J Surg Res 1982;32:214.
8. Norgard O, Rais O, Angquist KA. Familial occurrence of abdominal aortic aneurysms. Surgery 1984;95:650.
9. Tilson MD, Seashore MR. Human genetics of abdominal aortic aneurysms. Surg Gynecol Obstet 1984;158:129.
10. Johansen KW, Koepsell T. Familial tendency for abdominal aortic aneurysms. JAMA 1986;256:1934.
11. Webster MW, St Jean PL, Steed DL, et al. Abdominal aortic aneurysm: results of a family study. J Vasc Surg 1991;13:366.
12. Webster MW, Ferrell RE, St. Jean PL, et al. Ultrasound screening of first-degree relatives of patients with an abdominal aortic aneurysm. J Vasc Surg 1991;13:9.
13. MacSweeney STR, Powell JT, Greenhalgh RM. Pathogenesis of abdominal aortic aneurysm. Br J Surg 1994;81:935.
14. Powell J, Greenhalgh R. Cellular, enzymatic and genetic factors in the pathogenesis of abdominal aortic aneurysm. J Vasc Surg 1989;9:297.
15. Szilargyi DE, Smith RF. Contribution of abdominal aortic aneurysmectomy to prolongation of life. Ann Surg 1966;164:678.
16. Cohen JR, Mandell C, Chang JB, Wise L. Elastin metabolism of the infrarenal aorta. J Vasc Surg 1988;7:210.
17. Cohen JR, Mandell C, Wise L. Characterization of human aortic elastase found in patients with abdominal aortic aneurysms. Surg Gynecol Obstet 1987;165:301.
18. Cohen JR, Mandell C, Margolis I, et al. Altered aortic protease and antiprotease activity in patients with ruptured abdominal aortic aneurysms. Surg Gynecol Obstet 1987;164:355.
19. Anidjar S, Saltzmann J-L, Gentric D, et al. Elastase-induced experimental aneurysms in rats. Circulation 1990;82:973.
20. Menashi S, Campa JS, Greenhalgh RM, Powell JT. Collagen in abdominal aortic aneurysm: typing, content and degradation. J Vasc Surg 1987;8:578.
21. Ostergaard JR, Oxlund H. Collagen type III deficiency in patients with rupture of intracranial saccular aneurysms. J Neurosurg 1987;67:690.
22. Powell JT, Adamason J, MacSweeney STR, et al. Influence of type III collagen genotype on aortic diameter and disease. Surg Forum 1993;33:58.
23. Busuttil RW, Abou-Zamzam AM, Machleder HI. Collagenase activity of the human aorta. A comparison of patients with and without abdominal aortic aneurysms. Arch Surg 1980;115:1373.
24. Strachen DP. Predictors of death from aortic aneurysm among middle age men: the Whitehall study. Br J Surg 1991;78:401.
25. Strong JP, Richards ML. Cigarette smoking and atherosclerosis in autopsied men. Atherosclerosis 1976;23:451.
26. Crawford JL, Stowe CL, Safi HJ, et al. Inflammatory aneurysms of the aorta. J Vasc Surg 1985;2:113.
27. Moosa HH, Peitzman AB, Steed DL, et al. Inflammatory aneurysms of the abdominal aorta. Arch Surg 1989;124:673.
28. Pennell RC, Hollier LH, Lie JT, et al. Inflammatory abdominal aortic aneurysms: a thirty-year review. J Vasc Surg 1985;2:859.

29. Lieberman J, Scheib JS, Googe PB, et al. Inflammatory abdominal aortic aneurysm and the associated T-cell reaction: a case study. J Vasc Surg 1992;15:569.

30. Brophy CM, Reily JM, Smith GJ, Tilson MD. The role of inflammation in nonspecific abdominal aortic aneurysm disease. Ann Vasc Surg 1991;5:229.

31. MacSweeney STR, Young G, Greenhalgh RM, Powell JT. Mechanical properties of the aneurysmal aorta. Br J Surg 1992;79:1281.

32. Imura T, Yamamoto K, Kanamori K, et al. Non-invasive ultrasonic measurement of the elastic properties of the human abdominal aorta. Cardiovasc Res 1986;20:208.

33. Plecha FR, Avellone JC. A computerized vascular registry: experience of The Cleveland Vascular Society. Surgery 1979;86:826.

34. Miller DC, Myers BD. Pathophysiology and prevention of acute renal failure associated with thoracoabdominal or abdominal aortic surgery. J Vasc Surg 1987;5:518.

35. Cunningham AS. Anesthesia for abdominal aortic surgery—a review (Part I). Can J Anaesth 1989;36:426.

36. Yeager MP, Glass DD. Anesthesia for Abdominal Aortic Reconstruction: One Approach at Dartmouth Medical School. In M Roizen (ed), Anesthesia for Vascular Surgery. New York: Churchill Livingstone, 1990;285

37. Bush HL, Huse JB. Prevention of renal insufficiency after abdominal aortic aneurysm resection by optimal volume loading. Arch Surg 1981;116:1517.

38. Lampe GH, Mangano DT. Anesthetic Management for Abdominal Aortic Reconstruction. In M Roizen (ed), Anesthesia for Vascular Surgery. New York: Churchill Livingstone, 1990;265.

39. Tomatis LA, Fierens EE, Vergrugge GP. Evaluation of surgical risk in peripheral vascular disease by coronary arteriography. Surgery 1972;71:429.

40. Hertzer N, Young JR, Kramer JR, et al. Routine coronary angiography prior to elective aortic reconstruction. Arch Surg 1979;114:1336.

41. Isaacson IJ, Lowdon JD, Berry AJ, et al. The value of pulmonary artery and central venous monitoring in patients undergoing abdominal aortic reconstructive surgery: a comparative study of two selected, randomized groups. J Vasc Surg 1990;12:754.

42. London MJ, Hollenberg M, Wong MG, et al. Intraoperative myocardial ischemia: localization by continuous 12-lead electrocardiography. Anesthesiology 1988;69:232.

43. Gilbert HC, Vender JS. Cardiovascular Monitoring. In RR Kirby, N Gravenstein (eds), Clinical Anesthesia Practice. Philadelphia: Saunders, 1994;360.

44. Thys DM. The Normal ECG. In DM Thys, JA Kaplan (eds), The ECG in Anesthesia and Critical Care. New York: Churchill Livingstone, 1987;14.

45. Roizen MF, Beaupre PN, Alpert RA. Monitoring with two-dimensional transesophageal echocardiography: comparison of myocardial function in patients undergoing supraceliac, suprarenal-infraceliac or infrarenal aortic occlusion. J Vasc Surg 1984;1:300.

46. Smith JS, Cahalan MK, Benefiel DJ, et al. Intraoperative detection of myocardial ischemia in high-risk patients: electrocardiography versus two-dimensional transesophageal echocardiography. Circulation 1985;72:1015.

47. Cahalan MK. Pro: transesophageal echocardiography is the "gold standard" in detection of intraoperative myocardial ischemia. J Cardiothoracic Anesth 1989;3:372.

48. Crawford ES, Mizrahi EM. The impact of distal aortic perfusion and somatosensory-evoked potential monitoring on prevention of paraplegia after aortic aneurysm surgery. J Thorac Cardiovasc Surg 1988;95:357.

49. Hands LJ, Collin J, Lamont P. Observed incidence of paraplegia after infrarenal aortic aneurysm surgery. Br J Surg 1991;78:999.

50. Laschinger JC, Izumoto H, Kouchoukos NT. Evolving concepts in prevention of spinal cord injury during operations on the descending thoracic and thoracoabdominal aorta. Ann Thorac Surg 1987;44:667.

51. McCullough JL, Hollier LH, Nugent M. Paraplegia after thoracic aortic occlusion: influence of cerebrospinal fluid drainage. J Vasc Surg 1988;7:153.

52. Drenger B, Parker SD. Spinal cord stimulation evoked potentials during thoracoabdominal aortic aneurysm surgery. Surgery 1992;76:689.

53. Berendes JN, Bredee JJ, Schipperheyn JJ, Mashour YAS. Mechanisms of spinal cord injury after cross clamping of the descending thoracic aorta. Circulation 1982;78(Suppl 3):198.

54. Mutch WAC, Thomson IR, Tskey JM, et al. Phlebotomy reverses the hemodynamic consequences of thoracic aortic cross clamping: relationships between central venous pressure and cerebrospinal fluid pressure. Anesthesiology 1991;74:320.

55. Bower TC, Murray MJ, Gloviczki P, et al. Effects of thoracic aorta occlusion and cerebrospinal fluid drainage on regional spinal cord blood flow in dogs: correlation with neurologic outcome. J Vasc Surg 1989;9:135.

56. Woloszyn TT, Marini CP, Coons MS, et al. Cerebrospinal fluid drainage and steroids provide better spinal cord protection during aortic cross clamping. Ann Thorac Surg 1990;49:79.

57. Symbas PN, Pfaender LM, Drucker MH, et al. Cross clamping of the descending aorta. J Thorac Cardiovasc Surg 1983;85:300.

58. Marini CP, Grubbs PE, Toporoff B, et al. Effect of sodium nitroprusside on spinal cord perfusion and paraplegia during aortic cross clamping. Ann Thorac Surg 1989;47:379.

59. Gelman S, Reves JG, Fowler K, et al. Regional blood flow during cross clamping of the thoracic aorta and infusion of sodium nitroprusside. J Thorac Cardiovasc Surg 1983;85:287.

60. Nylander WA, Plunkett RJ, Hammon JW. Thiopental modification of spinal cord injury in the dog. Ann Thorac Surg 1982;33:64.

61. McCombs PR, Roberts B. Acute renal failure following resection of abdominal aortic aneurysm. Surg Gynecol Obstet 1979;148:175.

62. Breckwoldt WL, Mackey WC, Belkin M, O'Donnell TF. The effect of suprarenal cross clamping on abdominal aortic aneurysm repair. Arch Surg 1992;127:520.

63. Donahue JG, Munoz A, Ness PM. The declining risk of post-transfusion hepatitis C virus infection. N Engl J Med 1992;327:369.

64. Hallet JW Jr, Popovsky M. Minimizing blood transfusions during abdominal aortic aneurysm surgery: recent advances in rapid autotransfusion. J Vasc Surg 1987;5:601.

65. Modig J. Regional anesthesia and blood loss. Acta Anaesthesiol Scand 1988;89(Suppl):44.

66. Rosberg B, Fredin H, Gustafson C. Anaesthetic techniques and surgical blood loss in total hip arthroplasty. Acta Anaesthesiol Scand 1982;26:189.

67. Rosenfeld BA, Beattie C, Christopherson R, et al. The effects of different anesthetic regimens on fibrinolysis and the development of postoperative arterial thrombosis. Anesthesiology 1993;79:435.

68. Yoshihara H, Yamamoto T, Mihara H. Changes in coagulation and fibrinolysis occurring in dogs during hypothermia. Thromb Res 1985;37:503.

69. Colon R, Frazier OH, Cooley DA, McAllister HA. Hypothermic regional perfusion for protection of the spinal cord during periods of ischemia. Ann Thorac Surg 1987;43:639.

70. Berguer R, Porto J, Fedoronko B, Dragovic L. Selective deep hypothermia of the spinal cord prevents paraplegia after aortic cross clamping in the dog model. J Vasc Surg 1992;15:62.

71. Gelman S, McDowell H. The reason for cardiac output reduction after aortic cross clamping. Am J Surg 1988;155:578.

72. Hummel BW, Raess DH. Effect of nitroglycerin and aortic occlusion on myocardial blood flow. Surgery 1982;155:159.

73. Zaidan JR, Guffin AV. Hemodynamics of intravenous nitroglycerin during aortic clamping. Arch Surg 1982;117:1285.

74. Bjoraker DG, Knight PR. Intravenous nitroglycerin administration during infrarenal aortic clamping. Can Anaesth Soc J 1984;31:44.

75. Meloche R, Pottecher T, Audet J, et al. Haemodynamic changes due to clamping of the abdominal aorta. Can Anaesth Soc J 1977;24:20.

76. Silverstein PR, Caldera DL, Cullen DL, et al. Avoiding the hemodynamic consequences of aortic cross clamping and unclamping. Anesthesiology 1979;50462.

77. Gregoretti S, Gelman S, Henderson T, Bradley EL. Hemodynamics and oxygen uptake below and above aortic occlusion during crossclamping of the thoracic aorta and sodium nitroprusside infusion. J Thorac Cardiovasc Surg 1990;100:830.

78. Gelman S, Rabbani S, Bradley EL Jr. Inferior and superior vena caval blood flows during crossclamping of the thoracic aorta in pigs. J Thorac Cardiovasc Surg 1988;96:383.

79. Gelman SG. The pathophysiology of aortic cross clamping and unclamping. Anesthesiology 1995;82:1026.

80. Lunn JK, Dannemiller FJ. Cardiovascular responses to clamping of the aorta during epidural and general anesthesia. Anesth Analg 1979;58:372.

81. Attia RR, Murphy JD, Snider M, et al. Myocardial ischemia due to infrarenal aortic cross clamping during aortic surgery in patients with severe coronary disease. Circulation 1976;53:961.

82. O'Toole DP, Broe P, Bouchier-Hayes D, Cunningham AJ. Perioperative hemodynamic changes during aortic vascular surgery: comparison between occlusive and aneurysm disease states [abstract]. Br J Anaesth 1988;60:322.

83. Roberts AJ, Nora JD, Hughes A, et al. Cardiac and renal responses to cross clamping of the descending thoracic aorta. J Thorac Cardiovasc Surg 1983;86:732.

84. Peterson A, Brant D, Kirsh MM. Nitroglycerin infusion during infrarenal aortic cross clamping in dogs: an experimental study. Surgery 1978;34:216.

85. Harpole DH, Clements FM, Quill T, et al. Right and left ventricular performance during and after abdominal aortic aneurysm repair. Ann Surg 1989;208:356.

86. Gooding JM, Archie JP, et al. Hemodynamic response to infrarenal aortic cross clamping in patients with and without coronary artery disease. Crit Care Med 1980;8:382.

87. Rittenhouse EA, Maixner BA, Knott HW, et al. The role of prostaglandin E in hemodynamic response to aortic clamping and declamping. Surgery 1984;119:1332.

88. Graham LM, Stanley JC, Gewertz BL, et al. Prostaglandin F2 alpha attenuation of aortic declamping hyperemia and hypotension. J Surg Res 1976;20:413.

89. Krausz MM, Utsunomiya T, McIrvine AJ, et al. Modulation of cardiovascular function and platelet survival by endogenous prostacyclin release during surgery. Surgery 1983;93:554.

90. Golden MA, Donaldson MC, Whittemore AD, Mannick JA. Evolving experience with thoracoabdominal aortic aneurysm repair at a single institution. J Vasc Surg 1991;13:792.

91. Paterson IS, Klausner JM, Pugatch R, et al. Noncardiogenic pulmonary edema after abdominal aortic aneurysm surgery. Ann Surg 1989;209:231.

92. Kainuma M, Nishiwaki K, Shimada Y. Rise in pulmonary artery pressure following release of aortic crossclamp in abdominal aortic aneurysmectomy. Anesthesiology 1988;69:257.

93. Mathieson MA, Dunham B, Huval WV, et al. Ischemia of the limb stimulates thromboxane production and myocardial depression. Surg Gynecol Obstet 1983;157:500.

94. Anner H, Kaufmann RP Jr, Kobzik L, et al. Pulmonary hypertension and leukosequestration after lower torso ischemia. Ann Surg 1987;206:642.

95. Welbourne CRB, Goldman G, Paterson IS, et al. Neutrophil elastase and oxygen radicals: synergism in lung injury after hindlimb ischemia. Am J Physiol 1991;260:1852.

96. Bengston A, Lannsjo W, Heideman M. Complement and anaphylatoxin responses to cross clamping of the aorta. Br J Anaesth 1987;59:1093.

97. Joob AW, Harman PK, Kaiser DL, Kron IL. The effect of renin angiotensin system blockade on visceral blood flow during and after thoracic aortic crossclamping. J Thorac Cardiovasc Surg 1986;91:411.

98. Gamulin Z, Forster A, Simonet F, et al. Effects of renal sympathetic blockade on renal hemodynamics in patients undergoing major aortic abdominal surgery. Anesthesiology 1986;65:688.

99. Szilargyi DE, Hageman JH, Smith RF, Elliott JP. Spinal cord damage in surgery of the abdominal aorta. Surgery 1978;83:3856.

100. Doppman JL, Chiro G. Arteriographic identification of spinal cord flow prior to aortic surgery. JAMA 1968;204:174.

101. Grundy BL. Intraoperative monitoring of sensory-evoked potentials. Anesthesiology 1983;58:72.

102. Coles JG, Wilson GJ, Sima AF, et al. Intraoperative detection of spinal cord ischemia using somatosensory cortical evoked potentials during thoracic aortic occlusion. Ann Thorac Surg 1982;34:299.

103. Takaki O, Okumura F. Application and limitation of somatosensory evoked potential monitoring during thoracic aortic aneurysm surgery: a case report. Anesthesiology 1985;63:700.

104. Cheng MK, Robertson C, Grossman RG, et al. Neurological outcome correlated with spinal evoked potentials in a spinal cord ischemia model. J Neurosurg 1984;60:786.

105. Levy WJ. Spinal evoked potentials from the motor tract. J Neurosurg 1983;58:38.

106. Levy WJ, York DH, McCaffrey M, Tanzer F. Motor evoked potentials from transcranial stimulation of the motor cortex in humans. J Neurosurg 1984;15:287.

107. Lim RC, Bergentz SE, Lewis DH, et al. Metabolic and tissue blood flow changes resulting from aortic cross clamping. Surgery 1969;65:304.

108. Brant B, Armstrong RP, Vetto RM. Vasodepressor factor in declamp shock production. Surgery 1970;67:650.

109. Lefer AM, Martin J. Origin of myocardial depressant factor in shock. Am J Physiol 1970;218:1423.

110. Frank RS, Moursi MM, Podrazik RM, et al. Renal vasoconstriction and transient declamp hypotension after infrarenal aortic occlusion: role of purine degradation products. J Vasc Surg 1988;7:515.

111. Grindlinger GA, Weisel RD, Mannick JA, Hechtman HB. Volume loading and nitroprusside in abdominal aortic aneurysmectomy. Surg Forum 1978;29:234.

112. Grindlinger GA, Vegas AM, Manny J, et al. Volume loading and vasodilators in abdominal aortic aneurysmectomy. Am J Surg 1980;139:480.

113. Falk JL, Rackow EC, Blumenberg R, et al. Hemodynamic and metabolic effects of abdominal aortic cross-clamping. Am J Surg 1981;142:174.

114. Baue AE, McClerkin WW. A study of shock: acidosis and the declamping phenomenon. Ann Surg 1965;161:41.

115. Bayliss WM. On the local reactions of the arterial wall to changes of internal pressure. J Physiol (Lond) 1902;28:220.

116. Barcroft H. The mechanism of vasodilation in the limbs during and after arrest of the circulation. Angiology 1972;23:595.

117. Lewis T, Grant R. Observations upon reactive hyperemia in man. Heart 1925;12:73.

118. Fry WJ, Keitzer WF, Kraft RO, De Weese MS. Prevention of hypotension due to aortic release. Surg Gynecol Obstet 1963;116:301.

119. Thomas TV. Aortic declamping shock. Am Heart J 1971;81:845.

120. Perry MA, Wadhwa SS. Gradual reintroduction of oxygen reduces reperfusion injury in cat stomach. Am J Physiol 1988;254:366.

121. Gamulin Z, Forster A, Morel D, et al. Effects of infrarenal aortic cross clamping on renal hemodynamics in humans. Anesthesiology 1984;61:394.

122. Kountz SL, Tuttle KL, Cohn LH, et al. Factors responsible for acute tubular necrosis following lower aortic surgery. JAMA 1963;183:447.

123. Cronenwett JL, Lindenaauer SM. Distribution of intrarenal blood flow following aortic clamping and declamping. J Surg Res 1977;22:469.

124. Port FK, Wagoner RD, Fulton RE. Acute renal failure after angiography. American Journal of Roentgenology, Radium Therapy and Nuclear Medicine 1974;121:544.

125. Bush HL. Renal failure following abdominal aortic reconstruction. Surgery 1983;95:107.

126. Abbott WM, Cooper JD, Austin WG, et al. The effect of aortic clamping and declamping on renal blood flow distribution. J Surg Res 1973;14:385.

127. Flores J, DiBona DR. The role of cell swelling in ischemic renal damage and the protective effect of hypertonic solute. J Clin Invest 1972;51:118.

128. Abbott WM, Austen WG. The reversal of renal cortical ischemia during aortic occlusion by mannitol. J Surg Res 1974;16:482.

129. Pass LJ, Eberhart RC, Brown JC, et al. The effect of mannitol and dopamine on the renal response to thoracic aortic cross clamping. J Thorac Cardiovasc Surg 1988;95:608.

130. Paul MD, Mazer CD, Byrick RJ, et al. Influence of dopamine and mannitol on renal function during elective infrarenal aortic clamping in man. Am J Nephrol 1986;6:427.

131. Bush HL, Logerfo FW. Assessment of myocardial performance and optimal volume loading during elective abdominal aortic aneurysm resection. Arch Surg 1977;112:302.

132. Moffitt EA, Sethna DH. Nitrous oxide added to halothane reduces coronary flow and myocardial oxygen consumption in patients with coronary disease. Can Anaesth Soc J 1983;30:5.

133. Moffitt EA, Scovil JE. The effects of nitrous oxide on myocardial metabolism and hemodynamics during fentanyl or enflurane anesthesia in patients with coronary disease. Anesth Analg 1984;63:1071.

134. Roizen MF, Hamilton WK. Treatment of stress-induced increases in pulmonary capillary wedge pressure using volatile anesthetics. Anesthesiology 1981;55:446.

135. Eisele JH, Smith NT. Cardiovascular effects of 40 percent nitrous oxide in man. Anesth Analg 1972;51:956.

136. Benefiel DJ, Roizen MF, Lampe GH, et al. Morbidity after aortic surgery with sufentanil versus isoflurane anesthesia [abstract]. Anesthesiology 1986;65:516.

137. Bovil JG. Opioid analgesics in anesthesia: with special reference to their use in cardiovascular surgery. Anesthesiology 1984;61:731.

138. Reier CE, George JM. Cortisol and growth hormone response to surgical stress during morphine anesthesia. Anesth Analg 1973;52:1003.

139. Friesen RM, Thomson IR, Hudson RJ, et al. Fentanyl oxygen anesthesia for abdominal aortic surgery. Can Anaesth Soc J 1986;33:719.

140. Thomson IR, Putnins CL, Friesen RM. Hyperdynamic cardiovascular responses to anesthetic induction with high dose fentanyl. Anesth Analg 1986;65:91.

141. Roizen MF. Does Choice of Anesthetic (Narcotic Versus Inhalational) Significantly Affect Outcome After Cardiovascular Surgery? In F Estafamous (ed), Opioids in Anesthesia. Boston: Butterworth, 1984;180.

142. Rao TKL, El-Etr AA. Anticoagulation following placement of epidural and subarachnoid catheters: an evaluation of neurologic sequelae. Anesthesiology 1981;55:618.

143. Yeager MP, Glass DD, Neff RK, Brinck-Johnsen T. Epidural anesthesia and analgesia in high risk surgical patients. Anesthesiology 1987;66:729.

144. Baron HC, LaRaja RD, Rossi G, Atkinson D. Continuous epidural analgesia in the heparinized vascular surgical patients: a retrospective review of 912 patients. J Vasc Surg 1987;6:144.

145. Rosseel P, Marichal P, Lauwers LF, et al. A hemodynamic study of epidural versus intravenous anesthesia for aortofemoral bypass surgery. Acta Anaesthesiol Belg 1985;36:345.

146. Baron J-F, Bertrand M, Bavre E, et al. Combined epidural and general anesthesia versus general anesthesia for abdominal aortic surgery. Anesthesiology 1991;75:611.

147. Bunt TJ, Manczuk M, Varley K. Continuous epidural anesthesia for aortic surgery: thoughts on peer review and safety. Surgery 1987;101:706.

148. Kelleher SP, Robinette JB, Congen JD. Sympathetic nervous system in the loss of autoregulation in acute renal failure. Am J Physiol 1984;246:379.

149. Myers BD, Miller DC, Mehigan JT, et al. Nature of the renal injury following total renal ischemia in man. J Clin Invest 1984;73:329.

150. Ottinger LW. Ruptured arteriosclerotic aneurysms of the abdominal aorta. Reducing mortality. JAMA 1975;233:147.

151. Snow N. Hemopericardium from retrograde dissection of an abdominal aortic aneurysm. Ann Surg 1980;46:589.

152. Wakefield TW, Whitehouse WM Jr, Wu SC, et al. Abdominal aortic aneurysm rupture: statistical analysis of factors affecting outcome of surgical treatment. Surgery 1982;91:586.

Chapter 11

Postoperative Care of the Aortic Surgery Patient: Cardiopulmonary Management

Meir Chernofsky and Ruth S. Spector

For the anesthesiologist and the surgeon, much of the excitement of caring for the aortic surgery patient is played out in the operating room (OR) itself. As far as the patients and their families are concerned, when the dressing goes on, the risk and discomfort of the surgery have barely begun. After all, most complications and deaths occur in the postoperative period.

The postoperative care of aortic surgery patients as a group is no less complex than the care of cardiac surgery patients. Although young and healthy aortic surgery patients exist, they are not the norm.[1] The typical aortic surgery patient has one or more systemic diseases, e.g., coronary artery disease, hypertension, chronic lung disease, or diabetes.[2] Decreased functional reserve of the left ventricle may be related to any of the preceding conditions. Various degrees of renal insufficiency are also not uncommon in these patients.[2] In addition, there is the possibility of newly acquired organ dysfunction (e.g., central nervous system injury, acute renal failure, and mesenteric ischemia). In fact, the risk of failure of at least one organ system after aortic surgery may be as high as 20%.[3] An examination of Table 11-1 shows the most frequent factors associated with postoperative mortality in patients who underwent surgery for ruptured abdominal aortic aneurysm. Although patients who are lucky enough to undergo repair under elective conditions have much lower mortality, the causes of death are similar to those patients undergoing emergency abdominal aortic aneurysm repair.

This chapter and the two that follow focus on a number of postoperative issues that commonly arise after aortic surgery. Most of these issues are not unique to the aortic surgery patient and much of what is learned from aortic patients can be applied to both peripheral arterial surgery patients and other high-risk surgical patients.[4,5] The basics of postoperative care are well covered in general texts of anesthesiology.[6,7]

The voluminous literature of aortic surgery, which forms the basis of this book, often comprises postoperatively acquired data in the context of decisions made in the OR.[8,9] Studies that attempt to assess the results of management decisions made in the postoperative period were uncommon until recently. The acceptance of intensive care as a separate discipline, as well as the current interest in postoperative analgesia and postoperative myocardial ischemia are some of the factors that have enriched our understanding of the postoperative period. Additionally, the current focus on cost in health care highlights the postoperative period. Apparently, the postoperative period is the source of most variation in cost between individual patients and between various institutions and geographic areas.[10] Just when health policy planners would like to see the duration and intensity of postoperative care decrease, our colleagues are busy demonstrating that some patients can benefit from increased postoperative monitoring. Much of the work published by Mangano et al. in the last 5 years fits into this category.[11] It will take good outcome studies to demonstrate that increased expenditures are justified by decreased long-term cost and by gains in quality of life.

Table 11-1. Causes of Early and Late Mortality After Emergency Surgery for Ruptured Abdominal Aortic Aneurysm: Multivariate Analysis of Deaths in Patients with Ruptured Aortic Aneurysm

Risk Factor	Risk Factor Present (Number of Cases)	Mortality (Percentage)	Risk Factor Absent (Number of Cases)	Mortality (Percentage)	P value
Early deaths					
Cardiac arrest	21	81	96	26	<0.01
Loss of consciousness	29	72	88	23.8	<0.01
Acidosis (pH <7.3)	49	53	65	21.5	<0.1
Operating room hypotension (systolic blood pressure <80 mm Hg)	32	62.5	83	24.4	<0.1
Late deaths					
Reoperation	23	65	51	29	NS
Respiratory failure	32	69	42	19	<0.01
Renal failure	34	75	40	7.5	<0.01
Cardiac arrest	4	75	71	38	NS
Loss of consciousness	7	71	65	35	NS
Acidosis	22	55	51	33	NS
Operating room hypotension	12	41.6	63	39.7	NS
Massive transfusion (>18 units/24 hours)	18	50	56	36	NS

NS = not significant.
Source: Modified from LM Harris, GL Faggioli, R Fiedler, et al. Ruptured aortic aneurysms: factors affecting mortality rates. J Vasc Surg 1991;14:812.

Oxygen Delivery Goals

Many of the characteristic preexisting medical conditions as well as the acute perioperative complications that plague the aortic surgery patient are ischemic in nature. Ischemia is basically the process of cellular dysfunction and breakdown that results from failure of oxygen delivery to vulnerable tissues. Oxygen allows tissue to function under aerobic conditions, thus more efficiently supporting the process of oxidative phosphorylation.

While the function of hemoglobin (Hb) in oxygen transport and the role of cardiac output (CO) in Hb transport have been understood for quite some time, the modern era of oxygen delivery goals began about 25 years ago. Clowes and Del Guercio observed that survivors of major surgical trauma tended to deliver more oxygen to tissues and consume oxygen more efficiently than nonsurvivors.[12] Shoemaker expanded those observations to identify a subpopulation of surgical patients who tended not to do well. These patients seemed to have diminished oxygen delivery.[13] On this basis he and his group suggested that augmentation of oxygen delivery may affect the mortality of high-risk patients.[14] This suggestion was something of a leap, since the patients who had been observed to do better had often self-generated the excellent COs necessary to augment oxygen delivery. Therapeutic augmentation of oxygen delivery is, after all, balanced against the risks associated with driving the circulation too hard. Subsequently, a number of clinical trials seemed to demonstrate that improved oxygen delivery was beneficial even when therapeutically induced.[15–20]

The Achilles' heel of much of the early work on oxygen delivery is that the subjects, who were previously healthy, were victims of major trauma. One may legitimately ask what such patients have to do with aortic surgery patients, who are typically elderly with advanced atherosclerotic disease.[2] The study performed by Boyd and colleagues is therefore the most exciting of the trials of oxygen delivery augmentation for our purposes.[17] This study is contemporary and relatively large, and it addresses a patient population sicker and older than the trauma patients originally studied by Shoemaker. Boyd et al. limited their interventions by augmenting cardiac performance only to the extent that this could be achieved without undue increases in heart rate. (They accepted a maximum of 120% increase in resting heart rate.) Although their study protocol was designed such that they were not always able to boost the oxygen delivery of their study patients to the well-known Shoemaker goals (see following discussion), they were able to show improved outcomes for the augmented patients. Berlauk et al. expanded our knowledge by defining a hemodynamic picture that, when pursued in the preoperative patient, apparently improves outcome (Figure 11-1).[19] The trial by Yu and colleagues entered patients after a complication had occurred, so their patients were sick.[20] Like Boyd et al., they were able to boost oxygen delivery, but usually not to the preestablished "supranormal" goal. Yu et al. were not able to show a difference between their experimental and control groups, but they did show that patients who achieved supranormal hemodynamics, whether self-generating or by intervention, had decreased mortality. Hayes and coworkers also studied an already sick patient population. They were not able to show any benefit to boosting oxygen delivery.[21] However, they were much more aggressive than other authors in their use of inotropic agents. Not surprisingly, when the cardiovascular system is pushed hard enough, patients can lose the benefits of increased oxygen delivery. In the Hayes trial, patients who were able to elevate their oxygen delivery substantially with fluids alone did well.

Oxygen delivery (DO_2) is defined as the product of CO and arterial oxygen content (CaO_2). It is the volume of oxygen delivered to the body each minute.

Equation 11-1

$$DO_2 = CaO_2 \times CO$$

In equation 11-1, DO_2 is customarily expressed in milliliters per minute. Since CO is usually expressed in liters per minute, a conversion factor of 1,000 must be introduced on the right side of the equation. The CaO_2 term is expressed in ml per 100 ml of blood. When the conversion factor of 1,000 is

multiplied by the CaO_2 term expressed in these units, the result is a correction factor of 10.

Equation 11-2

$$DO_2 = CaO_2 \times CO \times 10$$

CaO_2 is determined by adding the amount of oxygen dissolved in plasma to the amount of oxygen carried by a unit amount of fully saturated Hb. The amount of oxygen dissolved in plasma is proportional to the partial pressure of oxygen (pO_2) in arterial blood. The proportionality constant is approximately 0.0031. The amount of oxygen carried by 1 g of Hb is approximately 1.39 ml, and the concentration of Hb is expressed in grams per 100 ml (g/dl).

Equation 11-3

$$CaO_2 = 1.39 \times Hb \times \text{arterial oxygen saturation} + 0.0031 \times PaO_2$$

It follows from equations 11-2 and 11-3 that anemia, abnormal Hb, airway obstruction, pulmonary failure, ventilation perfusion mismatch, right-to-left shunting, and circulatory failure from any cause all lead to failure of oxygen delivery.

The arterial oxygen saturation is by definition the percentage of Hb occupied with oxygen transport. This value is available clinically as the saturation measured by the pulse oximeter; the saturation thus obtained is known as the SaO_2. Arterial oxygen saturation is reported by blood gas laboratories; this reported value may have been directly measured by a laboratory oximeter or derived from a table that relates oxygen saturation to pO_2.

An examination of equation 11-3 with normal values inserted reveals that, under usual conditions, the contribution of dissolved oxygen to total oxygen is trivial. For most patients, providing an inspired percentage of oxygen higher than necessary to maintain a normal SaO_2 introduces the potential for oxygen toxicity without significantly improving DO_2.

The CO is the product of heart rate and stroke volume; the latter is in turn affected by the former, as well as by preload, afterload, and contractility. DO_2 is sometimes expressed as a raw number but is more commonly indexed to body surface area. By dividing DO_2 by body surface area (expressed in square meters) one obtains the oxygen delivery index (DO_2I).

Shoemaker et al.[18] have not only proposed the strategy of augmenting DO_2I in the critically ill

Preoperative Patient

Baseline CV Measurements

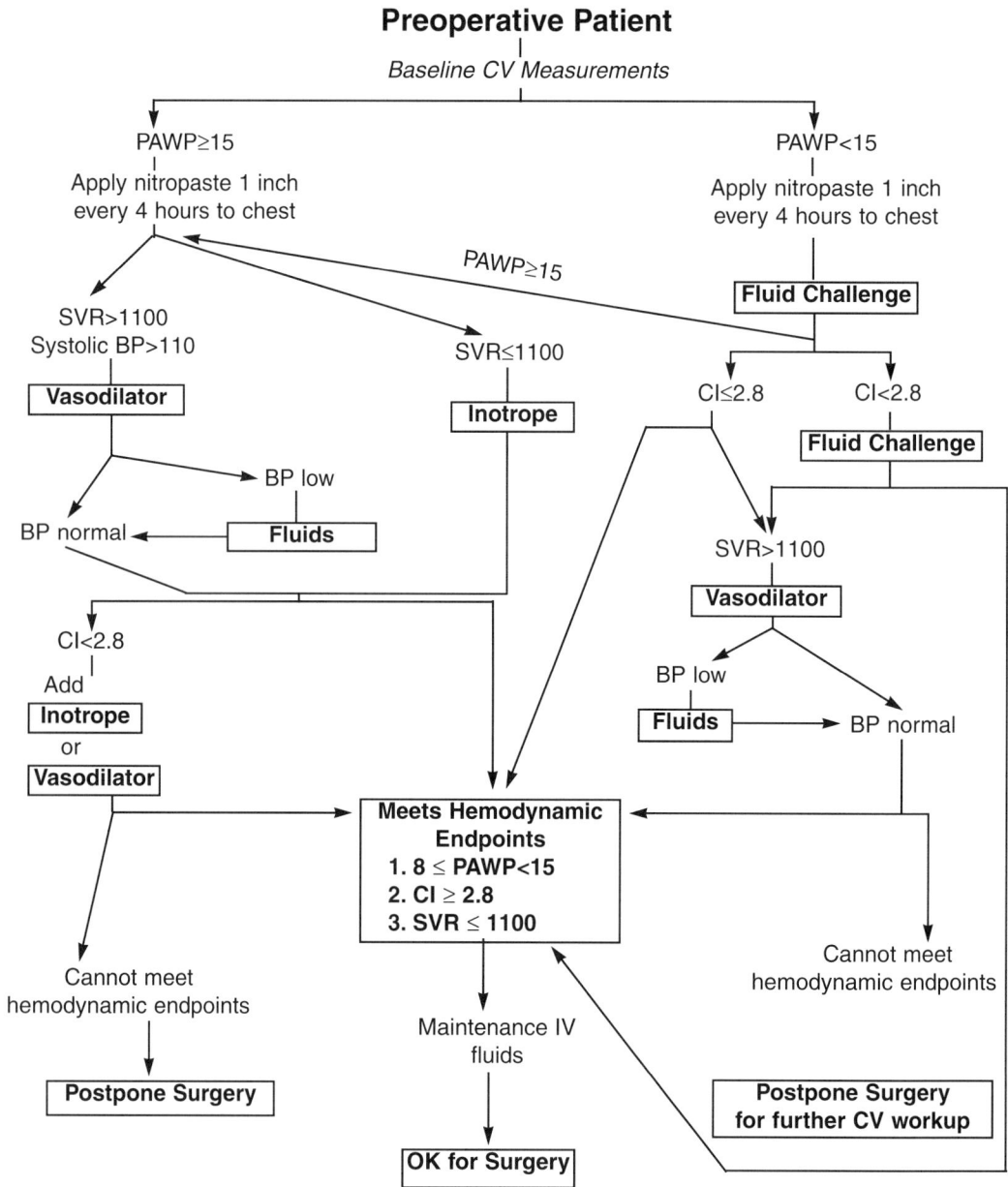

Figure 11-1. The algorithm used by Berlauk and colleagues in their clinical trial of preoperative hemodynamic optimization of vascular surgery patients. Inotropes are dobutamine or dopamine. Vasodilators are nitroglycerin or nitroprusside. (CV = cardiovascular; PAWP = pulmonary artery wedge pressure; SVR = systemic vascular resistance; BP = blood pressure; CI = cardiac index.) Units are mm Hg for pressure, dyne/sec/cm^5 for resistance, and liters/min/m^2 for CI. (Reprinted with permission from JF Berlauk, JH Abrams, IJ Gilmour, et al. Preoperative optimization of cardiovascular hemodynamics improves outcome in peripheral vascular surgery. Ann Surg 1991;214:289.)

surgical patient, but they have also contributed to establishing a specific endpoint of therapy. Their often-quoted goal of delivery of 600 ml/min/m^2 of oxygen has been dubbed a "supranormal hemodynamic goal." In terms of healthy patients, this goal is neither supranormal nor hemodynamic. An individual with a normal Hb of 14 g/dl and a normal CO of 5 l/m, is often delivering considerably more than 600 ml/min/m^2 of oxygen to his or her tissues, although only 25–30% of DO_2I is normally extracted. Normal oxygen delivery is being accomplished not only by a particular hemodynamic state, but also by a particular Hb concentration.

For the population of sick patients, however, Shoemaker et al. found, and others have confirmed, that a DO_2I of 600 ml/min/m^2 is indeed supranormal. Critically ill surgical patients commonly have an Hb concentration of 10 g/dl or lower. Even in an era when transfusion was performed far more readily than today (see Chapters 5 and 12), red cells were inconsistently administered to patients whose Hb was 10 g/dl or greater. Likewise, a diminished CO is common in the critically ill. As we have seen, although a self-generated DO_2I greater than 600 ml/min/m^2 may be a marker for survival, this particular goal may be hard to achieve with therapeutic interventions. Nevertheless, boosting DO_2I, even from low- to middle-range numbers, seems to improve outcome.

We focus first on oxygen delivery rather than use because we are better able to evaluate delivery. As a matter of fact, our evaluation of oxygen delivery, as we have defined it, is far from perfect. Our definition is global; it does not take into consideration regional differences in perfusion. For example, the effect of a low-flow state on the central nervous system may be somewhat less devastating if concomitant high levels of endogenous catecholamines are causing a greater percentage of CO to be delivered to the brain. Our measurement of DO_2I would not reflect such a redistribution of CO. (A number of new organ-specific technologies, such as transcranial Doppler blood flow velocity measurement and near-infrared spectroscopic analysis of intracerebral Hb saturation, are as yet incompletely developed and not in common clinical use.) Furthermore, our definition of DO_2 is precellular. The final stages of DO_2 in-

volve unloading of oxygen molecules from Hb and passive transport of these molecules through the capillary endothelium, extracellular fluid, and cell membrane to the mitochondria. That process is not addressed by measuring CaO_2 and CO. Capillary endothelial swelling, increased extracellular fluid, and cellular edema are all well-understood consequences of ischemic and metabolic insults. All of these processes can compromise cellular oxygen use with a normal DO_2I. Metabolic acidosis and elevations of blood lactate are useful for making inferences regarding the adequacy of cellular oxygen delivery in the face of adequate CO and arterial oxygen saturation.

The use side of the equation is just as critical as the delivery side. In patients, use, like delivery, can be evaluated only in global terms. We rarely measure the oxygen use of specific organs, and that is the value that really counts. If we accept this limitation, however, we can use the mixed venous oxygen saturation to make inferences regarding global oxygen use. Septic patients and other patients in critical stress states appear to extract more oxygen as more is made available, rather than using a limited amount as healthy patients do. Increased extraction is also one of the compensatory mechanisms available when DO_2 decreases.

The oxygen extraction ratio, or use coefficient, is the fraction of delivered oxygen that is actually consumed. Total body oxygen consumption (VO_2) is expressed in milliliters per minute.

Equation 11-4

The oxygen extraction ratio (O_2ER) = VO_2/DO_2

Fever, sepsis, thyrotoxicosis, malignant hyperthermia, and stress due to pain are all examples of conditions that increase oxygen use.

The final common pathway of circulatory failure is dysfunction of the microcirculation. When oxygen demand exceeds supply at the cellular level, anaerobic metabolism occurs. The resulting lactic acidosis is a marker of depletion of the high-energy phosphate bonds needed for cellular integrity and function.

A cellular defect in the ability to extract oxygen has essentially the same implication for cellular dysfunction as does a failure of DO_2.

Patients not subject to the stress of critical illness extract only the oxygen they need, without extracting the maximum. In this normal state, if extra oxygen is delivered, it will be left over. Augmenting DO_2 does not increase consumption. This state is referred to as *oxygen independence.*

Oxygen independence can be contrasted with the way the critically ill patient processes oxygen. For the critically ill patient, as more oxygen is delivered, more is extracted and consumed. This, at times, seems to be true no matter how much DO_2 is augmented. This state is referred to as *oxygen dependence.* Oxygen-dependent patients are grossly hypermetabolic. Left alone, their cardiopulmonary system is sometimes not able to meet the increased demand. These are the nonsurvivors who originally caught the attention of the investigators in this field.[12,13]

The means of monitoring DO_2 and VO_2 are discussed below in the section on hemodynamic monitoring.

Supranormal DO_2 goals make sense, but as noted they are not achieved without a price. The judgment required as to when the price is worth paying is what modern critical care is all about. Given the results of the trial by Hayes and colleagues, it is hard to argue that aggressive boosting of DO_2 is the standard of care for all patients.[21] However, the aortic surgery patient is more similar to the patients in the Berlauk and Boyd trials than the patients studied by Hayes et al. In aortic surgery patients, the interventions can usually be initiated before critical illness has supervened. In addition, most of the complications in aortic surgery patients are, as is discussed, ischemic processes that are potentially improved by increasing oxygen delivery.

Hb augmented beyond a certain value increases the viscosity of blood such that DO_2 to the microcirculation may fail to increase. In fact, a low Hb concentration may be adaptive in advanced shock states, which are characterized by obstructed flow in the microcirculation. Additionally, transfusion itself is not without risk, although the blood supply is safer today than ever before.

CO can be augmented by manipulating any of its contributory values, i.e., preload, afterload, contractility, or heart rate (Figure 11-2). The potential price paid by manipulating any of these parameters is discussed below.

Reduction of afterload is the most efficient means of increasing CO without directly increasing cardiac work. The problem with afterload reduction,

usually achieved with vasodilators, is that if hypotension results it may compromise perfusion of vulnerable atherosclerotic arterial beds such as the coronary vasculature. Additionally, most of our clinically useful vasodilators are not pure arterial dilators. Accompanying dilatation in the capacitance circulation may reduce venous return and thereby decrease CO. Augmentation of preload by fluid loading will usually increase CO with a moderate (often acceptable) increase in myocardial oxygen demand. The limiting factor with fluid loading is the need to avoid increases in lung water, especially in the patient vulnerable to acute lung injury. Preload augmentation complements afterload reduction in that it can limit hypotension by keeping the vasculature full.

Increases in heart rate have a limited ability to increase CO because tachycardia reduces diastolic filling time and stroke volume. Since tachycardia has a deleterious effect on myocardial oxygen supply and demand, it should generally be avoided. Afterload reduction and inotropic support are often provided by the same agent, and this is currently a common method of augmenting DO_2I. The question of how much to demand of a compromised myocardium is currently a focus of investigation.

Attention given to the adequacy of DO_2I is always a high priority in the critically ill surgical population. How hard to push the patient is a judgment call, but DO_2 should never be ignored, and it is safe to say that abnormally low DO_2 should rarely be tolerated.

Proper attention to DO_2I actually dictates most of the monitoring and management plan we adhere to in our patients. It will also be noted that to follow DO_2I properly, a pulmonary artery catheter (PAC) is necessary. Once in place, the PAC allows for monitoring of mixed venous oxygen saturation, a parameter that, when considered together with DO_2I, gives a glimpse of total body oxygen use. In the general sense, the efficacy of the PAC has not been proven. However, most of the work that leads to this conclusion predates (or ignores) the emphasis on supranormal DO_2I goals. Therefore, to claim that supranormal hemodynamic goals should not be pursued because the PAC has not been proven beneficial is circular reasoning of the worst kind.

Other than acute lung injury, which is an organ failure syndrome characterized by both systemic in-

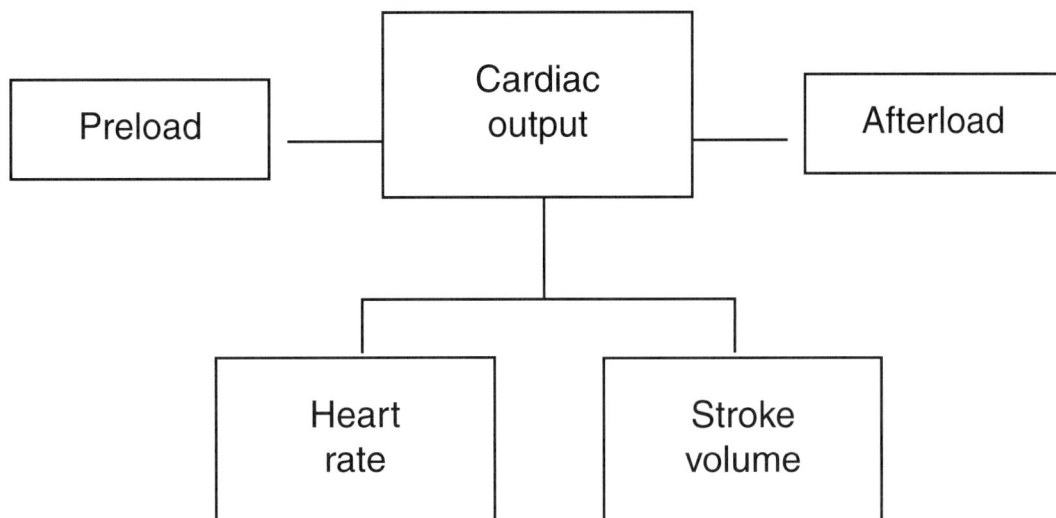

Figure 11-2. Determinants of cardiac output.

flammatory response and ischemia, all of the characteristic organ failure syndromes seen in the aortic surgery patient are ischemic syndromes. A generalized failure of DO_2 is obviously not the only cause of ischemia; in fact, diminished DO_2 is sometimes not a factor at all. Atherosclerotic plaque, thrombus, embolism, reperfusion-related endothelial dysfunction, and edema are all major causes. However, augmented DO_2 can compensate for ischemia caused by other factors. Therefore, augmentation of a normal DO_2I, subject to the tolerance of the myocardium, should be considered in almost all organ failure situations encountered in these patients. Low DO_2I should certainly be augmented. For purposes of discussion, when we talk about inadequate DO_2I and low output syndromes, we are talking about closely related issues.

Gastrointestinal tonometry, which is a relatively noninvasive continuous measurement of gastric mucosal pH, can detect ischemia to the gastrointestinal mucosa within minutes of its occurrence. An instructive review of the significance of this technique by one of its pioneers cites restoration of DO_2 to current tissue need as the best therapeutic response to the detection of mucosal acidosis.[22] No matter how one interprets the literature to date, management of DO_2 is central to the well-being of aortic surgery patients.

The Stress Response

Most management issues surrounding the aortic surgery patient are related to the stress response. The stress response sets up conditions favorable to the development of myocardial ischemia, hypertension, and congestive heart failure. The development of acute lung injury may be related to humoral cascades initiated by the stress response (Figures 11-3 and 11-4). Ischemic renal injury is exacerbated by vasospasm induced by trauma and sustained by the humoral stress response. Gastrointestinal complications, including hypomotility, gastric ulceration, and bowel ischemia, are probably exacerbated by the stress response. The hypercoagulable state, which characterizes the response to major vascular surgery, may be blocked by stress modulation. The issue of supranormal hemodynamic goals, which dominates our approach to critical care, addresses this issue of establishing new normal values for the stressed patient. The nutritional catabolic state, which develops in most patients, is stress related.[23] Finally, postoperative pain management is really a stress response issue. Nociception, the neurologic process associated with pain sensation, appears to go hand in hand with stress. Good postoperative pain management contributes to modulation of the stress response (see Chapter 13).

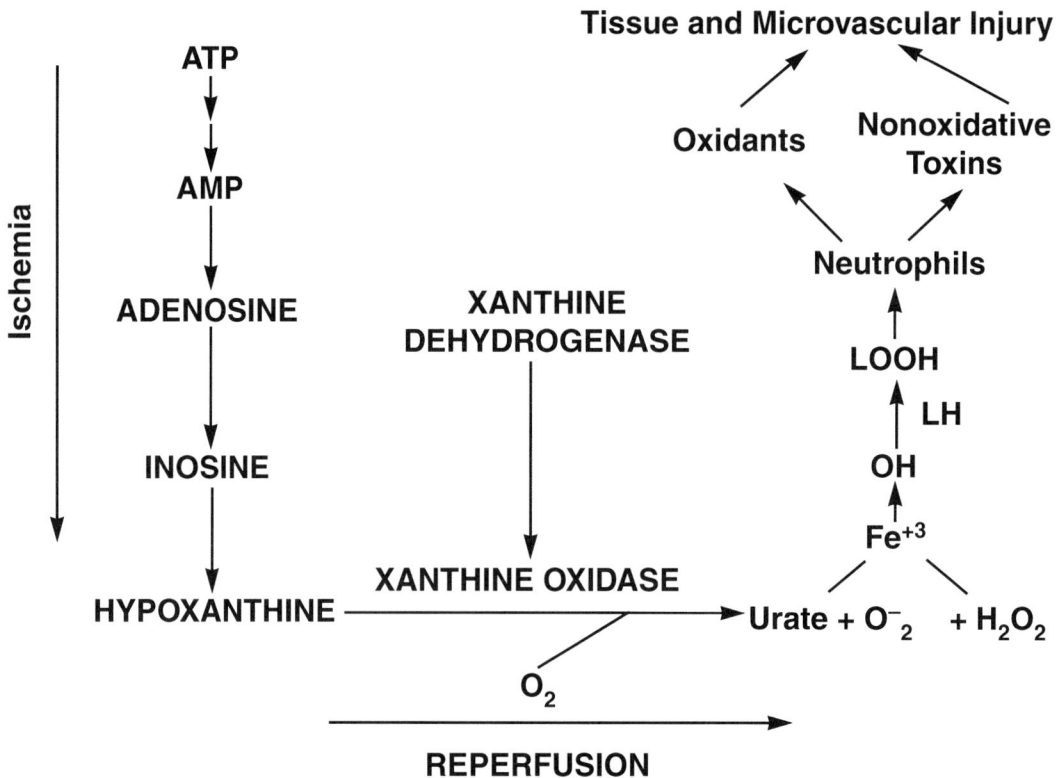

Figure 11-3. The proposed pathway by which the ischemia-reperfusion phenomenon results in widespread microvascular and tissue injury. (ATP = adenosine triphosphate; AMP = adenosine monophosphate.) (Reprinted with permission from EA Deitch. Multiple organ failure, pathophysiology and potential future therapy. Ann Surg 1992;216:117.)

Stress is an adaptive process when a young healthy individual is seriously injured. In such cases, it may tip the scales in favor of survival early in the trauma process. The stress response accomplishes this by taxing organ function to the limit, drawing on physiologic reserve. The time course of the surgical stress response, as described by Chernow and coworkers, is usually defined by common serologic markers such as cortisol and endogenous catecholamines.[24] These markers increase within 1 hour of incision and remain elevated for hours to days. In the past decade atrial natriuretic peptide has been studied extensively. The serum level of atrial natriuretic peptide follows a time course similar to more classical chemical markers of the surgical stress response, and atrial natriuretic peptide may modulate the vaso-

constrictor effects of catecholamines.[25] Stress markers have also been studied with regard to effects of aortic cross clamping.[26] While the stress response is far too complex to be fully represented by a few serum markers, Bassey et al. have shown that infusing such substances into healthy volunteers reproduces several aspects of the response.[27] They were able to induce increases in metabolic rate in the range of 30% within several hours, with CO and oxygen consumption showing similar increases.

Since the stress response must still be considered an incompletely defined entity, it is hard to assert in a rigorous manner that any particular intervention is modifying it. A number of studies have attempted in the last decade to demonstrate outcome differences with stress modification.[11,28–36] Although the

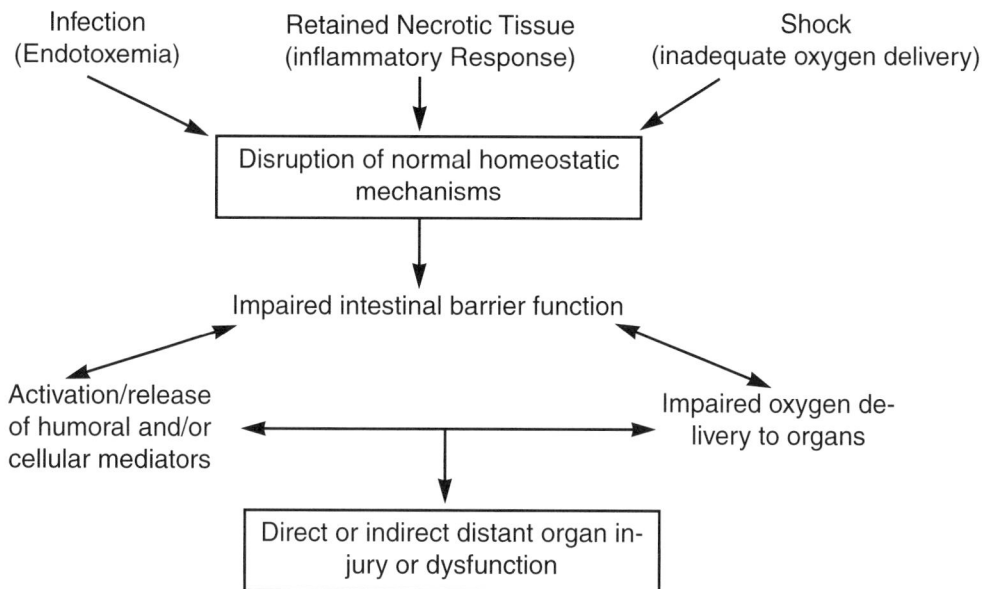

Figure 11-4. Pathways whereby hypoperfusion from any cause may lead to systemic inflammatory response syndrome associated with multiorgan system failure and septic shock. (Reprinted with permission from EA Deitch. Multiple organ failure, pathophysiology and potential future therapy. Ann Surg 1992;216:117.)

studies cited and many more present varied factors (epidural versus general anesthesia, prevention of myocardial ischemia, postoperative thromboembolism), they all are part of the stress story. The authors all study an intervention touted to alter the stress response and then look for differences in some aspect of stress or outcome.

Our relative ignorance about stress is highlighted by the fact that many of the good studies find improvements in outcome without expected changes in intermediary variables, or vice versa. In other words, our studies consistently fail to confirm causality even as they demonstrate association. For example, Yeager and coworkers, in what is their most widely quoted study, evaluated several potential effects of epidural anesthesia and analgesia in high-risk surgical patients.[30] They looked for and found an outcome advantage for epidural anesthesia. They looked for and did not find a difference in stress hormone levels between the study and control groups. This result contrasts with the findings of Mangano et al., who studied the potential effects of postoperative opioid infusion in myocardial revascularization patients.[11]

Their treatment group showed a lower incidence of ischemia than control patients, but no outcome differences could be detected by their methodology. Rosenfeld and coworkers infused stress hormones into healthy volunteers. This infusion failed to mimic the changes in coagulation parameters after vascular surgery.[37]

There are several gaps in our understanding of stress. It is, nevertheless, a central issue that, along with oxygen delivery, unites the otherwise fragmentary approach we are forced to take in discussing postoperative care.

Facility Issues

Transport

The first critical stage of postoperative care is the journey from the OR to the initial postoperative care location. The literature in this area is so sparse that a Society of Critical Care Task Force charged with formulating patient transport policy decided to consider articles without reference to study design.[38] It is certainly a common clinical impression that transport is a dangerous time. Most literature published to date reports on intensive care unit (ICU) patients being transported to diagnostic tests.[39,40] Although the consensus of these studies is that transport of critically ill patients is fairly safe, the postoperative transport is likely to be a higher risk maneuver. The patient is subject to the stress of being turned, uncovered, cleansed, and moved during a time when the level of effective anesthesia is not necessarily known. Should the patient express his or her discomfort by elevating his arterial or pulmonary pressures, the message may be missed or attributed to a transport-related problem, such as a transducer located below cardiac level. During transport the quality of monitoring is suspect; a transport monitor is frequently banged around and may not accommodate the number of waveforms needed. The transducer may not be properly calibrated, and the lines may be kinked, stretched, or partly disconnected. Arrival in the ICU is followed by a period of reattaching and zeroing monitors, changing infusions, unraveling lines, connecting the ventilator, disposing of soiled linens, giving reports to a new care team, and so on. It is only at the end of this critical period that the quality of monitoring and care that characterized the intraoperative period is reestablished. If the initial period of ICU chaos is included in the transport time, the duration of transport commonly exceeds 1 hour. Not many aortic surgery patients can afford 1 hour of hemodynamic instability.

The transport should be considered a procedure in itself and should be characterized by the same vigilance shown during induction of anesthesia. The OR is a relatively safe place when compared with the elevator.

The main areas of concern during transport are circulatory stability, avoidance of the "spaghetti" of tangled lines, securing of tubes and lines, visual contact with monitors and lines, temperature stability, and continued precise administration of vasoactive agents.

Disturbances of heart rate and blood pressure have the same differential diagnosis during transport as at any other time. Left to themselves, unstable vital signs will generally not improve in the elevator. A hyperdynamic circulation is a significant risk factor for bleeding and myocardial ischemia, and the consequences of hypovolemic hypotension are likewise serious. The patient is more likely to remain stable if precise administration of vasoactive medications is ensured with volumetric infusion pumps.

The common mistake of allowing infusion tubing to become tangled is as dangerous as it is sloppy. When the patient becomes unstable, bystanders tend to try to rearrange the lines or demand confirmation that particular medications are being delivered to the patient rather than the floor. Additionally, tangled lines prolong the transition to ICU monitoring on arrival. Tangled lines are easier to avoid if one port is chosen for all infusions along with a carrier, one large line is chosen for infusion of volume, and all unnecessary lines are flushed and capped off. An injection port or stopcock should be taped down to the mattress near the patient's head where it can be readily accessed by the anesthesiologist. The volume line is best used for this purpose; it can be sped up to rapidly deliver an emergency drug without giving a "bolus" of an infused agent. An assortment of emergency drugs (e.g., epinephrine, norepinephrine, nitroglycerin, sodium nitroprusside, esmolol, atropine, lidocaine, and thiopental) drawn up in syringes should accompany the patient.

The original tape securing lines and tubes may be bloodied and loose by the end of surgery. All taped areas should be inspected and resecured if necessary. High-pressure monitoring lines should be at least partly visible during transport to provide an extra visual clue of accidental disconnection with resulting massive bleeding.

If a second arterial line was used during surgery to provide simultaneous upper and lower extremity monitoring, the discontinuation of the extra arterial access is a judgment call. This decision need not be made before transport as long as both lines are secured against disconnection. Since few transport monitors will allow both lines to be transduced, the unmonitored line should be visible along much of its course during transport. When cardiac surgery patients have an extra arterial access in the groin, it is commonly continued in the early postoperative period against the possibility that aortic balloon counterpulsation will be necessary. For the aortic surgery patient, the use of the intra-aortic balloon pump is a last resort.

If one arterial line is to be retained, it seems preferable to retain the radial arterial line for postoperative monitoring. Access to dressing care is easier on the wrist, the infection rate may be lower for a radial line compared with a femoral arterial line, and the radial artery is less prone to arteriosclerotic change. However, if there is any question as to the quality of the radial artery catheter, the lower extremity arterial catheter should be retained.

If an epidural or subarachnoid catheter is in place, the dressing should also be checked before transport. Intraspinal catheters should be clearly marked to avoid the accidental intraspinal injection of a substance intended for intravascular administration. The subarachnoid catheter may be discontinued early or retained as an access for the administration of analgesic agents (see Chapter 13).

Hypothermia should be prevented by ensuring that warm, dry linen is in contact with the patient and that the patient is well covered prior to transport. Wet linen allows for the rapid loss of heat from the patient via conduction and evaporation, while exposure permits heat loss via radiation and convection.

The ideal transport monitor will display all parameters monitored during surgery. The monitors in common use are capable of much less. Often, transport monitors display digital readouts of all critical data but cannot accommodate as many waveforms as an OR monitor. We would sacrifice waveform displays in the following order from most expendable to critical: (1) central venous pressure, (2) electrocardiogram channel, (3) end tidal gas, (4) oximeter plethysmograph, (5) arterial pressure, and (5) pulmonary artery pressure. Assuming a digital readout of the arterial pressure is retained, displaying the pulmonary artery waveform may be more helpful than the arterial because the reliability of pulmonary pressures is contingent on a trained observer noting a satisfactory waveform. Furthermore, the common problem of overwedging of the tip of the PAC can be readily diagnosed if the waveform is observed.

Postoperative Care Unit

The well-established clinical practice of caring for all aortic surgery patients in an ICU setting is not likely to be examined by a prospective controlled study in the near future, because the ethics of such a study could not be defended. Retrospective studies that demonstrate the need for intensive care, such as that of Campbell et al.,[1] are useful in defending

the expense of intensive care when scrutinized by the health policy community.

The modern postanesthesia care unit should be, and is in most medical centers, comparable to a surgical ICU. Both settings should provide the potential for invasive hemodynamic monitoring, intensive pulmonary monitoring, controlled ventilation, intensive care by specially trained nurses, and timely implementation of changes in therapy. Decisions as to whether to transfer patients from the OR to a recovery facility or directly to a surgical ICU, as well as timing of transfer from recovery to the surgical ICU if a recovery type of facility is initially used, are made based on administrative, nursing, and staffing considerations. If one facility or the other is lacking in any of the areas mentioned previously, it is not appropriate for care of the aortic surgery patient, and no decision is necessary. The intensive postoperative care area will be referred to in this chapter generically as the ICU.

For the more unstable patients, every effort should be made to avoid an unnecessary second transport. If possible, such patients should be transferred from the OR to their ultimate destination. The most stable patients, particularly those who are candidates for early extubation and a shorter ICU stay, may benefit from the airway vigilance skills, which are the province of recovery room nurses. Aortic surgery patients, who are usually the recipients of an artificial graft, deserve to be as far as possible from any endemic focus of surgical infection. In many institutions, the recovery room is less likely to host resistant hospital flora.

Pulmonary Management

Among the earliest clinical decisions made in the postoperative period are those regarding mechanical ventilation and the timing of extubation. Although there is some evidence that preoperative pulmonary disease is a predictor of postoperative pulmonary morbidity in aortic surgery patients (see Chapter 2),[41–43] the preoperative pulmonary status is only one factor among many to be considered. Decisions regarding ventilatory management usually reflect the general welfare of the patient rather than the pulmonary status in isolation. The maintenance of adequate DO_2 without excessive work of breathing is the bottom line.

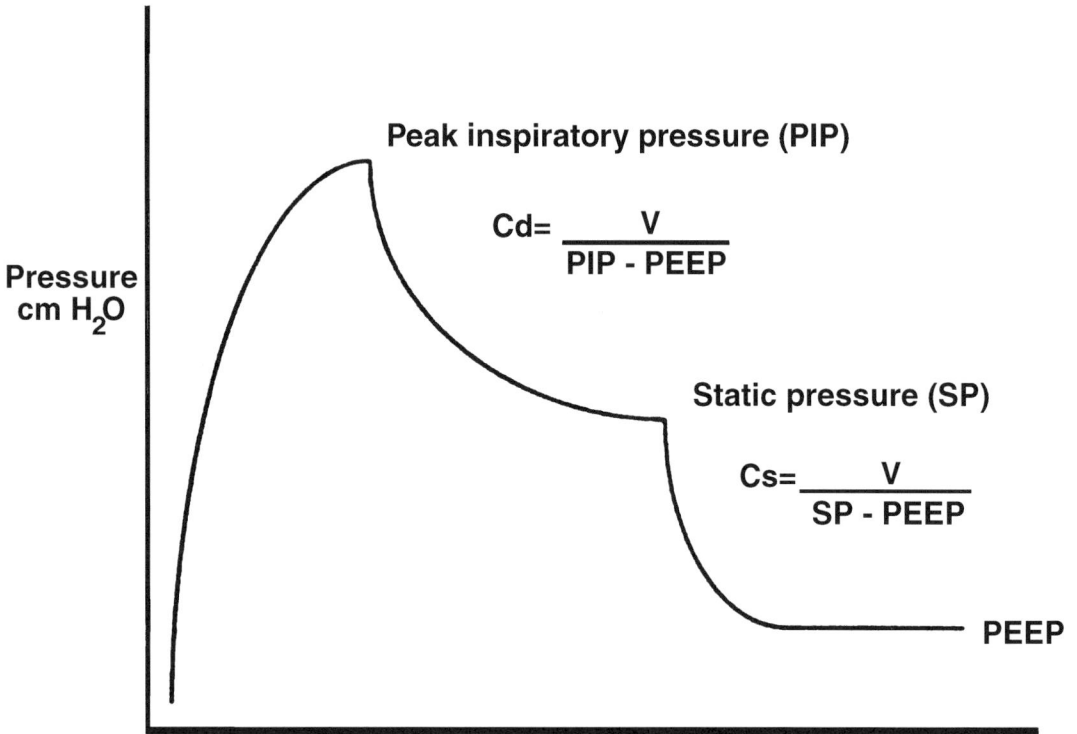

Figure 11-5. Airway pressure trace with equations for dynamic and static compliance. Normal static compliance for mechanically ventilated patients is approximately 50–85 ml per cm H_2O, depending on degree of recovery from neuromuscular blockade. Normal dynamic compliance is about 15–20% higher than static compliance. By definition, airway resistance is a factor in dynamic but not static compliance, since the pressure differential for static compliance is measured at a point at which air flow varies less abruptly. (Cd = dynamic compliance; Cs = static compliance; V = tidal volume; PIP = peak inspiratory pressure; PEEP = positive end-expiratory pressure.) (Reprinted with permission from A Perel, MC Stock. Handbook of Mechanical Ventilatory Support. Baltimore: Williams & Wilkins, 1992. Copyright Murray R. Abell.)

Initial Assessment

On arrival in the ICU the airway and chest are examined. Initial assessment also includes review of the airway and pulmonary management in the OR. Data from pulse oximetry and capnography are confirmed by an arterial blood gas analysis. Airway pressures and tolerance to ventilation are assessed (Figure 11-5). Pulmonary compliance, both static and dynamic, can be deduced from the inspiratory pressures and the expired tidal volume. The level of consciousness will suggest the need for sedation and paralysis as well as corroborate the adequacy of oxygenation and ventilation. An initial chest radiograph is performed. Flexible fiberoptic bronchoscopy should be available.

The proper placement of the endotracheal tube has often not been verified with a chest radiograph prior to arrival in the ICU. In the case of the thoracic aortic surgery patient, the single-lumen tube that the patient arrives with in the ICU will often have been inserted at the end of the surgery after removal of a double-lumen tube. Such a tube will have been secured at a time when numerous other distractions were pressuring the anesthesia team. Therefore, after resecuring the endotracheal tube, assessing the pressure in the pilot bag, and clinically verifying the proper placement of the endotracheal tube, a chest radiograph should be obtained. The only bedside tests that reliably exclude an esophageal intubation are flexible fiberoptic bronchoscopy and capnography. Although many ICUs do not have the equipment for continuous capnography, single-use disposable indicator units have been available for several years. These are reliable in verifying the presence of carbon dioxide in the expired gas. The presence of carbon dioxide in the expired gas does not exclude the possibility that the tube tip is in the larynx and the cuff is outside the trachea. In the presence of this disaster, the patient may move the tube with his or her tongue into the posterior pharynx at any time. Chest radiography and physical examination therefore complement the assessment of expired carbon dioxide.

The most reliable examinations for verifying proper depth of endotracheal intubation are flexible fiberoptic bronchoscopy and chest radiography. A proper depth of insertion as measured at the mouth suggests that a main stem intubation is not present, as does the ability to palpate the cuff over the proximal trachea when the cuff is rapidly inflated. The latter maneuver often elicits a pain response with bucking, hypertension, and tachycardia; such responses should be anticipated. Although movement of the chest may be helpful, auscultation is notoriously unreliable for assessment of endotracheal tube position. There has never been a convincing study that supports the accuracy of auscultation of breath sounds in either ruling out esophageal intubation or excluding a deep main stem intubation.

The initial chest film will also allow the assessment of central line placement and chest tube position. Pneumothorax, hemothorax, and gross fluid overload can be excluded. Evidence of acute lung injury may be present, although radiographs obtained 24–48 hours later are more sensitive for detecting this complication. (The diagnostic criteria for acute lung injury do not include radiologic findings.)

Occasionally, patients arrive in the ICU with a double-lumen endotracheal tube still in place. This is because exchanging the double-lumen tube with a single-lumen tube at the conclusion of surgery may be a bad idea for a number of reasons. There may have been concern that an indication for differential ventilation, such as a bronchopleural fistula, was present. It is also possible that deflation of the cuff of the double-lumen tube may have failed to produce a leak. In this case, there is a concern of overwhelming airway edema and this may have contraindicated a tube change. Double-lumen tubes may be retained for short periods (hours to days) if necessary. In managing these patients, tracheobroncheal suctioning will be more difficult due to the narrow diameter of each lumen. Special suction catheters are available for this and are supplied by the manufacturers of double-lumen tubes. Ventilation of these patients may also require higher than normal airway pressures. These pressures may reflect turbulent flow at the connector, and the alveolar pressures may be acceptable despite high peak inspiratory pressures registered at the gauge on the ventilator. Overinflation of the double-lumen tube cuffs must be avoided because it can lead to pressure necrosis of the airway mucosal lining, compression of the lumen, and herniation of the cuff over the tube tip.

Support of Ventilation

Rationale for Postoperative Support of Ventilation

Cardiac patients are now commonly extubated within hours of surgery. The aortic surgery patient is usually sicker than the cardiac surgery patient. With current surgical techniques, progress toward earlier extubation in the aortic surgery patient will not be dramatic.

The management and discontinuation of ventilator support become simpler if one remembers why ventilation is controlled in the first place (Table 11-2). The goals of mechanical ventilation are to assist in maintaining an acceptable alveolar ventilation achieved at a reasonable energy cost appropriate to the patient's cardiopulmonary reserve.

The patient with a ruptured aortic aneurysm is never a candidate for extubation within 24 hours of surgery. The high mortality of these patients in all reports (see Table 11-1) and the high incidence of postoperative organ system failure mandate that ventilation be controlled until stability is ensured. A group of patients to whom less attention is paid in the literature is those whose aortic aneurysms are not yet ruptured, but who have symptoms indicating the possibility of rupture. These are patients with a known abdominal aortic aneurysm who present with abdominal pain and in whom the presumption is that the aneurysm will soon rupture if not excised. At surgery, a hematoma of the aortic wall or a contained rupture may be found. It turns out that in this group of patients with expanding aneurysms, leaking aneurysms, or imminent rupture, the predicted mortality is midway between the disastrous prognosis of ruptured aneurysms and the favorable outlook for elective aneurysmectomy.[44,45] In this group caution is advised regarding early extubation.

Table 11-2. Etiologies of Postoperative Hypercapnea

Central respiratory depression
    Residual intravenous anesthetics or analgesics
    Residual inhaled anesthetics
Respiratory muscle dysfunction
    Upper abdominal or thoracic incision site
    Residual neuromuscular blockade
Physical factors
    Obesity
    Tight dressings
    Gastric dilatation
Increased carbon dioxide production
    Shivering
    Hyperthermia
    Systemic inflammatory response syndrome
Preexisting disease
    Pulmonary disease
    Skeletal deformities (e.g., kyphoscoliosis)
    Neuromuscular disease

Source: Modified from TW Feeley. The Recovery Room. In RD Miller (ed), Anesthesia (2nd ed). New York: Churchill Livingstone, 1986;1921.

For the patient operated under elective conditions, the rationale for a period of ventilator support is related to variable anesthetic recovery, obligatory pulmonary changes, incision type, cardiovascular stability, the possibility of unstable coagulation findings, and sometimes the poor general medical condition of these patients (see Table 11-2). The advantages of a safe early extubation include a shortened stay in the ICU, conservation of resources, simplification of hemodynamic management, patient satisfaction, and, possibly, the ability to better evaluate for neurologic changes.

The anesthetic chosen for the aortic surgery patient is often opioid based. While such an anesthetic is a good way to provide exceptional hemodynamic stability, it is sometimes slow to wear off. The neuromuscular blocking agent chosen may have been one that depends on renal or hepatic elimination, both of which may be sluggish in the early postoperative period (Table 11-3). In the case of the aortic aneurysmectomy performed via the transperitoneal approach, full neuromuscular blockade will often have been continued until the very end of surgery. A short period of ventilator support permits full recovery from the anesthetic. It must not be forgotten

that changes related to the anesthetic are only a fraction of the myriad perioperative changes that increase the work of breathing (Figure 11-6).

Most aortic surgery patients have some degree of increased capillary permeability in the lung as well as in other tissues.[46] This change results from the systemic inflammatory response syndrome induced by aortic cross clamping and reperfusion, as well as from any other period of hemodynamic compromise associated with the perioperative process. Figure 11-4 outlines the process as a generalized phenomenon. Concerning the lung, this process is called acute lung injury or adult respiratory distress syndrome when it meets certain criteria related to compromise of oxygenation and pulmonary mechanics. However, even if the criteria for acute lung injury are not met, it is not to be assumed that the aortic surgery patient has normal lungs. Commonly, decreased pulmonary compliance will

Table 11-3. Etiologies of Prolonged Neuromuscular Blockade

Depolarizing neuromuscular blocking agents
    Decreased pseudocholinesterase
    Abnormal pseudocholinesterase
    Hypermagnesemia
    Local anesthetics, high serum levels
Nondepolarizing neuromuscular blocking agents
    Unusually intense neuromuscular blockade
    Renal failure (depending on agent used)
    Hepatic failure (depending on agent used)
    Inadequate pharmacologic antagonism
    Hypothermia
    Residual inhalational anesthetic
    Abnormal acid–base status
    Hypokalemia
    Hypermagnesemia
    Drug interactions
        Antibiotics
        Antidysrhythmics
        Loop diuretics
        Dantrolene
        Local anesthetics
    Underlying neuromuscular disease
        Myasthenia gravis/myasthenic syndrome
        Other muscular disease

Source: Modified from RD Miller, JJ Savarese. Pharmacology of Muscle Relaxants and Their Antagonists. In RD Miller (ed), Anesthesia (2nd ed). New York: Churchill Livingstone, 1986;889.

LOAD (VS) N-M Competence

Resistive Loads

Chest Wall Elastic Loads

Lung Elastic Loads

Increased Metabolic Demands

Muscle Weakness

Impaired Neuromuscular Transmission

Depressed Drive

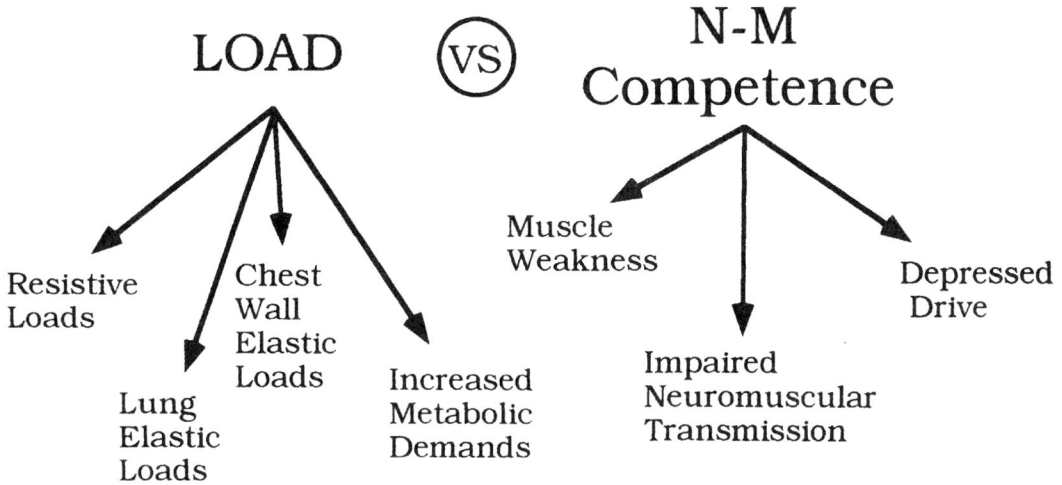

Figure 11-6. The balance between workload and neuromuscular (N-M) competence determines the ability to sustain alveolar ventilation and the related energy cost. All of these factors are subject to change for the worse during the perioperative period. (Modified from VF Murray, VA Nadel. Textbook of Respiratory Medicine [2nd ed]. Philadelphia: Saunders, 1994;2614.)

lead to increased work of breathing even in the absence of acute lung injury.

The aortic surgery patient invariably has a large, painful incision that causes splinting and contributes to respiratory impairment. Chest wall and diaphragmatic function will be abnormal. Some thoracic aortic surgery patients have a chest drain. One goal of the early recovery period is to maintain a state of analgesia profound enough to permit deep breathing, while permitting neurologic examination, cooperation with nursing care, and maintenance of the airway. Until this balance is established, ventilator support provides a margin of safety (see Chapter 13).

Major vascular surgery patients are prone to various kinds of hemodynamic instability, including ischemic myocardial dysfunction, hypertension, and volume disturbances. Wide fluctuations in these parameters are best managed if the patient has a protected airway and if the work of breathing can be modulated with a ventilator. In aortic surgery patients with low-output cardiac failure and pulmonary hypertension, as well as those who have had cardiac surgery in the past, ventilator support is usually indicated for about 24 hours after stability has been achieved.

Anticoagulants and their antagonists are almost always administered to vascular surgery patients at some point, and clotting homeostasis may not have

been achieved by the end of surgery. If a patient is extubated and then becomes frankly coagulopathic, reintubation may become urgent. Bleeding and edema, however, can make the procedure of reintubation traumatic and technically difficult. Patients should be extubated only when the probability of subsequent bleeding complications is judged to be low.

While it is certainly easier to do a neurologic examination on an patient without an endotracheal tube, the need for serial neurologic examination is a poor excuse for extubating a patient before his or her time. By judicious titration of analgesics and sedatives, most intubated patients can be maintained in an awake cooperative state when necessary. On the other hand, the problem in the central nervous system will only get worse if oxygenation and carbon dioxide elimination are compromised.

Ventilator Settings and Weaning

In the vast majority of aortic surgery patients, the specific ventilator mode chosen and the specific way the patient is weaned do not matter. In fact, weaning implies gradual discontinuation of a therapeutic modality such that the deconditioned patient can slowly take over an increased part of the workload. This is not applicable to the majority of aortic surgery patients, in whom mechanical ventilation is discontinued hours to days after surgery. Developing and following a consistent plan for each patient and closely monitoring his or her response is probably far more important than is the ventilator mode in which the patient is weaned. In fact, what we commonly do is better described as controlled sudden discontinuation rather than weaning.

The initial ventilator settings depend on the anticipated duration of ventilatory support as well as the general condition of the patient and type of ventilator available. For the vast majority of our patients, the initial settings use the synchronized intermittent mandatory ventilation (SIMV) mode with a positive end-expiratory pressure (PEEP) of 3–5 cm of H_2O and pressure support (PS) of 5–7 cm of H_2O. The initial SIMV rate is 9–10 breaths per minute. Tidal volume is generally initially set at 8–10 ml per kg of body weight. Somewhat lower volumes on a per kilogram basis are delivered to the obese patient because "the lungs are not fat" and the metabolic rate of fat tissue is somewhat lower than that of many other tissues. Inspired oxygen (FIO_2) is initially set at 100%. The advantages of this setting are that weaning can be accomplished without a change in the ventilator mode and that only rarely will there be other indications for a mode change.

The FIO_2 is titrated down immediately; to do this all that is required is reliable pulse oximetry. In the absence of any specific indication of organ failure, FIO_2 is rapidly reduced (over a period of 30 minutes or less) to the lowest value at which oxygen saturation is still 96–97%. There is no reason to reduce FIO_2 to less than 30%. An oxygen saturation below 90% is virtually never acceptable, but the goal of saturation above 90% is a matter of clinical judgment. In the rare patient in whom pulmonary failure is the predominant pathology, one may consider tolerating a saturation of 93–94%, providing for the possibility of ventilating with the lowest effective FIO_2. For the patient who may be suffering from myocardial ischemia or other organ failure pathology, one may elect to maintain a saturation of 98–99% even if a higher FIO_2 is required. (Some would argue that all aortic surgery patients automatically fall in this category.) The role of higher levels of PEEP in allowing for adequate oxygenation at lower FIO_2 values is well known. Higher levels of PEEP are used in the face of pulmonary injury and organ

system failure and are not used in patients who are candidates for extubation.

Once the target saturation is achieved, the accuracy of the oximetric saturation and the adequacy of ventilation are confirmed by an arterial blood gas (ABG) measurement. If pulse oximetry is unavailable, either because the patient is cold and peripherally vasoconstricted or the equipment is not present, the FIO_2 titration will be guided by ABG only and will be more cumbersome. When a pulse oximeter is not used, one may elect to use a slightly higher FIO_2 value than necessary to give the patient more reserve between routine ABG measurements. For a number of patients with severe vascular pathology, the peripheral pulse waves will be distorted so as to preclude pulse oximetry. In the case of the hypothermic patient, a careful digital block with 2–3 ml of lidocaine 1% may restore the ability to monitor saturation on a finger.

The importance of achieving the lowest FIO_2 possible at an early stage is related to the prevention of oxygen toxicity, avoidance of absorption atelectasis, and awareness of the patient's pulmonary reserve. If patients are maintained at an FIO_2 that is higher than necessary, then the saturation will remain at 99–100%. At this level the patient will register on the flat portion of the oxygen Hb dissociation curve, and moderate decreases in oxygenation between ABG measurements will not be evident. Such decreases are red flags, in that they are early warning signals for congestive heart failure, embolic phenomena, and a host of other problems. In fact, since most surgical patients have an intrapulmonary shunt that is greater than physiologic, decreased arterial saturation may signal a decrease in venous saturation. This situation requires further evaluation.

The first major question to address in the ICU is that of cardiac stability. The initial ventilator settings suggested previously will greatly reduce the work of breathing if the ventilator is well tolerated. For the patient who has myocardial ischemia, is in cardiac failure, or is otherwise very ill, the initial goal may be to completely take over the work of breathing rather than reduce it. This is achieved by increasing the breathing rate, adding a high level of PS, or by using the assist control mode. Sedatives to suppress the respiratory drive are important adjuncts, as are muscle relaxants. The plan for weaning and extubation in these patients is deferred until the patients achieve their optimum level of hemodynamic stability.

For patients with some degree of hemodynamic stability the total elimination of the work of breathing is undesirable. Atrophy of the inspiratory muscles, which may make weaning more difficult, may become a factor if extubation is not accomplished in the first few days. Habituation of the ventilatory control center in the brainstem does not seem to be a major factor even with very long periods of mechanical support. Therefore, we reduce the rate of mechanical ventilation (SIMV rate) to achieve, if possible, several spontaneous breaths per minute. The level of PS can be increased, if necessary, to allow spontaneous breaths to continue while preventing fatigue. PS at about 7 cm of H_2O will permit most patients to do much of the work of breathing by themselves, while eliminating the extra resistive load imposed by the endotracheal tube and breathing circuitry. Higher levels of PS will proportionately reduce the work of breathing. The initial level of PS is a matter of clinical judgment; it depends on the general condition of the patient and the state of recovery from general anesthesia. The ability to finely manipulate the workload on a breath-by-breath basis is a major advantage of PS mode. (Pure PS mode without SIMV may be unsafe in the early stages of recovery because it does not offer much protection against apnea. Some ventilators offer an apnea alarm and backup mechanical breaths in case of apnea even in the pure PS mode.)

Preparation for extubation may begin when the patient is awake and seems to be making progress toward meeting extubation criteria, including hemodynamic stability, successful pain control, and intact coagulation. A number of useful ventilation-oriented criteria for weaning are reviewed in Table 11-4. Weaning may be accomplished by reducing the SIMV rate, the level of PS, or both. A common error is to reduce settings too slowly. The only patients who benefit from a slow wean are those with poor cardiopulmonary reserve and those who are deconditioned after prolonged ventilator support.

Although in most patients it probably does not matter, it makes more physiologic sense to reduce the IMV rate to 4–6 per minute before reducing the level of PS; in this way nonphysiologic breaths, which are volume cycled, are eliminated first. The patient then may be observed to determine the native respiratory rate, while support for these breaths is reduced in a controlled fashion. It is currently believed that the PS mode allows relatively functional,

Table 11-4. Various Criteria Helpful for Determining Readiness to Wean from Mechanical Ventilation*

Traditional criteria	
Tidal volume	>5 ml/kg
Respiratory rate	<30 breaths/min
Maximum inspiratory force	> –25 cm H_2O
Vital capacity	>10–15 ml/kg
Successful pre-extubation trial	
Arterial pH	7.35–7.45
Arterial pCO_2	35–45 mm Hg
Arterial pO_2	>60 mm Hg
Effective unlabored breathing	
Rapid shallow breathing index	Respiratory rate/ tidal volume (liters) <50
Respiratory effort	Patient does not appear distressed (subjective)

*Such criteria are suggested guidelines; slight deviations are often acceptable when based on clinical judgment and preoperative baseline studies.

physiologic breaths. These breaths may resemble the natural length-tension relationship of the muscles of inspiration more closely than an SIMV breath.[47] On the other hand, SIMV breaths at a low rate are also useful because they guarantee an adequate tidal volume and thereby expanding borderline alveoli.

Therefore, a reasonable approach is to initiate weaning by decreasing the SIMV rate. Once a rate of 4 breaths per minute is achieved, the PS level is gradually reduced until 5 cm per H_2O is reached. Patients may be extubated without further reductions if other extubation criteria are met (see Table 11-4). Some intensivists wean the sicker, more frail patient to a setting of 2 breaths per minute before extubation.

Some clinicians may feel strongly about the need to completely discontinue SIMV and to terminate PS and PEEP, thus creating a T-tube trail. There is no reason, however, to withhold low-level PEEP (3–5 cm per H_2O) in the preextubation period, and the practice of a PEEP-free trial before extubation is discouraged. In the nonintubated patient, the vocal cords probably provide "physiologic PEEP," which is bypassed by the endotracheal tube. Therefore, a period without PEEP will prove nothing and may allow progression of atelectasis.[48]

Special considerations are necessary for the patient with severe chronic obstructive pulmonary disease, acute lung injury, multiple organ failure, or bronchopleural fistula. Such patients require an individualized approach to mechanical ventilation and weaning. The short text by Perel and Stock[47] is an excellent guide to the practice of ventilatory support. The critical care community is currently struggling to introduce science into what has previously been an art. Cohen has reviewed several papers that suggest that the management of ventilator therapy by a team approach decreases duration of ventilator therapy regardless of which specific modes are used.[49] Such a result is not surprising if one considers that problems with interdisciplinary communication, changed orders, and inconsistent implementation are common afflictions of the teaching hospital. Such problems are well addressed by protocols and a team approach.

Sedating the Ventilated Patient

Indications and Choice of Sedatives

While the provision of postoperative analgesia is an absolute requirement in all aortic surgery patients (see Chapter 13), the provision of sedation is not. The patient who fights the ventilator is in danger of injury, accidental self-extubation, and a deleterious increase in the work of breathing and oxygen consumption. However, most patients who arrive in the ICU after an anesthetic for aortic surgery are not struggling.

In fact, there are distinct advantages of an awake, cooperative patient. For any patient at risk of spinal cord damage (see Chapters 8 and 12), the ability to obtain cooperation for a neurologic examination is desirable. A certain percentage of patients who end up with spinal cord injury still have a normal neurologic examination at the conclusion of surgery. Ongoing clinical monitoring may uncover ischemia in its earliest stages, at which time it still may be reversible.[50,51] If extubation within several hours of arrival in the postoperative care area is anticipated, as is practical with relatively healthy abdominal aortic surgery patients, an awake, comfortable patient is essential. Amnesia may be provided with small doses of a benzodiazepine. Patients who are candidates for early extubation will benefit from moderate sedation, and such a choice must be indi-

vidualized. Both low-dosage midazolam (0.5–1.0 mg given intravenously repeated as needed) and propofol (boluses of 0.3–0.5 mg/kg followed by continuous infusion of 0.010–0.075 mg/kg/minute) are good options when the need for sedation is temporary. If the need for sedation becomes more prolonged, propofol may be continued. Propofol provides the advantage of excellent controllability of the sedated state, with weaning and extubation possible soon after a sedative dose of propofol has been discontinued.[52,53] Alternatively, any one of the longer acting benzodiazepines may be used.

The patient who is not a candidate for early extubation usually requires sedation. The sedation resulting from the residual anesthetic agent or from opioid analgesics may be initially adequate. If it is obvious that anxiety is leading to increased stress and consequent overuse of oxygen, the provision of sedation through specific drugs becomes desirable. In this situation, the benzodiazepines with a longer duration of action (e.g., diazepam and lorazepam) are effective and easy to titrate. There are data in aortic surgery patients that demonstrate decreased VO_2 with sedation.[52] In the large subgroup of patients with decreased myocardial reserve, this is beneficial.

If the patient is bucking and coughing on the endotracheal tube, additional opioid analgesia should be the next step, as opioids are efficient suppressors of the cough reflex. Lidocaine by intravenous bolus or infusion is a reasonable alternative; however, lidocaine infusion must be monitored carefully to avoid toxicity. Most patients with a history of either chronic benzodiazepine use or recent habitual use of alcohol should have benzodiazepines continued throughout the postoperative period to moderate the stress of withdrawal and prevent seizures.

It is difficult to demonstrate major outcome differences between various general anesthetic agents. Similarly, it is unlikely that the choice of a particular sedative agent will affect the outcome of postoperative care, and most familiar drugs perform well.[53]

The primary pharmacologic effect of opioids is analgesia. Opioids are, as noted previously, also useful in suppression of the cough reflex; however, they also have some preload reducing effect and are excellent sedatives. While sedation is usually provided with the sedative hyponotics discussed previously, there should be no hesitation to use opioids as sedatives if they are indicated for one or a combination of their other pharmacologic effects.

A relative overdose of propofol can cause hemodynamic instability, as can benzodiazepines when administered in the presence of opioids. All sedatives must be carefully titrated with repeated assessment of the hemodynamic profile.

The aortic surgery patient demonstrates altered pharmacokinetics of both opioids, such as fentanyl, and sedatives, such as midazolam.[54–57] Pharmacokinetics, however, when taken out of context, do not reliably predict prolonged duration of action, at least for anesthetic, analgesic, and sedative medications.[58,59] Furthermore, the goals of management for aortic patients are not inconsistent with the more gradual offset of sedative action. The time frame to awaken these critically ill patients is not measured in terms of minutes.

The advent of flumazenil, a specific antagonist at the benzodiazepine receptor, appears to offer a new dimension of controllability. At this point, there does not appear to be an excessive risk to antagonism of benzodiazepines in the nonhabituated patient. However, physicians should not forget that at one time we thought the same of naloxone's ability to reverse opioids. Anesthesiologists now recognize that pulmonary edema, severe hypertension, and tachycardia can result from opioid antagonism even in the healthy patient, and most anesthesiologists would not dare to administer naloxone to the typical aortic surgery patient. Flumazenil is contraindicated in the alcoholic patient, the patient with a seizure disorder, and the patient habituated to benzodiazepines. When used in other patients, flumazenil should be titrated in small boluses (0.05–0.10 mg) with frequent evaluation of the hemodynamic profile.

Role of Neuromuscular Blockade

No anesthesiologist should underestimate the need to remind our surgical colleagues that neuromuscular blocking drugs (i.e., muscle relaxants) are not sedatives. They are not indicated as first-line treatment of patient movement, regardless of how disturbing such movement is to the staff. It is nevertheless understood that in some situations neuromuscular blockade will be useful in the postoperative period. If a patient who, for whatever reason, is not a candidate for further sedative medications is either dangerously combative or fighting the ventilator, neuromuscular blockade as a temporizing measure seems reasonable. The same is true if a

procedure that can be performed under local anesthesia (e.g., an arterial cutdown) is necessary in the combative, unstable patient.

When neuromuscular blockade is necessary, the question of correct endotracheal tube position should be considered. Neuromuscular blockade negates any chance the patient has of surviving an unrecognized ventilator disconnection or accidental extubation. As discussed previously, any one method of verifying tube placement can be misleading.

Before neuromuscular blockade is administered, a minimal degree of amnesia and sedation should be ensured unless cardiovascular collapse makes this impossible. The use of scopolamine as an amnesiac agent (0.3–0.4 mg/70 kg) is relatively benign even in the unstable patient.

All muscle relaxants are capable of myriad drug interactions and pharmacokinetic variations (see Table 11-3). Prolonged neuromuscular blockade may occur in the acidotic patient or in the patient receiving certain antibiotics. In addition to the well-known risks and side effects of muscle relaxants, including the disastrous consequences of a ventilator disconnection during chemical paralysis, there is the relatively new concern of residual myopathy.[60–63] A number of reports of myopathic weakness after reversal of neuromuscular blockade in asthmatic patients on corticosteroids have been followed by similar reports of the same problem in nonasthmatics and patients who did not receive corticosteroids. Other studies searched for and did not find such problems.[64] It appears that use of relaxants for some critical duration can result in a myoneuropathy that outlasts the drug effect and can make a difficult weaning even more problematic. It is not yet clear what this critical duration is, or which drugs or modes of delivery place which patients at risk. It is possible that this complication can be minimized when the minimum effective dosage of drug is used and the state of neuromuscular blockade is monitored.[64] For most ICU applications, absolute paralysis is neither necessary nor desirable.

Extubation

Extubation Criteria

In addition to the extubation criteria that ensure adequate oxygenation and ventilatory function, there are a number of other aspects that should always be considered. Examination of dressings, chest tube drainage, and coagulation parameters should ensure that the possibility of emergency reoperation is remote.

The hemodynamic profile of the patient and examination of a recent chest film should confirm that severe fluid overload and congestive heart failure are not present. Positive pressure ventilation provides critical support to the patient in heart failure by reducing preload, afterload, and the work of breathing, while preventing fluid transudation across pulmonary capillary membranes.

When all other factors are favorable for extubation, occasionally recovery from the opioid anesthetic extends the duration of ventilatory support. There is virtually no justification for the use of the opioid antagonist naloxone to hasten awakening. The short duration of action of naloxone would mandate a continuous infusion. Constant careful titration would be necessary to antagonize the opioid sedation without antagonizing analgesia, and even then this goal would not always be achieved.[65]

Since the earliest study suggesting the possibility that the opioid agonist-antagonist nalbuphine can be useful in the postoperative setting, it has been difficult to put this topic to rest. The idea was that nalbuphine could potentially reverse the anesthetic effect of high-dose opioids, while protecting the patient with its own inherent analgesic properties. It was thought that the adverse effects seen with naloxone reversal may be avoided with nalbuphine. Unfortunately, the safety of this technique has not been proven. The case report of Blaise and coworkers raises serious questions regarding the safety of nalbuphine reversal in aortic surgery.[66]

Airway Safety

The ultimate goal of a safe extubation is to avoid the need for reintubation while having a realistic plan for how to reintubate if it should become necessary. Obesity, edema, and arthritis, among other conditions, may increase the incidence of difficult intubations in the aortic surgery population. A review of the anesthesia record or conferral with the anesthesiologist who intubated the patient should confirm that the intubation was not difficult. If there is any question as to the ease of intubation, a tracheal tube exchanger can be used. This device allows for a trial of extubation while retaining access to the trachea. Although various devices, such as nasogastric tubes, can be used to retain access to the trachea and facilitate reintubation if necessary, there are advantages to using the exchangers manufactured specifically for this purpose. Such exchangers are of adequate length and are stiff enough to facilitate reintubation without being so rigid as to injure the airway. Additionally, the dedicated exchanging catheter can be used as a conduit for jet ventilation if attempted reintubation does not go well. Some of the softer tube exchangers on the market can be left in situ for 1–2 hours. When multiple sizes are available, the selection of the proper exchanger is a judgment call. A larger exchanger will make reintubation less traumatic but at the same time will be more stimulating and more difficult for the patient to "breath around" and to tolerate for a brief period after extubation. Tracheal tube exchangers are not perfect. The softer tracheal tube exchangers, which are better tolerated, are easily dislodged, the reintubation may be very traumatic, and jet ventilation can be complicated by fatal barotrauma. Lidocaine 4% (3 ml) can be injected through the endotracheal tube before extubation to help the patient better tolerate the exchanger. The exchanger, when properly used, is advanced well beyond the end of the endotracheal tube: this can stimulate the bronchial mucous membrane causing bronchospasm and cough. The exchanger in place will initially touch the carina, a structure that is most sensitive to stimulation. Once the endotracheal tube is removed, the exchanger is pulled back using the numbers as a guide. These correspond to the markings on an endotracheal tube. By positioning the exchanger 2 cm deeper than the endotracheal tube was taped, one can often prevent prolonged stimulation of the carina while avoiding accidental dislodgment. The exchanger may be taped to the corner of the mouth and left in place for 10–15 minutes after extubation to ensure a good natural airway. Ideally, a satisfactory postextubation ABG will precede the removal of the exchanger. If jet ventilation via the exchanger is necessary, a number of precautions can minimize the incidence of barotrauma. A pressure-reducing valve and the shortest puffs possible should be used and adequate exhalation must be ensured.

Aggressive fluid administration may lead to generalized edema in the aortic surgery patient, as can a host of other processes that affect capillary integrity.

Airway edema may result, usually at the level of the larynx. The use of a double-lumen tube during surgery with its larger size, greater challenge of correct insertion, and need for a tube exchange at the end of surgery can also predispose to airway edema. This possibility can be investigated directly by extubating such patients over a flexible fiberoptic bronchoscope, with immediate reintubation if edema is visible. Where the level of suspicion is lower, it is still prudent to deflate the cuff of the endotracheal tube and demonstrate the presence of a leak with positive pressure breaths or the ability of the patient to breath around an occluded tube with the cuff down. In case of any doubt, the tracheal tube exchanger may be used. Known upper airway edema is best treated with short-term steroids (e.g., dexamethasone, 10–12 mg repeated once at 12 hours), upright positioning of the head and neck, avoidance of excessive neck movement, and delay of extubation for 24–48 hours.

It is not unusual for aortic surgery patients to become agitated while still intubated within the first several hours after the surgery. This agitation is sometimes interpreted as readiness for extubation. If a formal survey of extubation criteria has not yet demonstrated readiness for extubation, agitation and delirium should be managed with a review of the adequacy of oxygenation and ventilation, a hemodynamic assessment, and the judicious use of sedatives or analgesics. A state of partial paralysis due to residual muscle relaxation is not an infrequent cause of postoperative agitation. This can be dealt with by pharmacologic antagonism of the relaxant, sedation through the period of partial paralysis or readministration of relaxants. The choice of which option to use will depend on what relaxants were administered, the renal function of the patient, and the state of hemodynamic stability. Reversal of relaxants as usually practiced often results in a tachycardia, which can cause ischemia and confuse the management of the patient. Therefore, for all but the longest acting relaxants, the safest option may be to sedate the patient and allow the relaxant to be metabolized and excreted. The third option, that of continued chemical restraint, is rarely justified unless either severe hemodynamic instability makes the use of any sedation at all impractical or the patient's agitation is compromising mechanical ventilation.

The circumstances that usually prevail in the aortic surgery patient sometimes justify the prophylactic use of supplemental oxygen for days after extubation, especially during periods of sleep. Reeder et al. identified several episodes of desaturation in this setting and found a possible role for preoperative saturation monitoring to identify high-risk patients.[67–69] Their studies extend through the fifth postoperative night. They also found an association between desaturation and ischemic episodes.[70]

Pulmonary Complications

As noted previously, all aortic surgery patients acquire a pulmonary abnormality in the guise of a low-grade (often subclinical) capillary leak syndrome. In fact, Smith et al. found that increased urine protein loss predicted pulmonary dysfunction.[46] Protein is lost from the kidneys by a capillary leak mechanism similar to the endothelial failure seen in the lungs. This process is associated with acute lung injury when it develops to a degree that interferes with oxygenation and ventilation. (Adult respiratory distress syndrome is an older term that is still in common use. Its formal definition differs from that of acute lung injury.) The pO_2 in this condition is less than 60 mm Hg on an inspired percentage of oxygen greater than 0.6 (PEEP 0–5 mm Hg). At this point oxygen toxicity becomes a real risk. The chest radiograph is initially normal but may show pulmonary edema in a matter of hours. Multiorgan failure syndrome often accompanies acute lung injury. It is induced by the generalized defect in vascular endothelial integrity and the ensuing poor diffusion of oxygen-to-target tissues.

Other postoperative pulmonary complications are similar to the general population of sick surgical patients. They include aspiration pneumonia, pneumonia from other causes, congestive heart failure, transfusion associated lung injury, bronchitis, bronchospasm, atelectasis, pulmonary embolism, and pneumothorax.

Svensson and colleagues applied logistic regression analysis to data from their large series of thoracoabdominal aortic surgery patients.[42] They were able to identify chronic lung disease, history of smoking, and cardiac and renal complications as independent predictors of respiratory failure. The elderly, the obese, those with abnormal pulmonary function and those with complex operations are at increased pulmonary risk.[71] Studies such as these are not surprising, but they can contribute to surgical planning. Knowledge of such associations can also be helpful in the postoperative period, e.g., when deciding to prolong mechanical ventilation in a patient who is technically ready for extubation. Kispert et al. found preoperative spirometry to be highly predictive of pulmonary complications in the broader setting of major vascular surgery.[72] With such data, preoperative spirometry can be helpful in predicting and establishing weaning goals.

In addition to the preoperative status and the issue of subclinical capillary leak, there are other issues related to aortic surgery that put the lungs at risk. The finding in the study of Calligaro et al. that use of greater than a certain amount of crystalloid is an independent predictor of pulmonary morbidity is not a blanket endorsement of colloids; it is possible that use of large fluid volumes is a marker of a complex surgical procedure.[43] Paterson et al. showed that reperfusion of the lower limbs after aortic cross clamping is associated with increased synthesis of thromboxane A_2, a possible mediator of pulmonary hypertension and acute lung injury.[71]

The most sensitive early monitors for pulmonary complications seem to be the arterial oxygen saturation and the peak inspiratory pressure. Changes in either quantity, which are not explained by a recent ventilator adjustment, require investigation. The advent of pulse oximetry has superseded the warning value of the ABG, which is still useful in confirmation of the accuracy of the saturation as well as in the assessment of ventilation and acidosis.

Repeated chest radiographs were once a traditional part of the ICU care, but it is difficult to pinpoint their role, if any, as a routine (i.e., daily or twice daily) study. In the presence of stable online respiratory variables and a chest tube drainage system that is properly functioning, a routine chest radiograph should rarely contain surprises. Additionally, while most clinicians consider the chest radiograph to be a gold standard (because of near perfect sensitivity, specificity, and predictive value) for lung consolidation, this turns out not to be the case.[73] Variations in technique, interpretation, projection, and fluid status are partly responsible for these inconsistencies.

Circulatory Management

Interrelationship of Hemodynamic Variables

Circulatory management of the aortic surgery patient consists of maintaining adequate oxygen delivery against a background of circulatory disease typical of these patients, all the while adjusting for perioperative developments.

The most common etiologic factor in aortic disease is atherosclerosis, which is the same systemic disorder that is responsible for most coronary artery disease. Hypertension, an important risk factor for atherosclerosis as well as aortic dissection, is also a systemic disease with multiple pathologic consequences for the heart and vasculature. Diminished cardiac reserve, characteristic of the aortic surgery population, complicates the circulatory management of these patients in the postoperative period.

In this chapter individual aspects of the circulation are discussed one at a time, but this division is highly artificial. There is no individual section below addressing the low-output syndromes. Such sydromes are the topic of this entire section. Low-output syndromes often result in shock, which is the syndrome of inadequate DO_2, leading to microcirculatory failure, metabolic acidosis, coagulopathy, systemic inflammatory response with cellular membrane failure, and a host of organ-specific consequences.

By focusing on individual components of the hemodynamic picture, this chapter does not intend to ignore the excellent work that has established endpoints for multiple variables and then examined outcome. For example, Berlauk and colleagues investigated preoperative hemodynamic interventions designed to achieve a pulmonary artery occlusion pressure (PAOP) of 8–15 mm Hg, a cardiac index of 2.8 l/min/m^2 or greater, and a systemic vascular resistance (SVR) of 1,100 dyne/sec/cm^5 or less (see Figure 11-1).[19] Patients in whom these criteria could be achieved experienced fewer intraoperative events and less postoperative cardiac morbidity.

Years ago, medical students were taught that shock can be classified as cardiogenic, hypovolemic, distributive, or obstructive, with neurogenic and anaphylactic shock falling in the latter category. This scheme is still useful in the differential diagnosis of the initial cause of shock and planning of initial therapy. Almost always, one of these processes will have initiated the low-output syndrome. Unless immediately reversed, however, the fully developed syndrome of shock will ultimately involve many or all of these processes. Myocardial failure can lead to a stiffer myocardium that requires a higher preload to function. In this situation volume replacement will be part of the therapy. Hypovolemic shock often leads to decreased mean arterial pressure and decreased coronary perfusion, provoking ischemia and cardiac dysfunction. All shock syndromes other than septic shock can lead to a septic shock picture if, for example, intestinal hypoperfusion allows the systemic inflammatory response to be activated (see Figure 11-4). Spinal cord damage can result from marginally perfused tissue being further compromised by hypovolemic shock; this results in spinal shock that exacerbates the circulatory failure. The earlier a complete hemodynamic profile is obtained and analyzed, the greater the chance of being able to identify the initiating cause before a mixed picture has developed. Of course, often the initial cause will be obvious.

The diagnosis of the low-flow state involves considering the initial hemodynamic profile and the rapidity of onset of the change. Change is established with reference to the patient's optimal values, not the normal values listed in a book. This evaluation must be done in clinical context—is there bleeding, sepsis, or neurologic damage? The sudden onset of a low-flow state can indicate rupture of an anastamosis under the hypovolemic category of shock or ruptured papillary muscle or ruptured septum under the cardiogenic shock or anaphylactic shock, which is part of the distributive category. Rapid, but not necessarily sudden, onset of shock is consistent with bleeding gastric ulcer, surgical bleeding, pancreatitis, sepsis, and any of the other well-known causes of shock.

The initial hypothesis of the initiating cause of shock is just that, a hypothesis. It is confirmed by evaluating the response to therapy.

Hemodynamic Monitoring

Right-Sided Heart Catheterization

The PAC has been in common clinical use for over two decades. Aortic surgery, however, has been practiced successfully for far longer than that. In 1980, Grindlinger and colleagues published a study on hemodynamic optimization involving a protocol that can be implemented without the data acquired from a PAC.[74]

Have researchers been able to demonstrate improved outcomes with PAC use? In the narrow sense, the answer appears to be no.[75] Interestingly, the clinicians of the world do not agree. The difficulty proving outcome differences with the PAC is widely believed to be due to study design, sample size, and variations in the implementation of this less than perfect tool. A responsible panel of clinical scientists recently provided cautious support for the possibility that the PAC is useful, in an article whose bibliography is an excellent tour of PAC literature.[76] They concluded that any across-the-board statement regarding the usefulness of the PAC is premature.[76] The original trials of supranormal oxygen delivery indices by Shoemaker and colleagues[18] have been supplemented by a number of studies, most recently that of Boyd et al.[17] The precise optimization advocated by these trials is currently possible only with the data provided by a PAC, and the use of the PAC deserves a complete reevaluation in light of the current emphasis on DO_2.

Many aortic surgery patients, perhaps all at some institutions, arrive in their postoperative care area with a PAC. However, this is not a universal practice.[77] Many responsible anesthesiologists limit intraoperative monitoring to a central venous pressure line, and some insert a PAC toward the end of the surgery, believing it to be most useful for postoperative care. Adams et al. recently demonstrated the overall safety of monitoring certain low-risk patients only with a CVP catheter.[78] In a study of similar magnitude and design, Joyce and coworkers also showed no outcome differences between patients monitored with a central venous pressure line and with a PAC when the preoperative left ventricular ejection fraction was greater than 50%.[79] However, in each of these studies fewer than 50 patients were followed. In any study group of less than 100 patients, the incidence of any particular complication is not expected to be high enough to reach a conclusion about the influence of different monitoring modalities. Nevertheless, the absolute usefulness of the PAC in aortic surgery is not established beyond a reasonable doubt. Some aortic surgery patients in some institutions will continue to arrive from the OR without a PAC (see Chapter 4).

With the advent of transesophageal echocardiography (TEE) as an intraoperative monitor, even some anesthesiologists who formerly espoused the universal use of a PAC for aortic surgery now believe that the information available from TEE allows the safe conduct of anesthesia without a PAC. The quality of information, particularly regarding preload, may be better with TEE than with filling pressure measurements.[80,81] Contractility can be roughly estimated from TEE but cannot be directly assessed at all with a standard PAC. As a practical matter, intraoperative TEE does little for us in the postoperative period. Therefore, the TEE has created a new group of patients who may arrive in the ICU after aortic surgery without a PAC.

Until good data are available to the contrary, most if not all postoperative aortic patients suffering the beginnings of a major complication should have a PAC inserted for circulatory management and DO_2 optimization.

It has been said that the most common complication of PAC monitoring is underuse or misuse of the data. While many excellent texts and reviews cover the proper collection and use of PAC data (see Chapter 4), it is worth emphasizing that when faced with virtually any of the complications discussed in this chapter and the next, it is crucial to obtain an entire hemodynamic profile, including mixed venous oxygen saturation (SVO_2), CO, the gradient between pulmonary diastolic pressure and the PAOP, and derived indices. Newer catheters now available have the capability of measuring right ventricular ejection fraction and CO on a continuous basis.[82,83]

Most other complications of PACs are not unique to the aortic surgery setting. Vascular graft infection related to the use of a PAC appears to be rare.[76]

Mechanical ventilation and PEEP should not be discontinued even for short periods while cardiac filling pressures are measured. The numbers obtained while the patient is subject to positive intrathoracic pressures may not conform to normal pressures, but they are the only pressures that matter to the patient. Furthermore, discontinuation of PEEP may be dangerous in the face of lung injury.

The classical way of monitoring SVO_2 is to slowly withdraw a blood sample from the distal (pulmonary artery) port of a PAC for analysis of pO_2. This process is tedious and not free of sampling error. In particular, a partly overwedged catheter tip can easily yield an "arterialized" specimen, giving the clinician a false-negative result. For years now, the oximetric PAC has been available. This device processes a signal from infrared sensors to yield an on-line ratio of oxygenated to deoxygenated blood. Continuous SVO_2 analysis has its own set of problems, including calibration errors, high cost, and the same sampling error that plagues venous blood gas analysis. It is, however, more convenient than intermittent blood gas analysis.

When continuous SVO_2 became available, there was an expectation that it would serve as a marker of CO and patient well-being. This does not hold true, at least for abdominal aortic surgery patients.[84,85] Mixed venous oxygen saturation is not a simplistic stand-alone indicator of well-being: It is a reflection of how much oxygen the body has extracted. This is related to how much was made available (the DO_2) and how much was used at the tissue level (the VO_2).

Clearly, CO and SVO_2 are only two of the many variables involved, and they show a simple correlation only in patients who hold the other variables constant. The extraction ratio relates all variables involved and provides a more complete picture. Bleeding, emerging from anesthesia, shivering, fever, sepsis, sodium nitroprusside toxicity, and arterial desaturation are examples of disturbances that complicate any simplistic relationship between CO and venous saturation. Peripheral shunting, sometimes caused by the use of vasodilators, can lead to an increase in SVO_2 that does not reflect improved well-being. Intracardiac left-to-right shunting can also affect the interpretation of venous saturation in the same way, while right-to-left shunting will directly affect the delivery side.

Mixed venous oxygen saturation, when decreased, should prompt a search for the many possible causes. In particular, the venous saturation, when considered in the context of hematocrit and Hb and CO, provides a rational basis for difficult decisions involving transfusion and manipulation of CO. It should also be remembered that just as decreased arterial saturation is an important cause of decreased venous saturation, the reverse is also true. This is because the fraction of arterial blood, which comes from intrapulmonary shunts, is increased in the surgical patient. The saturation of shunted blood is a direct product of venous saturation.

Perhaps the most glaring weakness of SVO_2 monitoring is the fact that it is mixed. A change in

SVO_2 is nonspecific and tells us nothing about individual organ vascular beds. An unchanging mixed venous saturation does not guarantee that decreases in one area are not being canceled out either by increases in another or by changes in delivery.

When should the PAC be removed in the patient with a stable postoperative course? Patients who have undergone thoracic aortic surgery should have PAC monitoring continued for at least 36 hours. If, after this time, the patient is hemodynamically stable and the volume of sanguineous chest drainage is minimal, barring other major organ system complications, hemodynamic monitoring may be safely discontinued.

In the abdominal aortic surgery patient, the PAC often remains useful through the third postoperative day. Many of these patients experience substantial redistribution of fluid from the intravascular space to the tissues (termed *third spacing*) on the first postoperative day, resulting in a hypovolemic picture. Third spacing is primarily related to surgical trauma in the retroperitoneal space as well as the intestines. We actively warm most of our aortic surgery patients to prevent coagulopathy in the postoperative period, and the resulting vasodilatation may exacerbate the intravascular hypovolemia. Decreased urine output and diminished CO on the first postoperative day are often related to hypovolemia and are best addressed with fluid to replace the redistributive loss. The PAC is of obvious help in guiding fluid replacement. When oliguria is accompanied by normal or low filling pressures on the first postoperative day, fluid therapy is better than the use of inotropic vascular support because fluid addresses the real problem, intravascular hypovolemia. Furthermore, fluid replacement is associated with neither the tachycardia nor the substantial increase in myocardial oxygen demand that are common consequences of inotropic support. However, this fluid must eventually be mobilized into the central circulation and eliminated. Some patients with poor preload reserve may experience difficulties during this mobilization phase, which often occurs after mechanical ventilation has been discontinued. The management of mobilization difficulties includes preload reduction with nitrates and diuretics: the guidance provided by pulmonary artery pressure monitoring is very helpful at this point.

Echocardiography

Imaging modalities are usually thought of as techniques that produce a visual representation of internal pathologic anatomy. Monitoring modalities are those that provide a continuous reflection of physiology. Echocardiography falls into both categories.

We have already made reference to the intraoperative use of TEE. At present TEE is not a practical continuous monitor in the postoperative period. The data of Poterack indicate that TEE is already a fixture in the ORs of U.S. academic institutions where anesthesia residency training is conducted.[86] However, there are currently not enough monitors available in the United States to cover all the ORs in which they would be useful, much less the postoperative units. Given the realities of modern health economics and the high price of a TEE machine (i.e., about $200,000), one would expect the continued penetration of TEE to be slow. The safety of long-term esophageal intubation with current TEE probes has not been demonstrated. Furthermore, at this time TEE is useful only when a specially trained physician is in attendance to interpret the images. This too is an unrealistic expectation for the postoperative period.

It is likely that in the near future, microprocessors incorporated into echocardiographic equipment will be able to automatically process images and yield semiquantitative information useful to nurses and physicians who are not in constant attendance at the bedside. If these developments are accompanied by a smaller, softer probe and a more reasonable price, we may see the "grandchild" of today's TEE functioning as a routine continuous monitor.

In the meantime, the usefulness of echocardiographic examination in the ICU should not be underestimated. The use of transthoracic examination in the ICU is limited by the presence of dressings, wounds, and drains. Additionally, it may be difficult to turn a sick patient to the lateral decubitus position, and mechanical ventilation itself interferes with imaging from the surface. TEE bypasses all of these difficulties and is currently established as a useful tool in the ICU.[87,88] In capable hands, TEE can (1) resolve questions of volume status when the PAC is inconsistent or nonfunctional, (2) confirm the probability of ischemia when the electrocardiogram is unhelpful, (3) diagnose pericardial problems, and (4) clarify functional or structural changes in the aortic valve related to procedures on the ascending aorta. TEE with biplane or multiplane imaging capability provides superb images of aortic pathology, often obviating the need for a dangerous transport and angiographic procedure.[89,90] Echocardiographic examination to answer specific questions should be encouraged.

Hypertension

Assessment

Hypertension is especially dangerous in aortic surgery patients because it may overwhelm a compromised myocardium, disrupt a vascular anastamosis, increase surgical bleeding, increase third-space loses, or induce a new dissection. Cardiac consequences of hypertension include increased myocardial oxygen demand with ischemia, compromised left ventricular function, and the induction of dysrhythmias. The possibility exists that spinal cord tissue that has undergone an ischemic insult may be further compromised by hypertension in the presence of postischemic hyperemia. Likewise, renal and mesenteric tissue have often been subject to a period of intraoperative ischemia; these tissues may be more prone to edema and dysfunction resulting from hypertension. Pulmonary edema, cerebral edema, intracerebral bleeds, and malignant dysrhythmias are also possible sequelae of severe postoperative hypertension.

The approach to the hypertensive postoperative patient involves four stages: (1) verification that hypertension is indeed present, (2) detection and treatment of any underlying cause, (3) establishment of a therapeutic goal, and (4) selection of the specific antihypertensive agent that will do the least harm. *Least harm* in this context refers mainly to the least compromise of DO_2.

Before embarking on the treatment of hypertension, one should ensure that both the invasive arterial pressure and the noninvasive blood pressure determination agree. If they do not, the reliability of both systems should be checked.

Postoperative hypertension in the aortic surgery patient is commonly related to pain, anxiety, primary postoperative hypertension, or preexisting hypertension. Treatment of anxiety and pain are covered in both this chapter and in Chapter 13. The aortic

surgery patient who has undergone concomitant renal artery repair requires special considerations regarding the management of hypertension in the postoperative period.[91,92] Hypertension also occurs after coarctation repair in children (see Chapter 9).

For the patient who is still intubated, both pain and anxiety are treated empirically with supplementation on the occurrence of hypertension. If the treatment of pain and anxiety does not bring the blood pressure down to the target level, it does not mean that analgesia and sedation were not necessary. Administration of analgesics and sedatives should be continued while specific antihypertensive therapy is instituted.

The entity of primary postoperative hypertension is common. It is thought to be due to a surge in plasma catecholamines, which is easily demonstrated in most of these patients.[93] This surge is a stress response. Although various anesthetic techniques are capable of modulating the stress response to various degrees, the complete elimination of this response in 100% of patients is not practical and may not even be desirable. As discussed previously, the stress response does have an adaptive aspect. Complete blockade of these changes may leave the patient without important homeostatic tools necessary to recover from major surgery.

The early postoperative treatment of the patient with preexisting hypertension and the patient without a hypertensive history is quite similar and is discussed in some detail. Diagnostically, in the patient without a hypertensive history one would be more concerned that a rare underlying cause for the hypertension has been missed. The only real management difference between these two situations is that in the previously treated patient there would be a tendency to use the agents that the patient had already been taking. Even when agents familiar to the patient are considered, common sense must prevail. If the patient has newly acquired impaired left ventricular function, a sensible clinician will probably avoid beta-adrenergic blockers or at least administer them with caution, even if the patient had done well with these in the past.

There are many other common etiologies of postoperative hypertension that should be sought and treated. Among these are hypercapnea, abnormally deep position of the endotracheal tube, fluid overload, inadvertent overdose of an inotrope, alcohol or drug withdrawal, undiagnosed pheochromocytoma, and obstruction of the urethral catheter.

Goals of Antihypertensive Therapy

Optimal arterial blood pressures are defined in terms of systolic, diastolic, pulse, and mean pressures, because different values are critical to different organ systems. The adequacy of mean arterial pressure is an important variable for perfusion of the central nervous system and other vital organs. Adequate diastolic pressure is necessary for coronary perfusion because the left ventricle is generally not well perfused during systole. The definition of adequate depends on the patient's underlying vascular health. Most harmful effects of acute hypertension are related to the systolic arterial pressure, the apex of the pressure wave that can put stress on suture lines, and compromised microvasculature. Diastolic hypertension is more closely related to cardiac afterload and wall stress and control of chronic hypertension.

There is, therefore, no single optimal blood pressure for all aortic surgery patients. The patient who is known to be free of coronary artery disease and cerebral vascular disease will do well with systolic arterial pressures of 100 mm Hg and diastolic pressures in the 50 mm Hg range. Of course, the central underlying assumption in caring for aortic surgery patients is that few are free of atherosclerotic disease. Therefore, the ideal blood pressure for most patients is probably their baseline pressure. If the pressure, mean or systolic, drifts below 30% of baseline, it should be supported by the appropriate drug or fluid intervention after determining the etiology by hemodynamic profile.

Systolic hypertension in the previously normotensive patient should probably be treated when it exceeds 140 mm Hg. It is also probably appropriate to treat the hypertensive patient who has been well controlled when his or her systolic pressure exceeds 140 mm Hg, although many would accept a slightly higher pressure, perhaps up to 160 mm Hg. For the poorly controlled hypertensive patient whose systolic pressure is in the 180–200 mm Hg range, individual judgment must prevail. The patients in whom the highest systolic pressures are tolerated are those with known cerebral vascular occlusive disease and uncontrolled hypertension. Conversely, systolic pressures in the 150 mm Hg range should be aggressively treated if it is suspected that this moderate hypertension contributes to myocardial ischemia.

Diastolic hypertension in the previously normotensive patient should usually be treated when it is above 105 mm Hg. As with the systolic pressure, the baseline pressure is a major determinant in the patient with chronic hypertension. Aggressive efforts to lower diastolic pressures may result in myocardial ischemia.

The pulse pressure should not be ignored. A patient with an arterial pressure of 120/95 mm Hg has systolic, diastolic, and mean pressures that are quite acceptable. Flow, however, may be compromised, and there is no real way to know this in the clinical setting. On the other hand, a low pulse pressure is desirable when an aortic dissection is being managed medically or preoperatively. Causes of decreased pulse pressure include aortic stenosis and the use of many beta-adrenergic blocking agents. That is one of the reasons beta-adrenergic blocking agents are the agents of choice for the medical management of aortic dissection.

The patient with new onset central nervous system injury (spinal cord damage or stroke) following aortic surgery presents probably the greatest challenge in terms of setting a goal for blood pressure control. A number of assumptions are operative that may point in opposite directions. One must assume that there is neurologic tissue that is ischemic but not yet infarcted. To this zone of reversible injury, adequate blood flow must be delivered. Although adequate blood flow does not necessarily dictate high arterial pressure, high pressures may be necessary to maintain flow past areas of vascular injury and edematous tissue. It is possible, however, that tissues that are edematous, whether infarcted or reversibly injured, can suffer extended injury in the face of hypertension. Finally, tissues whose arterial tree is in a state of postischemic hyperemia may suffer further injury with hypertension. The problems of hyperemia and edema are combined under the category of reperfusion injury.

In the patient with central nervous system injury, an arterial pressure in the middle range of normal for that patient should probably be maintained. This may be especially challenging if spinal shock is present.

It is only fair to obtain input from the surgical team regarding what blood pressures should be tolerated. They are the ones who know the potential for dissection or suture disruption in any individual patient, and their input is critical.

It is important to remember that for a large subgroup of aortic surgery patients, especially those with mild chronic hypertension or with no preoperative history of hypertension, postoperative hypertension may be a temporary problem and in 3–4 hours one may be battling hypotension and hypovolemia. There is no place for long-acting antihypertensive agents in this setting.

If the patient was on an antihypertensive medication preoperatively, the continuation of the same agent or use of a shorter acting or parenteral agent from the same class is often the best option.

Antihypertensive Agents

The selection of a specific antihypertensive agent is one of many areas in critical care for which physicians often have strong biases unsupported by data. Some of the data that have been published are supported by pharmaceutical companies and may be biased in favor of specific drugs.

Before an antihypertensive drug is used, one should check the patient's hemodynamic profile because the results may suggest a specific therapy. There is usually a choice of appropriate agents. If the filling pressures are high or normal, intravenous nitroglycerin, a venodilator and coronary artery dilator, is a good start. Nitroglycerin functions as a donor of nitric oxide. For this reason, it is effective in the presence of damaged or dysfunctional vascular endothelium.

Although nitrates will usually not be sufficient for the control of severe hypertension, their effect complements other medications, and they may have a favorable effect on the myocardial demand/supply ratio. Nitrates are therefore excellent if myocardial ischemia is suspected, or if reperfusion injury is an issue. Intravenous nitrates are very short acting; therefore, if they are administered and preload drops excessively and a low-flow state is induced, the effect of nitrates is readily reversed by discontinuing the infusion and elevating the patient's legs. Many physicians administer nitroglycerin in a low dose to all postoperative patients with coronary artery disease, even in the absense of hypertension, as long as hypotension is not present. Tachyphylaxis is common with nitrates but is not a problem

in the acute situation; by the time it develops, the hemodynamic conditions of the patient may be radically different.

Calcium channel blocking agents have not been shown to consistently decrease long-term morbidity in cardiac patients. For short-term control of hypertension they are excellent agents. They can be relied on to favorably affect myocardial oxygen supply and demand when the agent chosen is appropriate to the hemodynamic profile. The drugs in this class vary in their control of tachycardia as well as in their degree of direct myocardial depression. Nifedipine is well tolerated in sublingual boluses of 10 mg. This dose will control severe systolic hypertension within 20–30 minutes of administration, and hypotension is relatively rare.

Nicardipine is a new calcium channel blocker of the nifedipine (dihydropyridine) family. Nicardipine is light, stable, and more water soluble than nifedipine by two orders of magnitude, making it practical for continuous infusion. Its elimination half-life is less than 1 hour. Otherwise, its pharmacodynamics are similar to nifedipine. The drug is approved in the United States for the control of hypertension and has been shown to be safe and effective in the postoperative setting.[94] Hemodynamic effects include decreases in SVR and coronary vascular resistance, with increases in cardiac index and coronary blood flow. There is little increase in venous capacitance. Nicardipine is an especially good choice if the heart rate is normal or low because mild, transient increases in heart rate are occasionally seen with it.[95] Nicardipine is capable of producing ischemia by further elevating the heart rate of a patient whose resting rate is already high; the increase in heart rate should not be ignored. As is the case with other vasodilators, these heart rate increases are probably reflex mediated, because nicardipine does not seem to increase serum markers of adrenergic stimulation.[96] In our experience, nicardipine can cause significant decreases in blood pressure when boluses are administered; therefore, it should be administered only by continuous infusion. When boluses are avoided, hypotension is less common with nicardipine than with sodium nitroprusside.

The intravenous formulations of the calcium channel blocking drugs verapamil and diltiazem are not approved in the United States as antihypertensive agents at this time. While they both have an antihypertensive effect, this effect is achieved in part by myocardial depression. Therefore, if either of these drugs is administered to the hypertensive patient in single doses large enough to normalize the blood pressure, unacceptable decreases in CO or increases in cardiac filling pressures may occur. However, if small doses of either of these drugs are titrated to heart rate and hemodynamic profiles are checked frequently, then the point at which myocardial depression starts to occur can be identified and further antihypertensive control can be achieved with a vasodilator. This type of combination therapy is useful in the hypertensive patient with tachycardia, in whom administration of a vasodilator alone may result in further increases in heart rate. Unlike the beta-blocking agents, the calcium channel blocking drugs do not exacerbate bronchospasm.

Virtually all drugs of the calcium channel blocking group, including nifedipine and nicardipine, are negative inotropic drugs. The differences lie in to what degree this effect is evident at clinical doses. The angiotensin-converting enzyme (ACE) inhibitors or the vasodilators may be better choices for the patient with borderline cardiac function.

The beta-adrenergic blocking drugs are useful in the setting of hypertension with tachycardia and well-preserved ventricular function. They have an excellent myocardial supply/demand profile. For the patient with an aortic dissection, the main therapeutic goal is to diminish the rate and force of left ventricular contraction. The beta-blockers are drugs of choice in this setting. Contractility is not usually measured directly in patients; therapeutic goals are defined in terms of decreases in heart rate and pulse pressure.

For most patients almost all beta-blocking drugs are equally good choices. The beta$_1$-selective blocker esmolol is an excellent choice for initiation of therapy. Its short half-life of 9 minutes makes it easy to withdraw if the response is exaggerated. Labetalol, although not selective for the beta$_1$ receptor, has the advantage of having alpha-blocking properties. The predominant action of labetalol, however, is beta blockade. Labetalol is easy to titrate and relatively short acting. It may be administered in doses of 2.5–5.0 mg. The onset of action is rapid, so the bolus dose may be repeated every 2–3 minutes until the desired effect is achieved. Labetalol is conveniently administered by continuous infusion, but it is not an ultrashort-acting agent. If myocardial ischemia is present, it is important to maintain diastolic arterial pressure. Labetalol should be used only if an elevated

SVR is present. For patients with moderate-to-severe bronchospastic disease all beta-blocking agents should probably be avoided, because the selective beta$_1$-blockers are only partially selective.

Because tachycardia is detrimental to diastolic filling and coronary perfusion, there is a tendency to want to use beta-blocking agents in the setting of hypertension and tachycardia, even if the ejection fraction is mildly depressed. Le Bret and colleagues, working with Coriat's group, used TEE to evaluate myocardial function before and after labetalol was administered for postoperative hypertension in aortic surgery patients.[96] They found that as blood pressure decreased, left ventricular end-diastolic area increased. Although the dose of labetalol they used (0.75 mg/kg given over 2 minutes) is more aggressive than the dose we have suggested, the take-home message is clear. In the aortic surgery patient given labetalol (and probably any other beta-blocker), myocardial depression is very real. In some settings, such as with elevated CO or myocardial ischemia, moderate myocardial depression is not a bad thing. Certainly in the absence of frank pump failure, the patient previously treated with beta-blockers may continue to receive them. Stone and coworkers support the salutary role of these drugs in preventing ischemia.[97] Pasternack et al. also were interested in limiting ischemia and found beta-blockade to be well tolerated in abdominal aortic surgery patients.[98] If, on the other hand, one is attempting to support supranormal DO$_2$ to preserve renal and other organ function, the myocardial depression associated with beta-blockade may be best avoided.

The arterial vasodilator sodium nitroprusside is often the first choice agent of surgeons, and this agent still receives favorable reviews in anesthesia texts. It was once the standard against which new drugs were compared.[94,99] Attractive qualities of sodium nitroprusside include efficacy in controlling virtually any hypertensive situation, preservation of CO, and a short duration of action.

In most circumstances, we do not recommend the solo use of sodium nitroprusside. The reactive tachycardia sometimes observed with sodium nitroprusside is confusing and detrimental if coronary perfusion is problematic. There is also some suggestion that sodium nitroprusside, like adenosine, can cause a harmful redistribution of coronary blood flow referred to as steal.[100,101] Sodium nitroprusside and other pure arterial vasodilators may worsen hypoxemia in the patient with pulmonary disease by inhibiting hypoxic pulmonary vasoconstriction. Although cyanide toxicity is rare today, the presence of sodium nitroprusside can confuse the differential diagnosis of metabolic acidosis. Cyanide toxicity is particularly unlikely if the dose does not exceed 4–5 μg/kg/minute or 2 mg/kg in 24 hours.

Nitroprusside is more attractive in combination with nitrates, beta-blockers, or both. Beta-blockers may act synergistically with sodium nitroprusside by decreasing the renin-angiotensin release that occurs with the use of sodium nitroprusside alone. With combination use, the total nitroprusside dose will be lower, and in the case of beta-blockers, tachycardia will be minimized. Other than superb controllability, the most important advantage for nitroprusside is its lack of negative inotropic effect.

Hydralazine is not commonly used as a first-line agent for treating postoperative hypertension. Some of the problems involved with its use include reflex tachycardia, delay in onset time of up to 30 minutes, and a relatively long duration of action. It is not the best of agents in terms of impact on myocardial oxygen demand and supply. Nevertheless, the drug continues to be used in settings where the availability of newer, more expensive drugs is limited, as well as in units that have extensive experience with it. Hydralazine is most effective in settings in which tachycardia is unlikely (i.e., pacemaker-dependent patients, patients who are on beta-blockers, and patients with resting bradycardia), hypertension is moderate, and beta-blockers can be safely introduced if tachycardia develops. Hydralazine is also a reasonable follow-up drug for sodium nitroprusside. After the acute hypertension is controlled and hemodynamics are stabilized, hydralazine in small doses allows the sodium nitroprusside to be safely discontinued.

Phentolamine is a nonspecific alpha-adrenergic blocker. Its antagonism at the alpha$_1$- and alpha$_2$-receptors makes it a powerful vasodilator. It was one of the first vasodilators in use and is still used by some physicians as a specific agent for pheochromocytoma. Reflex tachycardia makes its solo use undesirable in the setting of aortic surgery. When combined with beta-blockade it is actually a good agent that is ignored today primarily because of newer drugs.

Prazosin was popular for a long time as an antihypertensive agent because its specificity as a blocker of the alpha$_1$-receptor allowed efficient mediation of endogenous catecholamine release. It is a long-acting agent that is rarely used in the ICU today.

The ganglionic blocker trimethaphan, still favored by some physicians, has a long record of safety. Compared with nitroprusside, trimethaphan causes little tachycardia and little increase in pulse pressure. Therefore, trimethaphan shares with beta-blockers and calcium channel blockers a special place in the treatment of real or potential aortic dissection. Disadvantages of trimethaphan include ileus, tachyphylaxis, potentiation of neuromuscular blockade, and pupillary dilatation, making neurologic examination more difficult.

The ACE inhibitors are excellent antihypertensives and vasodilators. Agents of this class, which are in common use, include captopril and enalapril. Enalapril is available in parenteral form. These drugs are preload and afterload reducers. While excellent for medical patients with congestive heart failure, these drugs must be used with greater caution in the aortic surgery population. They can cause prolonged hypotension and seem to do so on a regular basis in the OR when administered on the day of surgery.[102–105] Perhaps more serious is the acute reduction of renal function that can occasionally be seen with ACE inhibitors. Renal reserve can be markedly reduced in the aortic surgery population, and renal failure is of course not uncommon. It is probably not fair to blame ACE inhibitors unilaterally, for they can also improve renal blood flow by dilating intrarenal arteries. Currently, we limit the use of ACE inhibitors to stable patients who are already on the drug chronically. Even in these patients, we avoid reintroducing these drugs in the first 24 hours of the postoperative period. As one would expect, rebound hypertension, sometimes associated with the central alpha$_2$ agonist clonidine, is not a common problem for the patient treated preoperatively with ACE inhibitors.[101] The parenteral form of enalapril has only recently been introduced, and ongoing clinical trials with it may justify an increased role for ACE inhibitors in aortic surgery.

The use of epidural blockade, if available, may prevent the onset of hypertension or control postoperative hypertension effectively.[26] The mechanism of action is probably a combination of analgesia and partial sympathetic blockade. If the hemodynamic profile suggests that reduction of either preload or afterload would be beneficial, a bolus of opioid should be administered (or readministered) in an available epidural or intrathecal catheter.[34] If an adequate trial of opioids fails to control the hypertension, an epidural bolus of dilute local anesthetic such as bupivacaine 0.05–0.10% may be appropriate. Partial intrathecal local anesthetic blockade is more difficult to achieve. Neural blockade can exacerbate ischemia by decreasing diastolic arterial pressure. However, neural blockade can also favorably affect myocardial oxygen balance by treating pain and its resulting tachycardia and by lowering afterload if it is elevated.[106–108] The hemodynamic profile is the ultimate guide for therapy.

A number of new agents as well as familiar ones not previously used for postoperative hypertension are currently being evaluated. Fenoldopam, a peripheral dopamine agonist also being evaluated for afterload reduction in low-output syndromes and renal protection, is effective in the treatment of postoperative hypertension.[109] Incidentally, in the small study by Goldberg et al.,[109] placebo treatment significantly reduced blood pressure in 50% of the patients. This statistic should make anesthesiologists think twice about coming to definitive conclusions based on our own clinical experience. The downside of fenoldopam appears to be increased heart rate, which is the weakness of almost all pure direct vasodilators. Since its hemodynamic and renal profile is otherwise excellent, it may prove useful for combination therapy.

The calcium antagonist isradipine can be administered in multiple small boluses or by continuous infusion. It appears to be equivalent to other drugs of its class in treating postoperative hypertension. Increased heart rate can occur, but apparently this is not as common or as severe as the tachycardia seen with familiar agents.[110–112]

Ketanserin is a serotonin receptor antagonist and also a weak antagonist at the alpha$_1$-adrenergic receptor. When administered in the setting of hypertension, ketanserin acts as a balanced venodilator and afterload reducer. It appears to effectively control postoperative hypertension and for this indication can be administered as a bolus followed by an infusion. Although not yet widely studied in the postoperative aortic patient, ketanserin is attractive for use in vascular surgery patients because of its favorable effects on blood rheology. The mechanism of this effect is not completely understood, but ketanserin inhibits the effects of serotonin on platelets. Side effects include a dose-related prolongation of

the QT interval. Its arrhythmogenic properties are exaggerated in the hypokalemic patient, a property ketanserin shares with digitalis glycosides. Aortic surgery patients are especially prone to hypokalemia as some will have been taking potassium-depleting diuretics preoperatively and others will have had diuretics administered as part of the intraoperative renal protection effort.[113]

Adenosine is a powerful vasodilator that enjoys a cyclical revival as an investigational agent to treat hypertension and for use in induced hypotension.[99] It has a good hemodynamic profile and does not consistently increase heart rate. However, the question of benign coronary vasodilatation versus steal and the increased intrapulmonary shunt fraction caused by this agent will probably limit its use.[101,114] When continuously infused, adenosine can also induce intolerable conduction block and unacceptable hypotension. Additionally, there is some question as to whether adenosine may impair renal function.[115] Therefore, adenosine is not an appropriate antihypertensive for the vascular surgery population.

When reduction of SVR is a specific therapeutic goal, there are two broad classes of drugs that are used, vasodilators and inotrope vasodilators (inodilators). There is some crossover, since some drugs initially considered inodilators have been found to increase CO largely by afterload reduction. In practical terms, what separates such a drug from the pure vasodilators may be the relative lack of tachycardia with some of the inodilators. Drugs considered inodilators are discussed later in the section on inotropic drugs.

Just as it is important to consider information derived from the hemodynamic profile in selecting antihypertensive therapy, it is important to recheck a hemodynamic profile after therapy has been instituted. Likewise, ST-segment trending, if available, should be closely followed at this point. Although control of hypertension should prevent or improve ischemia, the determinants of coronary perfusion are complex. Ischemia may unexpectedly appear or worsen because of either increased heart rate or decreased diastolic pressure. Such changes have been reported after administration of nicardipine, a drug known to have a favorable coronary perfusion profile.[95] There is every reason to assume that depending on the hemodynamic profile, almost any antihypertensive drug can worsen ischemia.

Fluid Management and Preload

Fluid Status and Aortic Surgery

When a low-flow state is addressed, preload is the first component of the hemodynamic status to be assessed and treated. The reasons for this are discussed later in the section on myocardial ischemia. Accuracy in fluid management is critical in the aortic surgery patient because errors in too much or too little fluid can lead to compromised DO_2 and myocardial stress or ischemia. After fluid is displaced into the third space, it must be mobilized into the central circulation at a later time. Therefore, the patient who is a "little dry" may be extremely hypovolemic 6 hours postoperatively. He or she may also have congestive heart failure 3 days postoperatively. In the sicker aortic surgery patients, fluid management errors must be recognized and corrected before they trigger a vicious cycle of failure.

Volume Status Assessment

Classical Methods. The assessment of intravascular volume is difficult in the clinical setting. No one parameter is either sensitive or specific, and relying on a single parameter often leads to disastrous errors. Furthermore, cardiac preload and intravascular volume are not the same.

The only assessment that has a chance of leading us in the right direction is collection of as many parameters as possible and assimilation of the whole picture. When individual parameters are not consistent, upgraded information is needed. A central venous pressure line will need to be upgraded to a PAC, or an echocardiographic examination may be necessary.

Examination of fluid balance can be helpful if the patient undergoes elective surgery and has no major recent illness or diuretic therapy. Under these ideal circumstances, if the intraoperative blood loss is well estimated, an intraoperative fluid balance history is a good starting point. In examining fluid balance history, we are likely to err on the side of believing the patient to have a more volume expanded condition than he or she actually has. The reason for this is that on the "balance sheet," the "in" number may be accurately known, whereas the "out" number does not accurately reflect the ongoing third-space losses and low-grade bleeding, both

of which are difficult to measure. A history of recent administration of diuretics or radiographic contrast is a critical component of fluid balance data.

Urine output cannot be ignored, but it is far less helpful than is usually assumed. The hypovolemic patient may maintain adequate urine output if the fluid loss is acute, if diuretics (commonly administered intraoperatively for aortic surgery) or contrast agents are still on board, if serum glucose is above the renal threshold, or if a renal concentrating defect is present. Analysis of urine electrolytes and specific gravity may add some information.

Heart rate and arterial blood pressure may be altered by a host of factors, although the combination of a mid-high normal arterial pressure and a relatively low heart rate suggests that severe hypovolemia is not present. Opioids, calcium channel blockers, beta-adrenergic blockers, conduction system disease, and other vasoactive agents blur the responsiveness of vital signs to volume status.

The presence of generalized edema virtually assures that total body fluid is elevated but says nothing about intravascular volume. Tissue edema is not good for the surgical patient, but it is a fact of life. Tissue may not heal well or hold suture well in the presence of edema.

Laboratory values may not be very helpful in the assessment of volume status. The Hb and hematocrit are of limited usefulness in aortic surgery because bleeding, loss of plasma volume, and expansion of plasma volume may be occurring rapidly and simultaneously. The blood urea nitrogen, serum creatinine, and the ratio of these two may be insensitive in the face of acute renal dysfunction. Serum sodium is of even less value.

As discussed previously, cardiac filling pressures are the most well-accepted parameters for the trending of volume. In fact, filling pressures are influenced by vascular tone and cardiac function and therefore do not monitor volume status at all. As a rule, these parameters, when used correctly, present an accurate picture of right- and left-sided heart atrial pressure. The discussion of factors that disturb the correlation between PAOP and left atrial pressure is left to texts on anesthesiology and critical care. Instead, this chapter focuses on the fact that filling pressures, even when accurately known, do not have a linear or consistent relationship with ventricular preload.[81] The rigorous basic science definition of preload involves the tension and length of a cardiac muscle fiber before contraction.[116] In the clinical situation, preload is the size of the ventricle at end diastole and is related to filling pressure via the variable known as *compliance*. This variable is not constant, easily predicted, or easily measured. Compliance is dramatically altered by acute ischemic changes and chronic disease states. Nevertheless, cardiac filling pressures are helpful when considered in the total context and when their values are trended. As isolated numbers, filling pressures are only helpful when extremely high or low, and they can be misleading. Stable filling pressures do not imply unchanging ventricular loading conditions in the clinical setting.[80]

Newer Techniques. Left ventricular size can be assessed with echocardiography.[117] The reader should not get the impression that echocardiographic assessment of preload is flawless. This assessment is subject to a number of technical problems. Measurement of absolute ventricular volume is complex and imperfect. Estimation depends on proper imaging plane, anatomic variation, choice of geometric assumptions used, and compensations related to contractility.[80,117] When performed correctly, either from the chest wall or via TEE, echocardiography yields one of the best approximations we have of ventricular preload and functional volume status. While obviously not a practical routine continuous monitor, echocardiography is helpful for specific indications. Conflicting information regarding volume status in a critically ill patient and failure of a sick patient to respond to multiple fluid challenges are both reasonable indications for echocardiographic examination. Our clinical experience confirms a number of studies that demonstrate that data derived from a PAC often do not correlate with volume status as assessed by echocardiographic examination of the ventricle.[81]

Systolic pressure variation (SPV) analysis is an excellent indicator of preload and is practical in any mechanically ventilated patient with an arterial line.[118] SPV analysis correlates more directly with preload than with total volume status. In practice, SPV analysis contributes to fluid therapy decisions. The best discussion of this technique may be found in the monograph by Perel and Stock.[47] The physiology reviewed in their book is essential for any critical care physician to understand. Coriat and colleagues have applied SPV analysis to aortic surgery patients and

shown a correlation between the SPV and left ventricular size as assessed by echocardiography.[119]

The basic requirements for SPV analysis are positive pressure ventilation, a properly damped or underdamped arterial line tracing, and a freezable monitor display on which numeric scales can be appreciated directly on the arterial trace. If one uses a monitor without this capability, SPV can often be measured on a paper recording of the pressure wave. The presence of excessively high peak inspiratory pressures (over 30 mm Hg) and a nodal cardiac rhythm may bias the method, introducing the impression that hypovolemia is present when it is not. The use of ventilatory rates over 12 breaths per minute will complicate the assessment. Almost all patients can tolerate having the rate turned down to 10 breaths per minute for the 30 seconds necessary to assess the SPV.

In most patients, the arterial pressure varies with each mechanical breath and settles toward a stable baseline when positive pressure breaths are withheld for a short period of time (15 seconds). The effect of a positive pressure breath on this baseline consists of an initial increase in the systolic pressure followed by a decrease to below the baseline. The systolic pressure then recovers to baseline during the expiratory phase. The early increase is referred to as the delta up (Δ_{up}). The decrease from the former baseline is referred to as the delta down (Δ_{down}).

The sum of the Δ_{up} and the Δ_{down} is the SPV. This will usually be the difference between the highest and lowest systolic pressures seen over the course of one ventilator cycle including the expiratory phase. The Δ_{down} specifically correlates with left ventricular preload.

Subject to the limitations described previously, the complete absence of a Δ_{down} strongly suggests that the patient is either normovolemic or hypervolemic. (One cannot assess the degree of hypervolemia with this technique.) When Δ_{down} is present but is less than 10% of the systolic pressure, hypervolemia is extremely unlikely, and the patient is either normovolemic or slightly hypovolemic. We refer to this state as volume tolerant. The volume-tolerant patient should tolerate small fluid challenges, and in fact CO should improve with fluid. If the Δ_{down} is greater than 10% of the systolic pressure, the patient is significantly hypovolemic. The degree of Δ_{down} under these circumstances is roughly proportionate to the degree of hypovolemia, and successful volume repletion (or discontinuation of preload-reducing agents) should be accompanied by a decrease in the SPV.

It is easier to perform SPV analysis if the sweep rate of the arterial trace is temporarily decreased to the slowest setting allowed by the monitor. This allows one to freeze the display and view two to four times as many waves as one normally sees on the 25 mm/sec sweep speed commonly used. Incidentally, the adjustment of sweep speed also facilitates the measurement of pulmonary artery pressure and PAOP (wedge pressure), especially when attempting to interpret these pressures in light of respiratory variation.

While SPV can be roughly assessed from the plethysmographic tracing of some pulse oximeters, such an assessment is tricky and recommended only to those familiar with both monitors and SPV analysis.[120]

Volume Replacement

Routine Management.   After a complete assessment of fluid status has been made, rational treatment is planned. Hypervolemia is treated with diuretics, nitrates, and, rarely, dialysis or hemofiltration. Normovolemia is addressed by ordering continued maintenance and replacement fluids based on a realistic estimate of ongoing losses with frequent hemodynamic assessments. Maintenance fluid therapy should technically consist of hypotonic saline solutions with glucose and potassium.

For abdominal aortic surgery patients, the loss of fluid from the circulation via third spacing is substantial. Additionally, these patients are often actively rewarmed in the early postoperative period, and this process leads to vasodilatation. Therefore, the abdominal aortic surgery patient is commonly hypovolemic in the early postoperative period. Administration of substantial amounts of warmed fluid may be necessary. Oliguria in these patients is usually due to hypovolemia.

Content of Fluid Replacement.   When volume must be replaced in the aortic surgery patient, which fluid is best? If red cells are also needed then they are the obvious choice. In modern practice, blood or blood products are never given only for volume replacement. The only exception is albumin, which is technically a blood-bank product, but

carries no increased risk of infectious complications. The indications for transfusion and factor replacement are discussed in Chapters 5 and 12.

If blood-bank products are not indicated, the question is whether to use crystalloid or colloid. As has been stated by others, if there were an easy answer to the crystalloid versus colloid controversy, it would have been found by now. The problem with withholding crystalloid as part of the therapy is that as volume shifts in and out of the intravascular space occur, fluid is lost from the interstitial space. Microcirculatory and cellular integrity do not recover unless this fluid is replaced. Accordingly, most experts now agree that a colloid-only approach to fluid replacement is almost never acceptable, except possibly in cases involving severe head trauma with minimal coexisting injury.

Isotonic crystalloids, such as normal saline and lactated Ringer's solution, are acceptable as the sole asanguineous fluid, and many institutions use almost no colloids. Peripheral edema is common when a patient is resuscitated with crystalloids after volume loss, but pulmonary edema is not an automatic consequence of isotonic crystalloid fluid resuscitation. The lungs have excellent defenses against pulmonary edema, but when these are overwhelmed, colloid offers little protection. One may imagine that colloid would protect against washout of serum proteins, but it actually takes large volumes of crystalloid to reduce the concentration of proteins to critical levels.

Advocates of colloid therapy point out that their administration is more efficient because a greater proportion of administered colloids remains in the intravascular space. Additionally, colloids may minimize the problem of peripheral edema. Peripheral edema is usually considered to be a cosmetic issue, but edema may impair wound healing and contribute to skin breakdown. If there is no clinical lung injury, colloids may minimally assist in the defense against pulmonary edema.[121]

The replacement crystalloid of choice is almost always normal saline with varying amounts of potassium added as dictated by serum potassium and renal function. Lactated Ringer's solution is slightly hypotonic but this should not make a difference in moderate quantities. Although the lactate in Ringer's solution is metabolized by a healthy liver to bicarbonate ion, this solution should not be seen as a treatment for metabolic acidosis, which is best treated by addressing the underlying cause. Truly hypotonic crystalloids have a small role in fluid replacement.[122] They predispose to fluid overload, hyponatremia, and pulmonary edema. Some physicians now advocate the use of hypertonic saline, more or less as a routine component of volume replacement.[123]

The replacement colloid of choice depends in part on cost and availability. Albumin, the gold standard colloid, used to be expensive but is now priced competitively with 6% hetastarch (Hespan) in some areas. While albumin administration has been alleged to adversely affect protein synthesis in some medical patients, this does not seem to occur in aortic surgery patients.[124] Hetastarch allegedly contributes to clotting abnormalities, but there is no evidence that this occurs if the dosage is limited to 15–20 ml/kg. Gold and coworkers have shown that a dosage of 6% hetastarch in this range does not cause coagulopathy in aortic surgery patients.[125]

No intensivist needs to be taught the importance of monitoring and treating electrolyte disturbances. The occasional occurrence of severe hypocalcemia in aortic surgery patients is not always appreciated. Not so long ago, calcium was administered in grams during major surgeries as if it were a benign drug, because it was considered to be an inotrope with no negative side effects. As the role of calcium in cellular injury has become clear, most practitioners have become conservative with calcium, administering it only when its use is indicated. During aortic surgery, blood is likely to have been administered rapidly, and calcium-free fluids are likely to have been exclusively used so that all intravenous lines will be compatible with red cells containing the anticoagulant ethylenediaminetetraacetic acid. In many ORs, intraoperative laboratory examinations are done with portable on-site automated analyzers that do not always report serum calcium levels. Serum calcium, preferably ionized calcium, should therefore be assessed for every aortic surgery patient on admission to the ICU. Hypocalcemia should be treated gradually and conservatively.

Serum magnesium undergoes significant shifts in its distribution in aortic surgery patients. Hypomagnesemia is a well-known cause of cardiac dysrhythmias and can also contribute to cellular damage, especially in the face of ischemia and hypercalcemia.

The need for glucose replacement and the amount needed depend on many well-known factors. At one time, administration of large amounts of glucose-containing fluid was routine after aortic surgery. Interestingly, this tendency led to conclusions about optimal tonicity of fluids that are not accepted today but were at the time.[126] Today the implications of the stress response and the potential deleterious effects of hyperglycemia are better understood. Hyperglycemia is avoided for many reasons, including its diuretic effect, potential to compromise wound healing, and possible role in worsening the effects of central nervous system insults.

Preload Reduction

The reduction of preload should be undertaken with great caution, and it should not be assumed that reduction of PAOP to normal levels is required.

Truly high cardiac filling pressures (i.e., PAOP >22 mm Hg) should always be treated. Such high pressures result in pulmonary edema when transferred to the pulmonary vasculature and in fiber overstretch and increased myocardial oxygen consumption with decreased coronary perfusion when transferred to the myocardium.

Available maneuvers to reduce preload include positive pressure ventilation, venodilators, diuretics, inotropes, specific dopamine-receptor agonists, inodilators, and hemodialysis. None of these therapies is mutually exclusive. In some settings, combination therapy may be desirable.

Nitrates are fairly specific for venodilatation and preload reduction at low doses. They should be titrated carefully—if hypotension and tachycardia result, the patient is probably worse off, and therapy should be reassessed. Direct dilatation of coronaries cannot be assessed clinically and should be considered an added advantage, not the goal of therapy. Nitrates have the advantage of not directly causing a diuresis, so urine output remains a useful, if imperfect, indicator of renal perfusion and function. Nitrates do not directly increase myocardial oxygen demand.

Diuretics, particularly the parenteral loop diuretics such as furosemide, are useful if they fit into the plan for renal management. They alter the significance of urine output. Diuretics also decrease total body fluid, which is not a desired result unless the patient is clearly hypervolemic.

Inotropic support, if successful, will reduce preload by improving forward flow. If tolerated, inodilators are the preferred method of support. By increasing the vascular capacitance, inodilators optimize loading conditions at less energy cost to the myocardium than the typical inotrope.

Low-dose dopamine is discussed in Chapter 12 in the section on renal management. It is often helpful for the patient with fluid overload. Low-dose dopamine is an inotrope capable of increasing heart rate and myocardial oxygen consumption. Newer agents that stimulate the same receptors are becoming available. Dopexamine (already released for clinical use in the United Kingdom) is the most promising.

If renal function is severely compromised, hemodialysis should be considered at the first indication that fluid overload, acidosis, hyperkalemia, or hypernatremia are intractable to other methods.

Myocardial Ischemia

Definition of Risk

The aortic surgery patient shares with all vascular patients a high incidence of coronary artery disease as well as a concentrated exposure to events that may precipitate ischemia (see Chapter 2). It is clear that of all ischemic episodes in the perioperative period, those occurring postoperatively are the most significant. Furthermore, most perioperative infarctions occur in the postoperative period, and many of these are painless.[127]

Prevention and Monitoring

The process of preventing perioperative myocardial events begins with the preoperative evaluation (see Chapter 2). Paradoxically, advances in this area have led to an abbreviated preoperative evaluation for certain patients who are thought to be at lower risk.[128] Since the process of selecting patients for various regimens of preoperative screening is by definition statistical, individual patients who in fact have high-risk coronary artery disease may be missed and relegated to low-risk protocols. Vigilance in the postoperative period is a critical safety net for such patients. Awareness of the patient's history should include a review of the intraoperative events. Aortic surgery is, among other things, a well-monitored stress test.

As the importance of postoperative myocardial ischemia is firmly established, current research questions optimal postoperative monitoring and preferred treatment. Physicians need to know who to monitor, what monitors to choose, where to use them, how long to use them, and how to respond to abnormalities.

Details related to monitoring for myocardial ischemia are covered in Chapter 4. Briefly, the monitors used for ischemia detection in the OR include basic electrocardiography, ST-segment analysis, PAOP waveform analysis, and TEE. Symptom assessment is not available in the OR.

The postoperative period differs from the perioperative period in several ways. Although continuous electrocardiographic monitoring during the first postoperative days is almost universal, ST-segment analysis is available only on the newest of electrocardiographic monitors, and such equipment is more commonly available in the OR than in the ICU. Without ST-segment analysis, electrocardiographic monitoring is an insensitive ischemia monitor. Dysrhythmias are often associated with ischemia but are neither sensitive nor specific for it. TEE is not very practical in the ICU, as discussed previously. Symptom assessment should be helpful in the postoperative period. In fact, several factors conspire to make symptoms all but worthless in detecting postoperative ischemia. In the best of circumstances, fewer than 50% of episodes are symptomatic, and most frank perioperative myocardial infarctions (MIs) are asymptomatic. In aortic surgery patients, the patient is intubated for much of the early postoperative period, and aggressive analgesic regimens can hide any symptoms that would otherwise be reported. While analgesic regimens are favorable toward myocardial oxygen balance, they are not a panacea. Therefore, the PAC tracing may be valuable in the detection of subendocardial ischemia. This type of monitoring, however, is not automated and is practical only with exceptional attention to the quality of the tracing.

It would be nice to know which patients, if any, do not have to be monitored for ischemia in the postoperative period. From the plethora of data reviewed in Chapter 2 regarding preoperative evaluation, the following groups emerge: (1) patients in whom coronary artery disease has been excluded, (2) those in whom coronary artery disease has been confirmed and corrected, (3) those who have definite coronary artery disease that cannot be further treated, (4) those who probably do not have coronary artery disease but were not subject to testing because of a (well-justified) conservative philosophy,[128] and (5) those who may have coronary artery disease but were statistically likely to do well and did not require further evaluation. In the second group, the reality is that a majority of patients will still be at some risk, although perhaps lower than before their revascularization. Unfortunately, revascularization is neither perfect nor permanent.

Therefore, all patients, except those in whom coronary artery disease has been excluded, are candidates for monitoring. Ideally, this monitoring should consist of continuous electrocardiography with ST-segment analysis and should be continued for at least 3 days. This goal is practical in the many institutions in which the ICU stay for aortic surgery patients is 48–72 hours. The cost of upgrading old electrocardiographic monitors to instruments capable of ST trending is probably well worth it.

When ischemia is detected, the patient should have a hemodynamic assessment and should be optimized according to the principles outlined in the following section. Preoperative evaluation of coronary artery disease has been discussed in Chapter 2. It is important for the physicians involved in postoperative care to be aware of the results of any testing done. Not all ischemic changes are catastrophic. Longer episodes, lasting 20 minutes or more, have an increased risk of heralding an MI. Short episodes may also be ominous, but for some patients it is normal to suffer from frequent short-lived episodes of ischemia. Many of these episodes occur despite hemodynamics that suggest optimal myocardial oxygen supply-demand balance. It is not known at this time which self-limited ischemic episodes are important. Careful attention to the preoperative history and evaluation will sometimes reveal a pattern of ischemia that can be expected to continue into the postoperative period.

Hemodynamic Goals

Because ischemia monitoring is known to be imperfect, it is important to routinely control vital signs as a precaution against ischemia. By avoiding hemodynamic conditions that are known to upset the myocardial oxygen demand-supply ratio, ischemic changes can be prevented (Figure 11-7). By doing so, anesthesiologists may protect their patients despite their less-than-perfect ability to actually identify ischemia. As mentioned previously, some ischemic episodes continue despite excellent hemodynamic control. The significance of such episodes, particularly the ones lasting only minutes, is unknown at this point.

Coronary perfusion pressure, which should be maximized, is roughly described as the difference between the diastolic arterial pressure and the PAOP. Coronary perfusion itself is proportional to the coronary perfusion pressure integrated over time. Therefore, our goal is to maximize the time during which coronary perfusion takes place and to maximize the coronary perfusion pressure.

The supply side of the coronary oxygen balance is described in terms of perfusion pressure rather than coronary blood flow because the latter does not directly relate to anything that can be measured clinically. What really matters, of course, is oxygen delivery to the myocardium, which is the product of coronary artery flow and arterial oxygen content. The arterial oxygen content is in turn related to arterial oxygen saturation and Hb. When myocardial ischemia is a possibility, a less than adequate PaO_2 (e.g., a PaO_2 associated with an arterial oxygen saturation less than 95–96%) should not be tolerated. Neither can anemia be left untreated. There is a growing body of experimental evidence suggesting that mild anemia (hematocrit <27%) can cause ischemia.[129,130] The current practice of tolerating hematocrits close to 20% is, therefore, intended for healthy patients only. There are no data to support the safety of significant anemia in the patient at risk for myocardial ischemia.

Myocardial oxygen demand, which should be minimized, is elevated by tachycardia, increased afterload, increased stroke work, and, to a lesser extent, increased preload. Any stressor that increases metabolic rate will increase ventricular work. Fever should be aggressively treated. It is interesting to note that hypothermia is now also known to cause ischemia.[131,132] Coronary artery spasm, when present, is the principal reversible change in coronary blood supply related to the arteries themselves.

Coronary perfusion time is maximized by the avoidance of tachycardia, which is the single most devastating adverse condition for coronary perfusion. (This is true because tachycardia also increases myocardial oxygen demand substantially.)

O₂ Supply:

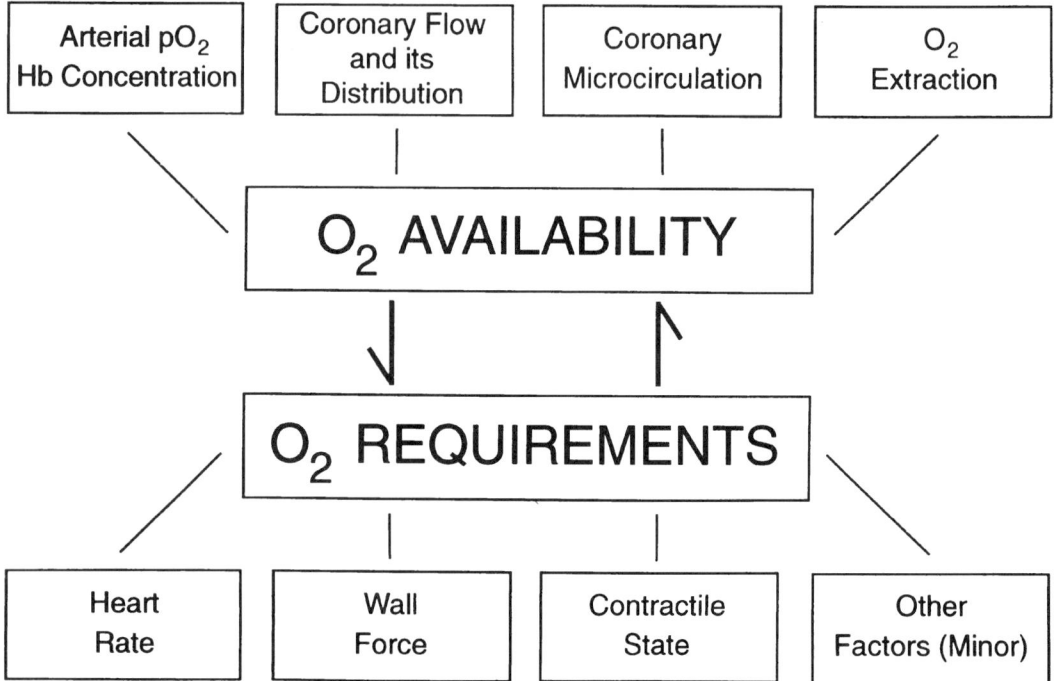

Figure 11-7. Schematic representation of the factors that regulate the demand and supply of oxygen in the myocardial cells. (pO₂ = partial pressure of oxygen; Hb = hemoglobin.) (Reprinted with permission from KT Weber, JS Janicki. The metabolic demand and oxygen supply of the heart: physiologic and clinical considerations. Am J Cardiol 1979;44:723.)

Beta-blockade, if tolerated, is the first-line approach in the treatment of ischemia-inducing tachycardia. Perfusion pressure is maximized by supporting arterial blood pressure when necessary and avoiding excessively high left ventricular filling pressures.

When the goal is ischemia prevention, arterial pressure is best supported by vasopressors rather than pure inotropic agents. Inotropes, by definition, will increase ventricular stroke work. They are also more likely to cause tachycardia. Vasopressors are not perfect; they do not augment CO directly and, in fact, they may compromise it. They also do not augment flow to specific tissue beds. However, they may prevent tachycardia via reflex mechanisms. Vasopressors, such as phenylephrine and norepinephrine, tend to favorably affect the distribution of myocardial blood flow, preserving flow to the vul-

nerable endocardium. If decreased CO is caused by ischemic pump failure, vasoconstrictors may indirectly augment CO by increasing coronary perfusion. Nevertheless, the effect of vasopressors on the coronary circulation cannot be monitored directly, so their use in this setting should be temporary. Known ischemia requiring vasopressor support should prompt cardiac consultation. When inotropic agents are necessary, the choice depends on the hemodynamic profile.

When vasoconstrictors are used in aortic surgery patients, particularly those with known peripheral vascular disease, the surgical team should be informed. Vasoactive agents such as phenylephrine and norepinephrine can potentially compromise flow to the distal arterial tree, usually in the lower extremities. The more distal the anastomosis, the higher the risk. Patients with disease of the renal or mesenteric artery are in the same category.

If arterial hypertension must be controlled, the choice of agents is important. The section on hypertension discusses the myocardial supply-demand profile of many agents in current use.

The physiology as presented previously suggests that low left ventricular filling pressures are good. After all, elevated filling pressures, like tachycardia, are culprits in increasing demand as well as in diminishing supply. In reality, the correction of apparently high filling pressures via preload reduction should be undertaken with caution. A stiff diseased ventricle may require high filling pressures to generate adequate output. In fact, the normal heart compensates for low filling pressures by increasing contractility.[80] This is a mechanism that is not necessarily healthy in the situation of ischemia and may not be available to the ischemic heart. Furthermore, the deleterious effect of high filling pressure on myocardial demand is minimal compared with the effect of tachycardia.

Attempting to improve myocardial oxygen balance by therapeutic reduction of preload is therefore not inappropriate, but it sometimes yields diminishing returns. For example, consider a patient with an arterial blood pressure of 110/60 mm Hg and a PAOP of 20 mm Hg. The patient may be thought to benefit from a lower preload. Assuming a chronically diseased ischemic ventricle, one would not want to lower PAOP too much (15–16 mm Hg is a reasonable goal). If one were to achieve this by infusion of nitroglycerin, assuming that the arterial pressure is not affected, the perfusion pressure would improve by only 4 mm Hg. In fact, most interventions that lower filling pressure also lower arterial pressure. If this occurs, the net gain in coronary perfusion pressure may be negative.

Afterload should be controlled by keeping SVR in the normal range. While modest improvement in myocardial oxygen demand may be achieved by further reductions in SVR, this is often at the expense of lowering diastolic arterial pressure and compromising coronary perfusion pressure.

Left ventricular work can be manipulated when hypertension is accompanied by adequate CO. In this situation, administration of a negative inotrope will modulate myocardial oxygen demand. Agents that accomplish this are discussed in the section on hypertension. Beta-blockers are the first-line ther-

apy but calcium channel blockers, particularly verapamil and diltiazem, also have the required profile. If CO is inadequate and afterload has been optimized, then the inotropic state of the heart must be either left alone or augmented. To avoid too much of an increase in myocardial oxygen demand, inotropic agents that are least prone to cause tachycardia and are most effective at unloading the heart should be chosen.

In patients who are chronically treated with calcium channel blockers, rebound spasm of the coronary arteries is possible. Therefore, these drugs should usually be continued throughout the postoperative period.

All of the previously mentioned hemodynamic goals, as well as aggressive analgesia, sedation, and temperature control are indicated as a routine in any patient at risk for myocardial ischemia. If an ischemic episode is detected, it is treated by more aggressive hemodynamic control and by some of the measures discussed in the next section on MI. One should not hesitate to obtain cardiac consultation if the response to therapy is not positive. This is especially true for the patient who had no cardiac consultation preoperatively.

Postoperative Myocardial Infarction

The diagnosis of postoperative MI is not radically different from the diagnosis of MI in other settings. Symptomatology may be limited by the often silent nature of these infarcts, and by sedation and analgesia. Electrocardiography may be less helpful because postoperative MI is often of the "non–Q wave" variety. Biochemical markers, including the myocardial band fraction of creatine kinase, may be moderately elevated in aortic surgery patients in the absence of any other evidence of infarction; therefore, the implication of moderate enzyme elevations is not straightforward.[133] Higher elevations are significant and may correlate with outcome.[134] Troponin may be more specific than the myocardial band fraction of creatine kinase.[135] Echocardiographic examination will define abnormal wall motion but will not confirm irreversibility. A battery of nuclear scans may be helpful in equivocal cases.

The process of MI should never be considered complete and irreversible. Between infarcted tissue and healthy tissue there is clearly a spectrum of myocardium that is potentially salvageable. Such myocardium is referred to as stunned (postischemic) or hibernating (reversibly ischemic). The intensivist should never give up attempts to improve myocardial oxygen balance and salvage myocardium. All measures discussed in the previous section regarding prevention and treatment of ischemia should be continued in the face of apparent MI.

For decades it has been recognized that perioperative MI often occurs several days postoperatively. Many, if not most, of these infarctions will be due to causes other than poor hemodynamic control. In the past, these infarcts were attributed to inadequate pain relief with increased patient activity, decreased vigilance as patients are transferred out of intensive care, and mobilization of third-space fluid into the central circulation. These factors, which speak to the issue of the hemodynamic aspects of the stress response, are all important.[127] Recently, the issues of pathologic platelet activation, abnormal increases in procoagulants,[136] and persistent elevations in plasma catecholamine levels[137] have received increased attention. The question of which of these factors are significant is relevant because they can all be addressed therapeutically if one is willing to embark on the necessary investigations and pay the respective price. The preventive maneuvers undertaken may address more than one of the possible causes, while the use of continuous epidural analgesia may address several.[11,31]

Aggressive pain management (see Chapter 13) usually pays off in terms of favorable myocardial oxygen balance. Increased attention to preload reduction during the period when third-space fluid is being mobilized may protect against ischemia on the second and third postoperative days. This can be accomplished by the routine use of nitrates.

Given that few studies have addressed the issue of treatment in the postoperative setting, clinical judgment must prevail when MI is suspected. All patients in whom MI is suspected should be treated with supplemental oxygen. Anemia should be treated,[129,130] and hypothermia should be treated by whatever means are available. Hypothermia may be protective of the myocardium when isolated by cross clamping and cardiopulmonary bypass, but hypothermia is poorly tolerated in the ischemic patient.[131] Shivering increases total body oxygen consumption with a concomitant increase in myocardial oxygen demand. Hypothermia also increases catecholamines and other stress hormones independent of shivering.[132] This ef-

fect can also increase myocardial oxygen demand, which may explain the ventricular dysrhythmias seen with progressive decreases in temperature.[132] Fever must also be treated for more obvious reasons.

The postoperative aortic patient with infarction or ischemia should almost always have invasive hemodynamic monitoring. In the postoperative patient with MI, there are too many conflicting influences on the circulation to predict hemodynamic variables. Analgesia should be ensured, usually with opioids. In the awake patient opioids can be titrated to analgesic effect with the cardiac filling pressures as a secondary guide. In the ventilated patient, opioids should be titrated to optimal hemodynamics. The newly adapted modality of thoracic epidural block for the treatment of unstable angina may have some application in this setting if coagulation is intact[106–108]; however, studies have not been performed in the aortic surgery population. Nitroglycerin has generally favorable effects on epicardial arterial tone, left ventricular preload, and collateral blood flow. Preload should not, however, be reduced to the point that CO is diminished. The preservation of renal function depends on adequate CO, as does patency of new vascular grafts and distal diseased arteries. Beta-adrenergic blockers have a favorable effect on myocardial oxygen balance, but again CO should not be sacrificed. The availability of the short-acting beta-adrenergic blocker esmolol allows a therapeutic trial with a short-term commitment.

It is not clear that the presence of ischemia or MI is an automatic indication for attempts at dilation of coronary arteries with calcium channel blockers. Their use is advisable, however, if another indication is present. Valid indications would be (1) the control of hypertension, especially if the patient had been on calcium channel blockers preoperatively, (2) the control of angina, especially angina refractory to nitroglycerin, beta-adrenergic blockers, and analgesics, (3) preexisting knowledge that vasospasm is a major factor, and (4) the control of tachycardia in the setting of adequate arterial pressure and a contraindication to beta-adrenergic blockade.

If the patient had been on calcium channel blockers in the recent past for any indication, it may be prudent to continue these to avoid a withdrawal syndrome. Of the drugs of this class, nifedipine is the only one that has actually been implicated in poor outcome in the setting of acute MI.[138] There is no evidence implicating calcium channel blocking agents in poor outcomes for aortic surgery patients.

There is currently some interest in the potential of calcium channel blockers to preserve myocardium and limit infarct size. This activity has been inspired in part by the advent of nicardipine, a calcium channel blocking agent reviewed previously as an antihypertensive. Currently, nicardipine is approved in the United States only for hypertension. Studies that claim myocardial-preserving or infarct-limiting effects for nicardipine have involved small numbers of patients. The drug is not an accepted infarct-limiting agent at this time.[139]

For the nonsurgical patient with MI, antiplatelet agents, anticoagulation, and thrombolytic therapy are important tools in the armamentarium. The excellent review by Bates concludes that "the increased risk of bleeding from the operative site precludes the use" of these modalities in the surgical patient, a statement that is no doubt true for surgical patients in general.[127] While intensivists are cautious about using thrombolysis in any surgical patient, antiplatelet therapy and heparin are not absolutely contraindicated, and a case-by-case judgment must be made. The surgeon should be part of any such decision. Aortic disease or surgery is a strong relative contraindication to the use of the intra-aortic balloon pump.

Medicine is on the threshold of a number of promising new therapies to limit myocardial infarct size and reverse myocardial stunning or hibernation. Many of these are based on new understandings of the potential mechanisms for various reversible forms of postischemic injury. These putative mechanisms include accumulation of white blood cells at the ischemic site with resulting microvascular dysfunction, free radical formation, increased platelet adhesion, and intracellular accumulation of calcium. The mechanism of leukocyte involvement in postischemic injury relates to the ability of activated white cells to adhere to vascular endothelium, penetrate it, and release injurious substances into vascular and cardiac muscle. Indeed, the malfunction of vascular endothelium in the coronary circulation is the focus of many of the recent advances in myocardial preservation.

Adenosine is widely recognized as an agent with a short in vivo half-life that causes conduction block. Adenosine is currently marketed to be administered as a single bolus as a therapeutic agent for supraventricular dysrhythmia. The conduction block, as well as marked vasodilatation with resulting coronary steal and hypotension, makes the continuous infusion of adenosine impractical. Released endogenously as a by-product of ischemic metabolism, adenosine does have some important myocardial-preserving properties. It appears to act as an antioxidant and also to limit accumulation of white blood cells at ischemic sites.

Acadesine is the most comprehensively investigated agent of a new class of drugs.[140–142] Acadesine is an adenosine-regulating agent. It appears to increase local adenosine levels in ischemic tissues while having no effect on normal tissues. Preliminary clinical trials support the potential of this agent to limit MIs. There are, of course, no data in aortic surgery patients. However, the example of acadesine is mentioned here to give the reader a hint of where the treatment of evolving ischemic injury may be headed.

Other potential therapies being investigated include xanthine oxidase inhibitors, such as allopurinol, and various free radical scavengers. The mortality of perioperative MI was once as high as 50%. Although current mortality is clearly lower, an aggressive approach to treatment is still warranted. If the symptoms or signs of further ischemia cannot be controlled with the therapy outlined, emergency cardiac catheterization is indicated. Angioplasty, when practical, is an attractive alternative to emergency surgical revascularization.

Tachycardia

A particularly vexing problem in the postoperative setting is persistent tachycardia. Tachycardia is common in postoperative vascular patients and is particularly malignant in the (coronary) ischemic patient because of the associated increase in myocardial oxygen demand and simultaneous decrease in supply. Most texts point out that sinus tachycardia is usually a marker of an underlying stress response rather than a primary dysrhythmia. The standard list of underlying causes includes hypoxemia, ischemia, pain, anemia, hypovolemia, hypercarbia, urinary obstruction, anxiety, sepsis, effect of catecholamines, and so on. A category of tachycardias that encompasses some of the previously mentioned items is failure to optimize hemodynamics and maximize oxygen delivery.

The problem is that, e.g., occasionally one has searched for and treated all possible underlying causes and the heart rate is still 138 bpm. In such a case, further treatment options are surprisingly limited. Tachycardia is difficult to treat because it is an appropriate response to low stroke volume and low output. CO must ultimately match metabolic demand, a variable that we cannot really control. Metabolic rate may be grossly elevated in the sick patient. If cardiac reserve is limited because of depressed ejection fraction, tachycardia may be the only way to match CO with systemic oxygen demand. While an honest assessment demands ambivalence regarding the treatment of tachycardia, it is probably deadly in the face of myocardial ischemia.

Fluid challenge is an obvious first step, but these patients are often in varying degrees of congestive heart failure and cannot tolerate further volume expansion. Still, one should be flexible regarding cardiac filling pressures. If PAOP is 19 mm Hg in the face of tachycardia, a fluid challenge to elevate PAOP to 21–22 mm Hg can be worthwhile. In this situation, opioids, especially the newer synthetic members of the fentanyl family, have the property of slowing heart rate in the perioperative setting and should be tried. They should be administered at least until pain is absent. In the ventilated patient, opioids should be aggressively administered titrating to hemodynamic variables. Opioids, however, are not effective in controlling tachycardia related to stress and hypermetabolism. The use of beta-adrenergic blockers may be prevented by left ventricular dysfunction. If CO is in the low normal range, a cautious trial of esmolol is acceptable. In situations in which beta-blockade is deemed too dangerous, digitalization with gradual loading and careful attention to electrolyte balance is an acceptable option. Renal function must be considered in the later stages of digoxin loading and in the determination of a maintenance dosage. If all else fails, a cautious trial of a calcium channel blocker can be considered. Although verapamil shares with beta-blockers the undesirable effect of cardiac depression, at low doses (increments of 0.01 mg/kg) it is often tolerated and can bring about impressive reductions in heart rate. Verapamil does not exacerbate bronchospasm in the patient with obstructive lung disease and serum levels can be maintained

with an infusion. Diltiazem, a drug with less negative inotropic effect than verapamil at clinical dosages, may be even more effective.

Blunt trauma and deceleration injuries are among the causes of disruption to the thoracic aorta and aortic dissections. The original presentation of these injuries may have been dramatic or insidious. Either way, a myocardial contusion may have been missed initially. Myocardial contusions are a consequence of the force transmitted to the heart from either a blunt collision or an abrupt change in velocity. They produce myocardial injury either directly or through ischemia induced by traumatic disruption of a coronary artery with thrombosis. The consequences of a myocardial contusion are not unlike the complications of an MI.[143] A high index of suspicion that myocardial contusion is present must be maintained in any trauma patient. The diagnosis is confirmed by elevation of the MB fraction of creatine kinase in the serum, changes in the electrocardiogram, and abnormalities of ventricular wall motion as demonstrated by a noninvasive cardiac examination. Supportive treatment may include antidysrhythmic therapy, pacing, and support of low CO by therapy outlined in a following section. It is the rare patient who requires surgical intervention for coronary disruption or ventricular aneurysm.

Myocardial Failure

Although cardiogenic shock may result from disasters involving the integrity of the valves, papillary muscles, and ventricular walls, the most common cause is failure of contractility. Contractility is the force that the ventricle is capable of generating independent of loading conditions.

Contractility is usually not monitored directly. The closest we come today to clinically evaluating contractility is to estimate the vigor of wall motion, which can be done by echocardiography. However, this estimate is actually quite sensitive to loading conditions. Our approach to contractility is therefore more pragmatic than it is scientifically rigorous. In a practical sense, when CO is inadequate after preload, afterload, and heart rate have all been optimized, contractility is what is left to improve.

Another way of approaching contractility is through ventricular function curves (Figure 11-8). Contractility is the variable that, when de-

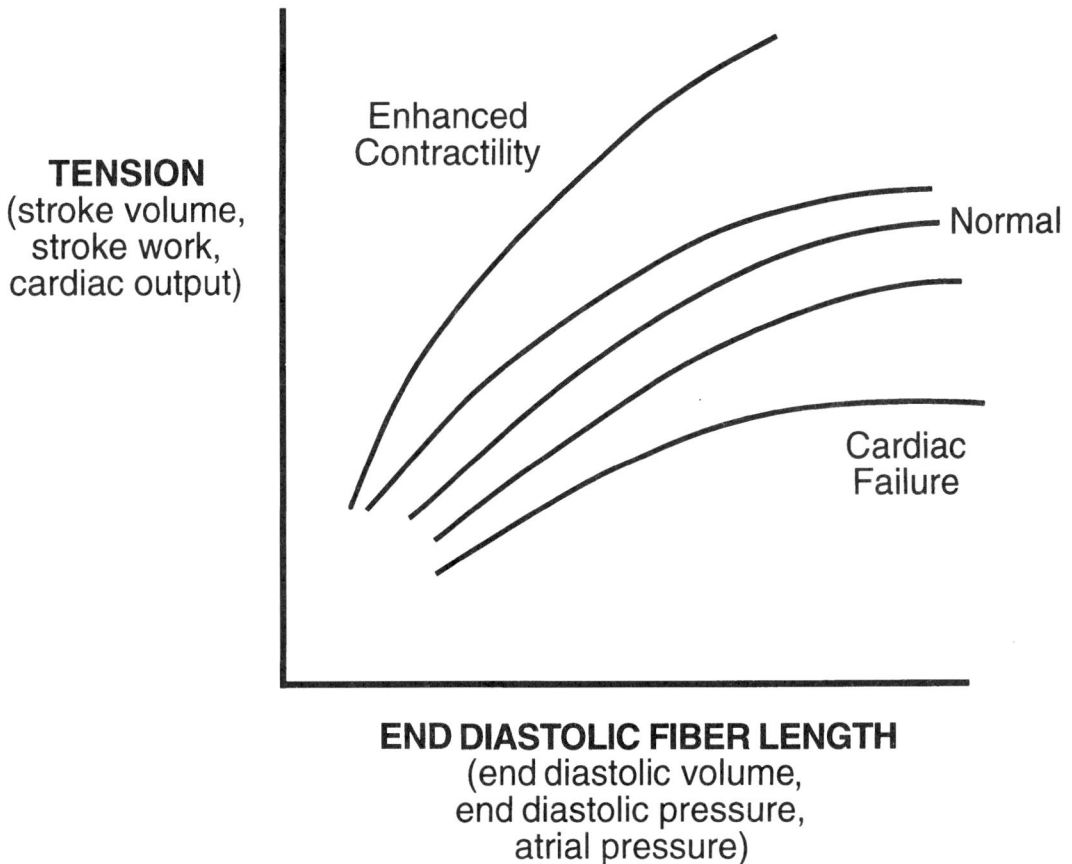

Figure 11-8. A "family" of ventricular function curves shows the relationship between ventricular wall tension and diastolic fiber length. Interventions that involve manipulation of venous return, via changes in intravascular volume or venous tone, tend to move the functional status of the heart along a particular curve. Interventions that affect contractility will tend to shift the curve. (Reprinted with permission from JN Cohn, JA Franciosa. Vasodilator therapy of cardiac failure. N Engl J Med 1977;297:27. Massachusetts Medical Society, Waltham, MA.)

pressed, is responsible for diminished CO at constant loading conditions.

Etiology and Diagnosis

The etiology of myocardial failure in the aortic surgery patient will not always be clear. Ischemia or related postischemic dysfunction must be assumed to be present unless the patient is among the few who have had coronary artery disease excluded by diagnostic studies. Ischemic syndromes can occur even in patients with normal coronary arteries by angiography results and may be related to a number of factors including coronary spasm and ischemic dysfunction of the smaller resistance ves-

sels. It is not uncommon for hypertensive patients to have anginal syndromes with normal coronary angiography. The ability of the patient with hypertensive cardiomyopathy to increase contractility to meet the demands of the stressed perioperative state is diminished; the same is true of severe or long-standing valvular heart disease, idiopathic cardiomyopathy, and congenital heart disease.

For the patient who underwent ascending aortic surgery, long cross clamp times and inadequate myocardial protection may result in myocardial dysfunction in the early postoperative period. In fact, some degree of myocardial dysfunction probably occurs after any period of cardiopulmonary bypass, regardless of how short and how aggressive the attempts at myocardial preservation are. The syndrome of *stunned myocardium* is a special case of postischemic reperfusion injury. With this syndrome, recovery generally takes hours to days and is probably facilitated by minimizing ventricular stroke work while avoiding further ischemic damage. Stunning is also seen with unstable angina and after non-surgical revascularization techniques such as angioplasty and fibrinolytic therapy. The term *hibernating myocardium* refers to myocardium that is ischemic but still partly functional. Recovery is possible for such tissue, but it takes longer than recovery from stunning and depends on meticulous attention to detail in optimizing the supply-demand balance. The differentiation between stunned and hibernating myocardium is not always possible in the clinical setting because it depends on evidence of ongoing ischemia such as ST-segment abnormalities.

The profile of any disease involving ventricular hypertrophy is similar to ischemia at the cellular level. Hypertrophied tissue is at a greater mean distance from nutrient capillaries, and ventricular hypertrophy does not involve a parallel increase in blood supply. Additionally, almost all causes of ventricular hypertrophy can be associated with abnormal vascular endothelial function, which involves poor vascular adaptability to stress states.

A dilated ventricle is also a dysfunctional pump. Such a ventricle is not only weaker than a normal ventricle, but it also functions at higher wall tension, which increases oxygen demand. Therefore, myocardial oxygen demand is almost always an issue that must temper our use of inotropic agents. One is tempted to cite the young, previously healthy patient as an exception, but even such a patient would have diminished reserves in terms of myocardial supply-demand balance if shock had been present for any length of time. This does not mean that inotropic agents are to be avoided when ischemia is a factor. Inadequate CO itself compromises coronary perfusion as well as other vulnerable tissues; therefore, it cannot be allowed to persist. Furthermore, inotropic agents may be helpful in recruiting stunned (postischemic) myocardium.

The differentiation of right- and left-sided ventricular failure is based on clinical data that physicians, for the most part, are constantly assessing. The main tool for ongoing evaluation, the PAC, is a right-sided heart catheter. Therefore, physicians are constantly deducing left-sided heart functional status from the PAC, and with the exception of PAOP, all data from the PAC directly reflect right-sided heart function. The two ventricles depend on one another and interact in all pathologic states. When the entity of right-sided heart failure is invoked, the reference is to primary right-sided pathology, which can be induced by mitral valve disease, right coronary ischemia, chronic pulmonary disease, and pulmonary hypertension.

The comprehensive treatment of isolated or dominant right-sided heart failure is beyond the scope of this chapter. The best source we know of is the chapter by Hines and Barash in Kaplan's *Cardiac Anesthesia*.[144]

Inotropic Support

The definition of myocardial failure depends on prior optimization of loading conditions. The heart must be functioning at optimal preload (venous return) before inotropic drugs will be effective, because, regardless of how vigorously it contracts, the ventricle will not increase output if there is no blood to squeeze against. However, it is the optimization (reduction) of afterload that can improve CO with a net decrease in myocardial oxygen demand. The drugs used for loading condition optimization have all been discussed previously. As is true for ischemia, the target preload must be on the high side. A failing myocardium will almost always be stiff and function high on its ventricular function curve.

Afterload should be manipulated, using short-acting vasodilators by infusion to experiment with various levels of SVR. Many patients will be found to be functioning at an abnormally high SVR. Patients who are septic and those in whom neural blockade has been instituted may need no vasodilators and may even require vasoconstrictors.

Nonpharmacologic Measures. In the face of apparent myocardial failure, oxygenation should be maximized by increasing the FIO_2 if necessary. For the short-term period of initial evaluation and optimization, oxygen toxicity is not a concern.

At all but the lowest end of the spectrum, CO should only be considered in relation to the body's need and cannot be considered inadequate in isolation. Therefore, analgesia and sedation should be ensured. The work of breathing should be minimized by adjusting the ventilator to provide virtually total ventilatory support.

Metabolic acidosis is one of the hallmarks of shock. It is both a marker and a modulator in that the myocardial response to catecholamines (both endogenous and pharmacologic) is diminished in the face of acidosis. Metabolic acidosis may not be totally correctable until the myocardial failure is treated, which is a no-win situation. However, metabolic acidosis should be compensated as much as possible by hyperventilation. If a pH greater than 7.22–7.25 cannot be achieved with hyperventilation, sodium bicarbonate should be administered with the goal of correcting the pH to 7.2 or higher.

Serum potassium should be corrected to the low-normal range, because the ischemic failing myocardium is already at increased risk of malignant dysrhythmia without help from electrolyte disturbances. Hyperkalemia is treated with sodium bicarbonate, infusion of insulin and glucose, and ion exchange resin if indicated. If necessary, hemodialysis should be instituted to address the acidosis and fluid overload, as well as the hyperkalemia.

As noted previously, low serum magnesium should be treated by intravenous magnesium sulfate, with 1–2 g repeated as necessary. Magnesium is a modulator of membrane stability as well as of calcium balance.

Frank hypocalcemia, measured as low ionized calcium, should be treated by intravenous calcium chloride or calcium gluconate. If myocardial failure is severe, infusion of calcium will result in increased blood pressure, but this is temporary. In terms of cellular damage, calcium may adversely affect cellular integrity; therefore, its administration should not be repeated indiscriminately.

One should double-check to be certain that no negative inotropes are being administered. Calcium channel blockers as well as beta-adrenergic blockers may fall in this category, as do barbiturates and some class 1 antidysrhythmic agents.

Inotropic Drugs.   When inotropic support is necessary, the important variables in choosing an agent are the heart rate and the SVR. Inotropic agents are broadly classified as those that come with vasodilatation and those that are also vasopressors. In the case of the catecholamines, the same drug may be in several categories depending on the dose. The inodilators include dopamine at low doses (in the

"renal dopamine" range), epinephrine at low doses, dobutamine, dopexamine, isoproterenol, amrinone, milrinone, and a number of investigational agents.

Isoproterenol is a sympathomimetic agent with a pure beta-receptor effect, affecting both $beta_1$ and $beta_2$ receptors. It consistently causes tachycardia and often causes dysrhythmia. Hypotension is also not uncommon. Today this drug is not a first-line inotrope.

The actions of dopamine are mediated by both direct receptor agonism and release of endogenous mediators. At low doses dopamine is excellent in that it may have a "double indication." Its possible use in the maintenance of renal function is discussed in Chapter 12. As an established drug it is cost effective and has a long record of safety. The original inodilator was a combination of dopamine and sodium nitroprusside. As an inodilator, the synthetic drug dobutamine is a more versatile agent. It maintains its vasodilator properties at higher doses and does not depend on intrinsic release of mediators for its action. Some clinicians believe that, when compared with dopamine, dobutamine is more of a pulmonary vasodilator. Both dopamine and dobutamine can cause tachycardia at higher doses, but not as readily as does isoproterenol. Dobutamine may fail to support arterial blood pressure in the face of hypotension even as it augments CO. Therefore, in the presence of hypotension, dopamine or norepinephrine may be better choices.

Epinephrine is a powerful inotrope but not reliable as a vasodilator. Dopexamine is discussed later in the context of its renal effects (see Chapter 12). It also has weak inotropic effects. Its role is not yet clear but it appears to be an inodilator with fewer side effects than older agents.

In the phosphodiesterase inhibitor (PDEI) class, amrinone and more recently milrinone are useful noncatecholamine inodilators. As PDEI agents, these drugs depend neither on intrinsic catecholamine release nor on adrenergic receptors for their action. The dilator effect of these drugs is potent, and hypotension sometimes limits their use. In the face of ischemia (confirmed or suspected), hypotension negatively affects coronary perfusion out of proportion to any decrease in cardiac work load. The hypotension is sometimes most acute after the loading dose of these agents. In the ICU, loading must be accomplished cautiously. These drugs may cause less tachycardia than the catecolamine analogues.

Because the site of action of PDEI drugs differs from the catecholamine agents, the two classes of drugs may be used in combination with synergistic effects. The combination of milrinone and norepinephrine is particularly useful when milrinone alone results in hypotension or an inadequate improvement in CO. Norepinephrine, via its alpha-agonist actions, counteracts the hypotension seen with milrinone, while the beta-agonist actions of norepinephrine add to the inotropic effects of milrinone. Like dobutamine, the PDEI drugs may show specific benefit if pulmonary hypertension is prominent.

The main inotropic vasopressors in current use are norepinephrine and epinephrine. Phenylephrine is a pure vasopressor that is discussed here for lack of a section on pure vasopressors.

Norepinephrine is a potent agonist at the $alpha_1$-adrenergic receptor, and it is a powerful $beta_1$ agonist. True to this profile, it is an inotrope with prominent vasoconstrictor properties. Patients with normal and elevated SVRs generally do not do well on norepinephrine for prolonged periods. In such patients, SVR increases further and organ blood flow decreases. While norepinephrine elevates arterial pressure in most patients, this is sometimes a cosmetic change not reflective of improved well-being. If hypotension and low flow are accompanied by low SVR and low CO despite adequate preload, norepinephrine may be the agent of choice. In this setting, it has a good anti-ischemic profile, improving coronary perfusion pressure while not usually causing tachycardia. Norepinephrine is also excellent in combination with inodilators. The type of hemodynamic profile appropriate for norepinephrine also occurs in sepsis, spinal shock, neural blockade, and circulatory failure secondary to acidosis, especially if tachycardia and myocardial failure are a problem.

Norepinephrine has been feared by some physicians for many years and seen as an agent of last resort. This is mainly because of the fact that its vasoconstrictor properties adversely affect flow to the kidneys and intestine. This is a legitimate concern and it should make us think twice regarding its prolonged use in the aortic surgery patient. For short-term use, this concern is less critical. In addition, low-dose dopamine may provide some protection against these adverse effects on renal and mesenteric blood flow.[145] Norepinephrine will certainly buy time in the setting of acute shock, pre-venting septic shock from evolving into combined septic-cardiogenic shock while other therapy is contemplated. There is long experience in cardiac surgery patients demonstrating that the vasoconstrictor effect of norepinephrine at least does not compromise coronary flow. While norepinephrine often does not cause tachycardia, it certainly is capable of elevating heart rate.

Epinephrine is useful both as a first-line inotrope and as an inotrope-vasoconstrictor. At low doses (e.g., 50 ng/kg/minute) the beta-receptor agonism of epinephrine predominates. Tachycardia is not inevitable at this low dose, and sometimes heart rate may actually decrease. This probably occurs because the VO_2 is being accommodated at a better stroke volume, requiring a lower rate. When tachycardia does occur, an alternate inotropic drug should be tried.

At higher doses (i.e., 100–300 ng/kg/minute) the combined stimulation of all adrenergic receptors with epinephrine yields a powerful inotropic effect, usually with chronotropy, along with arterial vasoconstriction and shunting of flow from splanchnic beds to heart and brain. This profile indicates that the drug is useful in acute vascular collapse. Epinephrine is also indicated for catastrophic bradycardia. Its complications are similar to norepinephrine, with the most prominent difference being that tachycardia is more common with epinephrine, probably because of a slightly different adrenergic agonism profile.

Phenylephrine is a pure peripheral vasopressor with no inotropic effect. It causes no tachycardia and, in fact, will usually decrease heart rate by reflex mechanisms. It is more consistent in this effect than norepinephrine. Phenylephrine, like epinephrine, can be administered by boluses or by continuous infusion. Its effect actually mimics that of fluid loading, but the effect is achieved faster and without the risk of fluid overload. Phenylephrine is often used to buy time while hypovolemic shock is treated. Its anti-ischemic profile is believed to be favorable, but this is not well established. Apparently, the induced vasoconstriction affects the coronaries but causes a favorable redistribution of flow to the most vulnerable areas rather than a net decrease in flow.

Digitalis glycosides allow for increased influx of intracellular calcium resulting in augmented contractility. These drugs are still considered to be excellent agents for supraventricular tachycardias, but they have a limited role as inotropes. Their effect is slow in onset compared with other drugs we have discussed, and they do not permit fine adjustment of inotropic support. While digitalis glycosides are not contraindicated, they do not play a role in acute inotropic support. For the patient already receiving it, digoxin may be continued in the postoperative period subject to judgments based on heart rate and possibly serum digoxin level.

Summary

The cardiopulmonary care of the postoperative aortic surgery patient focuses on balance. These patients, when suffering almost any postoperative complication, benefit from supporting the maximal CO and oxygen delivery that can be achieved without undue challenge to myocardial oxygen demand. Data provided by hemodynamic monitoring suggest the building blocks of this support.

Dysfunction of specific end organs in the setting of aortic surgery is usually ischemic dysfunction. When such a circumstance is present, the clinician may elect to risk working the myocardium harder to avoid a deadly organ failure syndrome. The particulars of these syndromes in their early stages are the subject of Chapter 12.

References

1. Campbell WB, Ballard PK, Goodman D. Intensive care after abdominal aortic surgery. Eur J Vasc Surg 1991;5:665.
2. Whittemore AD, Clowes AW, Hechtman HB, Mannick JA. Aortic aneurysm repair. Ann Surg 1980;192:414.
3. Olsen PS, Schroeder T, Agerskov K, et al. Surgery for abdominal aortic aneurysms. A survey of 656 patients. J Cardiovasc Surg (Torino) 1991;32:636.
4. Boucher CA, Brewster DC, Darling RC, et al. Determination of cardiac risk by dipyridamole-thallium imaging before peripheral vascular surgery. N Engl J Med 1985;312:389.
5. Krupski WC, Layug EL, Reilly LM, et al. Comparison of cardiac morbidity between aortic and infrainguinal operations. Study of Perioperative Ischemia (SPI) Research Group. J Vasc Surg 1992;15:354.
6. Rogers MC, Tinker JH, Covino BG, Longnecker DE. Principles and Practice of Anesthesiology. St. Louis: Mosby–Year Book, 1993.
7. Miller RD. Anesthesia (4th ed). New York: Churchill Livingstone, 1994.
8. Brimacombe J, Berry A. A review of anaesthesia for ruptured abdominal aortic aneurysm with special emphasis on preclamping fluid resuscitation. Anaesth Intensive Care 1993;21:311.
9. Verwaal VJ, Wobbes T, Koopman van Gemert AW, et al. Effect of perioperative blood transfusion and cell saver on the incidence of postoperative infective complications in patients with an aneurysm of the abdominal aorta. Eur J Surg 1992;158:477.
10. Rice K, Hollier LH, Money SR, et al. Financial impact of thoracoabdominal aneurysm repair. Am J Surg 1993;166:186.
11. Mangano DT, Silciano D, Hollenberg M, et al. Postoperative myocardial ischemia. Therapeutic trials using intensive analgesia following surgery. The Study of Perioperative Ischemia (SPI) Research Group. Anesthesiology 1992;76:342.
12. Clowes GHA Jr, Del Guercio LRM. Circulatory response to trauma of surgical operations. Metabolism 1960;9:67.
13. Shoemaker WC. Cardiorespiratory patterns of surviving and non-surviving postoperative surgical patients. Surg Gynecol Obstet 192;134:810.
14. Bland RD, Shoemaker WC, Shabot MM. Physiologic monitoring goals for the critically ill patient. Surg Gynecol Obstet 1978;147:833.
15. Deitch EA. Multiple organ failure, pathophysiology and potential future therapy. Ann Surg 1992;216:117.
16. Dahn MS, Lange P, Lobdell K, et al. Splanchnic and total body oxygen consumption differences in septic and injured patients. Surgery 1987;101:69.
17. Boyd O, Grounds RM, Bennett ED. A randomized clinical trial of the effect of deliberate perioperative increase of oxygen delivery on mortality in high-risk surgical patients. JAMA 1993;270:2699.
18. Shoemaker WC, Appel PL, Kram HB, et al. Prospective trial of supranormal values of survivors as therapeutic goals in high-risk surgical patients. Chest 1988;94:1176.
19. Berlauk JF, Abrams JH, Gilmour IJ, et al. Preoperative optimization of cardiovascular hemodynamics improves outcome in peripheral vascular surgery. Ann Surg 1991;214:289.
20. Yu M, Levy MM, Smith P, et al. Effect of maximizing oxygen delivery on morbidity and mortality rates in critically ill patients: a prospective, randomized, controlled study. Crit Care Med 1993;21:830.
21. Hayes MA, Timmins AC, Yau EHS, et al. Elevation of systemic oxygen delivery in the treatment of critically ill patients. N Engl J Med 1994;330:1717.
22. Fiddian-Green RG. Associations between intramucosal acidosis in the gut and organ failure. Crit Care Med 1993;21:103.
23. Faure H, Peyrin JC, Richard MJ, Favier A. Parenteral supplementation with zinc in surgical patients corrects

postoperative serum zinc drop. Biol Trace Elem Res 1991;30:37.

24. Chernow B, Alexander HR, Smallridge RC, et al. Hormonal responses to graded surgical stress. Arch Intern Med 1987;147:1273.

25. Blake DW, McGrath BP, Donnan GB, et al. Influence of cardiac failure on atrial natriuretic peptide responses in patients undergoing vascular surgery. Eur J Anaesthesiol 1991;8:365.

26. Kataja J. Thoracolumbar epidural anaesthesia and isoflurane to prevent hypertension and tachycardia in patients undergoing abdominal aortic surgery. Eur J Anaesthesiol 1991;8:427.

27. Bassey PQ, Watters JM, Aoki TT, Wilmore DW. Combined hormonal infusion simulates the metabolic response to injury. Ann Surg 1984;200:264.

28. Baron J, Bertrand M, Barre E, et al. Combined epidural and general anesthesia versus general anesthesia for abdominal aortic surgery. Anesthesiology 1991;75:611.

29. Cuschieri RJ, Morran CG, Howie JC, McArdle CS. Postoperative pain and pulmonary complications: comparison of three analgesic regimens. Br J Surg 1985;72:495.

30. Yeager MP, Glass DD, Neff RK, Brinck-Johnson T. Epidural anesthesia and analgesia in high-risk surgical patients. Anesthesiology 1987;66:729.

31. Tumen KJ, McCarthy RJ, March RJ, et al. Effects of epidural anesthesia and analgesia on coagulation and outcome after major vascular surgery. Anesth Analg 1991;73:696.

32. Christopherson R, Beattie C, Frank SM, et al. Perioperative morbidity in patients randomized to epidural or general anesthesia for lower extremity vascular surgery. The Perioperative Ischemia Randomized Anesthesia Trial Study Group. Anesthesiology 1993;79:422.

33. Quintin L, Bonnet F, Macquin I, et al. Aortic surgery: effect of clonidine on intraoperative catecholaminergic and circulatory stability. Acta Anaesthesiol Scand 1990;34:132.

34. Breslow MJ, Jordan DA, Christopherson R, et al. Epidural morphine decreases postoperative hypertension by attenuating sympathetic nervous system hyperactivity. JAMA 1989;261:3577.

35. Modig J, Borg T, Karlstrom G, et al. Thromboembolism after total hip replacement: role of epidural and general anesthesia. Anesth Analg 1983;62:174.

36. Rosenfeld BA, Beattie C, Christopherson R, et al, and the PIRAT Study Group. The effects of different anesthetic regimens on fibrinolysis and the development of postoperative arterial thrombosis. Anesthesiology 1993;79:435.

37. Rosenfeld BA, Faraday N, Campbell D, et al. Hemostatic effects of stress hormone infusion. Anesthesiology 1994;81:1116.

38. Guidelines Committee, American College of Critical Care Medicine, Society of Critical Care Medicine, and the Transfer Guidelines Task Force. Guidelines for the transfer of critically ill patients. Am J Crit Care 1993;2:189.

39. Cortes-Franco JE, Gamba-Ayala G, Aguilar-Salinas CA, et al. The transfer of critically ill patients. Rev Invest Clin 1991;43:323.

40. Hurst JM, Davis K Jr, Johnson DJ, et al. Cost and complications during in-hospital transport of critically ill patients: a prospective cohort study. J Trauma 1992;33:582.

41. Morishita Y, Toyohira H, Yuda T, et al. Surgical treatment of abdominal aortic aneurysm in the high-risk patient. Jpn J Surg 1991;21:595.

42. Svensson LG, Hess KR, Coselli JS, et al. A prospective study of respiratory failure after high-risk surgery on the thoracoabdominal aorta. J Vasc Surg 1991;14:271.

43. Calligaro KD, Azurin DJ, Dougherty MJ, et al. Pulmonary risk factors of elective abdominal aortic surgery. J Vasc Surg 1993;18:914.

44. Sullivan CA, Rohrer MJ, Cutler BS. Clinical management of the symptomatic but unruptured aortic aneurysm. J Vasc Surg 1990;11:799.

45. Cambria RA, Gloviczki P, Stanson AW, et al. Symptomatic, nonruptured abdominal aortic aneurysms: are emergent operations necessary? Ann Vasc Surg 1994;8:121.

46. Smith FC, Gosling P, Sanghera K, et al. Microproteinuria predicts the severity of systemic effects of reperfusion injury following infrarenal aortic aneurysm surgery. Ann Vasc Surg 1994;8:1.

47. Perel A, Stock MC. Handbook of Mechanical Ventilatory Support. Baltimore: Williams & Wilkins, 1992.

48. Annest SJ, Gottlieb M, Paloski WH, et al. Detrimental effects of removing end-expiratory pressure prior to endotracheal extubation. Ann Surg 1980;191:539.

49. Cohen IL. Weaning from mechanical ventilation—the team approach and beyond. Intensive Care Med 1994;20:317.

50. Crawford E, Mizrahi E, Hess KR, et al. The impact of distal aortic perfusion and somatosensory evoked potentials monitoring on prevention of paraplegia after aortic aneurysm operation. J Thorac Cardiovasc Surg 1988;95:357.

51. Crawford ES, Crawford JL, Safi HJ, et al. Thoracoabdominal aortic aneurysms: preoperative and intraoperative factors determining immediate and long-term results of operations in 605 patients. J Vasc Surg 1986;3:389.

52. Moritz F, Petit J, Kaeffer N, et al. Metabolic effects of propofol and flunitrazepam given for sedation after aortic surgery. Br J Anaesth 1993;70:451.

53. Chaudhri S, Kenny GN. Sedation after cardiac bypass surgery: comparison of propofol and midazolam in the presence of a computerized closed loop arterial pressure controller. Br J Anaesth 1992;68:98.

54. Hudson RJ, Thomson IR, Cannon JE, et al. Pharmacokinetics of fentanyl in patients undergoing abdominal aortic surgery. Anesthesiology 1986;64:334.

55. Hudson RJ, Bergstrom RG, Thomson IR, et al. Phar-

macokinetics of sufentanil in patients undergoing abdominal aortic surgery. Anesthesiology 1989;70:426.

56. Hudson RJ, Thomson IR, Burgess PM, Rosenbloom M. Alfentanil pharmacokinetics in patients undergoing abdominal aortic surgery. Can J Anaesth 1991;38:61.

57. Hudson RJ. Midazolam pharmacokinetics in patients undergoing abdominal aortic surgery. Anesth Analg 1994;79:219.

58. Hughes MA, Glass PSA, Jacobs JR. Context-sensitive half-time in multicompartment pharmacokinetic models for intravenous anesthetic drugs. Anesthesiology 1992;76:334.

59. Shafer SL, Stanski DR. Improving the clinical utility of anesthetic drug pharmacokinetics [editorial]. Anesthesiology 1992;76:327.

60. Segredo V, Caldwell JE, Mathay MA, et al. Persistent paralysis in critically ill patients after long term administration of vecuronium. N Engl J Med 1992;327:524.

61. Wokke JH, Jennekens FG, van den Oord CJ, et al. Histological investigations of muscle atrophy and end plates in two critically ill patients with generalized weakness. J Neurol Sci 1988;88:95.

62. Kupfer Y, Okrent DG, Twersky RA, Tessler S. Disuse atrophy in a ventilated patient with status asthmaticus receiving neuromuscular blockade. Crit Care Med 1987;15:795.

63. Rossiter A, Souney PF, McGowen S, Carvajal P. Pancuronium-induced prolonged neuromuscular blockade. Crit Care Med 1991;19:1583.

64. Khuenl-Brady KD, Reitstatter B, Schlager A, et al. Long-term administration of pancuronium and pipercuronium in the intensive care unit. Anesth Analg 1994;78:1082.

65. Michaelis LL, Hickey PR, Clark TA, Dixon WM. Ventricular irritability associated with the use of naloxone hydrochloride. Two case reports and laboratory assessment of the effect of the drug on cardiac excitability. Ann Thorac Surg 1974;18:608.

66. Blaise GA, Nugent M, McMichan JC, Durant PA. Side effects of nalbuphine while reversing opioid-induced respiratory depression: report of 4 cases. Can J Anaesth 1990;37:794.

67. Reeder MK, Goldman MD, Loh L, et al. Late postoperative nocturnal dips in oxygen saturation in patients undergoing major abdominal vascular surgery. Predictive value of pre-operative overnight pulse oximetry. Anaesthesia 1992;47:110.

68. Reeder MK, Goldman MD, Loh L, et al. Postoperative hypoxaemia after major abdominal vascular surgery. Br J Anaesth 1992;68:23.

69. Reeder MK, Goldman MD, Loh L, et al. Postoperative obstructive sleep apnea. Haemodynamic effects of treatment with nasal CPAP. Anaesthesia 1991;46:849.

70. Reeder MK, Muir AD, Foex P, et al. Postoperative myocardial ischaemia: temporal association with nocturnal hypoxaemia. Br J Anaesth 1991;67:626.

71. Paterson IS, Klausner JM, Pugatch R, et al. Noncardiogenic pulmonary edema after abdominal aortic aneurysm surgery. Ann Surg 1989;209:231.

72. Kispert JF, Kazmers A, Roitman L. Preoperative spirometry predicts perioperative pulmonary complications after major vascular surgery. Am Surg 1992;58:491.

73. Beydon L, Saada M, Liu N, et al. Can portable chest x-ray examination accurately diagnose lung consolidation after major abdominal surgery? A comparison with computed tomography scan. Chest 1992;102:1697.

74. Grindlinger GA, Vegas AM, Manny J, et al. Volume loading and vasodilators in abdominal aortic aneurysmectomy. Am J Surg 1980;139:480.

75. Ontario Intensive Care Study Group. Evaluation of right heart catheterization in critically ill patients. Crit Care Med 1992;20:928.

76. Raphael P, Cogbill TH, Dunn EL, et al. Routine invasive hemodynamic monitoring does not increase risk of aortic graft infection. Heart Lung 1993;22:121.

77. Sola JE, Bender JS. Use of the pulmonary artery catheter to reduce operative complications. Surg Clin North Am 1993;73:253.

78. Adams JG Jr, Clifford EJ, Henry RS, Poulos E. Selective monitoring in abdominal aortic surgery. Am Surg 1993;59:559.

79. Joyce WP, Provan JL, Ameli FM, et al. The role of central haemodynamic monitoring in abdominal aortic surgery. A prospective randomized study. Eur J Vasc Surg 1990;4:633.

80. Leung JM, Levine EH. Left ventricular end-systolic cavity obliteration as an estimate of intraoperative hypovolemia. Anesthesiology 1994;81:1102.

81. Douglas P, Edmunds H, St John Sutton M, et al. Unreliability of hemodynamic indexes of left ventricular size during cardiac surgery. Ann Thorac Surg 1987;44:31.

82. Dennis JW, Menawat SS, Sobowale OO, et al. Superiority of end-diastolic volume and ejection fraction measurements over wedge pressures in evaluating cardiac function during aortic reconstruction. J Vasc Surg 1992;16:372.

83. O'Dwyer JP, King JE, Wood CE, et al. Continuous measurement of systemic vascular resistance. Anaesthesia 1994;49:587.

84. Lind L, Skoog G, Malstam J. Relations between mixed venous oxygen saturation and hemodynamic variables in patients subjected to abdominal aortic aneurysm surgery and in patients with septic shock. Ups J Med Sci 1993;98:83.

85. Viale JP, Annat GJ, Ravat FM, et al. Oxygen uptake and mixed venous oxygen saturation during aortic surgery and the first three postoperative hours. Anesth Analg 1991;73:530.

86. Poterack KA. Who uses transesophageal echocardiography in the operating room? Anesth Analg 1995;80:454.

87. Oh JK, Seward JB, Khandheria BK, et al. Transesophageal echocardiography in critically ill patients. Am J Cardiol 1990;66:1492.

88. Oh JK, Sinak LJ, Freeman WK, et al. Transesophageal echocardiography in patients with shock syndrome. Circulation 1991;84(Suppl 2):127.

89. Erbel R, Engberding R, Daniel W, et al., and the European Cooperative Study Group for Echocardiography. Echocardiography in diagnosis of aortic dissection. Lancet 1989;1:457.

90. Seward JB, Khandheria BK, Edwards WD, et al. Biplanar transesophageal echocardiography: anatomic correlations, image orientation, and clinical applications. Mayo Clin Proc 1990;65:1193.

91. Hansen KJ, Starr SM, Sands RE, et al. Contemporary surgical management of renovascular disease. J Vasc Surg 1992;16:319.

92. Branchereau A, Espinoza H, Magnan PE, et al. Simultaneous reconstruction of infrarenal abdominal aorta and renal arteries. Ann Vasc Surg 1992;6:232.

93. Perry SM, Smith DW, Meacham PW, Wood M. Adrenergic response to nicardipine in the management of postoperative hypertension. J Cardiothorac Anesth 1990;4:707.

94. Halpern NA, Goldberg M, Neely C, et al. Postoperative hypertension: a multicenter, prospective, randomized comparison between intravenous nicardipine and sodium nitroprusside. Crit Care Med 1992;20:1637.

95. Goldberg ME, Halpern N, Krakoff L, et al. Efficacy and safety of intravenous nicardipine in the control of postoperative hypertension. IV Nicardipine Study Group. Chest 1991;99:393.

96. Le-Bret F, Coriat P, Gosnach M, et al. Transesophageal echocardiographic assessment of left ventricular function in response to labetalol for control of postoperative hypertension. J Cardiothorac Vasc Anesth 1992;6:433.

97. Stone JG, Foex P, Sear JW, et al. Myocardial ischemia in untreated hypertensive patients: effect of a single small oral dose of a beta-adrenergic blocking agent. Anesthesiology 1988;68:495.

98. Pasternack PF, Imparato AM, Baumann FG, et al. The hemodynamics of beta-blockade in patients undergoing abdominal aortic aneurysm repair. Circulation 1987;76:1.

99. Zall S, Kirno K, Milocco I, Ricksten SE. Vasodilatation with adenosine or sodium nitroprusside after coronary artery bypass surgery: a comparative study on myocardial blood flow and metabolism. Anesth Analg 1993;76:498.

100. Fremes SE, Wiesel RD, Baird RJ, et al. The effects of postoperative hypertension and its treatment. J Thorac Cardiovasc Surg 1983;86:47.

101. Gross GJ, Warltier DC. Coronary steal in four models of single or multiple vessel obstruction in dogs. Am J Cardiol 1981;48:84.

102. Colson P, Saussine M, Seguin JR, et al. Hemodynamic effects of anesthesia in patients chronically treated with angiotensin-converting enzyme inhibitors. Anesth Analg 1992;74:805.

103. Yates AP, Hunter DN. Anaesthesia and angiotensin-converting enzyme inhibitors: the effect of enalapril on perioperative cardiovascular stability. Anaesthesia 1988;43:935.

104. Selby DG, Richards JD, Marshman JM. ACE inhibitors. Anaesth Intensive Care 1989;17:110.

105. Coriat P, Richer C, Douraki T, et al. Influence of chronic angiotensin-converting enzyme inhibition on anesthetic induction. Anesthesiology 1994;81:299.

106. Blomberg S, Curelaru I, Emanuelsson H, et al. Thoracic epidural anaesthesia in patients with unstable angina pectoris. Eur Heart J 1989;10:437.

107. Blomberg S, Emanuelsson H, Ricksten SE. Thoracic epidural anesthesia and central hemodynamics in patients with unstable angina pectoris. Anesth Analg 1989;69:558.

108. Blomberg A, Emanuelsson H, Kvist H, et al. Effects of thoracic epidural anesthesia on coronary arteries and arterioles in patients with coronary artery disease. Anesthesiology 1990;73:840.

109. Goldberg ME, Cantillo J, Nemiroff MS, et al. Fenoldopam infusion for the treatment of postoperative hypertension. J Clin Anesth 1993;5:386.

110. Marty J. Role of isradipine and other antihypertensive agents in the treatment of peri- and postoperative hypertension. Acta Anaesthesiol Scand 1993;99(Suppl):53.

111. Lawrence CJ, Lestrade A, de Langes S. Isradipine, a calcium antagonist, in the control of hypertension following coronary artery bypass surgery. Am J Hypertens 1991;4:207.

112. Brister NW, Barnette RE, Schartel SA, et al. Isradipine for treatment of acute hypertension after myocardial revascularization. Crit Care Med 1991;19:33408.

113. Brogden RN, Sorkin EM. Ketanserin. A review of its pharmacodynamic and pharmacokinetic properties. Drugs 1990;40:903.

114. Becker LC. Conditions for vasodilator-induced coronary steal in experimental myocardial ischemia. Circulation 1978;57:1103.

115. Zall S, Milocco I, Ricksten SE. Effects of adenosine on renal function and central hemodynamics after coronary artery bypass surgery. Anesth Analg 1993;76:493.

116. Abbot B, Mommaerts W. A study of the inotropic mechanism in papillary muscle preparations. J Gen Physiol 1959;41:533.

117. Schiller N, Acquatella H, Ports T, et al. Left ventricular volume from paired biplane two-dimensional echocardiography. Circulation 1979;60:547.

118. Marik PE. The systolic blood pressure variation as an indicator of pulmonary capillary wedge pressure in ventilated patients. Anaesth Intensive Care 1993;21:405.

119. Coriat P, Vrillon M, Perel A, et al. A comparison of systolic pressure variations and echocardiographic estimates of end-diastolic left ventricular size in patients after aortic surgery. Anesth Analg 1994;78:46.

120. Partridge BL. Use of pulse oximetry as a noninvasive indicator of intravascular volume status. J Clin Monit 1987;3:263.

121. Dawidson IJ, Willms CD, Sandor ZF, et al. Ringer's lactate with or without 3% dextran 60 as volume expanders during abdominal aortic surgery. Crit Care Med 1991;19:36.

122. Bomberger RA, McGregor B, DePalma RG. Optimal fluid management after aortic reconstruction: a prospective study of 2 crystalloid solutions. J Vasc Surg 1986;4:164.

123. Croft D, Dion YM, Dumont M, Langlois D. Cardiac compliance and effects of hypertonic saline. Can J Surg 1992;35:139.

124. Nielsen OM, Thunedborg P, Jorgensen K. Albumin administration and acute phase proteins in abdominal vascular surgery. A randomized study. Dan Med Bull 1989;36:496.

125. Gold MS, Russo J, Tissot M, et al. Comparison of hetastarch to albumin for perioperative bleeding in patients undergoing abdominal aortic aneurysm surgery. A prospective, randomized study. Ann Surg 1990;211:482.

126. Boutros AR, Ruess R, Olson L, et al. Comparison of hemodynamic, pulmonary, and renal effects of use of three types of fluids after major surgical procedures of the abdominal aorta. Crit Care Med 1979;7:9.

127. Bates ER. Treatment of acute myocardial infarction: a cardiologist's perspective. Int Anesthesiol Clin 1992;30:237.

128. Suggs WD, Smith RB 3d, Weintraub WS, et al. Selective screening for coronary artery disease in patients undergoing elective repair of abdominal aortic aneurysms. J Vasc Surg 1993;18:349.

129. Christopherson R, Frank S, Norris E, et al. Low postoperative hematocrit is associated with cardiac ischemia in high risk patients. Anesthesiology 1991;75(Suppl):99.

130. Nelson AH, Fleisher LA, Rosenbaum SH. The relationship between postoperative anemia and cardiac morbidity in high risk vascular patients in the ICU. Crit Care Med 1993;21:860.

131. Frank SM, Beattie C, Christopherson R, et al. Unintentional hypothermia is associated with postoperative myocardial ischemia. Anesthesiology 1993;78:468.

132. Frank SM, Higgins MS, Breslow MJ, et al. The catecholamine, cortisol, and hemodynamic responses to mild perioperative hypothermia: a randomized clinical trial. Anesthesiology 1995;82:83.

133. Andersen PT, Nielsen LK, Moller-Petersen J, Egeblad K. Non-cardiac creatine kinase-B activity in serum after abdominal aortic bypass surgery. Acta Chir Scand 1988;154:359.

134. Rettke SR, Shub C, Naessens JM, et al. Significance of mildly elevated creatine kinase (myocardial band) activity after elective abdominal aortic aneurysmectomy. J Cardiothorac Vasc Anesth 1991;5:425.

135. Hamm CW, Ravkilde J, Gerhardt W, et al. The prognostic value of serum troponin-T in unstable angina. N Engl J Med 1992;327:146.

136. Gibbs NM, Crawford GP, Michalopoulos N. Postoperative changes in coagulant and anticoagulant factors following abdominal aortic surgery. J Cardiothorac Vasc Anesth 1992;6:680.

137. Riles TS, Fisher FS, Schaefer S, et al. Plasma catecholamine concentrations during abdominal aortic aneurysm surgery: the link to perioperative myocardial ischemia. Ann Vasc Surg 1993;7:213.

138. Held P, Yusuf S, Furberg C. Effects of calcium antagonists on initial infarction, reinfarction, and mortality in acute myocardial infarction and unstable angina. Br Med J 1989;299:1187.

139. Koolen JJ, van Wezel HB, Visser CA, et al. Nicardipine for preservation of myocardial metabolism and function in patients undergoing coronary artery surgery. Anesthesiology 1989;71:508.

140. Bullough DA, Zhang C, Montag A, et al. Adenosine-mediated inhibition of platelet aggregation by acadesine. A novel antithrombotic mechanism in vitro and in vivo. J Clin Invest 1994;94:1524.

141. Engler RL. Harnessing nature's own cardiac defense mechanism with acadesine, an adenosine regulating agent: importance of the endothelium. J Card Surg 1994;9(Suppl 3):482.

142. Leung JM, Stanley T 3rd, Mathew J, et al., and SPI Research Group. An initial multicenter, randomized controlled trial on the safety and efficacy of acadesine in patient undergoing coronary artery bypass surgery. Anesth Analag 1994;78:420.

143. Rothstein RJ. Myocardial contusion. JAMA 1983;250:2189.

144. Hines RL, Barash PG. Right Ventricular Performance. In JA Kaplan (ed), Cardiac Anesthesia. Philadelphia: Saunders, 1993.

145. Schaer GL, Fink MP, Parrillo JE. Norepinephrine alone versus norepinephrine plus low dose dopamine: enhanced renal blood flow with combination pressor therapy. Crit Care Med 1985;13:492.

Chapter 12

Postoperative Care of the Aortic Surgery Patient: End-Organ Integrity

Meir Chernofsky and Ruth S. Spector

Central Nervous System Injury

Aortic surgery patients have atherosclerotic and hypertensive diseases. These diseases contribute to the etiology of these patients' cerebrovascular diseases. The anterior spinal cord has no collateral source of perfusion and is highly dependent on descending aortic blood flow. Blood flow in the aorta is temporarily interrupted in virtually every type of aortic surgery. Therefore, aortic surgery patients, as a group, are at risk for central nervous system (CNS) injury, both in the spinal cord and brain.

Thoracic aortic surgery patients are at especially high risk for both stroke and spinal cord injury regardless of the etiology of their diseases. The act of opening and operating on the thoracic aorta introduces the risk of air and particulate emboli. The common pathologic processes requiring surgical correction, dissection, and aneurysm may involve the carotid or vertebral arteries and may predispose to cerebral embolism or thrombosis. Patients who undergo procedures on the aortic arch can be subjected to total circulatory arrest with its inherent risk of cerebral ischemia. Other potential insults relate to the use of cardiopulmonary bypass and to surgical complications. The application of the cross clamp itself can cause severe hypertension. Today this is usually well controlled by vasoactive agents and shunting techniques, but occasionally the increase in blood pressure may cause a stroke. Retrograde embolization from abdominal aortic disease is also a rare cause of stroke.

Spinal cord injury has been reported after surgery at all levels of the aorta, but it is more commonly associated with procedures performed between the aortic valve and renal arteries. It usually manifests as paralysis, because the anterior spinal cord, which carries the motor tracts, is most vulnerable to ischemia. Other than the site of cross clamping, risk factors include patient age, prolonged cross clamp time, the site and size of the aneurysm or dissection, and the occurrence of a ruptured aneurysm (Table 12-1).[1] The patient's vascular anatomy and the surgical technique also play a role.[2] The anterior radicular artery, which feeds the anterior spinal artery, is difficult to locate angiographically and surgically. It can originate anywhere between T7 and L4. Patients also differ in their ability to perfuse the anterior spinal cord with collateral flow; perhaps 50% of patients can tolerate having their anterior radicular artery severed. (The exact percentage is obviously unknown.) Cord injury may be complete at the end of surgery or may evolve during the postoperative period.[3]

Detection of injury at any level of the CNS is facilitated by achieving an awake, cooperative state early in the postoperative period. The greater the risk of neurologic injury, the greater the need for an early neurologic examination. An awake patient need not mean an extubated patient. If postoperative neuromuscular blockade is avoided and analgesic medications are carefully titrated, an intubated and ventilated patient may be cooperative enough to assist in excluding major neurologic injury. Conversely, an extubation done before its time may exacerbate

Table 12-1. Factors That Increase Risk of Spinal Cord Injury

Patient's age
Origin (level) of anterior radicular artery
Relationship of anterior radicular artery to site of aneurysm
   or dissection
Potential for collateral arterial flow
Site of aortic cross clamping (thoracic versus abdominal)
Duration of cross clamping
Presence of aortic dissection
Site and size of dissection
Presence of ruptured aneurysm
Associated low oxygen delivery state

---

neurologic injury by allowing the development of hypoxemia, hypercarbia, and hemodynamic instability.

Routine neurologic checks in the intensive care unit (ICU), which are the responsibility of the nursing staff as well as the physicians, are instituted postoperatively as soon as possible and repeated every 2–4 hours for the first 24–48 hours in all aortic surgery patients. Motor function of the upper and lower extremities needs to be followed because it is at particular risk.

Neurologic injury may be complete when detected; however, sometimes it is at least partly reversible. Because reversibility can only be determined in retrospect, it is critical to be aggressive with hemodynamic modulation, blood pressure control, and specific protective measures. The tendency to give up after initial discovery of such injury must be avoided. Early radiologic and neurologic consultation is almost always indicated.

All patients with suspected or confirmed CNS injury should have their fluid management strategy modified to avoid volume overload and hyponatremia. By maintaining normovolemia and normal to high osmolarity and tonicity, one can bias the Starling forces across capillary membranes to minimize localized CNS edema. When intravascular volume replacement is indicated and red cells are not needed, there may be some benefit to the use of colloids. In such cases there is also a role for hypertonic saline in limited amounts with serial analysis of serum sodium. Hyperglycemia (glucose > 180–200 mg/dl) should be aggressively treated to avoid localized lactic acidosis in ischemic areas of the CNS. If sedation is necessary, it should be achieved with agents such as barbiturates and benzodiazepines that have the potential for brain protection. While the sedative dosages of these agents are below the dosages that are considered brain protective, these agents are unlikely to adversely affect intracranial compliance. Mild hyperventilation (to a $PaCO_2$ of 32–33) should be induced if cerebral edema is likely. More aggressive reduction of $PaCO_2$ is appropriate if intracranial hypertension is demonstrated but should not be attempted when spinal cord injury is suspected because hypocarbia may reduce spinal cord blood flow.

Just as patients at risk for myocardial ischemia are approached with aggressive control of myocardial supply and demand before ischemia develops, patients at known risk for CNS injury should be, to some extent, treated as if they already have evolving injury. Patients at special risk include those who underwent total circulatory arrest, other aortic arch patients, patients with known cerebrovascular disease, and patients at risk for spinal cord injury (as discussed previously) (see Chapter 8).

Stroke

Strokes may be embolic, thrombotic, or hemodynamic in origin. Embolic strokes tend to cause infarcts in the distribution of the main arterial branches. Sources of emboli include the heart, aortic arch, carotid or vertebral arteries, and rarely the more distal aorta via a retrograde mechanism. Embolic material, in addition to atherosclerotic debris and thrombotic plaque, may include air and surgical debris. Thromboembolic disease of the carotid arteries is beyond the scope of this chapter but such strokes are in the differential diagnosis of any new postoperative neurologic deficit.

A cardiac or aortic source of emboli can be investigated with echocardiography. Transesophageal echocardiography is indicated to exclude embolic sources in the left atrial appendage as well as the aortic arch. Depending on the nature of the embolic source, heparin therapy may be indicated, antiplatelet therapy may be started, or surgical intervention may be required. The institution of heparin or antiplatelet therapy is partially a surgical decision because of the implications these agents have for postoperative bleeding.

Proper hemodynamic management of stroke is critical. In Chapter 11 we reviewed the issue of blood pressure control tailored to maximize oxygen delivery to injured neural tissue while avoiding possible reperfusion injury. This strategy is applied to achieve the best oxygen delivery index (DO_2I) possible at the safest arterial pressure for the individual.

The majority of patients who have had total circulatory arrest actually do very well. Tabayashi et al. reported that in their series, postoperative neurologic deficits could not be detected in any of their survivors, even when detailed mental status examinations were done.[4] Ergin and coworkers found that in patients who had undergone circulatory arrest, global neurologic dysfunction was almost always temporary.[5] In their series, most permanent neural injuries were thrombotic strokes. The incidence of stroke in this population is related to the site of surgery and not the method of cerebral protection used. The new technique of retrograde cold cerebroplegia has not been around long enough to evaluate its effect on the postoperative course (see Chapter 7).[6]

Spinal Cord Injury

Pathology and Risk Profile

The incidence of spinal cord injury in aortic surgery patients varies from under 0.1% for elective abdominal aortic reconstruction to as high as 6–30% or more for thoracoabdominal surgery, ruptured aneurysm, and traumatic rupture of the aorta.[3,7–10] Of the risk factors listed in Table 12-1, the duration of cross clamping and the site and size of the lesion are by far the most important. There are several intraoperative strategies aimed at prevention of spinal cord ischemia, including drainage of cerebrospinal fluid (CSF), total body hypothermia, tight control of glucose, high-dose corticosteroids, diuretics, cooling of the cord, and various bypass techniques. Diuretics such as mannitol are sometimes used for their potential as free radical scavengers. The bypass and shunt interventions such as the Gott shunt and left atrial to femoral artery bypass unload the ventricle, thus contributing to control of cross clamp–related hypertension. The use of these modalities varies from institution to institution. Although various centers report dramatic differences in the incidence of spinal cord damage, these differences do not always correlate with preventive strategies used. At this point, no single preventive measure is considered superior.[8,11] The current trend is to combine multiple strategies for spinal cord protection with meticulous surgical techniques, including careful handling of visible intercostal arteries and varying the position of the clamp to minimize ischemic time (see Chapter 8).

In many patients who suffer spinal cord injury, the evidence is already present by the end of surgery, but such injuries may or may not be permanent.[12] Postoperative spinal cord ischemia can also occur in patients who appear to have intact neurologic examinations at the end of surgery.[3,13,14] Late onset spinal cord injury may be related to reperfusion; in particular, neuroexcitatory amino acids can activate the N-methyl-D-aspartate (NMDA) receptors, thus inducing cellular damage. However, it is much more likely that these late injuries are ischemic in nature and are related to hypotension and low-flow states, which are often reversible.[3] Some patients who develop new onset postoperative spinal cord deficits may have had their anterior radicular artery compromised during surgery and may have tolerated this arterial interruption because of collateral flow. This collateral flow may then have been diminished by hypotension in the early postoperative period, due perhaps to bleeding or rewarming. Spinal cord injury can occur at any level, including the lumbosacral roots. Injuries that occur after infrarenal aortic cross clamping may be related to anatomic variation in the origin of the artery of Adamkiewicz, which can branch off the aorta as low as the mid-lumbar segments in 1% of patients.

Although perioperative spinal cord injury often cannot be fully reversed in the postoperative period, such injury shares with all ischemic infarcts the potential for a borderline area of reversible injury. Areas of borderline ischemia are often edematous. Such peri-infarct edema interferes with local perfusion, thus further compromising tissue that cannot afford more insult. Since any functional loss that can be prevented may improve the quality of life for the patient, attention to detail is critical in the patient with spinal cord injury. Aside from the issue of neurologic preservation, these patients have a much higher overall mortality than their neurologically intact peers.[7] As one would expect, the source of this mortality is primarily sepsis caused by concomitant visceral ischemia. Spinal shock is also a potential contributing factor.

Management

As is the case for any patient with an organ system complication, the first priority of therapy is the maintenance of adequate oxygen delivery and the aggressive treatment of low-flow states. Specific attention is directed at the spinal cord perfusion pressure, which is approximated by the difference between the mean arterial pressure and the CSF pressure (see Chapters 4 and 8). With regard to spinal cord perfusion pressure, there is more room for error in the postoperative period than during aortic cross clamping, when the perfusion is related to *distal* aortic pressure. Nevertheless, postoperative decreases in perfusion are dangerous. Therefore, mean arterial pressure should be maintained in the normal range even if excellent DO$_2$I is obtainable at lower arterial pressures. Oxygen delivery is, after all, measured with reference to right ventricular output, not flow to the CNS. When it comes to arterial pressure, however, more may not be better. Reperfusion injury is a major consideration, and excessive arterial pressure may exacerbate the edema-ischemia cycle. The optimal arterial pressure is unfortunately not known.

If hypertension occurs in a patient with spinal cord injury, it should be addressed with cerebral protective anesthetics, which tend to lower arterial pressure. If the patient's ventilation is still controlled, anesthetic agents of the barbiturate class are ideal. Thiopental, or the nonbarbiturate agent propofol, can be titrated to the point at which cardiac output begins to decrease. If further control of hypertension is necessary, or if it is clear that the circulatory depressant effects of intravenous anesthetics will not be tolerated, therapy is guided by the hemodynamic profile. When vasoactive agents are necessary, drugs that are capable of inducing precipitous decreases in arterial pressure, such as sodium nitroprusside, are not the first choice. Calcium channel blockers may be safer. Inodilators such as dobutamine, amrinone, and milrinone are worthwhile considerations in the hemodynamic management of hypertension with a low-flow state (see Chapter 11).

Spinal shock is a low-flow state that results from severe spinal cord injury. This low-flow state in-

duces a vicious cycle of inadequate perfusion of the CNS; therefore, oxygen delivery must be supported to limit the extent of damage. Spinal shock is neurogenic shock, a redistributive form of hemodynamic compromise that results from an acute increase in vascular capacitance. This increase results from the loss of sympathetic outflow and vasomotor tone. When such vasodilatation has occurred, a normal blood volume will not be able to maintain an adequate preload, and cardiac output will decrease.

Spinal shock is well known to anesthesiologists because the physiology is similar to that which occurs with high spinal and epidural neural blockade. Spinal shock is treated by fluid loading and discontinuation of vasodilators. Fluid therapy must be tempered by attention to osmolarity to avoid further edema of damaged neural tissue. Vasopressors such as norepinephrine and phenylephrine will partly reverse the acute vasodilatation. However, such agents may contribute to arterial vasospasm and may compromise flow to the extremities in the setting of peripheral vascular disease. It is also conceivable that vasopressors may contribute to cerebral vasospasm, although this is difficult to assess.

Ventilatory management in the setting of spinal cord injury involves apparently conflicting demands. Serial neurologic evaluation is best performed in an awake, cooperative patient. The neurologic injury will often have been detected with cooperation of the patient. Once the presence of neurologic injury is established, serial examination may not change the early clinical approach. While some patients may be awake and cooperative when still intubated, many will require sedation to tolerate the endotracheal tube and ventilator. One may be tempted to extubate to avoid the need for sedation. Nevertheless, early extubation in these patients may be a grave mistake. Patients with fresh neurologic injury must not be allowed to hypoventilate. Furthermore, these patients, as stated previously, often have concomitant organ system ischemia and sepsis. The hemodynamic and fluid interventions used for neurologic protection can further destabilize the patient. Therefore, controlled ventilation should be continued during the uncertain early stages of neurologic injury. Extreme hyperventilation should also be avoided.

Specific measures to protect the spinal cord are no longer limited to the operating room. Nor should they be, given the substantial incidence of new injury in the postoperative period as well as the potential reversibility of deficits already present. Administration of protective drugs, cord cooling, and continued spinal fluid drainage are all being studied in the postoperative period.[12,15]

CSF drainage appears to be safe, but its efficacy in the postoperative period is not established. Nevertheless, CSF drainage is sometimes continued into the postoperative period, and CSF pressure is occasionally monitored. These interventions are certainly worthwhile in the face of the postoperative onset of a neurologic deficit.

While a subarachnoid catheter will usually have been placed by the anesthesiologist, the preferences of the surgeon and neurologic consultant should be considered in terms of the postoperative use and removal of this catheter. The lumbar subarachnoid catheter, when present, can be used as a route of administration for analgesics. In the setting of spinal cord injury, common sense would suggest that analgesics administered by this route be given in a small volume and perhaps be infused only after withdrawal of an equal volume of CSF to avoid an acute increase in CSF pressure.

Moderate hypothermia will effectively reduce spinal cord metabolism. In our routine abdominal aortic surgery patients, we treat postoperative hypothermia to avoid coagulopathy. Mild hypothermia should be tolerated, however, in any patient at risk of spinal cord ischemia. Aggressive rewarming is potentially dangerous because it can increase spinal cord metabolism while simultaneously causing hypotension and decreased spinal cord perfusion. Fever, likewise, cannot be tolerated. Corticosteroids, barbiturates, calcium channel blockers, and osmotic diuretics may have a place in postoperative spinal cord protection. The systemic and neuraxial administration of agents that act on the NMDA receptor is currently being investigated. The NMDA receptor mediates the effect of excitatory neurotransmitters, which are released in excess during neural ischemia and are potentially damaging in that setting.

Coagulation and Red Cell Mass

Coagulation

Coagulation defects initiated in the intraoperative period may continue to pose a problem postoperatively. The coagulation cascade is a complex inter-

Table 12-2. Factors Involved in Normal Hemostasis

Primary hemostasis
Vessel wall integrity
Platelet number and function
Fibrinogen
Calcium
von Willebrand's factor
Secondary hemostasis
Serum coagulation factors
Protease inhibitors
Calcium
Phospholipids

Source: Modified from RI Parker, JC Farmer. Coagulation: Essential Physiologic Concerns. In JM Civetta, RW Taylor, RR Kirby (eds), Critical Care (2nd ed). Philadelphia: Lippincott, 1992;1700.

actional system of enzymatic activators and inhibitors (Table 12-2). The healthy human depends on a delicate balance of the clotting mechanism—clot forms when needed, never inappropriately, and dissolves when no longer useful. For the aortic surgery patient, disaster strikes if either clot formation or fibrinolysis is allowed to proceed unchecked. The building blocks of coagulation include platelets, the vessel wall, and the serum coagulation cascade. The latter is commonly divided into the intrinsic and extrinsic pathways and the common pathways of clot formation and lysis. In reality, all of the building blocks interact at many levels, and any conceptual separation is artificial.

Vascular anastomoses, suture lines, and pathologic processes related to atherosclerosis are all examples of vascular injury. Disruption of the intimal layer of a vessel triggers a multiphase response. Vascular smooth muscle contraction may curb bleeding by reducing the area of the disruption, but the first phase of the hemostatic mechanism is platelet deposition (primary hemostasis). This is followed by secondary hemostasis, a complex process in which serum proteins and platelets interact to form a fibrin clot. This process is in turn kept in check by fibrinolysis, allowing blood flow to continue past the point of injury (see Chapter 5).

Evaluation of Coagulation

Platelet number is routinely evaluated in the complete blood count. Assuming normal platelet

Normal	Hemophilia	Thrombocytopenia	Fibrinolysis	Hypercoagulability

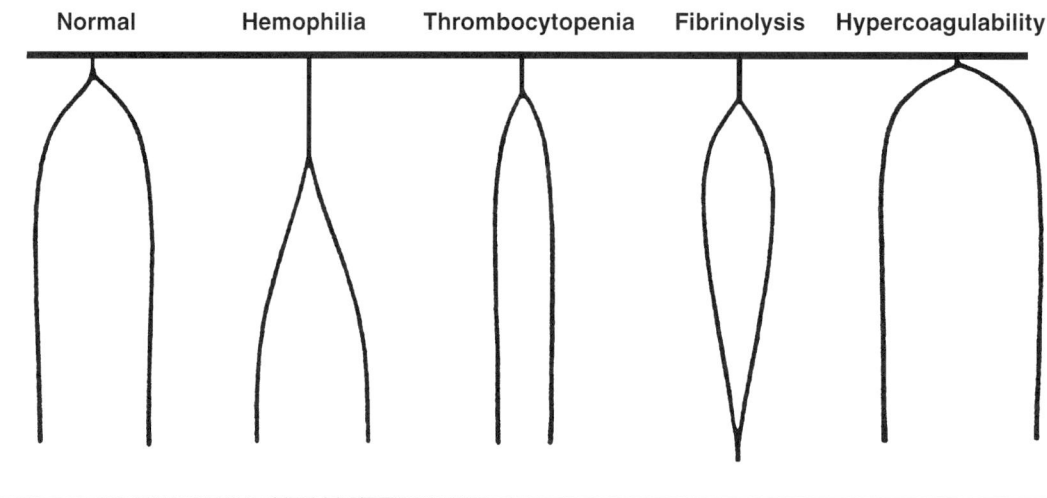

Figure 12-1. Schematic depiction of changes in coagulation that are reflected in the thromboelastograph. Platelet dysfunction or thrombocytopenia is characterized by a prolonged reaction time for initial fibrin formation (6–8 minutes) with decreased maximal amplitude (50–70 mm) and clot formation rate (>50 degrees), and fibrinolysis by decreased maximal amplitude and clot formation rate and whole blood clot lysis time. (Reprinted with permission from RK Stoelting, SF Dierdorf. Anesthesia and Co-Existing Disease [3rd ed]. New York: Churchill Livingstone, 1993;411.)

function, spontaneous bleeding is rare at a platelet count over 20,000 per ml, while counts in the 50,000–70,000 per ml range are usually adequate to support hemostasis in the face of trauma (recent surgery). In our setting the most common causes of thrombocytopenia are dilutional thrombocytopenia, disseminated intravascular coagulation (DIC), and drug-induced thrombocytopenia.

Platelet function is far more difficult to measure. The in vivo template bleeding time is neither specific nor sensitive in the surgical setting. Nevertheless, a severely prolonged template bleeding time with an adequate number of platelets is suggestive of platelet dysfunction. The thromboelastograph (TEG) can reflect some aspects of platelet number or function, but it does not reliably detect the presence of aspirin-related platelet malfunction (Figure 12-1). Conceptually, the TEG can be useful in providing insight into the cause of coagulation abnormalities. Originally used in liver transplant patients, the TEG measures clot strength and development over time (Figures 12-1 and 12-2). The TEG is a test performed at bedside run on whole blood. In its current form, the TEG does little to suggest specific therapies. However, the basic test can be modified by various additives to predict the response to certain interventions. For example, the abnormal TEG

can be repeated with heparinase added to the specimen. Common causes of platelet malfunction include recent aspirin use, some vasoactive drugs, hypothermia, heparin-associated dysfunction, bypass pump–related malfunction, and azotemia.

The extrinsic pathway is screened by the prothrombin time, while the partial thromboplastin time and activated clotting time reflect the adequacy of the intrinsic pathway. Abnormalities of the combined pathway are reflected in prolongation of both tests as well as the thrombin time. Clinically, the most common causes of prolonged coagulation time in the aortic surgery patient are residual anticoagulation, hypothermia, DIC, and dilutional coagulopathy. Abnormally low fibrinogen levels (below 150 mg/dl) and elevated fibrin split products both reflect the presence of DIC.

The activated clotting time and heparin levels are used to assess the presence and activity of residual heparin and the efficacy of heparin antagonism. Specific heparin-protamine titration instruments are available for bedside use.

Hemostasis After Aortic Surgery

In the postoperative aortic surgery patient, vessel wall trauma and abnormal flow are facts of life.

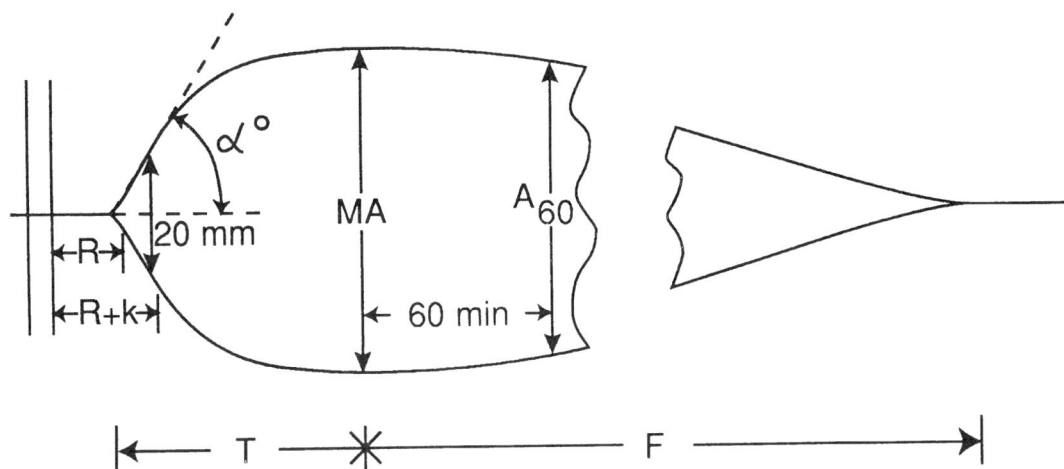

Figure 12-2. Variables derived from the thromboelastograph with normal values in parentheses. (R = reaction time for initial fibrin formation [6–8 minutes]; R + k = coagulation time [10–12 minutes]; α = clot formation rate [> 50 degrees]; MA = maximal amplitude [50–70 mm]; A_{60} = amplitude 60 minutes after MA; T = time; F = whole blood clot lysis time [> 300 minutes].) (Reprinted with permission from YG Kang, DJ Martin, J Marquez, et al. Intraoperative changes in blood coagulation and thromboelastograph monitoring in liver transplantation. Anesth Analg 1985;64:888.)

These are classical precursors to both bleeding and thrombosis. Aortic surgery patients may be further disadvantaged by a typical picture of acquired abnormalities of coagulation. Surgical bleeding and hypothermia-related coagulopathy are common, as is dilution of platelets and clotting factors. Residual heparin effect is most prominent after cardiopulmonary bypass. DIC is common after a ruptured abdominal aortic aneurysm and can also occur after elective procedures complicated by hypotension, excess volume loss, and circulatory arrest.

Hypothermia and Coagulopathy.   Coagulopathy secondary to postoperative hypothermia is a problem we should be able to prevent or at least treat once we accept its importance (Table 12-3). At low body temperatures, prothrombin time and partial thromboplastin time are prolonged even when all factor levels are normal.[16] Hypothermia retards enzyme function, slowing both clot formation and platelet activation.[17] Hypothermia explains in part the coagulopathies seen after cardiopulmonary bypass.[18,19] Paradoxically, hypothermia may enhance the fibrinolytic side of the cascade.[17] Reversible abnormalities in platelet number, shape, and function have been associated with hypothermia.[18,20,21] Platelets are usually infused at room temperature

Table 12-3. Possible Mechanisms by Which Hypothermia Compromises Normal Coagulatory Function

Prolonged prothrombin time and partial thromboplastin time
Retarded clot formation
Retarded platelet aggregation
Decrease in number of circulating platelets (sequestration)
Decreased platelet function
Contributing factor in initiation of disseminated intravascular coagulation
Imbalance in production of arachidonic acid metabolites

rather than body temperature, which can be partially responsible for the delayed functional recovery of transfused platelets.

Hypothermia may contribute to DIC.[19] Hypothermic tissue damage, specifically vascular endothelial injury, may lead to release of tissue thromboplastin. Although we usually think of hypothermia as being tissue-protective, myocardial dysfunction and severe dysrhythmias may also occur at low temperatures. It has been suggested that this may exacerbate the low-flow state that triggers DIC.[22,23]

Another mechanism of hypothermia-induced co-agulopathy, suggested by Valeri and colleagues, is an imbalance in arachidonic acid metabolite production.[21] Once massive transfusion is necessary, hypothermia may be exacerbated, which may lead to a vicious cycle.

Hypothermia may be intentional, such as residual hypothermia after bypass and after total circulatory arrest. Rewarming is often incomplete. When the prevention or treatment of CNS injury is an issue, mild hypothermia is preferable to overly aggressive rewarming. Unintentional hypothermia is far more common. It is seen frequently both in descending thoracic and in abdominal aortic aneurysm patients and is due mostly to exposure.

Bypass Procedures and Postoperative Coagulopathy.   Cardiopulmonary bypass with full heparinization is often used for ascending aortic and aortic arch aneurysms, with or without hypothermia or total circulatory arrest. Left atrial to femoral artery bypass and femoral-femoral bypass are examples of techniques used to provide distal perfusion during suprarenal descending thoracic and thoracoabdominal aortic surgery. Techniques like the latter do not always require full heparinization. Abdominal aortic surgery does not require cardiopulmonary bypass, but smaller doses of heparin (e.g., 5,000–10,000 U) are commonly administered. The degree of anticoagulation may or may not be monitored, and protamine reversal is avoided by many surgeons due to the potential hemodynamic complications of protamine.

Additionally, heparin rebound and heparin-induced platelet dysfunction are of concern in patients who have been on heparin for a prolonged period preoperatively as well as patients who have been on cardiopulmonary bypass.

Thrombocytopenia and low-grade DIC were commonly associated with bypass when bubble oxygenators were used, although both occur subclinically even with membrane oxygenators. DIC and platelet dysfunction can become manifest as significant problems, usually after long bypass times.[24] Platelet activation is probably inevitable with synthetic surface contact, and the trauma of suction and roller pumps can contribute to this process. Deposition of fibrinogen and other factors also occurs. The protein-platelet interactions lead to circulation and deposition of platelet aggregates,

triggering a syndrome similar to DIC. Independent of the DIC problem, platelets returned from bypass have been altered by plasmin adhering to mechanical contact surfaces. This interaction diminishes the ability of the platelets to normally aggregate and attach.[24] A more complete discussion of these issues may be found in Chapter 5.

Management of Coagulopathy

There can be no disagreement with administering indicated blood products in the face of clinical bleeding and a demonstrated laboratory coagulation abnormality. When abnormal laboratory values are not accompanied by bleeding, one is "treating the numbers rather than the patient." When is this appropriate? Conversely, when should one empirically treat bleeding with blood products (coagulation factors and platelets) in the absence of laboratory guidance?

The primary role of laboratory assessment of coagulation is to guide therapy of established clinical bleeding. In the nonsurgical patient who is not bleeding, abnormal laboratory values are often not treated unless they are extreme. In the surgical patient, however, there is clearly a role for treating laboratory abnormalities even when the deviation from normal is moderate. After all, surgical mortality increases if reoperation is necessary or if shock and DIC supervene. Prophylactic therapy with clotting factors and platelets is entirely appropriate in the setting of corresponding laboratory abnormalities.

When severe acute bleeding occurs, there may be no time to wait for a laboratory assessment of coagulation. If platelets, fresh frozen plasma, or both can be made available before laboratory test results arrive, and if one clinically suspects that these products are necessary, their empirical use is reasonable.

The current standard of care, however, does not support the "recipe" use of blood products when neither bleeding nor laboratory abnormality is present. There is no role for two units of fresh frozen plasma after a certain number of red cell units unless the prothrombin time is prolonged. Neither should 10 U of platelets be administered after a certain volume of red cells unless the platelet count is dangerously low. The misguided use of blood products leads to patient complications as well as a dangerously short supply of these products for patients who truly need them.

Factor deficiency is preferentially treated with specific replacement if the cause is a known chronic condition. Fresh frozen plasma contains all clotting factors and is useful in the acute situation. Current blood banking techniques can make fresh frozen plasma available in 20 minutes, so it should normally not be thawed unless it will definitely be used. Cryoprecipitate is an excellent source of von Willebrand's factor, fibrinogen, and factor VIII.

Platelets from stored red cell products, even whole blood, have no real viability. However, fresh whole blood that is less than 48 hours in vitro is a reliable source of active platelets in limited numbers. Most platelets administered in the United States are via concentrates.

A unit of platelets should increase the platelet count by 5,000–10,000 per ml. A single donor platelet concentrate transfusion will increase the platelet count by about 60,000 per ml. These concentrates decrease the number of donors to whom the recipient is exposed, thereby minimizing infectious complications. Transfused platelets do not have nearly the longevity of endogenously produced platelets. Furthermore, transfused platelets are often in a stunned state, and they may not function in vivo for up to 1 hour after transfusion.

As a very rough guide, protamine reverses heparin on a milligram for milligram of circulating heparin basis (not the total heparin dosage; 1 mg of heparin is roughly 100 U). Severe hemodynamic reactions to protamine are common, and there are several mechanisms, some of which are not dose related. Nevertheless, it is prudent to administer somewhat less than the calculated protamine dosage necessary and then reassess the state of reversal. The full protamine dosage is always preceded by a test dose of 10 mg, with a 5-minute observation period before further protamine administration. It is important to remember that hypothermia greatly slows the metabolism of heparin. Ideally, protamine dosage should be guided by automated protamine-heparin titration.

DIC is a symptom, albeit a dangerous one. It is properly treated by addressing the underlying cause, which is usually a low-flow state. Theoretically, one should not administer factors because they can further complicate the problem. However, if bleeding is allowed to persist, the underlying low-flow state will not be addressed and factors will be further reduced. Therefore, factors should be transfused guided by the laboratory examination and the presence of clinical bleeding.

The use of heparin in DIC continues to be controversial and has few advocates. Large dosages can complicate the bleeding picture and are probably contraindicated. However, in severe DIC, small dosages of heparin (1,000–2,000 U) can slow the DIC process.

If coagulopathy is thought to be due to primary fibrinolysis rather than DIC, therapy with epsilon-amino caproic acid is appropriate. DIC and primary fibrinolysis are differentiated by the platelet count, which is normal in the latter condition.

For most aortic surgery patients, hypothermia is the unintentional result of exposure, irrigation, a cool environment, and transfusion. Such patients should be rewarmed in the ICU by whatever means are available. Warming and humidification of inspired gases is most effective and is safe as long as heating of gases above 42°C is avoided. Damp linen should be changed promptly. External active rewarming devices such as the Bair-Hugger (Augustine Medical, Eden Prairie, MN) function by circulating warm air through an inflatable plastic blanket. Such devices have proven to be safe and effective. We apply a warming device to every abdominal aortic surgery patient on arrival in the ICU. During rewarming, vasodilatation may lead to hypotension; it is critical to maintain cardiac output by volume replacement. A postoperative low-flow state can exacerbate ischemic injury to the spinal cord, kidney, or intestine. When neurologic injury has occurred, one may wish to delay rewarming the patient. If in this setting rewarming is necessary because of coagulopathy, one may elect to rewarm more slowly and to a lower target temperature.

Intravenous fluid warming devices fall into two categories. Traditional blood warmers are variations on the theme of running the intravenous tubing through a hot water bath. Such devices are safe and inexpensive but are effective only at certain flow rates. If the fluid is flowing rapidly, it will not be in contact with the warm section of the tubing long enough to warm up. If the fluid flow is slow, it will emerge from the warmer and cool off before it gets to the patient. Effective flow rates differ according to the devices used. Rapid transfusion rewarming devices such as those manufactured by Level One Technologies (Rockland, MA) are engineered to be more flexible, effectively warming fluids even at high-flow rates. Some of these devices have a countercurrent warming device that is in contact with the entire length of intravenous tubing. These warmers are more expensive, as is the single-use dedicated intravenous tubing necessary for their use. Most of these devices are available with a rapid transfusion pump.

The fluids themselves can also be warmed by microwave or by standard warming cabinets. A number of recipes have been proposed for warming both fluid and blood products in the microwave but none of these are consistently reliable. If the fluid bottle is too warm to handle without discomfort, it is too warm to infuse. Blood products should probably not be warmed in a microwave oven at all.

Aprotinin reduces blood loss during major vascular surgery including aortic surgery. Its exact mechanism of action is unknown. Lord and coworkers address the possibility that aprotinin's effect may be related to modulation of neutrophil activation.[25] If this is determined to be important, it will speak to all systems that depend on intact white cell function. In the aortic surgery patient, this would include the occurrence of postoperative infection and acute lung injury. At present, aprotinin may not be indicated in thoracic aortic surgery in which hypothermic perfusion or circulatory arrest were used.[26] Furthermore, the possibility that aprotinin may be associated with an increased incidence of renal failure is alarming in the context of aortic surgery. Studies that demonstrate that this is not a major concern in the cardiac patient cannot be considered reassuring in the context of aortic surgery with its special renal risks.[27]

In a small prospective study, Lethagen and colleagues found possible benefit and no complications to the preoperative use of desmopressin.[28] In the postoperative coagulopathic patient in whom all correctable issues have been addressed, a trial of desmopressin is reasonable (see Chapter 5).

Anticoagulation and Antithrombotic Therapy

While the usual focus of attention in the early postoperative period is on coagulopathy, to some of our patients deep venous thrombosis (DVT) is more of a threat. The authors are unaware of any recent, large prospective study that assessed the risk of DVT or pulmonary embolism in unprophylaxed aortic surgery patients. Farkas et al. demonstrated an incidence of 7.5% of postoperative DVT in a population of aortic surgery patients treated throughout the perioperative period with either low-dose heparin or a new heparin fraction preparation.[29] Although 7.5% sounds like a high incidence, it should be remembered that Farkas and colleagues were looking very hard, and their goal was to compare two drugs and not to establish the incidence of clinically important DVT. Since this study did not contain an untreated control group, no statement can be made about the relative risk of perioperative bleeding events in aortic patients prophylaxed with a low-dose anticoagulant.

In view of the usual safety of low-dose heparin prophylaxis in general medical and surgical patients, treatment of the stable aortic surgery patient may be warranted if no bleeding is present. The timing of initiating this therapy must be discussed with the surgeon, because it depends on many factors including heparin and protamine use. When used, low-dose heparin will rarely be started before the 12th postoperative hour because during that first half-day the degree of hemostatic stability can change from minute to minute. Many centers avoid the use of even low-dose heparin because bleeding can be life-threatening when it does occur. Anti-DVT compression boots on the lower extremities are commonly continued in the postoperative period.

Red Cell Replacement Therapy

The goal of red cell replacement therapy is to provide adequate oxygen-carrying capacity per unit of circulating blood to promote optimal organ functioning, minimize myocardial work, and avoid metabolic acidosis. Decades ago, the goal of red cell transfusion was to maintain a hemoglobin of 10 mg per dl and a hematocrit of 30%, and a transfusion could not be questioned if the blood count showed lower numbers than these. In the early 1980s, the acquired immunodeficiency syndrome focused attention on the infectious complications of transfusion, including the more common risks such as non-A, non-B hepatitis (Table 12-4). Until recently, non-A, non-B hepatitis could not be detected at all in banked blood. Now that the so-called hepatitis C can be detected, it is clear that there are "non-A, non-B, non-C" viral agents. Additionally, according to current practice, in most patients hematocrits far lower than 30% are quite acceptable. A consensus conference of the National Institutes of Health suggested that hematocrits in the low 20% range are absolutely acceptable in healthy patients.[30]

The aortic surgery patient is clearly not a healthy patient. He or she lives with decreased functional reserve and, unlike the healthy patient, may not be able to compensate by maintaining adequate oxygen delivery (DO_2) in the face of anemia. There cannot be any universal transfusion trigger or arbitrary hemoglobin below which one transfuses. In fact, the very idea that transfusion should be undertaken at a specific hemoglobin must be considered primitive in the face of the sophisticated hemodynamic data one can obtain on ICU patients.

The need for additional red cells in the postoperative aortic surgery patient is best assessed by asking one basic question: Are there sufficient circulating red cells so that more than enough oxygen is delivered to the tissues at the optimal cardiac output? Optimal cardiac output is discussed in Chapter 11. Optimal does not mean maximal, because maximum cardiac output can usually be obtained only by overdriving the myocardium. There are two complementary yardsticks by which the adequacy of oxygen delivery is assessed. The first yardstick is by formal serial calculation of DO_2, which the reader will recall is defined as the product of cardiac output and the arterial oxygen content (see Chapter 11). Although there is no magic DO_2 correct for all patients, Shoemaker et al. did pinpoint the value of 600 ml/minute as one point above which critically ill patients were more likely to survive.[31] If cardiac output and arterial oxygen saturation are both optimized in the face of anemia, the only way left to improve DO_2 is by red cell transfusion.

If, after analyzing DO_2, it is unclear whether the individual needs more red cells, it is important to assess the second yardstick, mixed venous oxygen saturation (SVO_2). This parameter puts the DO_2 in the context of total body oxygen use.[32] As a determinant of red cell transfusion, SVO_2 is actually better than DO_2 because it allows the individual patient to indicate what he or she needs based on what he or she is actually using. The determinants of SVO_2 are DO_2 and oxygen demand (total body oxygen consumption). SVO_2 must be measured after a period during which the patient has been comfortable and undisturbed. Movement, turning, pain, and agitation can all lower the saturation temporarily even if baseline oxygen delivery is adequate. If the SVO_2 is abnor-

Table 12-4. Complications Associated with Transfusion of Blood Products

Immediate reactions
  Systemic
        Shock (acute hemolytic reaction, anaphylactic
            reaction)
        Fever, rigors (bacteremia, immunologic
            transfusion reaction, leukocyte-mediated)
  Hematologic
        Coagulopathy (dilution of platelets and clotting
            factors, acute hemolytic reaction, hypothermia,
            disseminated intravascular coagulation)
  Pulmonary and cardiac
        Fluid overload, congestive heart failure
        Transfusion-related acute lung injury (related to
            leukoagglutinin?)
        Bronchospasm (anaphylactic reaction)
  Renal
        Hematuria (transfusion reaction, coagulopathy)
        Oliguria (low cardiac output from any of
            previously mentioned reasons)
  Cutaneous
        Urticaria (isolated or associated with other
            manifestations)
Late complications
  Infectious
        Hepatitis (type B, non-A, non-B)
        Cytomegalovirus
        Human immunodeficiency virus
  Immunologic
        Acquired antibodies to red cell antigens
        Nonspecific immunocompromise
Complications that occur even with autologous blood
  (properly identified)
        Fluid overload, congestive heart failure, hypothermia,
            dilution of platelets and clotting factors, and
            bacteremia and its consequences

mally low (i.e., below 70%), optimization of both the supply and demand side is indicated. Excessive demand is addressed by optimizing sedation, analgesia, and hemodynamics, treating fever, treating any infection, and modulating the stress response. If all this has been addressed and the SVO_2 is still unsatisfactory, one may consider transfusing red cells.

The hemoglobin and hematocrit are therefore considered only as a single piece of input data in a complex algorithm. Red cells are sometimes indicated despite a hemoglobin that we have been conditioned to accept as adequate. Baxter et al. studied aortic surgery patients and demonstrated that a hemoglobin of up to 12 mg/dl may be necessary to meet accepted oxygen delivery goals.[33] As mentioned previously, there is no logical transfusion trigger for the aortic surgery patient, but if we had to indicate a specific hematocrit for transfusion, it would not be nearly as low as 21%. Cardiac ischemia, which appeared to be related to the anemia itself, has been demonstrated with hematocrits as high as 27%.[34,35] Therefore, the old 30% standard for hematocrit, discarded years ago for healthy patients, may be more reasonable for the aortic surgery patient.

To summarize the indication for transfusion in the postaortic surgery patient, transfusion should be guided by both the DO_2 and SVO_2. The hematocrit is a secondary guide, with values between 28% and 33% being reasonable goals. Transfusion is probably not indicated when the hematocrit is greater than 36%, even if DO_2 is inadequate. As hematocrit increases toward 40%, the increased viscosity of blood compromises microcirculatory flow and undermines any potential increase in DO_2.

It has been shown that in aortic surgery patients the hematocrit and hemoglobin values correlate poorly with the red cell mass.[36] While the red cell mass may be more relevant to long-term erythrocyte homeostasis, this value has limited applicability to the patient's acute status since it is rarely measured expeditiously and it includes an unknown fraction of the total blood volume in the capacitance part of the circulation.

If the patient has autologous predonated red cells available they should always be used first. Autologous blood will minimize many of the infectious and immunologic risks of red cell transfusion (see Table 12-4). However, even autologous red cells should not be considered totally benign and should be administered only on indication. Fluid overload, bacterial contamination, and clerical errors can all lead to deadly complications from autologous blood transfusion.

The first red cell products transfused in the postoperative period are sometimes salvaged autologous red cells. These are often harvested during surgery, but postoperative pleural drainage can also be reinfused. Salvaged autologous red cells are either washed or filtered but unwashed. (It is possible to safely transfuse filtered pleural blood without further processing because it is defibrinogenated.) Autotransfusion offers obvious benefits in terms of decreasing the viral infection risk and preserving the longevity of red blood cells. The literature supports the general safety of salvage autotransfusion, as well as its efficacy in reducing or eliminating the need for banked red cells.[37–40] The study of Long et al. failed to show any outcome difference between patients transfused with washed or unwashed autologous red cells.[41] They did, however, demonstrate transient coagulation abnormalities in patients treated with unwashed cells, but their small study population was relatively free of major complications. A larger study by Ouriel et al. compared autotransfusion of filtered unwashed pleural blood to homologous banked blood and found that the autologous filtered blood was safe and offered advantages in terms of cost, preservation of platelets, and coagulation factors.[42] Their study confirmed the clinical irrelevance of the transient laboratory abnormalities seen with unwashed red cells.

Washed red cells, such as those processed by the Cell Saver (Haemonetics Corp., Braintree, MA.), appear to be safe for use in aortic surgery patients. The use of filtered unwashed blood, while safe in most patients could theoretically be disruptive to a patient with an established coagulopathy. Even such a patient can benefit from unwashed blood, especially if it was filtered in a way that preserves functioning platelets.

Renal Management

Etiology, Epidemiology, and Risk

The combined activities of cardiac and vascular surgery are together the most common cause of acute renal failure. Renal failure is a major cause of morbidity and mortality in aortic surgery patients. In a series of elective aortic surgeries reported by Martin et al., renal failure was the most common complication.[43] The main culprit is decreased renal perfusion, and those who have undergone aortic cross clamping above the origin of the renal arteries are at the highest risk.[44] Patients who have undergone elective infrarenal aortic reconstruction, a much more common procedure, also develop postoperative renal failure at a rate higher than that seen after major nonvascular surgery.

Although the maintenance of adequate renal function in the aortic surgery patient is a major intraoperative issue, the consequences of renal damage often are manifested only postoperatively. Decreased urine output may have causes other than intrinsic renal compromise, and the serum creatinine level takes hours or days to increase significantly even if a patient is abruptly rendered anephric. Accordingly, renal damage in its early reversible stage is not as readily evident as is acute cardiac decompensation or CNS injury.

Etiologic Insults

Although the main culprit in acute renal failure is decreased perfusion, there are many factors that may contribute to or decrease the threshold for injury. Hypertension, diabetes, and the resulting atherosclerosis are the most common etiologies of aortic disease. These conditions are also risk factors for chronic renal failure. The intuitively pleasing idea that preoperative renal dysfunction is a predictor of further renal deterioration in the postoperative aortic surgery patient has been confirmed in some but not all studies.[45–48]

Chronic renal failure is a disease with a long asymptomatic phase, so the degree of preexisting renal failure is not always appreciated. During the long latent phase of chronic renal failure, renal function is adequate for everyday demands but lacks the reserve to withstand an insult such as a low-flow hemodynamic state.

Some aortic surgeries are preceded by an angiographic procedure. The osmotic contrast burden associated with such procedures can cause worsening of preexisting renal dysfunction, which is usually a reversible problem.[49] If several days or more elapse between angiography and the surgical procedure, the patient's volume status will usually have time to reequilibrate. If, however, the angiography is followed by surgery within 2–3 days, the contrast-related renal dysfunction can diminish reserve against further renal insult. The same is true if intraoperative contrast studies are necessary. Such adventures can cause impressive diuresis resembling diabetes insipidus.

All aortic surgery compromises renal perfusion to some degree. Aortic cross clamping anywhere between the aortic valve and the celiac artery reduces renal blood flow by directly interrupting renal perfusion for the period of cross-clamp application. It is not entirely clear that efforts to forestall renal ischemia by shunts or cardiopulmonary bypass improve renal outcome.[50] A large retrospective series reported that neither bypass strategies nor renalplegia with cold crystalloid seemed to decrease the risk of renal failure after thoracic aneurysmectomy.[47]

It is interesting that patients also develop ischemic renal failure after infrarenal aortic cross clamping. Gross perfusion of the kidneys continues if the clamp is distal to the renal arteries, yet changes in renal function apparently develop.[51] Infrarenal aortic cross clamping is known to cause intrarenal redistribution of blood flow away from cortical nephrons. The studies of Gamulin's group confirm that abnormal renal hemodynamics are common after infrarenal cross clamping, even when frank renal failure does not develop.[52,53]

Welch et al. measured renal artery blood flow during infrarenal aortic surgery and found it to be diminished in patients who later developed decreased renal function.[54] This decreased flow, whether a local phenomenon or related to cardiac output, is probably the main culprit. The changes in cardiac function related to declamping may tax the reserve of an unhealthy heart, causing decreased renal perfusion.

Other contributors to renal failure following infrarenal surgery are preexisting renal and atherosclerotic disease, nephrotoxins, mediator-related changes, and mechanical insults. The mediators are those of the systemic inflammatory response syndrome triggered by aortic cross clamping and reperfusion. Renal manifestations of this syndrome include vasoconstriction, redistribution of blood flow, and increased vascular permeability.[55] The ischemic process itself, regardless of how it was induced, triggers further elaboration of leukotrienes and other mediators.[56]

Many abdominal aortic surgery patients experience central hypovolemia in the early postoperative period secondary to the process known as *third spacing*. This decrease in circulating volume may be exacerbated by the early postoperative rewarming of a mildly hypothermic patient, which is accompanied by vasodilatation and redistributive hypovolemia. Diuretics administered during surgery to protect renal function can further deplete intravascular volume. The perioperative diuresis can mask renal dysfunction in its very early stages. As a matter of fact, the practice of using urine output as an indicator of incipient acute renal failure is clearly flawed.

In addition to the renal insults specific to the aortic surgery patient, these patients are not immune to the risks of renal dysfunction common to all ICU patients. Among these are fluid management issues, renal toxins, and the renal effects of controlled ventilation. The mention of renal toxins usually implies drugs such as aminoglycoside antibiotics and nonsteroidal analgesics. The use of nonsteroidal anti-inflammatory agents as adjuncts to pain management can contribute to renal failure, especially in the presence of hypovolemia. The potential role of myoglobin, whether from compartment syndrome, surgical trauma, or transfusion reaction, should not be forgotten.

As early as 1968, changes in renal function observed in critically ill patients were ascribed to mechanical ventilation.[57] Since then, changes observed in ventilated patients have included decreased urine output, concentrating defects, decreased glomerular filtration, water retention with decreased sodium excretion, decreased renal blood flow, and decreased hematocrit.[58] Multiple factors are operative in these patients; therefore, it is obviously difficult to separate those that may be related to mechanical ventilation and even more difficult to prove a causal relationship. The most obvious candidates for blame for these changes in renal function are the direct circulatory changes known to be caused by positive pressure ventilation and their effect on renal blood flow. A depressant effect of mechanical ventilation on atrial natriuretic hormone could also explain some of the observed abnormalities.[59]

Once the process of acute renal failure has been initiated by hypoperfusion, there are other factors that contribute to the maintenance of renal injury. These include redistrubution of blood flow away from the cortex and damage or obstruction of renal tubules.

Relative Risk of Renal Failure

One basic way to stratify renal risk is to divide patients into two groups: (1) those at normal risk and (2) those at increased risk because of preexisting renal dysfunction and suprarenal or juxtarenal pathology (see Chapter 2). In the thoracoabdominal group, Schepens et al. found that advanced age and elevated serum creatinine were both predictive of the need for postoperative dialysis.[60] Diffuse atherosclerosis and hemodynamic instability are also predictive of postoperative renal morbidity. Unlike the situation for spinal cord ischemia, duration of suprarenal cross clamping does not correlate with risk of postoperative renal failure.

Patients who have surgeries that directly involve the renal vessels carry increased renal risk compared with patients in whom the renal vasculature is normal and was not manipulated.[44,61] Concurrent repair of preexisting renal artery stenosis and aortic pathology delivers mixed results in terms of renal function.[62] Ligation of the left renal vein is sometimes carried out to improve exposure to a critical segment of aorta. Nypaver and coworkers found that the need to revascularize any major branch of the abdominal aorta was associated with an increased risk of both renal and intestinal major organ ischemic complications.[46] In contrast, the study by Allen et al. supports cautious optimism in the high-risk group.[63] Chaikof et al., in a study designed to assist in preoperative decisions regarding renal revascularization, also found that postoperative renal function was surprisingly good in this high-risk group of patients.[64] Their patients underwent combined abdominal aortic aneurysmectomy and renal revascularization, so the whole point of these operations was to preserve or improve renal function. Nevertheless, the patients did undergo the renal stress of aortic surgery. Good results (a relative term) such as those reported in these studies may be due in part to the increased vigilance that the high-risk patient is subjected to at every step. In contrast, the unexpected postoperative renal failure seen in aortic surgery patients is more vexing, partly because of our incomplete understanding of the specific risk factors.

The patients with end-stage renal disease who undergo aortic surgery are in a category by themselves. The management challenges they represent are formidable; however, they have little to loose in terms of renal function. If the patient is a candidate for renal transplantation, simultaneous aortic reconstruction is an option.[65]

Intraoperative efforts at renal protection are at least as relevant as any preexisting risk factors. In this vein, the usefulness of all measures other than careful hemodynamic support is controversial.[47,48,66–69] As in the issue of intraoperative spinal cord protection, most of the papers that support renal protective techniques are small trials that prove little.

Incidence of Renal Dysfunction

The incidence of frank postoperative renal failure has been reported as 3–18% in thoracoabdominal operations[66,70] and 40% after ruptured abdominal aortic aneurysms,[71] with intermediate numbers for urgent or elective treatment of various pathologies. In many of the same studies, mortality for postoperative renal failure has been reported as anywhere up to 90%. The least favorable figures generally apply to ruptured abdominal aortic aneurysm patients. In this population the development of renal failure may be the strongest predictor of death.[72,73] Furthermore, the mortality of renal failure in this population does not seem to be improving. This may be because physicians tend not to deny emergency surgery to anyone, or it is also possible that in the ruptured abdominal aortic aneurysm patient, renal failure is a marker of what is essentially irreversible shock.

Detection of Renal Injury.   There is no ongoing monitor of functional reserve for the kidneys with the responsiveness of ST-segment analysis for myocardial ischemia. Urine output is clearly an inadequate monitor. Low urine output is neither sensitive nor specific as an indicator of renal failure, although postoperative renal failure is less likely in patients who maintain a urine output of greater than 60 ml/hour.[74] While low urine output should never be taken lightly, it is a matter of common clinical experience that most patients who drop their urine output do not have abnormal renal function. The same is true of critically ill patients, and oliguria is commonly related to either hypovolemia or an excess of antidiuretic hormone (ADH).[75] In sicker patients, unending efforts to force the production of urine can be harmful. Conversely, some patients who have or are destined to develop renal failure, including those who have been given osmotic diuretics, produce urine volumes in the acceptable range.

Frank anuria can suggest an obstructed or kinked urinary catheter but, in the setting of an acute aortic dissection, it also can be a warning that the process has extended to the renal vessels. True obstructive uropathy after aortic surgery usually occurs after the early postoperative period.[76]

Despite the limitations of urine output as an indicator of renal well-being, it should not be ignored. Rather, changes in urine output should prompt urgent further evaluation of hemodynamics and other factors that affect renal well-being.

The limited use of blood urea nitrogen is well known. Blood urea nitrogen adds to the total picture of volume assessment and the differentiation of prerenal insufficiency and renal failure. Elevated serum creatinine, if not an early or sensitive indicator, is at least specific. Glomerular filtration rate can be assessed by a creatinine clearance based on a 2-hour measurement, which is almost as accurate as the same measurement made on a 24-hour collection.[77] In the absence of endogenous or exogenous osmotic diuretics, the bedside measurement of urine specific gravity is helpful. Specific gravity measurement is easily accomplished with a hand-held instrument, and this measurement should be routine. Diminished urine output with specific gravity greater than 1.016 suggests adequate concentrating ability and preserved renal function, possibly with ADH excess as the culprit. Specific gravity in the 1.010 range with oliguria suggests renal dysfunction. In the absence of diuretics or the syndrome of inappropriate ADH secretion, measurement of urine electrolytes is also helpful. Urine sodium greater than 30 mEq/liter is suspicious for compromised renal function, possibly suggesting early acute tubular necrosis. Urine sodium less than 20 mEq/liter suggests intact renal tubular function and a functioning renin-angiotensin-aldosterone axis. In the face of low urine output, a low urine sodium suggests intravascular hypovolemia or an alternative cause of decreased perfusion to the kidneys (Table 12-5).

The fractional excretion of sodium is a derived parameter. The ratio of the urine sodium to the serum sodium is divided by the same ratio for creatinine. The result is usually multiplied by 100 and expressed as a percent. When oliguria is prerenal and the kidneys are still functional, the serum creatinine would tend to be low with the urine creatinine tending to be higher. The urine sodium, as discussed previously, would tend to be lower, with the serum sodium being normal. Considering all of this information in the definition of fractional sodium excretion is seen to yield a lower number for the better functioning kidney (see Table 12-5). Thus, the fractional sodium excretion is no more than a way to combine information already available. This value has never been shown to be any more sensitive or specific than other parameters dis-

Table 12-5. Laboratory Parameters That Assist in the Differentiation of the Various Causes of Acute Renal Compromise

Measurement	Prerenal Azotemia	Acute Tubular Necrosis	Postrenal Cause
Urine Na (mEq/liter)	<20	>30	<30
Urine specific gravity	>1.020	1.009–1.012	1.009–1.012
Urine osmolarity (mOsm/liter)	>400	280–320	260–340
FENa	<1%	>1%	<1%

FENa = fractional excretion of sodium (see text for definition).
Source: Modified from RS Muther. Acute Renal Failure: Acute Azotemia in the Critically Ill. In JM Civetta, RW Taylor, RR Kirby (eds), Critical Care (2nd ed). Philadelphia: Lippincott, 1992.

cussed previously in the differential diagnosis of oliguria.[78] Today, fractional excretion of sodium is most useful in clinical research, typically to compare the renal effects of new drugs.

Bedside ultrasonography can assist in the investigation of postrenal causes of anuria. The use of ultrasonography to assess renal blood flow is still under investigation.[62]

In the absence of a urologic (postrenal) obstruction or a renal vascular problem, the best practical monitor of renal welfare is the pulmonary artery catheter. Renal protection is one of the best arguments for the routine use of a pulmonary artery catheter in aortic surgery.

Renal Protection and Optimization

In the general surgical patient, a fluid challenge is usually advised as the first assessment of oliguria. In the sophisticated monitoring environment advocated for the aortic surgery patient, physicians think in terms of DO_2 optimization, but a fluid bolus is still a common first step. In DO_2 optimization, preload is usually addressed first for reasons that are discussed in Chapter 11 whether or not the specific goal is renal protection. When urine output has actually fallen, augmentation of preload is often the first step unless frank fluid overload is present. Aortic procedures, particularly the abdominal variety, cause marked intestinal and retroperitoneal third spacing in the early postoperative period. The thoracic aortic surgery patient may be less tolerant of fluid boluses since such patients have less third spacing and are more vulnerable to the pulmonary

consequences of fluid overload. The hemodynamic profile is the best guide.

The administration of dopamine at renal dosages (i.e., 0.5–3.0 µg/kg/minute) is widely practiced when the kidneys are thought to be at risk, and in some units this is routine for all patients. However, there are reasonable arguments for more selective use.[79,80] Dopamine was reviewed as an inotropic agent in Chapter 11. The renal effect of dopamine is thought to be mediated by specialized receptors in the kidney, currently designated as DA-1 and DA-2 receptors. There is some evidence that dopamine is an in vivo mediator of natriuresis via these dopamine receptors, which affect electrolyte balance and renin release.[81] Marik has shown a role for the renin-angiotensin system in the diuretic action of dopamine.[82] Specialized dopamine receptors are also located in the mesenteric and renal arterial trees, where they mediate vasodilatation. The control of vascular tone in the kidney can potentially improve filtration fraction and distribution of blood flow between superficial and deeper nephrons.

Whether it is the vasoregulatory or natriuretic effects of dopamine agonism that are important for dopamine's renal effect in the clinical setting is not clear. In fact, it is no longer clear that there is any advantage to dopamine over other inotropic agents that are not agonists at specific intrarenal receptors. The question is important because in the aortic surgery setting the main concern is detection and prevention of ischemic renal damage. If the increased urine output seen with renal doses of dopamine is mediated only by a tubular mechanism, then no primary renal protection has resulted. Natriuresis maintains tubular flow of filtrate, but alone it does not provide protection from ischemia. If increased urine flow were all that was necessary for renal protection, there would be little concern associated with nonoliguric renal failure, and furosemide would be the best drug to use to protect renal function. If dopamine's renal effect is mediated mainly by increased cardiac output, then optimization of intravascular volume and hemodynamic support with any inotropic agent would provide equal benefit. However, if, as earlier studies have suggested, dopamine does increase glomerular filtration by direct effect on the renal vasculature, this may translate into true renal protection. Duke et al. recently compared the renal effects of low-dose dopamine and low-dose dobutamine in critically ill patients.[83] Under the conditions of their study, dopamine was nothing more than a diuretic, while dobutamine did not increase urine output but did increase creatinine clearance.

Early clinical studies showed that in certain settings low-dose dopamine increases glomerular filtration rate, a property not shared by other inotropic medications available at that time at the dosages studied.[84,85] Szerlip recently concluded that the evidence for benefit of renal-dose dopamine is strongest for short-term use in the case of the non-hypovolemic patient with near-normal renal function who is oliguric despite a trial of diuretics.[79] Dopamine is likewise effective as a natriuretic in the patient with congestive heart failure. Conversely, in the euvolemic aortic surgery patient in whom adequate urine output can be maintained, dopamine has not yet been shown to be of benefit.[86]

There is in fact little real evidence that dopamine has any protective role when administered prophylactically in humans. Myles et al. found prophylactic dopamine in the setting of coronary artery surgery not to be of benefit.[87] On the other hand, the setting of aortic surgery is unique in terms of renal risk, and there is animal evidence that dopamine protects against ischemic injury when administered prophylactically.[88] Additionally, low-dose dopamine is a low-risk intervention. Duke and Bersten, who do not encourage the routine use of renal doses of dopamine, argue that the biggest problem with its use may be that it masks a situation where the kidneys are still at risk of ischemic damage.[80] A similar argument is made against the administration of diuretics to oliguric patients. On the other hand, if the kidneys are already being protected as much as possible, the issue of masking is irrelevant. The wide dosage range for renal dopamine quoted in the literature suggests that tachycardia, should it occur, could be modified by a dosage decrease. It is true that hypovolemia would undermine any good that dopamine could do, since inadequate preload can cause low cardiac output and induce unhealthy renal compensations. However, in many ICUs the approach of supranormal hemodynamics (see Chapter 11) is well accepted, and avoidance of hypovolemia is part and parcel of this approach. Furthermore, the aortic surgery patient is also at risk for intestinal ischemia, and dopamine may benefit mesenteric blood flow. In the setting of aortic surgery, renal doses of dopamine are a reasonable short-term modality in the oliguric patient as long as normovolemia is maintained. Until better data are available, even prophylactic use (use in the patient with normal urine output) is reasonable. An old suggestion, that of using dopamine to modulate the adverse effects of positive end-expiratory pressure in the respiratory failure patient, may still be applicable.[89]

Given the current direction of the literature, the death knell of renal dopamine will be the advent of more specific agents. Such artificial dopamine analogues include dopexamine, fenoldopam, and ibopamine.[90,91] All are potential inodilators, none are officially indicated for renal treatment, and, with the exception of dopexamine, none are available clinically at this time.

Dopexamine, introduced in Chapter 11 as an inodilator, is an agonist at the DA-1 receptor and thus a potential renal-protective agent. Its apparent use in improving hemodynamics is such that a recent trial of supranormal hemodynamics used dopexamine to achieve the desired augmentation of cardiac output.[92] Dopexamine shares with dobutamine (thought not to stimulate renal dopamine receptors) a lack of $alpha_1$-receptor agonism. This means that dopexamine is less likely than dopamine to decrease renal perfusion at higher dosages. Human volunteer studies suggest that compared with dopamine, dopexamine is more of a vasodilator than a natriuretic.[93] Beneficial effects in patients with renal dysfunction have been confirmed.[94] No full study has yet compared dopexamine with renal doses of dopamine in the aortic surgery patient, but Gray et al. showed it to be at least as effective as dopamine for renal protection in the liver transplant patient.[95]

Fenoldopam shares with dopexamine the property of agonism at the DA-1 receptor. Fenoldopam can be administered parenterally or orally. Like dopamine, it can in some settings induce natriuresis, increase urine output, and enhance creatinine clearance. All of these actions have been demonstrated in a patient population similar to the aortic surgery patient.[96]

The most important therapeutic tool we have to protect the kidneys is hemodynamic optimization and maintenance of oxygen delivery. While hemodynamics must be optimized, the goal is not necessarily the highest cardiac output obtainable. If this were the only goal, we would push the heart to the limit, and many hearts would fail on an ischemic basis. The real goal is to achieve the best cardiac output obtainable with a reasonable cardiac workload. This balance, at our current level of knowledge, is a judgment call. The supranormal goals referred to previously provide a reasonable framework for this decision.

There is a classic problem in general internal medicine known as the *heart versus the kidneys*. Briefly, the question is whether to administer diuretics to the patient in chronic congestive heart failure to the point that blood urea nitrogen and serum creatinine are at levels that suggest chronic renal insufficiency (thus threatening the kidneys) or to administer diuretics less aggressively (thus settling for less cardiac preload reserve). A similar issue arises in the surgical situation of pneumonectomy. The desire to adequately hydrate the patient and preserve renal function is tempered by the fear that fluid overload may provoke postpneumonectomy pulmonary edema. (The relationship between overhydration and postpneumonectomy pulmonary edema remains unproven.)

In the setting of aortic surgery and renal risk, the same type of question exists. To protect the kidneys, one should push cardiac output a little harder, at the same time aiming toward a slightly higher preload than is otherwise desirable. Fluid is the most important modality in optimizing hemodynamics in this population. With good hemodynamic monitoring, the risk of fluid overload is minimal, and its consequences are usually correctable.

When choosing inotropic agents in the setting of renal compromise, it is advisable to avoid the vasoconstrictors such as phenylephrine and norepinephrine. The vasopressors tend to pacify physicians by providing good blood pressures while doing nothing to improve renal perfusion. Dobutamine, amrinone, and their younger relatives dopexamine and milrinone are better choices in the setting of increased renal risk.[83] One may also choose to avoid dopamine in dosages above the commonly accepted renal dosage if another agent will support the circulation equally well. On the other hand, low-dose dopamine should not be discontinued, because it may protect against adverse renal effects of vasopressors.[97]

If there are depressant effects of mechanical ventilation on renal function, it would seem that there is not much we can do about them. However, an examination of the possible mechanisms of this effect reveals that all of these effects can at least be moderated. Aggressive maintenance of volume status and adequate cardiac output, adequate treatment of pain, control of the stress response, and timely resumption of spontaneous ventilation when possible are all suggested as basic to the care of the aortic surgery patient.

Beyond hemodynamic optimization is the question of diuretics for renal protection. For several years the state of the art has been that diuretics do not offer primary renal protection. They increase urine flow and can convert oliguric renal failure to the easier-to-manage entity of nonoliguric renal failure. Diuretics may help prevent renal tubular damage and obstruction, processes that probably contribute to renal injury. However, the act of increasing urine flow by a tubular mechanism, as diuretics do, does nothing to prevent or reverse the initial renal ischemic insult. A good percentage of clinicians, however, continue to believe that diuretics are of value in acute oliguria, and these agents continue to be commonly administered to patients who do not respond to a fluid bolus. Diuretics are also commonly administered as prophylactic agents before aortic cross clamping, with the target organ for protection being either the spinal cord or the kidneys. There are some redeeming features to diuretics when cautiously administered. In the setting of early presumptive acute renal failure, response to diuretics may be a good prognostic factor and may simplify management.[98] Although not well investigated, it is also possible that diuretics decrease the oxygen use of renal tubular cells. Renal ischemia is, like myocardial ischemia, involved in both supply and demand. Diuretic administration must be followed by meticulous hemodynamic assessment. Loop diuretics can shift the cardiac preload lower on the Starling curve and compromise cardiac output. Osmotic diuretics can do the same if a diuresis is produced, and they can act as an acute fluid load and precipitate congestive heart failure.

Our current practice regarding the postoperative use of diuretics is to administer them mainly for neurologic, cardiac, and pulmonary indications. For absent congestive heart failure, fluid overload, or a CNS catastrophe we do not often administer diuretics with the goal of producing urine. For the patient who has undergone an aortic procedure that involved suprarenal cross clamping, it is unclear if there is any prophylactic benefit to diuretics as far as preservation of renal function. For the patient who has had only infrarenal cross clamping, there is certainly no evidence that diuretics are of any benefit to renal function. The most common cause of decreased urine output in the abdominal aortic aneurysm patient is decreased cardiac preload secondary to the third spacing that is so prominent in that procedure. The treatment of this situation is optimization of hemodynamics, usually with fluid replacement. Diuretics administered to produce urine output can turn latent hypovolemia into frank prerenal azotemia.

An important part of renal protection is the avoidance of potentially toxic drugs. Nonsteroidal anti-inflammatory drugs are known to have deleterious effects on renal blood flow. The importance of this effect in any individual patient is difficult to assess. In the hypovolemic patient, renal prostaglandins are thought to have a special role in maintaining optimal distribution of blood flow within the kidney.[99] In rats, vasodilator prostaglandins also effectively protect against ischemia.[100] The aortic patient is, of course, far more complex than a hypovolemic or pure ischemic model. For one thing, it is hoped that hypovolemia will be avoided in aortic patients and that a supranormal model of hemodynamics will be adapted. It may well be that nonsteroidal drugs are safe in aortic surgery patients. However, caution dictates that until the safety of nonsteroidal anti-inflammatory drugs can be confirmed in clinical trials, ketorolac be avoided as an analgesic. The use of nonsteroidal anti-inflammatory drugs for indications other than analgesia must be decided on an individual basis.

Among the antibiotics are several potential renal toxins, with aminoglycosides being the classic example. If their use is deemed necessary in the aortic surgery patient, the appropriate determination of serum drug levels allows accumulation of the drug to be avoided. Other precautions to minimize the toxicity of this class of drugs are identical to the general approach of adequate cardiac output and urine flow that have already been advocated.

The approach to renal protection has changed little in the last several years. What is on the horizon? In addition to new dopamine agonists mentioned, several other approaches show promise in early experimental work. Investigators have been successful to some extent at dissecting the neurohumoral response that occurs during and after aortic cross clamping, including distal cross clamping.[101-103] Specific modulators of many of the factors implicated are available. The possibility exists that manipulations of the sympathetic response, the prostaglandin cascade, or the kallikrein system may potentially improve renal function. However, the disappointing results with trials of antimodulator therapy in septic shock should remind us that these systems are extremely complex. In the absence of specific knowledge as to which responses are causative of renal compromise, which are epiphenomena, and to what extent these changes are adaptive, clinical application is not yet possible.

In the aortic surgery patient, renal damage is primarily ischemic, and calcium entry is a common marker for ischemic cell damage. Increased intracellular calcium ion can be demonstrated in experimental ischemic renal damage, and calcium entry blockers can modify this response. At a more functional level, ischemia-induced changes such as loss of renal autoregulation have been shown to be reversible by calcium channel blockers. A number of early studies suggested that calcium channel blockers can have renal protective effects.[104,105] The mechanism of their protection may of course have little to do with calcium accumulation in renal cells, and local hemodynamic effects may be more important. Recent work has confirmed the potential of calcium channel blockers to confer renal protection. For example, manidipine increased renal blood flow, glomerular filtration rate, and urine flow in a dog preparation. A natriuretic effect was also demonstrated.[106] While a study in hypertensive patients confirmed a favorable renal hemodynamic profile,

Table 12-6. Indications for Dialysis

Absolute
  Fluid overload, congestive heart failure refractory to
    other interventions
  Hyperkalemia, severe and refractory to medical
    management
  Hyperphosphatemia, hypernatremia severe and
    refractory to medical management
  Uremic pericarditis
  Central nervous system manifestations attributable to
    uremia (seizures, altered mental status)
Relative
  Blood urea nitrogen >100 mg/dl
  Creatinine >10 mg/dl
  Electrolyte disturbances in the moderate range
  Toxic levels of some drugs

the relative effects of manidipine on afferent versus efferent arterioles were not consistent with the dog data. Irzyniec et al. showed in a hypertensive rat model that the beneficial effects of nifedipine were similar to those of the sympatholytic agent moxonidine.[107] This would be significant if it held up for an ischemic model as well. Hemodynamic conditions often dictate the use of inotropic catecholamines, and simultaneous renal protection must not undermine the activity of the sympathomimetic agent.

Ischemic renal damage, like ischemic damage in other tissues, involves depletion of high-energy phosphate bonds as well as damage mediated by endogenous enzymes. Studies on the potential protective effects of adenine nucleotides are promising.[108,109] Investigations into the role of phospholipase A_2 in membrane deacetylation have shown that the effects of toxic enzymes are complex and possibly biphasic.[110] The complex question of differential vasoconstriction in the kidney raises the issue that the angiotensin system, and thus angiotensin-converting enzyme inhibitors, may play a role.[111]

While the status of atrial natriuretic peptide (ANP) is preliminary, the dynamics and kinetics of the synthetic form of the peptide are being worked out, as is the physiology of the native hormone.[112–114] Its potential as a specific renal protective agent is obvious. ANP is an endogenous peptide that is released in response to stretching of receptors in the atria. Its effects, in addition to the natriuresis for which it is named, include diuresis and systemic vasodilatation.

It appears that when ANP is infused into patients with acute renal failure, creatinine clearance can be increased, and the need for dialysis can be diminished.

The indications, techniques, and management of dialysis or ultrafiltration procedures are beyond the scope of this chapter (Table 12-6). There are now various ultrafiltration procedures available that are simpler and safer than hemodialysis. Ultrafiltration removes fluid as well as various products of the systemic inflammatory response, such as complement proteins and cytokines. The various ultrafiltration techniques are therefore not limited to renal indications.

Physicians are not able to predict who will survive acute renal failure and who among the survivors will recover significant renal function. Findings from experimental preparations suggest that a prior episode of acute renal failure provides resistance to the development of a recurrence after a new insult.[115] This finding, which is counterintuitive to say the least, shows how much there is to learn about renal pathophysiology.

Gastrointestinal Management

The gastrointestinal system is an active variable in the recovery of all aortic surgery patients, particularly those who have undergone abdominal or thoracoabdominal procedures. The insults to the intestines are mainly due to handling (mechanical trauma) and ischemia. The intestines are subject to the mechanical stresses of manipulation, retraction, lysis of adhesions, and displacement, especially with the transperitoneal approach in common use. The severity of the ischemic insult is related to preexisting disease, site of cross clamp application, duration of ischemia, collateral circulation, cardiac output, and regional blood flow. An additional factor that is yet to be completely elucidated is the relevance of increases in oxygen consumption of intestinal tissue in circumstances of stress and sepsis. Such increases may create a vicious cycle.[116]

Although the majority of aortic surgery patients do not suffer clinically obvious intestinal complications, apparently few are free of changes in intestinal function. Abnormal intestinal permeability has been demonstrated to occur almost routinely in aortic surgery patients, both in the elective and the emergency group.[117] Roumen et al. suggested that the constancy of this finding in patients who have had different hemodynamic courses indicates that reperfusion injury is the final common pathway.[117] Presumably, if the cause of changes in permeability was the early phase of the low-flow state associated with clamping, the extent of injury should vary from patient to patient because the ischemic insult is variable. The complexity of intestinal injury in this setting may defy simple explanation, and it is unclear how the clinically silent permeability changes described by Roumen and coworkers relate to complications. It is possible that the inflammatory mediators described as being important in the development of pulmonary and renal changes also play a role in gastrointestinal permeability (see Chapter 11).

Mesenteric Ischemia

Pathophysiology, Incidence, and Prognosis

Occasionally, mesenteric ischemia is the presenting complaint of the aortic surgery patient. When the symptoms are subacute, and surgery is directed at discreet atherosclerotic lesions of the mesenteric vasculature, the prognosis is actually favorable, even with simultaneous thoracoabdominal aortic reconstruction.[48,118–120] The prognosis is poor when the presentation is one of acute ischemia of the bowel. The patient who presents with ruptured abdominal aortic aneurysm also is burdened with an evolving bowel infarction.

For the majority of aortic surgery patients, bowel ischemia is a perioperative and postoperative risk. Mesenteric ischemia in the postoperative aortic surgery patient can occur as a surgical complication of a complex abdominal aortic reconstruction. It can also occur after more proximal aortic procedures. Cross clamping poses an ischemic risk because collateral circulation depends on individual anatomy, even when the level of clamp application is infrarenal. Systemic atherosclerosis and low-flow states, which exacerbate the ischemic insult, are also common in aortic patients.

In healthy individuals, the intestines assume the active function of excluding bacterial flora and their products from the circulation. By compromising this barrier function, intestinal ischemia often leads to sepsis, multiple organ failure, and death.[121,122]

This is also a common mechanism whereby shock states other than septic shock progress to sepsis.

While ischemic disease may occur anywhere in the intestine, colonic ischemia is most characteristic in the abdominal aortic surgery patient. Aortic surgery is, in fact, one of the most common antecedents to ischemic proctitis.[123] A review of the anatomy of the mesenteric vasculature readily demonstrates why this is so (Figure 12-3). The most common aortic surgery in the Western world is elective infrarenal aortic reconstruction for aneurysm. The blood supply to the small intestine, right colon, and transverse colon branches from the superior mesenteric artery, which branches off the aorta proximal to the renal arteries, safely above the usual site of infrarenal cross clamping. In contrast, the blood supply to the left colon comes from the inferior mesenteric artery (IMA). The IMA branches from the aorta well below the origin of the renal arteries and is often compromised by the reconstruction.[124] Although collateral supply from the superior mesenteric artery via the mesentery, as well as distal collateral circulation, permits ligation of the IMA in most patients, reliable collateral circulation cannot be guaranteed. Anatomic variability, low-flow states, and ischemia during cross clamping can all undermine the integrity of collateral circulation. The IMA can of course be reimplanted, but this procedure prolongs the operation, carries additional risk of bleeding and obstruction, and is not necessary in the vast majority of patients. IMA reimplantation is a matter of surgical judgment; it is practiced selectively or not at all at most centers.[44,125]

Although rare, rectal infarction may also occur. In one such case, this condition was diagnosed on abdominal radiography. Routine colonoscopy, which many advocate, would have been a more direct way to diagnose the problem.[126] For that matter, physical examination can yield clues to rectal ischemia, such as loss of sphincter tone.

Postoperative colonic ischemia has been related to perioperative intramucosal acidosis of the sigmoid colon and also to early increases and high peak levels of endotoxin, tumor necrosis factor, and interleukin 6.[127–129] These mediator elevations are in contrast to the less dramatic changes in the same factors seen after minor surgery and other surgical complications.[130,131] Most importantly, these mediators did not increase to the same degree in aortic surgery patients who developed no complications.

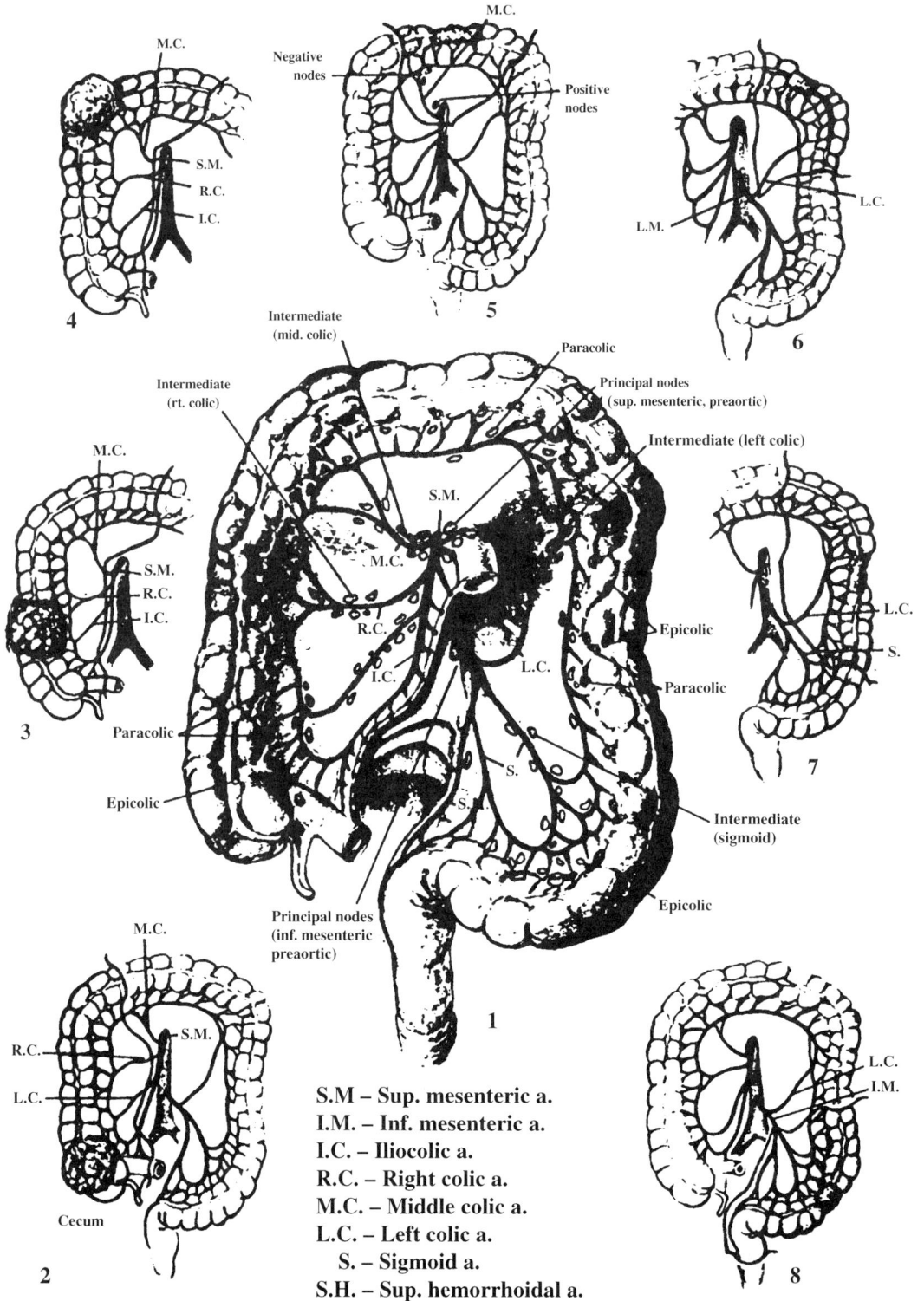

Figure 12-3. Vascular anatomy of the colon. It may be seen that the inferior mesenteric artery branches off the aorta in the middle of the usual area of reconstruction (and rupture) and that it supplies the distal colon. (Reprinted with permission from H Hodge. Surgical Anatomy [2nd ed]. Toronto: BC Decker, 1990;199. Copyright Mosby–Year Book.)

As these cytokines have been implicated in adult respiratory distress syndrome and in multiple system organ failure, the devastating nature of bowel ischemia is easily understood.

The incidence and mortality of bowel ischemia in aortic surgery patients depend on the definition of ischemia, the site of ischemia, the site and complexity of surgery, the urgency of the surgery, the surgical technique, the duration and level of cross clamping, the presence of a bypass technique, and the presence of a low-flow state.[44,46] The incidence ranges from 0.2–10.0%.[132] In the patient who presents with a ruptured aortic aneurysm, colonic infarction is obviously more common than in the elective patient. In the ruptured aneurysm population, colonic infarction is uniformly lethal when it does occur.[72] In a university hospital series, no patient whose aneurysm had been ruptured survived colonic ischemia, despite attempts to save some patients by resecting dead bowel.[133] The series of Bauer et al., while reporting comparatively good survival in the ruptured population, still identified colon ischemia as a strong predictor of early death.[134] Meissner and Johansen sought risk factors in the ruptured abdominal aortic aneurysm population and found that low cardiac output and the use of vasoconstrictors were predictive of colonic infarcts.[135] Two retrospective reviews of predominantly elective aortic procedures showed an incidence of 2.8% for intestinal ischemia with a 31% mortality in those afflicted.[124,136] A series studied prospectively showed that bowel ischemia in abdominal aortic surgery patients was more common if internal iliac flow had been interrupted bilaterally.[44] Seeger and colleagues showed in a series of abdominal aortic reconstruction procedures that the incidence of colon infarction was 2.7% during a period when the IMA was routinely ligated, with an 80% mortality. In contrast, in a later series of patients, the majority of whom had their IMA reimplanted, none suffered this complication.[125] Since the study by Seeger et al. involves the use of historical controls, the results suggest but do not prove an advantage for routine IMA reimplantation. The incidence of significant acute mesenteric ischemia in a closely related group of postoperative patients, those who have undergone cardiopulmonary bypass, is known to be at least 0.1%, with a 67% mortality.[137] The majority of those cardiac surgery patients suffered from a low-flow state, reminiscent of what Meissner and Johansen found in ruptured abdominal aneurysm patients.[135] Since some aortic surgery patients have had a cardiopulmonary bypass, and since all have had their vascular tree violated much closer to the mesentery than their cardiac surgery counterparts, one would expect the incidence of mesenteric ischemia in aortic surgery patients to be higher than the incidence in cardiac surgery patients.

Diagnosis and Management

Early diagnosis, which probably decreases the mortality of bowel ischemia, is extremely difficult, particularly in the abdominal aortic patient. In the thoracic aortic surgery patient, any abdominal symptoms should trigger a workup. However, in the abdominal aortic surgery patient, abdominal discomfort is expected. Usual bowel dysfunction, incisional abdominal pain, prolonged endotracheal intubation, sedation, analgesia, and nonspecific etiologies of fever and elevated white cell count all conspire to mask the signs of mesenteric ischemia. While the serum creatinine level has been reported to increase in cases of visceral ischemia, this is nonspecific.[124] In any case, once any of these signs are present, the process is already established. Once a picture of sepsis and abdominal rigidity is manifest, the ischemic process is advanced.

The data of Soong et al. suggest that the metabolic and inflammatory markers of the ischemic process can be detected with investigational techniques as early as the intraoperative period.[127] The suggestion by Cavaliere et al. that the creatine kinase isoenzyme pattern can warn of colonic infarction days before the event becomes manifest is clinically exciting and warrants further investigation.[138] Fiddian-Green et al. led the way in application of tonometry to early identification of patients at risk for sigmoid ischemia, suggesting that this complication is predictable even on the day of surgery.[128] Tonometry is basically a way of continuously measuring the pH of secretions in contact with a mucosal surface anywhere in the gastrointestinal tract.[129,139] The hydrogen ion content of these secretions is in equilibrium with that of the intracellular environment of the mucosal cells; therefore, a soft intramucosal catheter can serve as an intracellular pH probe. Intracellular acidosis is probably the earliest indicator of ischemia currently detectable by any technology. In the aortic surgery patient, postoperative diarrhea, bloody or not, is a common symptom of intestinal ischemia. Loss of anal sphincter tone has been described as an early finding of ischemic proctitis.

Currently, the colonoscope may be the best tool for early diagnosis. Some suggest that in the population of ruptured aortic aneurysm patients, colonoscopy should be routine to detect early ischemia.[133] Regarding patients who underwent elective abdominal aortic aneurysmectomy, Bast and coworkers found that routine colonoscopy yielded a 9% incidence of ischemic lesions of the colon.[140] This incidence is higher than the highest reported rates of symptomatic bowel ischemia in any series of elective surgery patients (several of their patients were asymptomatic). The colonoscope apparently is sensitive enough to detect a broad spectrum of patients with ischemic colitis, including those with mild or early disease. Among the symptomatic patients in the same series, the most common complaint was severe diarrhea.[140] One of the patients in the study by Bast and coworkers died (despite surgical intervention), yielding an 11% mortality for patients with colonic ischemia diagnosed by colonoscopy. That mortality seems relatively low for this serious complication. However, one must take into account that routine colonoscopy is an expensive and labor-intensive undertaking. It requires a change in position and sometimes sedation. Furthermore, bacteremia may occur during the procedure, and the possibility exists that an aortic graft may be seeded with bacteria. Therefore, the routine use of this procedure is an individual judgment. Jonung et al. and Laustsen et al. found that the sigmoidoscope, a more user-friendly tool than the colonoscope, was helpful in the diagnosis of post–aortic surgery ischemic colitis.[124,141] This is consistent with our understanding of the distal nature of this complication.

Once ischemic colitis has been identified, the direction of treatment is a surgical decision. The early mild cases are treated conservatively with antibiotics and bowel rest. In the series of Longo et al., conservative therapy was highly successful for properly selected patients.[142] As improved diagnostic methods identify patients earlier, conservative therapy may play more of a role. Patients with obvious necrotic bowel at the outset and patients whose disease is progressing despite conservative

care must undergo surgical exploration. Most important for the intensivist, all patients with suspected ischemic colitis should have aggressive hemodynamic management aimed at maximizing oxygen delivery. Although no clinical trial can prove it, the best use of the so-called supranormal hemodynamic goals is the preservation of an organ that is at risk of infarction. This is even more important when the organ at risk is the gut, which may be an important player in the development of multiple organ failure (see Chapter 11).[143]

Abnormal Intestinal Motility

The patient who has undergone a thoracic procedure is not immune from postoperative ileus, which, when present, is due usually to the nonspecific state of being critically ill. Serum hypoproteinemia and hypoalbuminemia are associated with impaired intestinal function, and decreased serum albumin is common in aortic surgery patients.[144] The functional ileus of postoperative patients is usually managed with nasogastric drainage continued until clinical evidence of bowel recovery appears. As we would expect, replacement of albumin does not seem to improve postoperative ileus, it appears that the decreased serum albumin is a marker and not a cause.[144]

The abdominal or thoracoabdominal aortic surgery patient has undergone extensive manipulation of the intestines, especially with the classic transperitoneal approach to the aorta. Ileus appears to be less of a problem with the retroperitoneal approach to abdominal aortic reconstruction.[145,146] Resolution of ileus usually parallels the patient's overall recovery. Gastric and colonic function often return later than small bowel function, which is the basis of jejunal tube feeding with elemental formulas.

Prolonged paralytic ileus (usually manifest as absence of bowel sounds or failure to pass stool or flatus) and mild abdominal distension and discomfort can prevent the resumption of normal enteral feeding. This situation is usually managed by instituting parenteral nutrition on the assumption that intestinal function is absent. However, the study of Barker et al. suggests that in many of these patients the small bowel is capable of peristaltic and absorptive function adequate to handle enteral feeding with low residue formulae.[147] Apparently, intestinal function is not an "all or nothing" proposition. In selected patients with ileus, a careful trial of enteral tube feeding with low residue formula may save the cost, risk, and clinical monitoring associated with central parenteral nutrition.

True intestinal obstruction is a rare complication of aortic aneurysm repair.[148,149] Presentation may be early or late, and reported causes include duodenal intramural hematoma, adhesions involving the Dacron graft, and superior mesenteric artery syndrome. Management may be surgical or expectant. Again, the possibility of mesenteric ischemia must never be ignored.

Abdominal distension is not normal after abdominal aortic surgery. When bleeding, perforation, ischemia, and ileus have been excluded, other etiologies must be sought.[150]

Gastric Ulceration and Bleeding

Gastric ulceration and related gastrointestinal bleeding were until recently approached as an isolated complication of the critically ill state. Early research attention was devoted to determining which histamine H_2-receptor blocker should be administered by what kind of infusion to keep the gastric pH at an arbitrarily high level as measured at some specific interval. The problem was seen as a local one, related to either excessively acidic gastric secretions or decreased resistance to ulceration. This approach was successful at lowering the incidence and severity of peptic ulceration and bleeding in the critically ill population.[151–153] Corresponding reduction in mortality has been harder to demonstrate.

The concept of tonometry was discussed previously in connection with colonic ischemia. Recent work with this tool applied to the stomach suggests that the significance of gastric pH may go way beyond the question of gastric ulceration. It appears that pH of gastric secretions may be a marker of perfusion and perhaps of adequacy of oxygen delivery.[154,155,143]

The relationship between mucosal gastric pH and patient welfare, if it exists at all, is certainly not a simple or linear function. The pH measured by a tonometer probe adjacent to gastric mucosa is not identical to the pH of aspirated gastric secretions. While intramucosal acidosis may be a marker of poor perfusion, the ability to acidify gastric secretions is an energy-requiring process that

cannot proceed in the face of inadequate perfusion.[154] Additionally, the process of acidification of gastric juice also has adaptive value. When intestinal flora move into the gastric area in the absence of acid secretions, microaspiration can more commonly result in pneumonia.

In addition to the adequacy of systemic perfusion and the impact of preventive strategies aimed at alkinization of gastric secretions, the integrity of coagulation also contributes to the incidence of upper gastrointestinal bleeding.[156,157]

Therefore, the armamentarium of measures to prevent gastric ulceration and bleeding consists of proper hemodynamic and coagulation management, management of the stress response, the administration of antacids or mucosal protectors by nasogastric tube, the administration of H_2-receptor blockers, and the use of agents that protect gastric mucosa by other means.[139,151,152,155,157] Prominent among newer drugs are the prostaglandin E_1 analogues such as misoprostol. Drug therapy may be administered empirically or titrated to gastric pH. Not surprisingly, a history of peptic ulcer disease is a major risk factor for postoperative bleeding ulcer.[48,156] Attention to detail, including aggressive treatment of coagulopathy, is indicated in the patient with a preoperative history of peptic ulcer disease. Among the alternatives to antacids (H_2-blockers, sucralfate, and prostaglandin analogues), it is hard to consistently show advantage for any one approach. There is little efficacy in combined therapy. The current trend seems to favor agents other than the H_2-blockers, at least in the postoperative period.[153]

Pancreatitis and Biliary Disease

Asymptomatic increases in amylase are common after aortic surgery.[158] These may reflect low-grade pancreatic inflammation. In contrast, acute pancreatitis is uncommon following aortic surgery.[159] Postoperative pancreatitis reflects a poor general condition. The gastrointestinal tract is indeed a barometer of systemic perfusion. Patients with postoperative pancreatitis are not necessarily alcoholics or patients with biliary disease. Diagnosis and treatment in the aortic surgery patient are no different than for other surgical patients.

Acute cholecystitis in the postoperative period can progress to gallbladder necrosis and sepsis.

Table 12-7. Some of the More Common
Potential Complications of Parenteral Nutrition

Associated with intravenous access
    Peripheral: phlebitis, cellulitis, compartment syndrome
    Central: line sepsis, pneumothorax, vascular trauma,
        chylothorax, parenteral solution in pleural space,
        disconnect with bleeding
Associated with nutritional solution itself
    Fluid overload
    Hyperglycemia
    Hypoglycemia
    Metabolic acidosis
    Electrolyte disturbances
    Renal, hepatic dysfunction
    Hypercapnea
    Bacteremia, sepsis

Source: Modified from RK Stoelting, SF Dierdorf. Anesthesia and Co-Existing Disease (3rd ed). New York: Churchill Livingstone, 1993;389.

This complication is difficult to diagnose because dressings, analgesic care, and expected abdominal findings can cover up the early warning signs. A high index of suspicion must therefore be maintained in any patient who has fever, an increase in white blood cell count, or any change in the abdominal findings.

Metabolic Management

Diabetes

The rationale for glucose control itself was described earlier. The general care of the diabetic patient for aortic surgery is not unique. Diabetics have a higher incidence of coronary artery disease, cerebral vascular disease, renal disease, and general atherosclerotic disease than nondiabetic controls. In the perioperative period diabetics have a higher incidence of infection and metabolic complications. Treiman et al. have confirmed that diabetics have more complications, but not in a way that would alter their management.[160] Most of their complications are issues that physicians already vigilantly look for in all aortic surgery patients.

Glucose balance in diabetic patients undergoing major surgical procedures is best managed with continuous infusions of insulin, glucose, and potassium, which are adjustable at independent rates. Diabetics with any degree of renal insufficiency are at high risk for hyperkalemia. All insulin-requiring diabetics are at increased risk of lactic acidosis, hyperosmolar state, and ketoacidosis.

Nutrition

There is no evidence that the nutritional needs of the aortic surgery patient are vastly different from those of other major surgery patients. The degree of surgical trauma to which the abdominal aortic surgery patient is subjected is often far greater than that experienced by the cardiac surgery patient. A significant postoperative condition of negative nitrogen balance can be expected. This can lead to mass wasting of vital organs, the resulting dysfunction of which can affect outcome. The goal of perioperative nutritional support is to minimize the tendency toward negative nitrogen balance. Positive nitrogen balance, in addition to preserving organ function, allows better healing of surgical wounds and appears to helps maintain immunocompetence.

Nutritional support, by whatever route is practical, should be instituted early in the postoperative period, preferably by the middle of the first postoperative week. Studies in surgical patients have shown that early nutritional support may shorten hospital stay and minimize morbidity and mortality.[161,162] Askanazi et al. demonstrated the salutary effect of immediate postoperative nutritional support following radical cystectomy.[163] The patients in their treatment group had shorter hospital stays (averaging 17 days) than the patients whose only source of calories was 5% glucose, whose hospital stays averaged 24 days.

Both the enteral and parenteral routes can be used to deliver calories and essential nutrients. There is no reason to favor the intravenous route if tube feedings are practical. Enteral support is just as effective as intravenous hyperalimentation at modulating surgically induced negative nitrogen balance.[164] By avoiding costly intravenous alimentation, the incidence of complications, such as line sepsis and hyperglycemia, can be minimized (Table 12-7). Additionally, the use of the gastrointestinal tract may decrease the translocation of bacteria and endotoxin through the intestinal mucosal barrier, which is a major mechanism of sepsis. Enteral feeding may also decrease the likelihood of gastric stress ulceration, prevent acalculous cholecyctitis, and better maintain the trophic state of the gut.

When the gastrointestinal tract does not tolerate sufficient volumes of nutrients for total support, combination therapy can allow the administration of more dilute parenteral alimentation solutions while maintaining many of the possible benefits of enteral nutrition. Additionally, some of the complications of intravenous nutrition may be minimized.

Nutritional support is managed by using mathematical formulas to predict quantitative requirements and then modifying these according to response. Initial route and formula content are reevaluated on a daily basis.

Basal metabolic rate (BMR) is the minimal caloric requirement necessary to maintain body function in an adult at rest. BMR can be determined from a chart that takes into account age, sex, and body surface area, which is in turn determined from a body surface area chart based on height and weight. BMR can also be determined by the Harris-Benedict formula.[165]

The surgical patient is not a healthy adult at rest. Actual energy expenditure, according to Long et al., is predicted by modifying BMR by an activity factor and an injury score.[166] A simpler approach is to estimate the stress level, which is shown in Table 12-8.

Nitrogen balance is often reassessed by determining the 24-hour urea nitrogen. A positive balance of 2 g per day is a reasonable therapeutic goal. Protein intake and sometimes calorie intake are increased if nitrogen balance remains negative.

Some degree of impairment in intestinal function is to be expected in a majority of aortic surgery patients. It is a matter of surgical judgment as to what evidence of bowel recovery must be present before enteral feedings are started, whether by tube or mouth. This also depends on the type of formula used. At the very least, for enteral feeding to commence, nasogastric drainage must be minimal, and there must be no suspicion of bowel ischemia. The feeding tube should be aspirated for residual formula every 2–4 hours when feedings are initially instituted.

The patient who ends up on nutritional support usually is fed (or infused with) a proprietary alimentation formula that provides most of the patient's nutritional needs, including supplementation of water-soluble vitamins and trace elements.

Table 12-8. Estimating the Stress Level and Caloric Requirements in the Surgical Patient

Level of Stress	Caloric Requirements
No stress	28 kcal/kg/day (117.6 kJ/kg/day)
Mild stress	30 kcal/kg/day (126 kJ/kg/day)
Moderate stress	35 kcal/kg/day (147 kJ/kg/day)
Severe stress	40 kcal/kg/day (168 kJ/kg/day)

These formulae are available with a variety of nutrient ratios. They have been adapted to the needs of patients who require fluid restriction (double concentrated) as well as the needs of patients with renal and hepatic disease.

When parenteral nutrition is required, the risk of line sepsis can be lowered by adhering to strict aseptic technique in insertion and maintenance of the dedicated central line. Calorie intake is supplemented with intravenous fat emulsions that also provide essential fatty acids. Basic calorie requirements are provided with concentrated glucose. Trace elements, insulin, and electrolytes are added as determined by frequent laboratory assessment. The ongoing individualization of the nutritional program should prevent overzealous feeding. Volume overload, hyperglycemia, electrolyte disturbances, and hypertriglyceridemia must be avoided.

The patient who seems to be ready for oral nutrition generally receives whatever he or she can hold down. We are currently learning more about the specifics of how changes in nutrient levels may accompany the stress response, and how such changes may affect wound healing.[167] Hospital dietitians and nutritionists as well as dedicated ICU nutritional support teams can be helpful in establishing protocols to minimize the mandatory state of malnutrition that develops in most patients after major surgery. The *Handbook of Total Parenteral Nutrition* is an excellent source for critical care nutrition.[168]

Emergency Reoperation

Aortic reoperation itself need not be a disaster.[169] Patients undergoing emergency reoperation have a dramatic increase in mortality as compared with patients not requiring it.[120] One would expect that

mortality in early reoperation would compare favorably with mortality for the ruptured abdominal
aneurysm patient because the catastrophe of the patient undergoing reoperation occurs in a setting of
intense monitoring and early diagnosis. Olsen et al.
found this to be the case, showing an 81% survival
rate for early reoperation.[45] Even relaparotomy after
ruptured abdominal aortic aneurysm repair carried
only a 50% additional mortality in one series.[170]
Not surprisingly, the main conditions that require
reoperation are bleeding and infection, with non-
bleeding graft occlusion a distant third. By comparison, reoperation for obstruction of grafts is much
more common after peripheral revascularization,
probably because of the smaller size and lower flow
in extremity arteries.

Common sense dictates that one should have an
organized approach to the resuscitation, transport,
and induction of these patients to favorably affect
the survival rate. Depending on the facility and the
staff, simple procedures can be undertaken in the
ICU to avoid transport to the operating room.
Wound exploration and debridement may fall into
this category. It is, however, a rare ICU that can
handle a procedure that involves brisk bleeding.
Furthermore, it is easier to minimize the risk of contamination and infection in the operating suite than
in the ICU.

While no blanket rules can cover the variety of
situations encountered, there are some special concerns regarding transport that need to be discussed.
The transport is likely to elicit a stress response
from the patient. Management of sedation in the
preoperative period depends on the hemodynamic
stability of the patient and the patient's mental status. For the patient who is hemodynamically stable
and awake, it is reasonable to start the administration of intravenous anesthetics before transport. If
this is done, sufficient time should be allowed for
each bolus of anesthetic to reach its peak hemodynamic effect before the patient is moved; therefore,
adequate hemodynamic adjustments may be made
under controlled circumstances.

If the surgeon believes that minutes count, or if
the patient is unstable, administration of large
dosages of anesthetic should obviously be deferred
until the patient is settled in the operating room. A
dosage of scopolamine before transport (i.e., 0.3–0.4
mg intravenously for amnesia) is reasonable, as are
small dosages of opioids or benzodiazepines.

If the patient has already developed some degree
of acute lung injury, decreased compliance may
make ventilation via Ambu bag ineffective. The in-
line valve of Ambu-like devices is such that inadequate tidal volumes can be delivered to the
noncompliant lung. Alternatives include a transport
ventilator and a Mapleson-type portable anesthesia
system. The Jackson-Reese system can be constructed from basic equipment and is also available
as a disposable unit. The simple operator-controlled
valve on such a system allows the necessary flexibility to ventilate the injured lung. Whatever system
is used, a few minutes verifying the adequacy of
ventilation before transport is time well spent.

A portable positive end-expiratory pressure
(PEEP) valve should be used to continue PEEP
therapy. In the severely injured lung, it can take 30
minutes to rerecruit atelectatic alveoli after even a
brief interruption of PEEP. Severe hypoxemia, as
well as pulmonary edema and stress, can occur in
the interim. This is one of the reasons why PEEP is
not interrupted to measure cardiac filling pressures
(see Chapter 11), and why unnecessary endotracheal suctioning is not performed in the hypoxic
lung-injured patient.

Most thoracic aortic patients have chest drains
during the recovery period. The vast majority of
these function as fluid drains, and the patient will
not deteriorate if suction is discontinued for the
transport period. For the patient with a persistent
leak of air into the pleura (indicating an early bronchopleural fistula), the ability to tolerate a clamped
chest tube must be tested before transport. If the patient is suction dependent, then another piece of
heavy equipment (portable suction device) must be
taken along.

The physician who thinks it is ridiculous to get
worked up about a transport has probably not partic-
ipated in many. The complexity of these adventures
justifies the growing literature in this area as well as
the attention now being paid to protocols and quality improvement for critical patient transport.[171–174]

While some catastrophic complications such as
massive bleeding or critical loss of perfusion to a
vital organ can be addressed with reexploration (either in the operating room or in the ICU itself), other
problems with a less acute presentation may be indications for radiologic evaluation. This commonly
involves angiographic study or computed tomographic scanning. Magnetic resonance imaging has

proven useful in answering a variety of postoperative questions in aortic patients.[175] The logistical nightmare of subjecting an unstable critical patient to magnetic resonance imaging can preclude its use in such patients except in centers with a plan for magnetic resonance imaging of the critical patient.

Conclusion

When things go well for our patients, many of the issues discussed in this chapter remain in the background. When things go poorly, we sometimes wonder why we bother at all; it is easy to feel that one is torturing hopelessly ill people with invasive and aggressive therapies. When we think of the future of our patients, we often imagine the worst. Unlike surgeons, intensivists and anesthesiologists do not have outpatient follow-up and do not regularly see the long-term results of their labor.

If one had to pick a simple descriptor to separate the complicated patients from those who sail through their postoperative course, it would be readiness for transfer out of the ICU within 36–72 hours of surgery. Gefke et al. found that even among patients who require more than 48 hours of ICU care, greater than half were still alive at 1 year, usually with a reasonable quality of life as judged by the patients.[176] Apparently, our efforts are well worth the price.

References

1. Crawford ES, Crawford JL, Safi HJ, et al. Thoracoabdominal aortic aneurysms: preoperative and intraoperative factors determining immediate and long-term results of operations in 605 patients. J Vasc Surg 1986;3:389.
2. Svensson LG, Hess KR, Coselli JS, Safi HJ. Influence of segmental arteries, extent, and atriofemoral bypass on postoperative paraplegia after thoracoabdominal aortic operations. J Vasc Surg 1994;20:255.
3. Crawford E, Mizrahi E, Hess KR, et al. The impact of distal aortic perfusion and somatosensory evoked potentials monitoring on prevention of paraplegia after aortic aneurysm operation. J Thorac Cardiovasc Surg 1988;95:357.
4. Tabayashi K, Ohmi M, Togo T, et al. Aortic arch aneurysm repair using selective cerebral perfusion. Ann Thorac Surg 1994;57:1305.
5. Ergin MA, Galla JD, Lansman SL, et al. Hypothermic circulatory arrest in operations on the thoracic aorta. Determinants of operative mortality and neurologic outcome. J Thorac Cardiovasc Surg 1994;107:788.
6. Bachet J, Guilmet D, Goudot B, et al. Cold cerebrolegia. A new technique of cerebral protection during operations on the transverse aortic arch. J Thorac Cardiovasc Surg 1991;102:85.
7. Gloviczki P, Cross SA, Stanson AW, et al. Ischemic injury to the spinal cord or lumbosacral plexus after aorto-iliac reconstruction. Am J Surg 1991;162:131.
8. Hollier LH, Money SR, Naslund TC, et al. Risk of spinal cord dysfunction in patients undergoing thoracoabdominal aortic replacement. Am J Surg 1992;164:210.
9. Cox GS, O'Hara PJ, Hertzer NR, et al. Thoracoabdominal aneurysm repair: a representative experience. J Vasc Surg 1992;15:780.
10. Schmidt CA, Wood MN, Gan KA, Razzouk AJ. Surgery for thoracoabdominal aortic aneurysms. Am Surg 1990;56:745.
11. Nugent M. Pro: cerebrospinal fluid drainage prevents paraplegia. J Cardiovasc Vasc Anesth 1992;6:366.
12. Hill AB, Kalman PG, Johnston KW, Vosu HA. Reversal of delayed-onset paraplegia after thoracic aortic surgery with cerebrospinal fluid drainage. J Vasc Surg 1994;20:315.
13. Salam AA, Sholkamy SM, Chaikof EL. Spinal cord ischemia after abdominal aortic procedures: is previous colectomy a risk factor? J Vasc Surg 1993;17:1108.
14. Samso-Sabe E, Valles-Esteve J, Gallart-Gallego L, et al. Spinal cord ischemia in the postoperative period of aortic surgery. Rev Esp Anestesiol Reanim 1990;37:234.
15. Davison JK, Cambria RP, Vierra DJ, et al. Epidural cooling for regional spinal cord hypothermia during thoracoabdominal aneurysm repair. J Vasc Surg 1994;20:304.
16. Rohrer MJ, Natale AM. Effect of hypothermia on the coagulation cascade. Crit Care Med 1992;20:1402.
17. Patt A, McCrosky BL, Moore EE. Hypothermia-induced coagulopathies in trauma. Surg Clin North Am 1988;68:775.
18. Khabbaz KR, Marquardt CA, Wolfe JA, et al. Reversible platelet dysfunction following cardiopulmonary bypass: a temperature-dependent defect in platelet membrane thromboxane A_2 synthesis. Surg Forum 1989;40:201.
19. Mahajan SL, Myers TJ, Baldini MG. Disseminated intravascular coagulation during rewarming following hypothermia. JAMA 1981;245:2517.
20. Reed RL, Johnston TD, Hudson JD, Fischer RP. The disparity between coagulopathy and clotting studies. J Trauma 1992;33:465.
21. Valeri CR, Feingold H, Cassidy G, et al. Hypothermia-induced reversible platelet dysfunction. Ann Surg 1987;205:175.
22. Paul J, Cornillon B, Baguet J, et al. In vivo release of a heparin-like factor in dogs during profound hypothermia. J Thorac Cardiovasc Surg 1981;82:45.

23. Yoshihara H, Yamamoto T, Mihara H. Changes in co-agulation and fibrinolysis occurring in dogs during hypothermia. Thromb Res 1985;37:503.

24. Spiess BD, Chang SB. Intraoperative Coagulation Disorders. In SJ Thomas, JL Kramer (eds), Manual of Cardiac Anesthesia (2nd ed). New York: Churchill Livingstone, 1993;517.

25. Lord RA, Roath OS, Thompson JF, et al. Effect of aprotinin on neutrophil function after major vascular surgery. Br J Surg 1992;79:517.

26. Westaby S, Forni A, Dunning J, et al. Aprotinin and bleeding in profoundly hypothermic perfusion. Eur J Cardiothorac Surg 1994;8:82.

27. Lemmer JH Jr, Stanford W, Bonney SL, et al. Aprotinin for coronary artery bypass grafting: effect on postoperative renal function. Ann Thorac Surg 1995;59:132.

28. Lethagen S, Rugarn P, Bergqvist D. Blood loss and safety with desmopressin or placebo during aorto-iliac graft surgery. Eur J Vasc Surg 1991;5:173.

29. Farkas JC, Chapuis C, Combe S, et al. A randomised controlled trial of a low-molecular-weight heparin (enoxaparin) to prevent deep-vein thrombosis in patients undergoing vascular surgery. Eur J Vasc Surg 1993;7:554.

30. National Institutes of Health. Consensus conference: perioperative red cell transfusion. JAMA 1988;260:2700.

31. Shoemaker WC, Appel PL, Kram HB, et al. Prospective trial of supranormal values of survivors as therapeutic goals in high-risk surgical patients. Chest 1988;94:1176.

32. Lind L, Skoog G, Malstam J. Relations between mixed venous oxygen saturation and hemodynamic variables in patients subjected to abdominal aortic aneurysm surgery and in patients with septic shock. Ups J Med Sci 1993;98:83.

33. Baxter BT, Minion DJ, McCance CL, et al. Rational approach to postoperative transfusion in high-risk patients. Am J Surg 1993;166:720.

34. Christopherson R, Frank SM, Norris EJ, et al. Low postoperative hematocrit is associated with cardiac ischemia in high-risk patients. Anesthesiology 1991;75:99.

35. Nelson AH, Fleisher LA, Rosenbaum SH. The relationship between postoperative anemia and cardiac morbidity in high risk vascular patients in the ICU. Crit Care Med 1993;21:860.

36. Cordts PR, LaMorte WW, Fisher JB, et al. Poor predictive value of hematocrit and hemodynamic parameters for erythrocyte deficits after extensive elective vascular operations. Surg Gynecol Obstet 1992;175:243.

37. McMahon AJ, McCormick JS. Combined predeposit and salvage autotransfusion in elective aortic aneurysm repair. J R Coll Surg Edinb 1993;38:71.

38. Tulloh BR, Brakespear CP, Bates SC, et al. Autologous predonation, haemodilution and intraoperative blood salvage in elective abdominal aortic aneurysm repair. Br J Surg 1993;80:313.

39. Duchateau J, Nevelsteen A, Suy R, et al. Autotransfusion during aorto-iliac surgery. Eur J Vasc Surg 1990;4:349.

40. Brown G, Bookallil M, Herkes R. Use of the cell saver during elective abdominal aortic aneurysm surgery—influence on transfusion with bank blood. A retrospective survey. Anaesth Intensive Care 1991;19:546.

41. Long GW, Glover JL, Bendick PJ, et al. Cell washing versus immediate reinfusion of intraoperatively shed blood during abdominal aortic aneurysm repair. Am J Surg 1993;166:97.

42. Ouriel K, Shortell CK, Green RM, DeWeese JA. Intraoperative autotransfusion in aortic surgery. J Vasc Surg 1993;18:16.

43. Martin LF, Atnip RG, Holmes PA, et al. Prediction of postoperative complications after elective aortic surgery using stepwise logistic regression analysis. Am Surg 1994;60:163.

44. Johnston KW, Scobie TK. Multicenter prospective study of nonruptured abdominal aortic aneurysms. I. Population and operative management. J Vasc Surg 1988;7:69.

45. Olsen PS, Schroeder T, Agerskov K, et al. Surgery for abdominal aortic aneurysms. A survey of 656 patients. J Cardiovasc Surg (Torino) 1991;32:636.

46. Nypaver TJ, Shepard AD, Reddy DJ, et al. Supraceliac aortic cross clamping: determinants of outcome in elective abdominal aortic reconstruction. J Vasc Surg 1993;17:868.

47. Svensson LG, Coselli JS, Safi HJ, et al. Appraisal of adjuncts to prevent acute renal failure after surgery on the thoracic or thoracoabdominal aorta. J Vasc Surg 1989;10:230.

48. Svensson LG, Crawford ES, Hess KR, et al. Thoracoabdominal aortic aneurysms associated with celiac, superior mesenteric, and renal artery occlusive disease: methods and analysis of results in 271 patients. J Vasc Surg 1992;16:378.

49. Parfrey PS, Griffiths SM, Barrett BJ, et al. Contrast material-induced renal failure in patients with diabetes mellitus, renal insufficiency, or both. A prospective controlled study. N Engl J Med 1989;320:143.

50. Livesay JJ, Cooley DA, Ventemiglia RA, et al. Surgical experience in descending thoracic aneurysmectomy with and without adjuncts to avoid ischemia. Ann Thorac Surg 1985;39:37.

51. Awad RW, Barham WJ, Taylor DN, et al. The effect of infrarenal aortic reconstruction on glomerular filtration rate and effective renal plasma flow. Eur J Vasc Surg 1992;6:362.

52. Gamulin Z, Forster A, Morel D, et al. Effects of infrarenal aortic cross clamping on renal hemodynamics in humans. Anesthesiology 1984;61:394.

53. Gamulin Z, Forster A, Simonet F, et al. Effects of renal sympathetic blockade on renal hemodynamics in patients undergoing major aortic abdominal surgery. Anesthesiology 1986;65:688.

54. Welch M, Knight DG, Carr HM, et al. Influence of renal artery blood flow on renal function during aortic surgery. Surgery 1994;115:46.

55. Smith FC, Gosling P, Sanghera K, et al. Microproteinuria predicts the severity of systemic effects of reperfusion injury following infrarenal aortic aneurysm surgery. Ann Vasc Surg 1994;8:1.

56. Klausner JM, Paterson IS, Goldman G, et al. Postischemic renal injury is mediated by neutrophils and leukotrienes. Am J Physiol 1989;256:794.

57. Sladen A, Laver M, Pontoppidan H. Pulmonary complications and water retention in prolonged mechanical ventilation. N Engl J Med 1968;279:448.

58. Annat G, Viale JP, Bui Xuan B, et al. Effect of PEEP ventilation on renal function, plasma renin, aldosterone, neurophysins and urinary ADH, and prostaglandins. Anesthesiology 1983;58:136.

59. Leithner C, Frass M, Pacher R, et al. Mechanical ventilation with PEEP decreases release of alpha-atrial natriuretic peptide. Crit Care Med 1987;15:484.

60. Schepens MA, Defauw JJ, Hamerlijnck RP, Vermeulen FE. Risk assessment of acute renal failure after thoracoabdominal aortic aneurysm surgery. Ann Surg 1994;219:400.

61. AbuRahma AF, Robinson PA, Boland JP, Lucente FC. The risk of ligation of the left renal vein in resection of the abdominal aortic aneurysm. Surg Gynecol Obstet 1991;173:33.

62. Aronson S, Wiencek JG, Feinstein SB, et al. Assessment of renal blood flow with contrast ultrasonography. Anesth Analg 1993;76:964.

63. Allen BT, Anderson CB, Rubin BG, et al. Preservation of renal function in juxtarenal and suprarenal abdominal aortic aneurysm repair. J Vasc Surg 1993;17:948.

64. Chaikof EL, Smith RB 3rd, Salam AA, et al. Ischemic nephropathy and concomitant aortic disease: a ten year experience. J Vasc Surg 1994;19:135.

65. Wright JG, Tesi RJ, Massop DW, et al. Safety of simultaneous aortic reconstruction and renal transplantation. Am J Surg 1991;162:126.

66. Torsello G, Kutkuhn B, Kniemeyer H, Sandmann W. Prevention of acute renal failure in suprarenal aortic surgery. Results of a pilot study. Zentralbl Chir 1993;118:390.

67. Awad RW, Barham WJ, Taylor DN, et al. Technical and operative factors in infrarenal aortic reconstruction and their effect on the glomerular filtration rate in the immediate postoperative period and 6 months later. J Vasc Surg 1990;4:239.

68. Bush HL Jr. Renal failure following abdominal aortic reconstruction. Surgery 1983;93:107.

69. Allen BT, Rubin BG, Anderson CB, et al. Simultaneous surgical management of aortic and renovascular disease. Am J Surg 1993;166:726.

70. Svensson LG, Crawford ES, Hess KR, et al. Experience with 1509 patients undergoing thoracoabdominal aortic operations. J Vasc Surg 1993;17:357.

71. Chawla SK, Najafi H, Ing TS, et al. Acute renal failure complicating ruptured abdominal aortic aneurysm. Arch Surg 1975;110:521.

72. Previti FW, Onopchenko A, Glick B. The ruptured abdominal aortic aneurysm in a community hospital. A 5 year study. Am Surg 1992;58:499.

73. Harris LM, Faggioli GL, Fiedler R, et al. Ruptured aortic aneurysms: factors affecting mortality rates. J Vasc Surg 1991;14:812.

74. Alpert RA, Roizen MF, Hamilton WK, et al. Intraoperative urinary output does not predict postoperative renal function in patients undergoing abdominal aortic revascularization. Surgery 1984;95:707.

75. Zaloga GP, Hughes SS. Oliguria in patients with normal renal function. Anesthesiology 1990;72:598.

76. Schein M, Saadia R. Ureteral obstruction after abdominal aortic surgery. Am J Surg 1991;162:86.

77. Sladen RN, Endo E, Harrison T. Two-hour versus 24-hour creatinine clearance in critically ill patients. Anesthesiology 1987;67:1013.

78. Zarich S, Fang LST, Diamond JR. Fractional excretion of sodium. Exceptions to its diagnostic value. Arch Intern Med 1985;145:108.

79. Szerlip HM. Renal-dose dopamine; fact and fiction [editorial]. Ann Intern Med 1991;115:153.

80. Duke GJ, Bersten AD. Dopamine and renal salvage in the critically ill patient. Anaesth Intensive Care 1992;20:277.

81. Casagrande C. Dopamine and the kidney in heart failure. Herz 1991;16:102.

82. Marik PE. Low-dose dopamine in critically ill oliguric patients: the influence of the renin-angiotensin system. Heart Lung 1993;22:171.

83. Duke GJ, Briedis JH, Weaver RA. Renal support in critically ill patients: low dose dopamine or low dose dobutamine? Crit Care Med 1994;22:1919.

84. Horowitz D, Fox SM 3rd, Goldberg LI. Effects of dopamine in man. Circ Res 1962;10:237.

85. McDonald RH Jr, Goldberg LI, McNay JL, Tuttle EP Jr. Effects of dopamine in man: augmentation of sodium excretion, glomerular filtration rate, and renal plasma flow. J Clin Invest 1964;43:1116.

86. Baldwin L, Henderson A, Hickman P. Effect of postoperative low-dose dopamine on renal function after elective major vascular surgery. Ann Intern Med 1994;120:744.

87. Myles PS, Buckland MR, Schenk NJ, et al. Effect of "renal-dose" dopamine on renal function following cardiac surgery. Anaesth Invensive Care 1993;21:56.

88. Lindner A, Cutler RE, Goodman WG. Synergism of dopamine plus furosemide in preventing acute renal failure in the dog. Kidney Int 1979;16:158.

89. Hemmer M, Suter PM. Treatment of cardiac and renal effects of PEEP with dopamine in patients with acute respiratory failure. Anesthesiology 1979;50:399.

90. van-Veldhuisen DJ, Girbes AR, de-Graeff PA, Lie KI. Effects of dopaminergic agents on cardiac and renal

function in normal man and in patients with congestive heart failure. Int J Cardiol 1992;37:293.

91. Carey RM, Siragy HM, Ragsdale NV, et al. Dopamine-1 and dopamine-2 mechanisms in the control of renal function. Am J Hypertens 1990;3:59.

92. Boyd O, Grounds RM, Bennett ED. A randomized clinical trial of the effect of deliberate perioperative increase of oxygen delivery on mortality in high-risk surgical patients. JAMA 1993;270:2699.

93. Olsen NV, Lund J, Jensen PF, et al. Dopamine, dobutamine and dopexamine. A comparison of renal effects in unanesthetized human volunteers. Anesthesiology 1993;79:685.

94. Atallah MM, Saied MM, el-Diasty TA, et al. Renal effect of dopexamine hydrochloride in patients with chronic renal dysfunction. Urol Res 1992;20:419.

95. Gray PA, Bodenham AR, Park GR. A comparison of dopexamine and dopamine to prevent renal impairment in patients undergoing orthotopic liver transplantation. Anaesthesia 1991;46:638. [Published erratum in Anaesthesia 1992;47:92.]

96. Poinsot O, Romand JA, Favre H, Suter PM. Fenoldopam improves renal hemodynamics impaired by positive end-expiratory pressure. Anesthesiology 1993;79:680.

97. Schaer GL, Fink MP, Parrillo JE. Norepinephrine alone versus norepinephrine plus low dose dopamine: enhanced renal blood flow with combination pressor therapy. Crit Care Med 1985;13:492.

98. Campise M. Acute renal failure: prevention and treatment. Arch Ital Urol Nefrol Androl 1990;62:25.

99. Murray MD, Brater DC. Adverse effects of non-steroidal anti-inflammatory drugs on renal function. Ann Intern Med 1990;112:559.

100. Kaufman RP Jr, Anner H, Kobzik L, et al. Vasodilator prostaglandins (PG) prevent renal damage after ischemia. Ann Surg 1987;205:195.

101. Larson CP, Mazze RI, Cooperman LH, Wollman H. Effects of anesthetics on cerebral renal and splanchnic circulations. Anesthesiology 1974;41:169.

102. Dunn MJ, Hood VL. Prostaglandins and the kidney. Am J Physiol 1977;233:169.

103. Margolius HS. The kallikrein-kinin system and the kidney. Ann Rev Physiol 1984;46:309.

104. Goldfarb D, Iaina A, Serban I, et al. Beneficial effect of verapamil in ischemic acute renal failure in the rat. Proc Soc Exp Biol Med 1983;172:389.

105. Wait RB, White G, Davis JH. Beneficial effects of verapamil on postischemic renal failure. Surgery 1983;94:276.

106. He H, Tamaki T, Aki Y, et al. Effects of the calcium antagonist manidipine on renal hemodynamics and function in dogs: comparison with nifedipine. Blood Press 1992;3(Suppl):68.

107. Irzyniec T, Mall G, Greber D, Ritz E. Beneficial effect of nifedipine and moxonidine on glomerulosclerosis in spontaneously hypertensive rats. A micromorphometric study. Am J Hypertens 1992;5:437.

108. Blanco J, Canela EI, Sayos J, et al. Adenine nucleotides and adenosine metabolism in pig kidney proximal tubule membranes. J Cell Physiol 1993;157:77.

109. Kartha S, Toback FG. Adenine nucleotides stimulate migration in wounded cultures of kidney epithelial cells. J Clin Invest 1992;90:288.

110. Zager RA, Schimpf BA, Gmur DJ, Burke TJ. Phospholipase A_2 activity can protect renal tubules from oxygen deprivation injury. Proc Natl Acad Sci U S A 1993;90:8297.

111. Dworkin LD, Benstein JA, Parker M, et al. Calcium antagonists and converting enzyme inhibitors reduce renal injury by different mechanisms. Kidney Int 1993;43:808.

112. Takagi T, Nishikawa M, Mori Y, et al. Effects of atrial natriuretic peptide infusion and its metabolism in patients with chronic renal failure. Endocrinol Jpn 1991;38:497.

113. Laragh JH, Atlas SA. Atrial natriuretic hormone: a regulator of blood pressure and volume homeostatis. Kidney Int 1988;25(Suppl):64.

114. Shenker Y, Port FK, Swartz RD, et al. Atrial natriuretic hormone secretion in patients with renal failure. Life Sci 1987;41:1635.

115. Honda N, Hishida A, Kato A. Factors affecting severity of renal injury and recovery of function in acute renal failure. Ren Fail 1992;14:337.

116. Dahn MS, Lange P, Lobdell K, et al. Splanchnic and total body oxygen consumption differences in septic and injured patients. Surgery 1987;101:69.

117. Roumen RM, van der Vliet JA, Wevers RA, Goris RJ. Intestinal permeability is increased after major vascular surgery. J Vasc Surg 1993;17:734.

118. Cunningham CG, Reilly LM, Rapp JH, et al. Chronic visceral ischemia. Three decades of progress. Ann Surg 1991;214:276.

119. Kieny R, Batellier J, Kretz JG. Aortic reimplantation of the superior mesenteric artery for atherosclerotic lesions of the visceral arteries: sixty cases. Ann Vasc Surg 1990;4:122.

120. Christensen MG, Loretzen JE, Schroeder TV. Revascularization of atherosclerotic mesenteric arteries: experience in 90 consecutive patients. Eur J Vasc Surg 1994;8:297.

121. Marshall JC, Christou NV, Meakins JL. The gastrointestinal tract, the "undrained abscess" of multiple organ failure. Ann Surg 1993;218:111.

122. Deitch EA. Multiple organ failure, pathophysiology and potential future therapy. Ann Surg 1992;216:117.

123. Nelson RL, Briley S, Schuler JJ, Abcarian H. Acute ischemic proctitis. Report of six cases. Dis Colon Rectum 1992;35:375.

124. Jonung T, Ribbe E, Norgren L, et al. Visceral ischemia following aortic surgery. Vasa 1991;20:125.

125. Seeger JM, Coe DA, Kaelin LD, Flynn TC. Routine reimplantation of patent inferior mesenteric arteries limits colon infarction after aortic reconstruction. J Vasc Surg 1992;15:635.

126. Mackay C, Murphy P, Rosenberg IL, Tait NP. Case report: rectal infarction after abdominal aortic surgery. Br J Radiol 1994;67:497.

127. Soong CV, Blair PH, Halliday MI, et al. Endotoxaemia, the generation of the cytokines and their relationship to intramucosal acidosis of the sigmoid colon in elective abdominal aortic aneurysm repair. Eur J Vasc Surg 1993;7:534.

128. Fiddian-Green RG, Amelin PM, Herrmann JB, et al. Prediction of the development of sigmoid ischaemia on the day of aortic operations: indirect measurements of intramucosal pH in the colon. Arch Surg 1986;121:654.

129. Bjorck M, Hedberg B. Early detection of major complications after abdominal aortic surgery: predictive value of sigmoid colon and gastric intramucosal pH monitoring. Br J Surg 1994;81:25.

130. Baigrie RJ, Lamont PM, Kwiatkowski D, et al. Systemic cytokine response after major surgery. Br J Surg 1992;79:757.

131. Baigrie RJ, Lamont PM, Dallman M, Morris PJ. The release of interleukin-1 beta (IL-1) precedes that of interleukin 6 (IL-6) in patients undergoing major surgery. Lymphokine-Cytokine Res 1991;10:253.

132. Ernst CB, Hagihara PF, Daugherty ME, et al. Ischemic colitis incidence following abdominal aortic reconstruction: a prospective study. Surgery 1976;80:417.

133. van-Vroonhoven TJ, Verhagen HJ, Broker WF, Janssen IM. Transmural ischaemic colitis following operation for ruptured aortic aneurysm. Netherlands Journal of Surgery 1991;43:56.

134. Bauer EP, Redaelli C, von Segesser LK, Turina MI. Ruptured abdominal aortic aneurysms. Predictors for early complications and death. Surgery 1993;114:31.

135. Meissner MH, Johansen KH. Colon infarction after ruptured abdominal aortic aneurysm. Arch Surg 1992;127:979.

136. Farkas JC, Calvo-Verjat N, Laurian C, et al. Acute colorectal ischemia after aortic surgery: pathophysiology and prognostic criteria. Ann Vasc Surg 1992;6:111.

137. Allen KB, Salam AA, Lumsden AB. Acute mesenteric ischemia after cardiopulmonary bypass. J Vasc Surg 1992;16:391.

138. Cavaliere F, Martinelli L, Guarneri S, et al. Creatine kinase isoenzyme pattern in colonic infarction consequent to acute aortic dissection. A case report. J Cardiovasc Surg (Torino) 1993;34:263.

139. Mythen MG, Webb AR. Intra-operative gut mucosal hypoperfusion is associated with increased post-operative complications and cost. Intensive Care Med 1994;20:99.

140. Bast TJ, Van-der-Biezen JJ, Scherpenisse J, Eikelboom BC. Ischaemic disease of the colon and rectum after surgery for abdominal aortic aneurysm: a prospective study of the incidence and risk factors. Eur J Vasc Surg 1990;4:253.

141. Laustsen J, Jensen BV, Jelnes R, et al. The value of sigmoidoscopy in the diagnosis of ischemic colitis following aortic reconstruction. Int Angiol 1990;9:117.

142. Longo WE, Ballantyne GH, Gusberg RJ. Ischemic colitis: patterns and prognosis. Dis Colon Rectum 1992;35:726.

143. Fiddian-Green RG: Associations between intramucosal acidosis in the gut and organ failure. Crit Care Med 1993;21:S103.

144. Woods MS, Kelley H. Oncotic pressure, albumin and ileus: the effect of albumin replacement on postoperative ileus. Am Surg 1993;59:758.

145. Darling RC 3d, Shah DM, McClellan WR, et al. Decreased morbidity associated with retroperitoneal exclusion treatment for abdominal aortic aneurysm. J Cardiovasc Surg (Torino) 1992;33:65.

146. Lacroix H, Van Hemelrijk J, Nevelsteen A, Suy R. Transperitoneal vs. retroperitoneal approach for routine vascular reconstruction of the abdominal aorta. Acta Chir Belg 1994;94:1.

147. Barker SG, Dodds RD, Middlemiss A, et al. Small bowel function after aortic surgery. Postgrad Med J 1991;67:757.

148. Lamont PM, Clarke PJ, Collin J. Duodenal obstruction after abdominal aortic aneurysm repair. Eur J Vasc Surg 1992;6:107.

149. Clyne CA, Kumar AS. Duodenal obstruction following reconstruction of abdominal aortic aneurysm. Eur J Vasc Surg 1993;7:98.

150. Pabst TS 3d, McIntyre KE Jr, Schilling JD, et al. Management of chyloperitoneum after abdominal aortic surgery. Am J Surg 1993;166:194.

151. Cook DJ, Witt LJ, Cook RJ, Guyatt GH. Stress ulcer prophylaxis in the critically ill: a meta-analysis. Am J Med 1991;91:519.

152. Shuman RB, Schuster DP, Zucherman GR. Prophylactic therapy for stress bleeding: a reappraisal. Ann Intern Med 1987;106:562.

153. Martin LF. Stress ulcers are common after aortic surgery. Endoscopic evaluation of prophylactic therapy. Am Surg 1994;60:169.

154. Higgins D, Mythen MG, Webb AR. Low intramucosal pH is associated with failure to acidify the gastric lumen in response to pentagastrin. Intensive Care Med 1994;20:105.

155. Haglund U. Intramucosal pH. Intensive Care Med 1994;20:90.

156. Konno H, Sakaguchi S, Hachiya T. Bleeding peptic ulcer after abdominal aortic aneurysm surgery. Arch Surg 1991;126:894.

157. Borrero E, Ciervo J, Chang JB. Antacid vs sucralfate in preventing acute gastrointestinal tract bleeding in abdominal aortic surgery. A randomized trial in 50 patients. Arch Surg 1986;121:810.

158. Goldstone J. Aneurysms of the Aorta and Iliac Arteries. In WS Moore (ed), Vascular Surgery: A Comprehensive Review. Philadelphia: Saunders, 1993.

159. McCombs PR, Mahon DE. Acute pancreatitis following aortic aneurysm repair: report of three cases. Ann Vasc Surg 1991;5:366.

160. Treiman GS, Treiman RL, Foran RF, et al. The influence of diabetes mellitus on the risk of abdominal aortic surgery. Am Surg 1994;60:436.

161. Mullen JL, Busby GP, Matthews DC, et al. Reduction of operative morbidity and mortality by combined preoperative and postoperative nutritional support. Ann Surg 1980;192:604.

162. Moghissi K, Hornshaw J, Teasdale PR, Dawes EA. Parenteral nutrition in carcinoma of the oesophagus treated by surgery: nitrogen balance and clinical studies. Br J Surg 1977;64:125.

163. Askanazi J, Hensle TW, Starker PM, et al. Effect of immediate postoperative nutritional support on length of hospitalization. Ann Surg 1986;203:236.

164. Fletcher JP, Little JM. A comparison of parenteral nutrition and early postoperative enteral feeding on the nitrogen balance after major surgery. Surgery 1986;100:21.

165. Harris JA, Benedict TG. Biometric studies of basal metabolism in man. Washington, DC: Carnegie Institute of Washington, Publication No. 279.

166. Long CL, Schaffel N, Geiger JW, et al. Metabolic response to injury and illness: estimation of energy and protein needs from indirect calorimetric and nitrogen balance. J. Parenter Ent Nutr 1979;3:452.

167. Faure H, Peyrin JC, Richard MJ, Favier A. Parenteral supplementation with zinc in surgical patients corrects postoperative serum zinc drop. Biol Trace Elem Res 1991;30:37.

168. Grant JP. Handbook of Total Parenteral Nutrition (2nd ed). Philadelphia: Saunders, 1992;78.

169. Najafi H. Dacron aorta. Ann Thorac Surg 1993;56:968.

170. Slootmans FC, van der Vliet JA, Reinaerts HH, et al. Relaparotomies after ruptured abdominal aortic aneurysm repair. Eur J Vasc Surg 1994;8:342.

171. Guidelines Committee, American College of Critical Care Medicine, Society of Critical Care Medicine, and the Transfer Guidelines Task Force. Guidelines for the transfer of critically ill patients. Am J Crit Care 1993;2:189.

172. Cortes-Franco JE, Gamba-Ayala G, Aguilar-Salinas CA, et al. The transfer of critically ill patients. Rev Invest Clin 1991;43:323.

173. Hurst JM, Davis K Jr, Johnson DJ, et al. Cost and complications during in-hospital transport of critically ill patients: a prospective cohort study. J Trauma 1992;33:582.

174. Sullivan N, Frentzel KU. A patient transport pilot quality improvement team. Quality Review Bulletin 1992;18:215.

175. Di-Cesare E, Di-Renzi P, Pavone P, et al. Postsurgical follow-up of aortic dissections by MRI. Eur J Radiol 1991;13:27.

176. Gefke K, Schroeder TV, Thisted B, et al. Abdominal aortic aneurysm surgery: survival and quality of life in patients requiring prolonged postoperative intensive therapy. Ann Vasc Surg 1994;8:137.

Chapter 13

Management of Pain in the Aortic Surgery Patient

Meir Chernofsky and Michael Hanania

Rationale and Theory of Analgesic Care

The prevention and treatment of pain after aortic surgery is a compassionate as well as a physiologic necessity. Aortic surgery incisions, which are large and truncal, impair spontaneous ventilation. Diaphragmatic and chest wall dysfunction, which results from the surgical incision, contributes to pulmonary impairment, and effective analgesia is beneficial to facilitate coughing and deep breathing. In fact, Pansard et al. have recently shown increases in diaphragmatic activity in aortic surgery patients after epidural block.[1] Newer surgical approaches such as the retroperitoneal incision do not seem to reduce postoperative pain.[2] The prevalence of coronary artery disease in aortic surgery patients suggests an important role for pain control in prevention of stress-related myocardial ischemia.

State-of-the-art postoperative analgesia is expensive. In addition to the extra procedures, specialized pumps, and monitors involved, as well as the ongoing in-service education and quality improvement work needed, the system must often support full-time physicians, pharmacists, and nurse-specialists. Mortality is already low in the general surgical population, and it is hard to demonstrate even lower mortality with high-tech postoperative pain management. Therefore, the extra cost of intensive pain management must be justified in terms of other outcome measures such as the length of the hospital stay. In the aortic surgery population, with its relatively high mortality, physicians have the potential to show real improvements in morbidity and even

mortality with control of pain and stress. This was done in a group of high-risk surgical patients in a widely cited study by Yeager et al.[3]

There are a number of factors operative in aortic surgery patients that modify the approach to analgesia. The frequent use of anticoagulation raises questions about the safety of intraspinal analgesia. (In this chapter *intraspinal* refers to epidural and intrathecal techniques.) At the same time, the goal of discontinuing mechanical ventilation makes regional analgesia desirable because sedation can be minimized and the ability to cough maximized. The use of opioid analgesics alone may delay the return of bowel function, an important determinant of recovery after abdominal aortic procedures. The risk of renal dysfunction as well as the disastrous consequences of postoperative bleeding calls into question the use of anti-inflammatory analgesics.

This chapter reviews some of the theory behind acute pain management. It goes into detail to the extent that such details help the practitioner make the many decisions that are the bread and butter of postoperative pain management. Finally, specific protocols are provided in table form. The regimens suggested are clearly not the only good options, but they provide a starting point for the practitioner who is not a specialist in pain management.

History of Pain Management

The standard of practice in pain management that prevailed until the early 1980s dated back 40 years or more and was a relative therapeutic failure. It was characterized by the as needed use of opioid analgesics. Meperidine was generally given intramuscularly at 50–75 mg every 4 hours. A number of studies indicate that this approach left a majority of patients in severe pain.[4,5] This widespread failure did not occur because meperidine is a horrible drug or because the intramuscular route is wrong. Rather, the main problems seem to have been the exaggerated fears regarding the potential for addiction to opioids, the side effects of opioids, and the supposed danger of the usually more effective intravenous route. Delay in opioid administration was also a factor. The reasons why ineffective therapy of acute pain and postoperative pain persisted for so long in otherwise modern medical facilities are presented here:

Absolute underdosing of opioid analgesics

Knowledge deficit regarding proper dose

Exaggerated fear of addiction and respiratory depression (both in fact are rare)

Relative underdosing of opioid analgesics

Poor matching of dose and route of administration

Drug absorbed slowly from intramuscular route, resulting in delayed onset

Exaggerated fears regarding the danger of intravenously administered opioids leading to underdosing by this route

Poor timing of administration

As needed use of opioids failed to *maintain* analgesic state

Acute pain-anxiety cycle; time delay associated with buildup of pain, calling the nurse, requesting medication, waiting for medication to be injected, and so forth

Lack of knowledge regarding the consequences of pain

Adverse physiologic consequences

Impression that pain serves a useful purpose

There is a complex relationship between adequate analgesia and respiratory function. Pulmonary toilet, resumption of independent respiratory function, and extubation are all facilitated by adequate analgesia. Overdosing of opioid analgesics in the nonventilated patient leads to oversedation and impaired pulmonary function. The exacting titration of analgesia is challenging but important for the patient. Conversely, during periods of ventilatory sup-

port, the most feared side effect of opioid analgesia is obviated and there is little reason to withhold additional opioids. In this circumstance the margin of error is greatly increased.

The provision of sedation early in the postoperative period is important to the patient's comfort as well as his or her hemodynamic stability. Sedation and anxiolytic therapy are discussed in Chapter 11.

Preemptive Analgesia

The idea that pain is better prevented than treated sounds humane and practical. However, the physiologic basis of the prevention of pain is not so obvious. The key words here are "preemptive analgesia" and "windup phenomenon." These two terms refer to distinct but related phenomena, and the clinical implications of both concepts are, for our purposes, similar. A painful stimulus, besides triggering transmission of impulses in specific pathways, seems to effect structural changes in postsynaptic receptors. This probably occurs in the so-called wide dynamic range neurons that receive the first central synapse of the pain pathway. These changes may render the patient in pain relatively resistant to analgesic therapy. If these receptor changes could be prevented either by a nerve block or by achieving adequate concentrations of opioid analgesics in the central nervous system before the painful stimulus occurs, then subsequent analgesic requirements may be lower. Stated another way, the windup phenomenon refers to structural changes at the receptor level that help to sustain the pain response and increase the opioid requirement. Preemptive analgesia refers to the modification of these structural changes by attenuating the early nociceptive impulses. The alleged benefit of such modification is eventual use of a lower total dose of analgesics with fewer side effects and a happier patient.

The more basic concept of pain prevention is important in sick patients who are undergoing aortic surgery, because the stress response that results from pain is undesirable, even if it is addressed fairly rapidly.

Study design for clinical research in analgesia is exceptionally delicate for many reasons, one of which is the difficulty of defining a control group. The concept of preemptive analgesia is especially hard to prove clinically, especially with regard to specific outcomes such as reduction in morbidity and hospital stay. Nevertheless, the concept is probably valid and should be kept in mind. Interesting work has been done in this area.[6–12] As one would expect, preemptive analgesia is not demonstrated under all study conditions.[12] The effect of preventive analgesia on the windup phenomenon may differ depending on the route, type of medication, and specific drug. In general, it seems that in pain management, as in so many other areas of medicine, prevention may be more satisfactory than treatment.

Patients can only benefit from the practical application of preemptive analgesia. For example, when an epidural catheter is inserted before surgery, many practitioners wait until the end of surgery to administer a long-acting opioid such as morphine into the epidural catheter. If one considers the concept of preemptive analgesia, and especially given the fact that the onset of action of epidural morphine is prolonged compared with morphine administered parenterally, it makes more sense to administer a generous dose of epidural morphine as early as possible.[11] Along these lines, the earliest decisions regarding analgesia are in the hands of the operating room anesthesiologist.

Perioperative Management and Postoperative Analgesia

Influence of Premedication on Postoperative Pain

Virtually all aortic surgery patients should be considered for premedication with opioids, much as one would premedicate the cardiac surgery patient. Morphine (0.10–0.14 mg per kg) is appropriate for the robust patient who is otherwise free of central nervous system disease, pulmonary disease, pulmonary hypertension, or cardiac failure. Dosages are decreased for the elderly and for those with coexisting organ failure.

The use of alpha$_2$-agonist medication as a supplement to traditional analgesics is still in its infancy. Practitioners may want to consider the preoperative administration of clonidine (0.1–0.2 mg) a few hours before surgery, particularly in the hypertensive patient. In this setting, clonidine may provide some analgesic-sparing effect both during and after the surgery. Attenuation of the hemodynamic response to laryngoscopy has been demonstrated in cardiac as well as noncardiac surgery.[13] Improved control of the sympathetic storm associated with the early postoperative period has also been demonstrated. The main risk of clonidine appears to be the possibility of bradycardia and hypotension.

Influence of Anesthetic Technique

The intraoperative management of the aortic surgery patient will have a major impact on postoperative pain management. The perioperative decisions most important to the postoperative management are whether to use a regional technique and whether to use a high-dose opioid technique as the basis of the general anesthetic.

Although some advocates seem to believe that one is providing inferior care by not adding a regional technique to a general anesthetic, there is no objective evidence that this is so. Regional anesthesia, which in the case of aortic surgery is usually a supplementary rather than a primary technique, must be analyzed in terms of its potential benefits. If all of the alleged benefits of regional techniques can be achieved with systemic agents, then the wisdom of adding a regional anesthetic is correct. Regional blocks are not without complications and are costly and time consuming.

Rationale for Regional Techniques

Regional techniques may be beneficial in at least seven important areas: (1) use of an intrathecal catheter in spinal cord protection, (2) control of the perioperative hemodynamic response, (3) modification of the so-called endocrine stress response, (4) improvement of postoperative pulmonary function, (5) prevention of the hypercoagulable perioperative state, (6) superior patient satisfaction, and (7) shortening the duration of the intensive care unit (ICU) stay.

Drainage of cerebrospinal fluid (CSF) is used in many centers as an adjunct for spinal cord protection. The catheter inserted for this purpose can, with some special precautions, be used for intrathecal administration of analgesic agents. The use of an epidural catheter to achieve moderate cooling of the cord has been recently described, and such a catheter could also be used for analgesia (see Chapter 8).[14]

To prove a unique benefit for regional anesthesia in terms of perioperative hemodynamic control, one would have to compare a study group that received combined regional and general techniques with a control group that received only general anesthesia but had hemodynamics rigorously controlled with systemic medications. If one then found that comparable hemodynamic control could not be achieved in the general anesthesia group or that the epidural group had fewer myocardial infarctions despite similar hemodynamics, then the superiority of regional anesthesia would be established. However, studies with this type of design have failed to show that supplemental regional anesthesia provides superior cardiac outcome compared to rigorous control of hemodynamics by systemic medications.[15,16] Davies et al., who also did not find a major outcome difference between their general anesthesia group and epidural-general group, confirmed the common clinical impression that full perioperative activation of an epidural increases the requirement for vasopressors, which is not necessarily a good thing.[17] Apparently, supplemental regional anesthesia is just one good way among many to control the hemodynamic response. A preoperative oral dose of clonidine, for example, may provide excellent hemodynamic stability without the need for constant adjustment of vasoactive medications and without the mess and fuss of a major regional anesthetic.[13]

Postoperatively, epidural blockade can provide excellent control of hypertension, and the decreased morbidity seen with epidural analgesia in high-risk patients may be in part a reflection of blunting of hyperdynamic responses.[3,18] It is possible that other interventions aimed at sympathetic modulation, such as systemic clonidine, would be just as effective.

It has been suggested, based on a case report in an aortic surgery patient, that postoperative epidural analgesia may mask anginal symptoms, and a postoperative myocardial infarction may go unnoticed.[19] Blomberg and coworkers have shown that thoracic epidural analgesia is an excellent symptomatic treatment for angina.[20] The studies of Blomberg and coworkers suggest that thoracic epidural anesthesia improves not just the symptoms of ischemia but also the actual demand-supply conditions of the myocardium.[21,22] All of their work was with local anesthetic block, and the results may or may not be applicable to techniques using opioids or opioid-local anesthetic combinations.

While most of the epidural catheters function at the lumbar level, opioid analgesics clearly circulate throughout the intrathecal space. Opioid is delivered to the CSF at dermatomal levels that mediate angina. However, postoperative myocardial infarctions are notoriously silent with or without an epidural. Furthermore, systemic opioids are also an excellent treatment for angina and can therefore mask it, but one would never withhold opioids entirely in a surgical patient based on the ridiculous concern of masking angina. The work of Blomberg et al. on epidural local anesthetic agents does not rule out the possibility that favorable changes in myocardial oxygen demand-supply balance may also result from epidural opioids.

There is some evidence that regional anesthesia can provide superior control of the endocrine stress response. This is often assessed by measurement of blood glucose, serum cortisol, and other stress markers (see Chapter 11).[23–25] These are all intermediary variables, and it is unclear if lower levels of stress hormones are good for all patients. The stress response is, after all, present for a reason, and critically ill patients are often treated by replacement of the very substances whose release we want to control. Nevertheless, control of the metabolic stress response often correlates with other effects that are clearly favorable, such as superior control of hemodynamic responses.

By providing superior analgesia with lower opioid doses and less sedation, regional analgesia may be unique in reducing pulmonary complications in aortic surgery patients.[1,24,26] Epidural analgesia has been shown to decrease pulmonary complications in the cholecystectomy patient.[27] The finding of many investigators that extubation tends to occur earlier in patients treated with epidural analgesia is probably related, although pulmonary status is only one determinate of duration of mechanical ventilation.

For the orthopedic surgery population, regional anesthesia has been shown to lower the incidence of postoperative thromboembolic complications.[28] For aortic and major vascular surgery, the demands made on the coagulation system are far more complex. Furthermore, the area of concern is the arterial circulation, where flow dynamics are entirely different. While no definitive data address the influence of regional anesthesia and analgesia on coagulation in aortic surgery patients, a number of studies suggest that regional anesthesia may prevent arterial thromboembolic complications. Christopherson et al. compared epidural and general anesthesia for lower extremity revascularization.[29] They found a fairly dramatic decrease in postoperative graft thrombosis in the epidural group. A postoperative thrombotic complication in major vascular surgery is not just a nuisance, it is a disaster associated with significant morbidity and mortality.[30] In an earlier study, Tuman and coworkers found that vascular patients in general were hypercoagulable on thromboelastographic examination.[31] In their study, patients who had epidural anesthesia (supplemented with general anesthesia) and postoperative epidural analgesia had better outcomes when compared with those treated with general anesthesia alone and postoperative intravenous opioid analgesia. Gibbs et al. found that in aortic surgery patients, epidural blockade did not modify the postoperative changes in procoagulant factors previously described by their group as well as others.[32,33] Their small study does not exclude the possibility that actual outcome in terms of thrombotic complications may be better in patients who received epidural blockade. After all, for hip surgery patients, the benefit for regional anesthesia was demonstrated in the absence of differences in coagulation factor levels.

It is interesting that the mechanism of the changes seen in coagulation function between epidural and general anesthesia is not understood. It does not appear to be mediated by a simplistic modification of the stress response.[34]

Even after data are collected, patient satisfaction requires that value judgments be made regarding how to use the data. There is little hard information to guide physicians in this area. Certainly the data of Breslow et al. among others suggest that pain scores may be lower with epidural analgesia.[24]

There are a number of studies that suggest that time to extubation, length of ICU stay, and length of hospital stay are shorter when an epidural catheter is used for anesthesia and analgesia. The study of Yeager et al. is in this category.[3] More recently, de Leon-Casasola et al. compared general anesthesia with an epidural-general technique for major (truncal) cancer surgery.[18] Their large study showed that all three time indices of recovery discussed previously were shorter for epidural-general anesthetics than for general anesthetics followed by intravenous patient controlled analgesia (IVPCA). Additionally, cost savings were significant in the epidural group.

Although there were methodology constraints on their study that may have limited the validity of their results, further study is definitely warranted. Katz et al. and Mason et al. are among the groups that have found earlier extubation times in aortic surgery patients when regional analgesia was used.[26,35]

Choice of Regional Technique

Regional analgesia for the aortic surgery patients is commonly administered via the subarachnoid (SA) and epidural routes. The epidural route has the advantage of catheter access so that multiple medications can be administered continuously or by repeat bolus in the intraoperative and postoperative periods. While we will argue that SA catheters are also practical, the use of the continuous SA catheter is certainly not as widely accepted as catheterization of the epidural space. The presence of a functioning epidural catheter provides the ideal opportunity for effective postoperative analgesia. The main issue of controversy with epidural catheters is the influence of heparinization on the complication of epidural hematoma.

Epidural veins are frequently contacted and traumatized, either by epidural needles or catheters. Such damage, which may be obvious on insertion or on catheter aspiration, is usually of no consequence. Epidural hematomas large enough to cause neurologic damage are extremely rare, probably because the clotting mechanism limits the size of most epidural hematomas.

Many epidurals have been done, on purpose or unknowingly, in anticoagulated patients. Even in this group, neurologic damage is not common. Tamponade of the bleeding vessel in the epidural space may control such low-pressure venous bleeds. In any case, a traumatic epidural should pose little risk for subsequent heparinization if enough time has passed for clot maturation to occur (1 hour is probably adequate). Heparin does not lyse clots that are already formed.

In keeping with the previously mentioned principles, numerous aortic surgery patients have had epidurals placed preoperatively, with large series confirming the safety of this technique.[36] Since the report of Rao and El-Etr included about 4,000 patients, it can be concluded that the incidence of problems in this setting is not more than about 1 in 1,300, and perhaps less.[36] The use of this technique has even been reported in cardiac surgery patients, in whom anticoagulation is more aggressive than in most aortic surgery patients.[37]

Therefore, when receiving a patient with an epidural catheter, it is important to ask if any problem with vein puncture was encountered. If the answer is affirmative, the patient deserves special vigilance against neurologic changes and continued bleeding via the catheter.

In the case in which no problem was encountered inserting the epidural catheter, there is still the question of the safety of removing a catheter while the patient is anticoagulated.[38] Based on the remote possibility that a clot in the epidural space may be sheared off during catheter removal, it is customary in some hospitals to remove catheters only after anticoagulation has been reversed. Complications of catheter removal in the anticoagulated patient should be so remote that if there is a good reason to pull a catheter (such as sepsis) it should be removed despite the continued use of anticoagulants. After all, catheters come out by themselves quite often without the benefit of intact coagulation. When anticoagulation must be continued in a patient with an epidural catheter, it would seem advisable to carefully monitor the extent of anticoagulation, so as to avoid an extent of induced coagulopathy that exceeds what the patient actually needs.

Due to the controversy surrounding the use of epidural catheters in anticoagulated patients and the occasional technical difficulty of inserting them, the single-shot SA block is frequently used. The small needles that can be used for SA injections make vein trauma less of a concern. SA injection may be technically easier and faster in a patient with difficult anatomy. Finally, there is no delay while the analgesic substances are penetrating the dura, and the smaller dosages of all agents necessary for effect in the SA space remove the concern of systemic toxicity.

The postdural puncture headache (PDPH), one of the historical disadvantages of the SA injection, is now of less concern than in the past. PDPH is less common in the elderly and in male patients. These groups comprise the majority of aortic surgery patients. PDPH, which is postural, is also less of an issue in major surgery, because the patients tend to remain in bed in the early postoperative period. In contrast, patients hope to be ambulatory soon after more minor surgery. Finally, today's pencil-point needles reduce the incidence of PDPH to less than 3% even in patients at high risk for PDPH.[39]

The use of indwelling subarachnoid catheters has been avoided, primarily because of concern for PDPH and infection. Until recently, the only suitable catheters were those manufactured for epidural use. These large-bore instruments are expected to cause a high incidence of severe PDPH in young patients. However, in the elderly and predominantly male population who undergo aortic surgery, many anesthesiologists have placed epidural catheters in the SA space, and PDPH seems in fact to be rare.

There are no data to define a maximum safe duration for intrathecal catheterization. The concern that infection may be more common with SA catheters than with epidural catheters leads many practitioners to discontinue SA catheters earlier than they would a continuous epidural catheter or to avoid SA catheters entirely beyond the actual operative period. In a recent prospective study by Bevacqua et al. there were no infections in 139 patients with indwelling SA catheters who were prospectively followed for a mean duration of 66 hours with a maximum duration of up to 218 hours.[40] Seventy-one of these patients underwent aortic reconstruction, and the rest were also vascular surgery patients. Catheter size varied. Invoking the statistical shortcut of Hanley, one may conclude that under the conditions of Bevacqua's study, the incidence of clinical infections in similar patients can easily be over 1% and may be as high as 2%.[41] This small study is therefore not an unqualified recommendation for indwelling SA catheters, but we may safely conclude that infection is not common. The epidural catheter inserted in the SA space is apparently a viable alternative. For those who use CSF drainage for cord protection, an epidural-type catheter is most often used. If such a catheter is used in a patient and the neurologic status is stable, there is no reason why it cannot, with some special precautions, be used for postoperative analgesia.

Recently, small-bore catheters were released specifically for SA use. Their tiny diameter makes PDPH less likely. Several cases of cauda equina syndrome were described with these catheters, and their production was discontinued. The neurologic damage described is thought to be due to neurotoxicity of repeated dosages of concentrated local anesthetics affecting the same nerve roots. These microcatheters are too small to allow reliable drainage of CSF. They may come back into use for administration of anesthesia and analgesia after the cause of the reported neurologic damage is better understood. For now, continuous SA catheterization is performed with fairly large needles and catheters designed for epidural use.

For several years now, some anesthesiologists have been performing a single-shot SA injection with morphine (and sometimes with local anesthetic) and then inserting an epidural catheter. This technique combines the exceptional reliability and low-dose requirement of SA analgesia with the superior acceptability of an epidural catheter. Special devices are marketed to facilitate this double procedure, which can also be performed postoperatively. These devices consist of a spinal needle that, when fully inserted into the epidural needle, protrudes beyond it by about 2 cm. One identifies the epidural space in the usual manner and then performs the spinal through the epidural needle before threading the epidural catheter. One problem with this double procedure is that initially the epidural catheter is truly untested and correct placement is not certain.

With the use of either kind of regional anesthetic, the postoperative management of pain is simplified. The single-shot SA injection does not provide the ongoing flexibility of the epidural catheter but does provide excellent analgesia for up to 24 hours, depending on the dosage.

Regardless of which regional technique was performed intraoperatively, the anesthesiologist had the option of using an opioid only, adding dilute local anesthesia, or doing a complete nerve block supplemented with only light general anesthesia. The latter approach is the true epidural general or spinal-general technique. Such a combination may be more effective in preventing the pain response from becoming established. Nevertheless, a complete neural blockade has its own problems in terms of sympathectomy. Given the common presence of atherosclerotic vascular disease, the accompanying hypotension can be dangerous and must be battled throughout the management of the case. As of this date, the technique of complete neural blockade has not been shown to clearly improve outcome. A middle position often taken is to use local anesthetic in the epidural space but in a volume lower than that which is required for complete neural blockade. Such an approach may lead to a less extensive sympathectomy with less hypotension with smaller dosages of systemic anesthetic agents. In the postoperative period, this may allow for a more awake patient who can cooperate with examinations and care, and who may be extubated earlier. There are endless permutations of combined techniques. Understanding the possibilities allows one to properly tailor the postoperative analgesic care.

Postoperative Analgesia

There are a number of alternatives for provision of analgesia for the aortic surgery patient in the early postoperative period (Table 13-1). A directed history should be obtained. This assists the anesthesiologist in choosing the route of administration, drugs, and dosages used (Table 13-2). The experience, expertise, and equipment availability at the physician's institution may place important limitations on the use of more advanced techniques.

Parenteral opioid analgesics may serve as the primary analgesic modality, or they may be used to supplement a partially effective neural blockade technique. Likewise, intrathecal and epidural techniques have the potential to serve as the primary modality, but one should not hesitate to supplement these modalities as needed. Often, intraspinal analgesia is completely effective for incisional pain but ineffective for discomfort related to factors such as the endotracheal tube and muscle strains due to positioning.

There are a number of other modalities that are useful supplements to systemic opioid administration, such as intrapleural analgesia. In specific circumstances, these techniques are capable of reducing the requirement for systemic opioid. The patient benefits in that he or she may be more cooperative and alert and may be spared some of the dose-related side effects of opioid analgesics.

Parenteral and intraspinal analgesics can be delivered by intermittent bolus, continuous infusion, patient-controlled analgesia (PCA), or a combination of techniques. In the case of intraspinal blocks, opioid mixtures to which local anesthetics have been added are also routinely delivered by PCA. The principles of prescribing a PCA program are similar for all routes of administration. The differences between PCA programs for the various routes include the obvious differences in dosing as well as the time after each patient demand before which some relief is expected. This time interval is shortest for intravenous use, quite a

Table 13-1. Range of Options for Postoperative Analgesic Care of the Aortic Surgery Patient

Order of management decisions*
    Primary technique
        Route of administration
        Choice of opioid, additives, adjuncts
        Mode: PCA, continuous, bolus, combination
        Dosage and timing
    Breakthrough pain management: route, drug, and dose
    Management of nonincisional pain
    Management of discomfort related to endotracheal tube
    Treatment of anxiety
    Treatment of underlying substance abuse or chronic pain
Intravenous techniques: opioid analgesics
    As needed intravenous opioids; nurse and physician controlled*
    IVPCA (see Table 13-6)*
    Nurse-assisted IVPCA (see text discussion)*
    Continuous intravenous infusion of opioids; nurse and physician controlled*
    Combination IVPCA and continuous infusion of opioids (see Table 13-6)*
Other techniques for systemic opioid delivery
    Transdermal delivery system for fentanyl (almost never appropriate)
    Intramuscular delivery of opioids (almost never appropriate)
Techniques of neural blockade
    Intrathecal single injection; opioid, with or without local anesthetic
    Continuous intrathecal analgesia (see Table 13-11)*
        Repeat boluses
        PCA
        Continuous infusion
        PCA plus continuous infusion (intrathecal techniques can be supplemented by a very limited dose of local anesthetic)
    Continuous epidural analgesia (see Table 13-9)*
        Repeat boluses
        PCA
        Continuous infusion
        PCA plus continuous infusion (all epidural techniques may be supplemented by local anesthetic)
    Intercostal blocks
    Continuous intrapleural analgesia with local anesthetics
        Via dedicated catheter
        Via chest drain
    Local wound infiltration
Transcutaneous electrical nerve stimulation

*Techniques that are practical as the sole modality for analgesia during the first 3 postoperative days. All other options must be supplemented to various degrees. Although neural blockade techniques can often provide complete analgesia for the surgical incision, one should not hesitate to use systemic opioids or sedative-hypnotics if needed for sedation and to assist the patient in tolerating an endotracheal tube (see Chapter 11). These options provide for an infinite number of combinations that may be tailored to the patient's needs and the capabilities of the facility.
PCA = patient-controlled analgesia; IVPCA = intravenous patient-controlled analgesia.

bit longer for intrathecal use, and still longer for epidural administration.

Pharmacokinetics of Acute Pain Therapy

There are two components to an analgesic program, the base component and the adjustable component. The base component provides just that, a continuous insurance against periods without analgesia and control of the pain that is constant. The adjustable component enables the nurse (or patient) to respond to changing needs such as awakening, dressing changes, movement, and so on. The adjustable component also allows for temporary compensation if the basal component proves inadequate. While this

Table 13-2. Information Helpful in Designing an Individualized Postoperative Pain Management Program for the Aortic Surgery Patient

Medication history
    Use of opioids and sedatives, aspirin
Pain history
    Preexisting chronic pain conditions
Past medical history
    Cardiac, pulmonary, renal, gastrointestinal, hepatobiliary disease
Neuropsychiatric history
    Premorbid mental status, depression, personality disorder, substance abuse disorder, peripheral neuropathy, back pain, seizure disorder
Drug sensitivities/allergies
    Details: what was the specific reaction to each medication?
Coagulation status
    Preexisting problems, intraoperative use of anticoagulants, plan for continued anticoagulation
Anesthetic premedication
    Opioid administered? Alpha$_2$-agonist administered?
Consent
    If neural blockade has not as yet been done, was the possibility discussed with the patient?
Surgical management
    Size and location of incision
    Nature of procedure
    Segment and branches of aorta involved
    Risk to spinal cord
    Location of chest drains
    Mechanical stress to bowel
Anesthetic management
    Neural blockade; catheter present?
    Problems with block procedure: Difficult? Traumatic?
    Intraspinal medications
    Total dose of systemic opioid
    Residual neuromuscular blockade
    Intraoperative complications
General status of the patient
    Best guess as to timing of extubation
    Is sepsis likely to be an issue?
    Is acute renal or hepatic compromise likely?
Physical examination
    Heart rate, arterial pressure, and pulmonary artery pressure
    Signs of respiratory distress, tachypnea, retractions, elevated peak inspiratory pressure
    Surgical dressings, dressings on intraspinal catheters
Laboratory examination
    Chest radiograph: atelectasis, consolidation
    Coagulation profile

distinction between basal and adjustable analgesia is really just a restatement of basic pharmacokinetics, it is useful. For example, an epidural bolus dosage of morphine, although effective, represents a guess at the correct dose. If one has guessed low, some type of supplementation will be needed. Furthermore, a single dosage of intraspinal morphine, as the basal analgesic, will not always block episodic pain. If 4 mg is administered epidurally, and the patient is found to have breakthrough pain, this pain can be effectively treated with a bolus of a rapidly acting opioid administered into the epidural by nurse or patient control, with or without local anesthetic. The pain can also be addressed by an intravenous bolus of any opioid, again administered under patient or nurse control. While a repeat dosage of epidural morphine may be administered to increase the baseline analgesia, it will not treat the immediate breakthrough pain nearly as fast as the other options described previously.

The distinction between basal analgesia and breakthrough relief implies that analgesic orders should almost always contain an analgesic that is administered by the clock, and an additional component that is administered on an as-needed basis.

Long-acting drugs administered by bolus are appropriate for basal analgesia, and shorter-acting analgesics are administered by continuous infusion via any route. Breakthrough pain is treated by boluses of a short-acting drug, administered by the provider or the patient. These boluses can also take the form of increases in the rate of infusion of a short-acting opioid.

Drugs of intermediate duration of action may be appropriate for both functions, and their tendency to accumulate is a factor in the provision of basal analgesia. An order for an initial loading dosage of morphine followed by morphine at 2–4 mg every 20 minutes intravenously as needed for pain appears to violate the principle that basal analgesia must be provided. However, in the hands of a skilled nurse who is not afraid to administer small frequent doses prophylactically and who responds immediately to any suggestion of pain with additional morphine, the patient may do fine.

The basal analgesic plan is continuously reassessed in terms of the need for breakthrough analgesics. In the ideal situation, breakthrough dosages would not be necessary because the goal is perfect analgesia. However, if the patient is less than alert, the need for no breakthrough medications may suggest that the administration of basal analgesics be decreased slightly. Even if the patient is alert, pain-free, and without side effects, one should anticipate a decreasing need for analgesia after the first 2–3 days by attempting a slight dosage decrease in the basal analgesia and assessing the effect.

When the patient requires the administration of breakthrough medications more than once in a 1- to 2-hour period with intravenous PCA, the possibility is investigated that a particular circumstance, such as suctioning, a dressing change, or a related procedure, was the cause of the increased pain. If no such circumstance is found, the basal analgesic dosage is increased by 20–40%.

Intramuscular Opioid Analgesia

Intramuscular (IM) therapy does not figure prominently in these recommendations. In the best of worlds, opioids would not be administered IM. While we have all met patients who like their shots, most people find them painful. Additionally, as discussed previously, IM opioid injections can lead to delayed onset of adequate blood levels, which then may decline rapidly. Even when opioids are administered every 4 hours regardless of patient request, it is possible to have adequate blood levels of opioid for only 25% of the 4-hour interval. Conversely, IV opioid injections are not in themselves any less safe than IM injections. Of course, if one is aware of the pharmacokinetic factors and adjusts dosages accordingly, and especially if adequate doses are administered around the clock, IM therapy can be successful. Some readers may practice in settings in which resources are limited. In such institutions patients may be transferred out of the ICU early, PCA devices may not be available, and IV opioid use may not be accepted on the regular hospital ward. In such a setting, IM injections may be the best option until oral medication is tolerated. IM opioids are also useful for breakthrough pain in the patient who is already on oral analgesics.

Considerations for specific drug choice for IM therapy are no different than those for IV administration of opioids. Given an understanding of the relative potencies, most of the older mu-receptor agonists such as morphine, meperidine, methadone, and hydromorphone perform well (Table 13-3). Some special problems with meperidine are discussed here. Opioids of the agonist-antagonist class are not recommended for the aortic surgery patients because of their "ceiling effect" and the risk of adverse hemodynamic consequences of mu-receptor antagonism. The partial mu-receptor agonists such as buprenorphine may be safer, but there are few data to prove this.

Intravenous Opioid Analgesia

The administration of opioids by the IV route is the standard to which other analgesic options are compared. Intravenous therapy is briefly reviewed as an example of the principles that promote the success of any analgesic plan.

Table 13-3. Types of Endogenous Opioid Receptors with Examples of Agonists and Actions*

Type	Agonist Examples	Some Probable Actions
Mu		
Mu_1	Morphine, fentanyl	Supraspinal analgesia
	Several endogenous opioid peptides	Central acetylcholine turnover
		Catalepsy
Mu_2	Morphine	Respiratory depression
		Gastrointestinal tract motility
		Cardiovascular effects, e.g., bradycardia
		Central dopamine turnover
Delta	Met-enkephalin	Spinal analgesia
	Leu-enkephalin	Central dopamine turnover
		Regulation of mu-receptors
Kappa	Ketocyclazocine dynorphins	Spinal analgesia
		Inhibition of antidiuretic hormone release
		Sedation
		Miosis
Epsilon	Beta-endorphin	In vivo effect unclear
Sigma	SKF10,047	Psychological effects, dysphoria
		Linked to N-methyl-D-aspartate receptor actions
		Mydriasis
		Tachypnea
		Tachycardia

*Clean separation of actions by agonism of specific subtypes is possible only to a limited extent in the clinical situation. For example, there is no pure mu_1-agonist available; such a drug could potentially eliminate the risk of respiratory depression. Naloxone is a reversible antagonist at all opioid receptor types.

Source: Modified from GW Pasternak. Multiple morphine and enkephalin receptors and the relief of pain. JAMA 1988;259:1362.

Intravenous opioids are available worldwide, and even the older drugs in this class are safe, effective, and inexpensive. High-tech equipment such as infusion pumps and PCA pumps may simplify the administration of opioids, and PCA facilitates the use of opioids on the general surgical ward. However, in an ICU setting aggressive intermittent bolus administration of opioid by a nurse can provide analgesia that cannot be improved on with PCA. This is not surprising, because a skilled, attentive nurse can do everything a PCA pump can do.

For opioid analgesia via intermittent bolus administration to have the best possible result, the critical care nurse must be skilled at assessing the need for a bolus. Both patient input as to the presence of pain and signs of sympathetic stimulation, such as hypertension and tachycardia, are important. For that matter, these factors must be constantly assessed regardless of what analgesic plan is followed.

The physician's orders for opioid administration should include a range of as needed dosages and the possibility of repeat doses fairly often. If the order

reads "morphine 2–4 mg q2h IV prn pain," then even the best nurses will not be able to facilitate adequate analgesia because their hands are tied by an inadequate maximum dosage. A reasonable order for the typical patient would read "morphine 2–4 mg IV q10–15 min prn pain." (A maximum dosage should be indicated to prompt physician evaluation before administration of unlimited dosages of opioid.) With such a plan, underdosing is still possible. Small dosages given hourly with additional generous dosages ordered on an as needed basis may be the best compromise.

Orders to call the physician in case of inadequate pain relief or persistent tachycardia or hypertension should be routine regardless of what the analgesic plan consists of. Frequent in-service education of nursing personnel regarding pain assessment and therapy, as well as a mandatory pain score recorded on the vital sign flow sheets, is useful in maintaining a high standard of pain awareness.

Choice of the specific opioid for intravenous therapy is for most patients and physicians a matter

Table 13-4. Relative Potencies of Systemic Opioids*

Drug	Parenteral Dose	Oral Dose	Parenteral Potency (Relative to Parenteral Morphine)
Morphine	10 mg	30–60 mg	1
Meperidine	75 mg	Not suggested	0.15
Methadone	10 mg	20 mg	1
Hydromorphone	1.5 mg	6–8 mg	6
Codeine	130 mg	200 mg	0.08
Fentanyl	100 μg	Not available	100
Sufentanil	10 μg	Not available	1000
Alfentanil	500 μg	Not available	20
Butorphanol	2 mg	5	—

*All of the doses are approximately equipotent. The values apply to the acute effect of a single dose of opioid. These relative potencies are not by themselves useful in predicting opioid requirements over time. To predict the daily requirement of an opioid other than the one being used, one must take into account the duration of action of the drug and its metabolites in the individual patient, as well as the relative potency. Codeine demonstrates an analgesic ceiling and is therefore not really equipotent with the other opioids.

of price, familiarity, and local custom. Some patients have a true allergy to a specific agent. Many more patients report allergies to specific opioids, when in fact they suffered a nonallergic pharmacologic side effect (e.g., nausea, itching) that can occur with any and all drugs of this class. Most of the commonly used opioids are capable of inducing nonallergic histamine release.

For most patients, successful analgesia is achieved with any agent of the opioid class as long as the relative potencies are considered and the proper dosage is ordered (Table 13-4). No opioid is completely clean, i.e., free of unwanted side effects. We consider morphine to be the first-line agent. It is widely available, relatively inexpensive, and its duration of action is long enough so that continuous infusion is not mandatory. Disadvantages of morphine include occasional hemodynamic side effects, occasional allergic or histamine release phenomena, and the accumulation of a sedating (but not toxic) metabolite in renal failure. Hydromorphone is more potent than morphine by a factor of six, which, in the final analysis, is not an advantage. It is shorter-acting than morphine and may be appropriate for breakthrough analgesia, or if one desires close control of the level of sedation.

The popular opioid meperidine was the first synthetic opioid used clinically. It was invented by scientists in Nazi Germany during the period between the two World Wars, possibly in anticipation of their being cut off from sources of naturally occurring opiates. However, meperidine presents several problems and the authors use it only if there is a good reason (e.g., patient preference, allergy or nausea with other opioids) and no contraindication. Meperidine is not our first-line parenteral opioid because its nonanalgesic metabolite, normeperidine, is neuroexcitatory. Normeperidine is renally excreted and accumulates in renal failure. Aortic surgery patients routinely require opioid analgesia for many days, their renal function may be diminished, and accumulation can cause seizures and other neuroexcitatory phenomena. Even a patient with normal kidneys can suffer a toxic central nervous system reaction from metabolite accumulation if high dosages of meperidine are necessary (e.g., >15 mg/kg/day). This dose is not excessive from the analgesic point of view and is often inadequate. Therefore, meperidine is unique among the opioids in that it has a practical maximum dosage above which serious side effects can be seen even in the patient on mechanical ventilation, in spite of inadequate analgesia. Finally, there are a number of hemodynamic problems with meperidine. It is potentially a negative inotrope. Additionally, meperidine occasionally causes tachycardia, which is diagnostically confusing and not good for most patients.

When used, meperidine can be considered about one-eighth as potent as morphine, which is not in itself a disadvantage. It can be administered by all routes. However, some believe that its weak local anesthetic activity renders it more easily tolerated as an IM injection.

Methadone is a long-acting opioid that is particularly well suited to the provision of basal analgesia. In terms of initial dose, it is about as potent as morphine. However, the total daily equianalgesic dose of methadone often needs to be reduced over time, because the longer half-life of methadone leads to drug accumulation.

Codeine is a relatively weak opioid with an analgesic ceiling. It appears to cause a higher incidence of gastrointestinal upset than other agents. The authors can think of no good reason to select codeine for the aortic surgery patient in the early postoperative period. Oxycodone, which is often administered to patients in combination with acetaminophen after they are able to tolerate pills, is superior to codeine in its efficacy and has no analgesic ceiling. When administered in a combination tablet with acetaminophen, the acetaminophen component is the limiting factor that determines the maximal safe dose. It is currently available in a slow-release formulation. Neither of these opioids play a role in intravenous therapy.

Fentanyl is effective and potent and has a rapid onset of action relative to the previously discussed drugs. It is also remarkably clean of hemodynamic side effects such as tachycardia, hypotension, and hypertension that occasionally occur with the older agents. Its major downside is its relatively brief duration of action. Although the terminal elimination half-life of fentanyl is not all that different from that of morphine, its high lipid solubility leads to rapid redistribution out of the central compartment. Fentanyl is an excellent agent to achieve rapid control in a painful crisis, but its pharmacokinetics make it less practical as the primary intravenous opioid unless it is administered as a continuous infusion with additional boluses for pain. Everything discussed for fentanyl is even more true for its analogues sufentanil, alfentanil, and the ultra–short-acting agent remifentanil. These expensive and potent opioids are excellent to provide analgesia for procedures but at this point cannot be considered cost effective for routine analgesic care of the postoperative patient. As was discussed for IM injection, the use of opioid agonist-antagonists is not recommended for aortic surgery patients.

The common side effects of systemic opioid analgesics are easily treated. In addition to the standard pharmacologic measures used, almost all opioid side effects respond to antagonism at the opioid receptor by naloxone. For reasons discussed in the section on safety considerations of intraspinal analgesia and in Chapter 11, it is recommended that this be used selectively and with caution in the aortic surgery patient. Additionally, if opioid administration is to continue systemically, it is difficult to antagonize a side effect by naloxone without antagonizing the analgesia. Nonspecific antipruritics and antiemetics are therefore preferred.

When side effects occur, one must decide not only how to treat them but whether to continue the specific opioid or whether to change to another drug or route of administration. Urinary retention is not likely to improve with a change to a second opioid even if it is delivered by another route, so urinary retention is treated by continued bladder catheterization. Nausea is treated by antiemetics, and if it does not respond to these, it may improve with a change of opioid. Nausea may occasionally improve with a change from systemic to intraspinal administration. A surgical or ischemic complication is always in the differential diagnosis of severe nausea and vomiting in the postoperative patient (see Chapter 12). Pruritis is evaluated, and if it appears to be anaphylactic, a change of opioid is indicated in addition to specific treatment. However, pruritis of the face and upper body, not associated with a rash or with bronchospasm, is a common side effect of opioids. Such pruritis is nonallergic and responds to naloxone. Such itching will sometimes occur no matter which opioid is used, and it is treated by antipruritics such as diphenhydramine. A transfusion reaction, as well as a reaction to another drug, must be considered in the differential diagnosis of pruritis. Excessive sedation will usually improve if the route of administration can be changed to intraspinal. There is also an idiosyncratic variation between the various opioids in some patients regarding the degree of sedation they cause, so a trial of an alternative systemic opioid may be worthwhile.

Respiratory depression with systemic opioids indicates a relative overdose. Catastrophic respiratory depression must be addressed, as discussed in the following section on safety considerations of intraspinal analgesia. Respiratory depression that is apparently mild can be assessed with an arterial blood gas, and it can be treated by oxygen adminis-

Table 13-5. Differential Diagnosis of Inadequate
Analgesia with Intravenous Patient-Controlled
Analgesia

Delivery and access
    Disconnection or obstruction of intravenous access
    Infiltrated intravenous line
    Error in pump programming
    Pump malfunction (rare)
    Demand button not connected to pump
    Carrier intravenous delivery rate too slow
Patient selection and cooperation
    Patient not pushing demand button
        Lack of understanding
        Confusion or dementia
        Family attempting to modulate patient's use
        Frustration (inadequate loading dose, PCA dose too
          small, poor results with initial demands)
        Physical problem (arthritis, loss of button, mistaking
          nurse call button for PCA button)
        Unacceptable side effects (pruritis, nausea)
        Psychological profile that renders patient a poor can-
          didate for PCA (external locus of control)
    Patient pushing demand button but still in pain
        Dose too low; opioid-naive patient
        Dose too low; patient tolerant to opioid analgesics
        Chemical dependency; withdrawing from alcohol,
          sedative hypnotics, etc.
        Psychological factors: chronic pain history, depres-
          sion, personality disorder

PCA = patient-controlled analgesia.

tration, encouragement to breathe, and close observation while the effect of the opioid clears.

Patient-Controlled Analgesia

PCA is most readily adapted for intravenous use. Over the last decade its role in epidural therapy has become well established, and it is practical for intrathecal, intrapleural, and even subcutaneous administration. However, the potential for almost immediate gratification of the patient's need for analgesia is realized with opioid IVPCA more so than with other routes and uses. The positive reenforcement the patient experiences with IVPCA is an important factor in its success.

The PCA pump is a modified computer chip–controlled infusion pump with a button for the patient to press. This button is the only patient interface. A lockable compartment contains the medication. A lockable provider interface allows the care team to program the pump, i.e., to decide how much the patient gets on demand (by pressing the button), how frequently the button will be effective, and what other safety limits should be imposed.

PCA encourages adequate analgesia by removing health providers from the loop of administration of analgesic substances. Consider two patients in pain, one with intravenous PCA morphine and one with an order for morphine 5–7 mg every 4 hours as needed for pain. Both patients start the process of getting relief by pressing a button. The first patient gets a bolus of morphine that boosts the serum level within 1 minute and perhaps provides analgesia within 8 minutes. By this time, a second dosage can be demanded if needed. For the second patient, the ward clerk answers the nurse call button, the nurse is located and responds, the nurse checks the chart, looks for the keys to the narcotic locker, signs out the drug, and administers the injection. Any one of these steps is subject to interruption and delay. The dose achieves significant serum levels of morphine only 30 minutes after injection. The utter failure of this time-consuming approach is obvious as is the advantage of PCA. Had the second patient been administered the morphine intravenously, the results would occur earlier, but the patient would still be limited to an arbitrary dosage for a 4-hour period.

There are many situations in which it is not desirable to remove the health care provider from the decision process. Examples include certain critically ill patients and patients who for one reason or another will not be successful with PCA (Table 13-5). The vast majority of patients, including most ICU patients, can do well with PCA. Even in the ICU, where delayed nurse response is, it is hoped, not an issue, the use of the PCA pump is advantageous. Advantages of the IVPCA in the ICU are presented here.

- Need to complain of pain to the nurse obviated in the cooperative patient
- Immediate source of opioid frees up the nurse for other duties
- Technique has good continuity for use after transfer from the ICU
- Automatic electronic record of opioid use
- Potential for some pumps to provide continuous infusion

- Potential for successful use with nursing assistance even in some sedated and ventilated patients

In the ICU the nurse may press the demand button initially, so it is technically not patient controlled. During the early postoperative period, when the patient is mechanically ventilated and not yet alert, the nurse can and should assist the patient by pressing the demand button as needed. Particularly at this time, a continuous infusion is safe and helpful no matter what opioid is selected. Such infusion prevents the nurse from having to push the button constantly.

The inherent safety of PCA is related to the self-titration of dosages so small that one to two doses should not take the patient from the awake state to respiratory arrest. Rather, after a relative overdose that is not yet lethal, the patient will go to sleep and stop using the device while the drug can be metabolized and the providers can address the problem. This safety feature can be readily overridden if doses are too large, the interval between doses is too small, or the drug and the route are a bad match. An example of the latter problem would be the epidural PCA use of a long-acting opioid in relatively large dosages with a short lockout interval. Since no timely relief would occur after one or even two doses, the patient may titrate himself or herself into a delayed respiratory arrest.

Proper prescription of PCA requires standardized terminology. The concepts are the same regardless of the route of administration. The drug concentration is an important variable; depending on the pump, concentration error can lead to disastrous consequences. There is a large range of acceptable drug concentrations; local custom and consistency are the most important factors. *Demand* is the act of pressing the PCA button. The first decision made regarding PCA is what medication(s) and in what concentrations should be loaded. The *loading dose* is any one-time dose of medication programmed and controlled by the provider for immediate delivery. It is used when the bolus needed by the patient is beyond what can be safely programmed into the machine for patient use. Intraoperative opioids count as part of the loading dose to the extent that they are still present. The loading dose may be administered in increments by the

physician or nurse, titrating to effect. Repeat loading doses are often required in conjunction with increases in PCA dose when analgesia is inadequate. The loading dose must be large enough to establish a blood level of drug that exceeds the therapeutic threshold. Subsequent PCA doses then maintain this level.

The *bolus dose* or *dose volume* is the amount the patient self-delivers when he or she pushes the button. This dose must be large enough so that at least minimal improvement is perceived by the patient after each demand. It must be small enough so that any one demand will not take the patient from alert to unresponsive, or from a normal minute ventilation to severe respiratory depression. The *continuous infusion rate* is the rate at which drug is delivered continuously, independent of patient demand. This feature, not available on some older PCA pumps, is optional for most drugs; it is neither necessary nor desirable in most alert cooperative patients using intermediate duration drugs. Continuous infusion is often necessary when drugs with short effective half-lives, such as fentanyl and its relatives, are used. The continuous infusion rate modality is helpful for patients on mechanical ventilation, patients with opioid tolerance, and patients with high and predictable drug requirements. The *lockout interval* is the time period after a successful patient request during which subsequent presses of the button will have no effect. On most machines, a 1-hour maximum or 4-hour maximum lockout interval is available. This feature, when used, renders further self-dosing impossible if a preset maximum is reached. This interval must be long enough to allow a PCA dose to be delivered to its active site and affect some change. The purpose of the lockout interval is to prevent adverse cumulative effect of the drug. This interval is shortest for intravenous PCA using a rapidly running intravenous carrier line in a patient with normal circulation times. It is generally longest for epidural PCA.

Restricted-dose PCA is a PCA program in which limits other than the dose volume and lockout interval are imposed. An example of such a limit is the 4-hour limit. Four-hour limit is an optional feature on some PCA pumps. When activated, and when the programmed 4-hour limit is reached, further demands will be unsuccessful for the duration of the 4-hour period, and the pump may alarm. The 4-hour limit is useless unless it is substantially less than the total amount to which the PCA dose and lockout interval restrict the patient. Most pumps provide a history of how much drug was used and at what intervals the patient used the PCA. Some "smart" pumps can analyze the patient's use pattern and adjust many of the settings described previously if the provider so programs it.

Each PCA model is unique, especially in terms of whether it is programmed in volume or concentration. Every machine is potentially dangerous in the hands of a practitioner not familiar with its operation. Although the ICU patient should be safer because of the monitoring provided, model-specific in-service education is essential for all staff.

Although PCA provides more flexibility than provider-administered opioids, the program chosen is still a guess. The initial program may deliver too much drug, in which case sedation is commonly seen, or too little drug, in which case the pain is inadequately controlled. If the patient had not been adequately loaded with opioid initially, the same result will occur. One might expect that if the dose were too small, or if a loading dose had not been administered, the patient would compensate by pressing the button more frequently. In fact, what many patients do is press a few times, fail to perceive even partial relief, and give up. When such patients are assessed, they are found to be complaining of pain, having used little of the total opioid available to them.

Frequent evaluation allows for midcourse corrections. The most commonly adjusted parameter is the PCA dosage. It is usually changed by 20–40% and the effect is reassessed after 4–8 hours. If the change made was an increase in PCA dose, consider a small bolus to quickly establish the needed blood level of opioid. Too small a dose volume is only one item in the differential diagnosis of inadequate pain relief with a PCA (see Table 13-5).

The patient-controlled bolus must be large enough so that one or two doses will provide some change perceivable by the patient; otherwise the patient will give up and remain in pain. The bolus must also be small enough so that one to three doses will not take the patient from the awake state to total respiratory arrest. The lockout interval's only purpose is to allow enough time after a dose request so that the drug reaches the circulation and begins to take effect. This prevents "stair casing" several requests before any are effective, which can lead to a sudden overdose. The maintenance infusion, when used,

must be low enough so that overdose with this infusion alone is almost impossible. This component is potentially more dangerous because it is not under patient control. In fact, in post–cesarean section patients on intravenous PCA, Parker et al. and Sinatra et al. have shown increased side effects and no additional benefit to a basal infusion.[42,43]

While the PCA is intended primarily for use in the awake extubated patient, there are many ventilated patients who can benefit from it. As mentioned previously, for a well-educated nursing staff, there is nothing wrong with the nurses pressing the button for ventilated patients who cannot do so for themselves. In so doing, the nurse is titrating intravenous opioid as is traditionally done. However, it must be clearly understood that in the patient without ventilator backup, even if he or she is still intubated, if the button is pressed by someone other than the patient, the most important safety feature of PCA has been bypassed.

Virtually all of the opioids that are appropriate for intravenous bolus administration have been administered successfully by PCA, and the same pharmacologic principles apply. Morphine, meperidine, hydromorphone, and fentanyl are commonly used. Table 13-6 presents suggested dosages and PCA-program settings for these agents. These protocols are to be viewed only as starting points. They apply to the opioid-naive postoperative patient of average size and must be modified for other situations. The patient who is tolerant of opioids may require quite a bit more than these protocols suggest, while the very obese patient may (on a per kilogram basis) require quite a bit less. As adjustments are frequently required, it is obvious that while IVPCA gives the appearence of placing the patient on autopilot for short periods, it does not obviate the need for repeated reassessment of analgesia.

Computerized Infusion of Analgesics

In the early postoperative period when patients are ventilated and sedated and for patients who for other reasons are not good PCA candidates, the administration of systemic opioid by computerized infusion system can provide excellent analgesia. Such a system is particularly well adapted for use with short-acting opioids such as alfentanil. The plasma level of such drugs declines too quickly for bolus

Table 13-6. Typical Patient-Controlled Analgesia Regimens for Intravenous Opioid Analgesic Use in the Postoperative Adult Patient*

Drug	Concentration	Loading Dose	PCA Dose	Lockout Interval	Continuous Rate	Further Dose Restriction
Morphine sulfate	1–5 mg/ml	0.05–0.15 mg/kg	0.8–2.0 mg	6–12 minutes	0.5–2.0 mg/hour; usually unnecessary outside of ICU, useful in early postoperative period, especially while intubated	0.25 mg/kg every 4 hours
Meperidine	10 mg/ml	0.5–1.5 mg/kg	8–20 mg	6–12 minutes	10–20 mg/hour; usually unnecessary	2.5 mg/kg every 4 hours
Hydromorphone	1–2 mg/ml	0.02–0.04 mg/kg	0.2–0.5 mg	6–15 minutes	0.1–0.4 mg/hour; usually unnecessary	0.05 mg/kg every 4 hours
Fentanyl	10–50 µg/ml	2–4 µg/kg	10–25 µg	5–10 minutes	20–50 µg/hour; often necessary to prevent painful breakthrough	3–6 µg/kg every 4 hours

*These regimens apply to patients who are not on controlled ventilation. For patients still on controlled ventilation, doses may be increased almost arbitrarily, and the continuous infusion feature may be used with impunity. Where dose ranges are given, the lowest apply to frail elderly patients with poor organ reserve, and the highest to healthy young and middle-aged adults. Inadequate analgesia may be addressed with incremental 20–30% increases in the PCA dose, after considering the differential diagnosis of failed intravenous PCA analgesia (see Table 13-5).
PCA = patient-controlled analgesia.

administration of any type to be effective in maintaining analgesia. Davies et al. have studied a computerized system in aortofemoral surgery patients with good results.[44] The ultimate development, which is not yet available, will be a computer-driven PCA pump that adjusts the continuous administration rate of opioid as well as the PCA bolus dose to reflect a particular target serum level as well as the patient's response to it. The outcome gains of such expensive hardware to deliver expensive proprietary opioids are likely to be minimal for the average patient when compared with the now traditional PCA delivery of morphine.

Transdermal Opioid Delivery

The transdermal delivery system for fentanyl (fentanyl patch) is presently approved in the United States only for chronic pain. To date, the hesitancy regarding acute pain management with this modality relates to the relentless release of a potent respiratory depressant regardless of monitoring and patient input. In a general surgery population, Sandler et al. in fact found that transdermal fentanyl caused a high incidence of respiratory depression and did not obviate the need for supplemental opioid.[45]

The fentanyl patch is currently available to release 25, 50, 75, or 100 µg/hour of drug. Higher doses are readily delivered by mixing and matching patches. The delivery systems appear to function reliably but not without some degree of interpatient variability.[46–49] The patch is equivalent to a continuous infusion providing a base of analgesia. "Valleys" of pain are avoided, and supplementation can be provided by any intravenous opioid of choice, ideally by PCA. Increases in baseline analgesia are provided by simultaneous application of an extra patch and administration of boluses of longer acting opioids such as morphine or methadone. Episodic variations in pain can likewise be managed by PCA. This is especially convenient if a particular facility has invested in PCA equipment without a continuous infusion feature.

The application of transdermal fentanyl is limited by the fact that while the release is consistent in most patients over the 2–3 days following application of a new unit, the absolute equilibrium serum concentration is subject to individual variation. Therefore, the necessary dosage is not completely predictable. Neither, however, are our other modalities so predictable that their effect does not have to be frequently reassessed. The most important limitation of the fentanyl transdermal delivery system is that therapy can be neither initiated nor terminated abruptly. When a new delivery system is applied, the drug molecules, after being released from a permeable membrane, must transit the skin to reach the blood vessels in the subcutaneous tissues and be taken up systemically. Therefore, a new patch does not deliver its equilibrium blood level for about 12 hours. Even after a patch is removed (and even a 3-day-old patch must, for this purpose, be assumed to have the potential for 1 more day of drug release) a several hour supply of drug is in transit, having been released into the skin but not yet taken up by subcutaneous vessels. Therefore, the patient will maintain significant blood levels of fentanyl for as long as 12 hours. If either of these two circumstances is unacceptable, the patch should not be used.

Regional Analgesia

Postoperative Initiation of Regional Technique

If a regional technique was not used during surgery but is thought to be indicated for postoperative analgesia, an epidural (or intrathecal) catheter can be inserted at any time (depending on why one was not inserted initially). In fact, if the patient has a normal coagulation profile, is afebrile, and is reasonably stable, he or she should not be deprived of a regional technique just when he or she can benefit the most. However, some patients arrive in the postoperative care area without an epidural catheter because initial attempts failed. In such a case, it may be better to proceed with intravenous analgesia. If epidural placement was initially difficult, postoperative conditions may make it impossible. Tubes,

drains, and bandages make positioning harder than it was at the beginning of the procedure.

Not all epidural catheters function properly. The ideal way to be assured of a functioning epidural catheter is to insert the catheter while the patient is awake and demonstrate that analgesia is present below a particular dermatomal level. The history that a catheter was used as a major component of the anesthetic with only light general supplementation is also reassuring. In either case, a small percentage of catheters will have been accidentally displaced. A catheter that is reported to be intrathecal may also not function properly, but the return of clear fluid on aspiration is reassuring.

When a patient is received from the operating room with an epidural catheter, the catheter should be retested (Table 13-7). The goals of a test dose are to exclude three types of malplacement: intravascular, intrathecal, and "nowhere." While the return of blood or CSF on aspiration will diagnose the first two problems (positive aspiration is 100% specific), the lack of blood or fluid return does not reliably exclude intrathecal or intravenous placement (aspiration is not sensitive).

Anatomic and Physiologic Considerations in Regional Analgesia

Lipid Solubility of Opioids. Useful concepts that allow rationale selection of epidurally administered drugs include the location of the catheter in relation to the origin of pain and the relative potency and lipid solubility of the opioids used. Basically, the epidural catheter can be either near the dermatomes that are painful (e.g., a high lumbar or low thoracic epidural catheter for an abdominal operation, or a thoracic epidural catheter for a thoracotomy) or it can be fairly remote from the painful incision (e.g., a lumbar catheter for a thoracotomy). The opioids can be either relatively lipid insoluble (e.g., morphine, hydromorphone) or lipid soluble (e.g., fentanyl group, meperidine).

Morphine, as the prototypical lipid-insoluble agent, penetrates the dura slowly and, once in the CSF, remains there and circulates with it. A relatively small fraction will cross into the systemic circulation. Morphine is our most flexible agent for epidural use and is an excellent drug to use with a catheter that is remote from the nerve roots supplying the incision. If morphine is administered into a

Table 13-7. Procedures for Testing an Epidural Catheter for Malplacement

---

Excluding intravascular placement

1. Aspirate. If blood comes back, the catheter is intravascular. If blood does not come back, there is no conclusion.
2. After establishing adequate monitoring (electrocardiography, arterial line, pulse oximetry), inject lidocaine 1.5% with epinephrine, 15 μg. An increase in heart rate of >10 beats per minute within 60 seconds, an increase in systolic blood pressure of >15–20 mm Hg within 60 seconds, or a subjective feeling of tinnitus, dizziness, or metallic taste, constitutes a positive test result. Remove a definite intravascular catheter immediately. If a borderline test result occurs, the test may be repeated in several minutes.
3. This test is insensitive if beta-adrenergic blockade, deep calcium channel blockade, or conduction system disease is present.

Excluding intrathecal placement

1. Aspirate. If clear or serosanguineous fluid comes back, the catheter is intrathecal. Use the catheter as you would an intrathecal catheter. If there is no aspirate, there is no conclusion.
2. After establishing adequate arterial pressure monitoring and ensuring that the patient is not hypovolemic, inject lidocaine 1.5%, 3 ml, with epinephrine, 15 μg. Development of profound motor or sensory block within 5–10 minutes means the catheter is intrathecal. You may attempt to use the catheter as you would an intrathecal catheter (recommended) or you may remove it.
3. If the patient is noncooperative because of residual anesthetic, sedation, or neuromuscular blockade, intrathecal placement cannot be excluded.
4. Treat hypotension resulting from this test dose with fluid and vasopressors.

Excluding malplacement other than intrathecal or intravascular.

Proceed as for poorly functioning epidural (see Table 13-10).

---

lumbar catheter for a thoracotomy, it will be effective, with a delay of 1–3 hours depending partly on the volume in which the dose was administered. Morphine remains in the CSF as it circulates up to the brain stem and is prone to cause dangerous respiratory depression. Of course, if a thoracic epidural catheter is inserted for a thoracotomy patient, morphine will be effective more quickly at a lower dose. The risk of respiratory depression with a relatively low dose is probably unchanged, although adequate studies are lacking.

Fentanyl, as a very lipid soluble agent, may not always be as effective as morphine for thoracotomy pain when administered into a lumbar epidural catheter. The lipid solubility of the fentanyl class of opioids explains their rapid diffusion into the CSF and their rapid onset of effect compared with morphine. (The target site of action of epidural opioids is thought to be identical to that of intrathecal opioids, and epidural opioids are effective only after penetrating into the CSF.) It has traditionally been taught that high lipid solubility also causes fentanyl and related opioids to diffuse out of the CSF near the level at which they were injected. This, it was argued, explains the alleged lower incidence of respiratory depression with epidural fentanyl compared with morphine. By the time the CSF circulates up to

the brain stem, the putative site of respiratory depression, it will contain low concentrations of fentanyl. This rapid outward diffusion was also invoked to explain the sometimes disappointing results seen when fentanyl is infused into a lumbar epidural catheter to treat thoracotomy pain.

There are three problems with the preceding formulation. The first is that the incidence of respiratory depression is in reality very low with epidural morphine and has not been proven to be any lower with epidural fentanyl. In fact, Weightman recently found that in terms of respiratory depression after epidural administration, morphine and fentanyl may be equivalent.[50] The second problem is that for some patients lumbar epidural fentanyl is quite effective for thoracotomy pain. Reasons for this include systemic absorption, effective delivery to the thoracic CSF, cephalad transport within the cord, or some unknown mechanism. The third weakness is that if the explanation proposed previously is true, then when lipophilic drugs are administered epidurally they should not be detected in high levels in CSF obtained from cephalad sites. Furthermore, lipophilic drugs should not elicit hypalgesia to pinprick in cephalad dermatomes. However, D'Angelo et al. found hypalgesia at thoracic and cervical levels in some parturients after lumbar intrathecal sufentanil.[51] While epidural is not intrathecal and aortic surgery is not labor, the possibility exists that the lumbar epidural administration of lipophilic opioids may yield effective analgesia for high abdominal and thoracic pain.[51] Hansdottir et al. studied the kinetics of SA sufentanil in thoracotomy patients.[52] They found a mean residence time of sufentanil in CSF to be about 1 hour. This is shorter than the mean residence time for morphine, but more than long enough to account for significant cephalad spread. In dogs, Stevens and coworkers found that cisternal CSF contained high concentrations of sufentanil 22 minutes after a lumbar epidural injection.[53] Studying fentanyl after lumbar epidural administration in humans, Gourlay et al. found significant concentrations in cervical CSF 30 minutes after injection.[54] Finally, Coda et al. demonstrated finger analgesia in volunteers about 20 minutes after epidural fentanyl, sufentanil, or alfentanil through a lumbar catheter.[55] Although the quality of analgesia in the finger was not the same as in the toe, rapid penetration of the meninges, as well as rapid spread from lumbar to cervical levels, was elegantly demonstrated. Dosages were administered in a small enough volume that epidural spread to cervical levels cannot be invoked in the Coda study.[55]

Therefore, one can conclude the following from the location of an epidural catheter tip in relation to the surgical incision: (1) it is important regarding the use of local anesthetics for analgesia, and (2) it may explain superior analgesic efficacy of morphine compared with the fentanyl opioids in some patients. When the catheter is near the site of surgery and sometimes when it is not, many find fentanyl an effective epidural analgesic. The reader must therefore realize that the relationships between opioid solubility, catheter location, dosage, and specific dermatomal origin of pain are too complex for simple recomendations to be practical.

The closely related question of epidural versus intravenous fentanyl has also been examined by a number of recent investigations. Many of these have shown that epidural fentanyl and intravenous fentanyl at similar dosages are similar in their efficacy.[56–60] While a superficial acceptance of these fine studies would suggest that fentanyl should never be administered epidurally, there is in fact much more work to be done before epidural fentanyl is excluded from use. First, many of these studies have not looked at the addition of local anesthetic to epidural fentanyl. It is possible that local anesthetic agents such as bupivacaine, even in dilute concentrations, are synergistic with fentanyl in the epidural space to yield a quality of analgesia not obtainable with the intravenous route. The few studies done with combination therapy show a trend toward increased efficacy with the fentanyl-bupivacaine combination.[61] Second, most of these studies have compared equal dosages of fentanyl administered by the epidural and intravenous routes with the double-blinded placebo-controlled design. If the dosage response curve for opioids were linear, then one could deduce that at other dosages of fentanyl than those used in these studies, the equivalence of the two routes would hold up. Linear dosage response curves are not characteristic of opioids by either the epidural or intravenous route. Epidural morphine, for example, really shows a threshold response for analgesia, with dosages that produce CSF levels below the threshold providing little analgesia, and dosages above the threshold improving the duration of the analgesia more than the quality of analgesia. As for intravenous morphine, any recovery room nurse who frequently titrates morphine will testify that a patient receiving 2 mg every 3 minutes may still complain of severe pain after 10 mg and yet be awake and comfortable after only an additional 2 mg. Third, small improvements in the quality of analgesia with epidural fentanyl compared with systemic fentanyl can be hard to demonstrate in a study but real to the patient. Pending further study, fentanyl still holds a place in the epidural armamentarium.

Relative Potency of Intraspinal Opioids. The idea of relative potency in the context of intraspinal opioids can refer to the potency of an opioid in the neuraxis compared with the potency of the same opioid when administered systemically (Figure 13-1). The same idea can be expressed by comparing equipotent dosages of different opioids in the epidural or intrathecal space with reference to the systemic potencies discusssed earlier (Table 13-8). Either way, the relative potency of intraspinal opioids bears no direct relationship to the relative potency of systemic opioids. If anything, it appears that the most lipophilic opioids, some of which are among the most potent opioids, gain the least in potency when administered intraspinally rather than systemically.

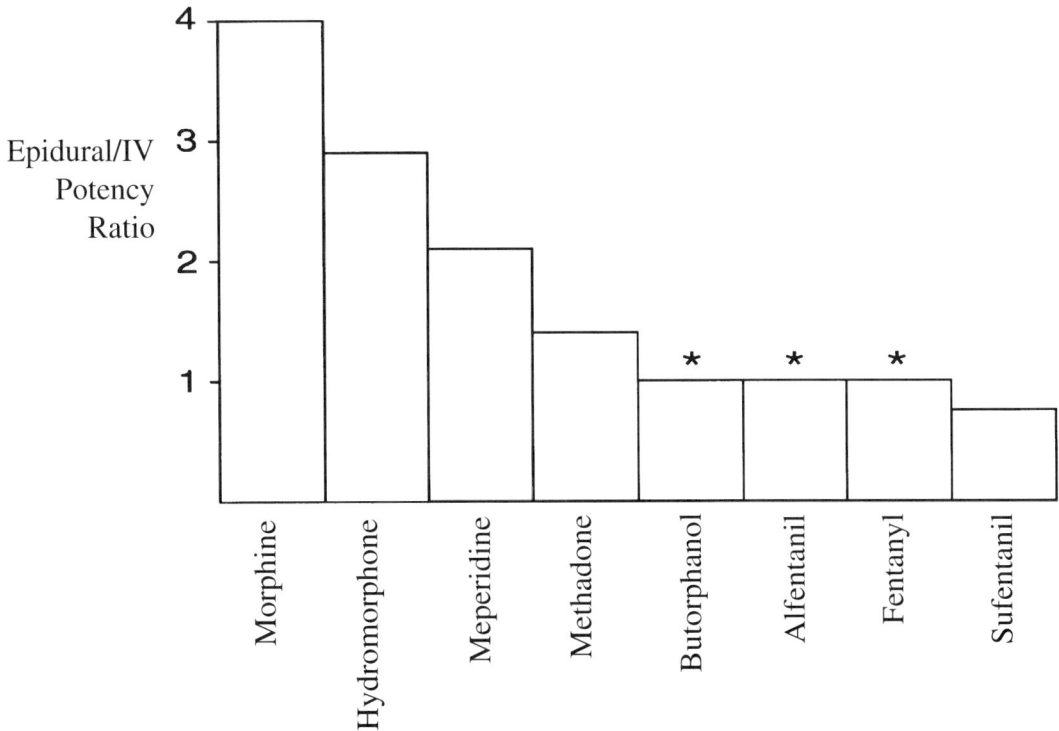

Figure 13-1. Bar graph illustrates the approximate potencies of representative opioid analgesics when administered epidurally compared with equianalgesic doses administered systemically. The most lipophilic opioids gain the least in potency when administered epidurally compared with systemically. The asterisks indicate agents that have apparently identical potency whether administered in the epidural space or systemically. (Modified with permission from JC Eisenach. Annual ASA Refresher Course Lectures 1994, Lecture 521:4, American Society of Anesthesiologists, Inc. A copy of the full text can be obtained from ASA, 520 N. Northwest Highway, Park Ridge, IL 60068-2573.)

The intraspinal administration of morphine is characterized by a tremendous gain in potency. If one were to manage the postoperative pain of a large abdominal incision with intravenous morphine for 18 hours in a middle-aged man, a total dosage of 30–50 mg would not be unusual. Analgesia of better quality is often obtained with 4 mg of morphine administered epidurally, a seven- to ninefold potency gain compared with systemic administration. Therefore, we can say that compared with parenteral administration, epidural morphine allows a lower total dosage with perhaps less sedation. If the SA route is chosen, the same results may be obtained with more rapid onset using a dose in the range of 0.5 mg, a 60- to 100-fold potency gain compared with systemic administration.

In contrast, the intraspinal use of fentanyl allows no such gain in potency. With reference to the same patient with an abdominal incision, a sys-

temic infusion of fentanyl may provide adequate analgesia at a rate of 100 μg/hour. Administered epidurally, 50–100 μg/hour of fentanyl may be required, which is a maximum potency gain of only twofold (see Table 13-8). It is no wonder that the preponderance of studies have been unable to show an advantage for epidural as compared with intravenous fentanyl administration. SA fentanyl is effective at a dosage of about 20 μg/hour, a sixfold gain over systemic administration.

For sufentanil, the most potent systemic opioid in common use, the potency gain of intraspinal administration is even less than that of fentanyl. When considering sufentanil, the interesting paradox that more drug may be required epidurally than would be needed systemically to produce analgesia is encountered. For sufentanil it is only when one considers intrathecal administration that one encounters a dosage that is in the same range as systemic

Table 13-8. Relative Potencies of Opioid Analgesics: Intraspinal Administration*

Drug	Epidural Opioids (Equipotent Doses/ Expected Duration of Action)	Intrathecal Opioids (Equipotent Doses)
Morphine	3–4 mg/12–18 hours	0.4 mg
Hydromorphone	0.25–0.5 mg/10–18 hours	—
Fentanyl	100 μg/2–3 hours	20 μg
Sufentanil	20 μg/2–3 hours	10 μg
Meperidine	40 mg/3–4 hours	Hard to compare because of weak local anesthetic activity that contributes to effect

*Duration of action of intrathecal opioids is similar to that for epidural opioids. Relative potencies of intraspinal opioids apply only to the acute effect of a single dose. To make predictions regarding repeat doses or continuous infusion requirements, one must be familiar with the usual duration of action of the various opioids. The standard dose in this table may be expected to provide adequate postoperative analgesia to an elderly adult after abdominal surgery and is unlikely to cause significant respiratory depression. Individual variation may necessitate increases of 20% or more for an individual patient. Compare potencies with those for systemic use in Table 13-4. See Tables 13-9 and 13-11 for actual protocols for intraspinal analgesia using patient-controlled analgesia equipment.

dosages. In fairness to sufentanil, when studied clinically in aortic surgery patients it has proven equivalent to fentanyl when administered in the appropriate dosage in the epidural space.[62]

Most of the issues reviewed in this chapter that relate to the use of intraspinal analgesia have been pharmacokinetic issues. It may well be that the explanation for the differences between various opioids in potency gain for intraspinal use is related to pharmacodynamics. Apparently, morphine agonism at supraspinal sites may be synergistic with its action at spinal receptors, whereas fentanyl's central agonism may only be additive with its spinal actions.[63] For intrathecal opioids, doses are lower than those used in the epidural space. Depending on the drug, systemic absorption may be minimal. However, intrathecal agents gain fairly rapid access to supraspinal sites via CSF circulation. All epidural opioids are absorbed systemically and presumably gain access to supraspinal receptors via the circulation, although rates of absorption differ for the various drugs. The experiment of Roerig and colleagues does not duplicate the clinical situation for either epidural or intrathecal use.[63] Further work in this area is needed.

Volume of Epidural Agents. All epidural medications should be delivered in adequate volumes. When dilute local anesthetics are administered as part of an epidural infusion, volume becomes critical because these agents function only at the roots to which they are applied. Unlike the opioids, local anesthetics generally do not penetrate the dura in sufficient concentrations to circulate in the CSF and provide analgesia to remote dermatomes. Rather, local anesthetics act on nearby nerve roots via the arachnoid granulations.

To determine the proper volume for a local anesthetic bolus, one must note at what vertebral level the epidural catheter has been inserted. Because epidural catheters are generally inserted 4–6 cm into the epidural space, the catheter tip may be located several centimeters caudal or cephalad. (When inserting an epidural, one has only limited control over which direction the catheter goes.) Additionally, the volume needed to fill the epidural space at any level and achieve blockade varies from patient to patient. For the purposes of postoperative pain management, where very dilute solutions are useful, it often pays to use higher volumes. Slade studied postoperative aortic surgery patients receiving epidural infusions of bupivacaine. He showed that identical milligram doses of bupivacaine were more effective when administered in a larger volume, despite the lower concentration that resulted.[64]

To summarize epidural pharmacology, thoracic epidural catheters are optimal for thoracic operations, although the initial placement is technically demanding and carries more risk than a lumbar epidural catheter. Morphine use may or may not carry more risk of severe respiratory depression than lipid-soluble opioids. The risk of severe respi-

Table 13-9. Suggested Regimens for Continuous Lumbar Epidural Analgesia After Abdominal Aortic Surgery*

Drug	Loading Dose	Infusion Concentration	Continuous Rate	PCA Dose	Lockout Interval
Morphine sulfate	3–5 mg in concentration of 1 mg/ml	100 µg/ml in saline	1.5–3.0 ml/hour, optional, especially in non-ventilated patient	4–7 ml	30–45 minutes with 4-hour lockout of 30 ml; or boluses of 1.5–3.5 mg administered every 3–4 hours by nurse/physician titrated to effect (Morphine does accumulate; successive doses should be reduced to avoid respiratory depression.)
Fentanyl	75–100 µg	5 µg/ml	3–6 ml/hour	4–7 ml	20–30 minutes with 4-hour lockout of 50 ml
Fentanyl/ bupivacaine	Fentanyl 50–100 µg in bupivacaine 0.08%, 5–12 ml	Fentanyl 5 µg/ml in bupivacaine 0.03–0.07%	5–8 ml/hour	5–8 ml	30–60 minutes with 4-hour lockout of 50–70 ml

*Morphine sulfate is available as a preservative-free preparation and this should be used if available. For fentanyl, the standard preparation is acceptable. Modifications for different procedures and catheter placements are presented here. For lumbar catheter after a thoracic procedure, morphine is the best choice. For thoracic catheter after a thoracic procedure, all of above are appropriate; use same concentrations and reduce volumes (loading, PCA, and infusion) by 30–50%. For high lumbar and low thoracic catheters with a high abdominal procedure, use the same protocol as for thoracic catheter and thoracic procedures.
PCA = patient-controlled analgesia.

ratory depression with morphine use is low, ranging from 0.1–0.5%.[65] Moreover, this section discusses patients in an intensive care area, and no such patient should ever suffer severe sequelae from respiratory depression. Morphine and hydromorphone are at the same time more flexible, less prone to be absorbed systemically, and perhaps more effective in almost all settings. Fentanyl and similar drugs may be safer and are also effective, and when sedation is beneficial, fentanyl may be more useful.

Management of Continuous Epidural Analgesia

There is tremendous flexibility with continuous epidural analgesia as long as the previously mentioned principles are kept in mind (Table 13-9). The lumbar epidural catheter for the abdominal aortic surgery patient is dosed, preferentially in the operating room, with a 3- to 5-mg loading dose of morphine repeated every 12–18 hours. If subsequent dosages are administered in a timely manner, dosages somewhat less than the initial dosage are appropriate. Alternatively, the loading dose can be

followed by an infusion at a rate of 150–300 µg/hour, with or without a PCA dose of 400–700 µg, with a lockout of 30–90 minutes. If the PCA feature is not used, breakthrough pain is treated with epidural or intravenous boluses of opioid. The addition of a dilute local anesthetic such as bupivacaine (0.05–0.08%) is reasonable for boluses and as the vehicle for continuous infusion. Our experience confirms the finding of George and coworkers that bupivacaine provides added analgesic benefit when added to epidural analgesic infusions.[61] We prefer bupivacaine over lidocaine for all acute pain applications because the longer duration of action of bupivacaine is useful, and it may be less subject to tachyphylaxis than lidocaine. Dilute local anesthetics can reduce the dose of opioid necessary and increase its effectiveness. In the absence of hemodynamic instability, the use of dilute local anesthetics is desirable. A liposome-associated formulation of bupivacaine under development may prolong the duration of analgesia after a single bolus compared with the conventional formulation.[66] The addition of epinephrine in concentrations of 2–5 µg/ml may also prolong the duration of action of dilute bupivacaine, but the advantage of this prolongation must be balanced against the possible harm of infusing epinephrine in patients at risk for coronary artery disease.

If one is moved to increase the concentration of the local anesthetics, there are several factors that influence the upper limit concentration that may be used. Sympathectomy should be avoided. In the patient who is capable of movement, motor block should be avoided. This occurs in the myotomes to which bupivacaine is applied when the concentration exceeds 0.1–0.2%. The avoidance of motor block facilitates neurologic examination and may avoid venous congestion. Alert patients are often disturbed by the sensation of numbness, which can occur with bupivacaine at or above concentrations of 0.1%. Finally, one wants to avoid systemic toxicity of local anesthetic. This rarely occurs below a total hourly dose of bupivacaine, 0.3 mg/kg, or lidocaine, 3 mg/kg/hour. In the case of lidocaine, serum levels are easily monitored in most centers.

As an alternative to morphine, fentanyl is used with or without bupivacaine. When fentanyl is used, the addition of local anesthetic is strongly recommended. Either way, basal analgesia with fentanyl requires continuous infusion, at least initially. Options are otherwise similar to those for morphine.

For the thoracic aortic aneurysm patient with a thoracic epidural catheter, starting doses and infusion rates are reduced by 30–50% from the doses listed previously. Otherwise, management options, including the addition of a local anesthetic, are similar. We initially choose fentanyl for our patients with thoracic catheters because its shorter half-life in the CSF may decrease the likelihood of respiratory depression and undesired sedation. However, there is no overwhelming evidence that fentanyl is safer than morphine, and the use of morphine is also reasonable. As mentioned previously, the use of fentanyl alone in an epidural may be no better than an IV infusion of the same dose. Therefore, the addition of local anesthetic is desirable at the same concentrations as suggested for the abdominal aortic patient. Local anesthetic delivered through a thoracic epidural catheter may more readily cause sympathetic blockade, and we have occasionally seen severe hypotension after even small volumes of local anesthetics, particularly when higher concentrations than recommended are used (see Table 13-9).

The patient who has undergone thoracoabdominal aortic surgery is managed best with a thoracic epidural catheter but can also do well with a high lumbar catheter. Doses and particularly volumes in which the doses are delivered are increased 20–30% over those recommended for thoracic catheters. Increasing the infused volume applies the analgesics to more dermatomes, providing adequate coverage for these large incisions. At most centers, no attempt should be made to extubate the thoracoabdominal aneurysm patient before 24 hours postoperatively, and there is no reason to be conservative with the dosage of epidural opioids; the dosage of epidural local anesthetics is limited by sympathectomy.

The situation of a thoracic aortic surgical patient with a lumbar epidural catheter, particularly one inserted in a lower lumbar interspace, is best managed with morphine that is administered by the delivery mode of choice. Traditionally, the addition of local anesthetics has not been considered effective in this scenario, because the tip of the catheter may be remote from the painful dermatomes, and the volumes necessary may therefore be large. In order to obtain effective thoracic analgesia, unnecessary abdominal anesthesia must be accepted. However, there will be the occasional patient whose lumbar catheter was inserted in a higher lumbar interspace and then threaded cephalad quite a distance. Such a catheter may be located close to thoracic dermatomes, and local anesthetic block may be helpful and is worth trying. Furthermore, there is relatively little risk of anesthetic overdose with the use of a dilute local anesthetic such as bupivacaine (0.03%), even in the large volumes (20 ml) needed to secure thoracic analgesia with an epidural catheter. Such dilute mixtures usually do not produce significant sympathectomy with its decreased cardiac preload and low cardiac output. Individual judgment must prevail. The theoretic disadvantage to the use of fentanyl in this situation was discussed previously, and it is not the first choice. In practice, fentanyl often produces acceptable analgesia.

If spinal cord injury is present or suspected, or if the surgeon has reason to believe that the patient is at high risk of such injury, the use of epidural analgesia must be called into question (see Chapter 12). Any volume increase in the epidural space will pressure the dura and increase intrathecal

Table 13-10. Protocol for Troubleshooting Poor Analgesia with an Epidural Catheter*

1. Inspect the entire infusion system for pump malfunction, disconnect, or accidental catheter removal. If a disconnect has resulted in the system being open, there may be an increased risk of infection and the catheter should be removed. Inspect the catheter entrance site for a depth of insertion that is consistent with epidural placement (at least 6 cm at the skin in thin patient, and preferably 8–15 cm). Inspect the infusion mixture for possible medication error.
2. Ensure hemodynamic stability. The next step will often cause hypotension if the patient is hypovolemic, especially for a thoracic catheter. Have phenylephrine or norepinephrine ready (see Chapter 11). Ensure adequate electrocardiographic monitoring.
3. Aspirate the catheter and ensure that no fluid or blood is returned.
4. Inject catheter with lidocaine 1.5% with epinephrine, 5 µg/ml (1:200,000), 3 ml.
5. Observe electrocardiographic tracing for 90 seconds. If heart rate increases by 10 beats/minute, and especially if arterial pressure increases simultaneously, the catheter is probably intravascular and should be removed. If the tachycardia persists it can be treated with esmolol. Go to an alternative analgesic scheme, usually intravenous patient-controlled analgesia. For the test dose to be specific, patient should be left quiet and unstimulated during test.
6. Examine the patient for decreased pain 5–10 minutes after injection. If pain is improved, administer a 4- to 10-ml bolus of whatever continuous infusion is being used and increase doses by 30–50%.
7. If patient does not report decreased pain after 10 minutes, examine for neural blockade in the dermatomal distribution of the probable catheter tip location. Ice testing is excellent for this. If a clear block is not present, administer 3–5 more ml of the same agent, with or without 50–100 µg of fentanyl, and wait 5 more minutes. If no block can be demonstrated, remove catheter and initiate parenteral analgesic regimen. If a good block is present, it is likely that the catheter is in the epidural space but the tip is remote from the painful dermatomes. Higher volumes may be necessary. Define where the block is in relation to the incision.
   In this situation, bolus and infusion volumes should be increased by 30–60%. If fentanyl is being used, consider switching to morphine, which may have a longer residence time in the cerebrospinal fluid. Bupivacaine is probably not appropriate if the block generated by the test dose is remote from the incision.
   Note: a continuous intrathecal catheter is evaluated by the ability to aspirate cerebrospinal fluid. If none can be aspirated and analgesia is inadequate, the catheter should be removed and an alternative plan pursued.
   The use of epinephrine to rule out intravascular injection is not 100% sensitive, and may fail with beta-adrenergic blockade or cardiac conduction disease. Therefore, all epidural local anesthetics are administered slowly.

*Inadequate analgesia is unacceptable in the aortic surgery patient. If an epidural catheter must be removed, it can be replaced. Alternatively, parenteral opioid analgesia via patient-controlled analgesia can be instituted.

pressure, thereby decreasing spinal cord perfusion pressure. Furthermore, if local anesthetic is added, resulting sympathetic blockade may decrease cardiac output (a low-flow state is undesirable in the patient with spinal cord injury). If epidural analgesia is used in a situation in which the risk to the spinal cord is present but not high, the goal should be to infuse as little volume as possible to the epidural space. In such situations, the use of undiluted morphine is best.

The situation of poor pain relief with attempted epidural analgesia has a differential diagnosis that must be evaluated systematically (Table 13-10). It is a shame to remove a catheter that could be effective with a change in dosage, but it is equally unacceptable to expose a patient to risk by increasing the dose of analgesic without excluding dangerous malplacements.

The common side effects of epidural opioids are similar to those of intrathecal opioids and not qualitatively different from those associated with systemic opioids. There are two differences in the treatment of intraspinal opioid side effects and systemic opioid side effects: (1) the patient may experience the side effects of intraspinal opioids for a prolonged period, and (2) it is possible to antagonize certain side effects by low-dose naloxone without antagonizing spinal analgesia. Nevertheless, naloxone is not a first-line treatment for mild side effects of opioids. Its use may be considered for severe pruritis or nausea that is refractory to other measures since both these side effects can occasionally lead to complications. The dosage (1–2 µg/kg/hour) is slightly less than that used for respiratory depression. Naloxone infusion may need to be continued for several hours because of

Table 13-11. Infusion Compositions and Rates for Continuous Intrathecal Analgesia for the Aortic Surgery Patient*

Drug	Loading Dose	Infusion Composition	Continuous Infusion
Morphine sulfate	0.5 mg (up to 1 mg in the patient who is expected to remain on the ventilator for 24 hours). Re-bolus with 0.2–0.5 mg every few hours as needed for pain. (Morphine does accumulate; successive doses should be reduced to avoid respiratory depression.)	Morphine 50 µg/ml = 0.05 mg/ml	20–40 µg/hour = 0.4–0.8 ml/hour
Fentanyl	20–50 µg	10 µg/ml	10–20 µg/hour = 1–2 ml/hour

*The addition of local anesthetic to analgesic infusions for intrathecal use is tricky because there is a fine line between the minimal dose of local anesthetic needed for analgesia and the dose that will cause motor and sympathetic block. Addition of local anesthetics is usually not necessary. If used, bupivacaine, 1.25–2.0 mg as a bolus, may be given.

the long-lived effects of epidural opioids, particularly morphine.

Management of Continuous Intrathecal Analgesia

Continuous intrathecal analgesia catheters are almost always placed lumbar. Effective analgesia is produced via this route with opioids in dosages lower than those required for epidural analgesia (Table 13-11). Morphine and fentanyl are both acceptable choices.

If the intrathecal catheter was placed primarily for CSF drainage, its use as a conduit for analgesics depends on the postoperative assessment of risk to the spinal cord. If risk is thought to be high, or if injury has already been documented, one should avoid the use of intrathecal analgesia. If risk is thought to be low, undiluted opioids can be injected into the subarachnoid catheter, perhaps after an equal or greater volume of CSF has been removed.

Safety Considerations of Intraspinal Analgesia

When considering the dangers of intraspinal (epidural and SA) analgesic therapy, most physicians think first of the risk of respiratory depression, a potentially lethal complication. In fact, the risk of this complication on general surgical wards is low when proper precautions are taken.[65] In the ICU setting in which aortic surgery patients recover for

the first few days, respiratory depression should be recognized promptly and is easily managed if diagnosis is not delayed. The risk of respiratory depression increases in the extreme elderly, the small patient, the patient with central nervous system disease, the patient with respiratory disease, and perhaps with larger dosages of morphine administered into more cephalad catheters. Many of the patients at risk are of course those who also have the most to gain by intraspinal opioids.

It is widely believed that decreased mental status and decreased respiratory rate are reliable early signs of respiratory depression. Bailey et al. found that in volunteers the earliest indicator of respiratory depression after intrathecal morphine is a decrease in the hemoglobin oxygen saturation.[67] In their study, decreased mental status and decreased respiratory rate did not always correlate with respiratory depression.

Respiratory arrest can certainly occur soon after a normal respiratory rate was present. Short apneic intervals often precede the rare respiratory arrest, but these are hard to detect. As a practical matter in the ICU, pulse oximetry, detection of short apneas, close monitoring of respiratory rate, and mental status assessment are all available. On a surgical ward, if one had to pick a technology for detecting respiratory depression after administration of intraspinal opioids, pulse oximetry would be the one to use. Otherwise, sedation scale assessment and monitoring of respiratory rate are still recommended. One should not refrain from administering intraspinal opioids to otherwise stable patients who will be on a surgical ward because pulse oximetry is not available.[65] It is, however, strongly recommended that general wards on which such patients are cared for have adequate numbers of nurses who are supportive of this therapy and who have been equipped with special in-service education and protocols.

We make it a practice of having naloxone ready at the bedside of every patient who has had intraspinal opioids. Respiratory depression from opioids in the aortic surgery patient is often best treated with tracheal intubation and ventilation for several hours. Naloxone may be used if the airway cannot be easily secured or if the risk of securing the airway is judged to exceed the risk of complications with naloxone. Naloxone must be carefully titrated, because its use puts the patient at risk for reversal of necessary analgesia, as well as tachycardia, hypertension, and pulmonary edema with all of their sequelae. These risks can be minimized by restricting the naloxone dosage to 1–2 µg/kg/hour after loading with titrated boluses of 20 µg. This dosage will usually not reverse the analgesia produced by intraspinal opioids.

Local anesthetics are potentially lethal in minutes if administered accidentally in overdose. The definition of overdose is relative and depends on where one believes the needle or catheter is located. Doses of local anesthetics that exceed the accepted safe limits can produce seizures and cardiac arrest even when administered into the intended compartment. When administered by infiltration or for neural blockade, bupivacaine in a single dose of up to 2 mg/kg is considered unlikely to produce systemic toxicity, as is lidocaine at 4–5 mg/kg, or lidocaine with epinephrine 1/200,000 at 6–7 mg/kg. When administered by infusion or repeated infiltration, the bupivacaine dosage should never exceed 0.3–0.4 mg/kg/hour, and the lidocaine dosage should not exceed 3 mg/kg/hour without serum level monitoring. Likewise, doses that are acceptable in the epidural space can be toxic if accidentally administered as an intravenous bolus. An epidural dose that is accidentally given intrathecally can cause instant respiratory arrest and profound hypotension that progresses to cardiac arrest. In the patient who is less than totally alert, these events can occur with no warning.

Initially, local anesthetics should be mixed and ordered only by individuals who possess an anesthesiologist's or hospital pharmacist's knowledge of their usual dosages, toxicities, and side effects. Once a facility has experience with simple, consistent protocols for analgesia, which include local anesthetics, the risk of a medication error is reduced. All boluses containing local anesthetics should be administered slowly (5–10 ml/minute), with frequent questioning of the patient regarding any neurologic symptoms and careful observation of the vital signs. A prudent clinician considers every epidural catheter to have the potential for intravascular or intrathecal migration at any time.

Even assuming that the local anesthetic mixture is correct and the dosage is well below that which produces toxic serum levels, there is still a potential hemodynamic problem. Dilute local anesthetic mixtures can sometimes produce vasodilatation leading to decreased preload, decreased cardiac output, and hypotension. This hemodynamic effect may be welcome or dangerous depending on the patient's status, but the potential for problems must be considered. Although more rare than hypotension, bradycardia can also occur secondary to cephalad spread and blockade of the cardiac accelerator fibers. All of these physiologic circulatory effects of local anesthetics are more likely with a thoracic epidural catheter or with large doses into a lumbar catheter. When an epidural catheter is tested and the test dose is positive for accidental SA migration, acute hypotension can be expected. Even a test dose is a major undertaking and one must be ready to manage sympathetic blockade and hypotension.

The weak local anesthetic property of meperidine may render it especially effective in the neuraxis. The same property may introduce an increased risk of sympathetic blockade and hypotension compared with morphine when used intraspinally. Meperidine is currently not approved by the United States Food and Drug Administration for intraspinal use. (Morphine is in fact the only opioid currently approved by the Food and Drug Administration for this purpose.) Unlike morphine, meperidine is not supplied in a preservative-free formula. It should be noted, however, that the necessity of administering morphine or any other opioid as a special preparation for spinal use has not been supported by clinical studies. In several countries where the expense of purchasing preservative-free morphine is not practical, the standard parenteral preparation of morphine is injected into the epidural space with impunity.

Intercostal and Intrapleural Block

The most commonly seen aortic surgery patient will have an abdominal midline incision. For such an individual, there is little place for neural blockade at sites more peripheral than the epidural space.[68] However, for an incision that is other than midline, whether thoracotomy or abdominal, intercostal nerve blocks have the potential to greatly reduce the requirement for systemic analgesics. Intercostal blockade may be especially well suited to the patient who for one reason or another (e.g., preoperative anticoagulation, anatomic abnormalities) was not thought to be a candidate for intraspinal blockade. Continuous intercostal blockade can also be instituted after an epidural or spinal catheter has, for whatever reason, been removed.

The one-time blockade of multiple intercostal nerves can be accomplished after induction of anesthesia, or after surgery is complete, in either the operating room or the postoperative care area.[69,70] When administered percutaneously, intercostal blocks are more effective from a posterior approach. This may be inconvenient in terms of positioning in some postoperative patients. For the thoracotomy patient, intercostal blocks can be performed under almost direct vision by the surgeon before closing the chest.

The single-shot intercostal block is easy and relatively safe. It is well known that these blocks result in the highest systemic levels of local anesthetic among all commonly used nerve blocks. However, adverse consequences of these high levels are rare.

The obvious limitation to single-shot intercostal blocks is the duration of action, which does not exceed 8–12 hours. Even if administered at the end of surgery rather than the beginning, they wear off just when one wants them to be most effective. Between 4 and 12 hours postoperatively the patient will wake up from high doses of potent opioids, and at this time many patients will be considered for extubation.

These limitations can be overcome by the technique of continuous catheterization of the pleural space and the administration of intrapleural (also called interpleural) local anesthetics (IPLA), which was first described by Kvalheim and colleagues and Reiestad and colleagues.[71,72] The efficacy of IPLA is supported in the literature by studies such as that of McIlvaine.[73] At this point there are relatively few data regarding use of IPLA in aortic surgery patients. The patient who has had abdominal aortic reconstruction by a midline incision is not a candidate for IPLA. (Bilateral IPLA is not accepted as a clinical practicality because of the obvious fear of bilateral pneumothorax and local anesthetic toxicity.) Kambam et al. found IPLA to be useful in aortic surgery patients undergoing lateral thoracotomy for aortic disease.[68] In fact, the most common study patient for the postoperative use of IPLA has been the patient for open cholecystectomy, a procedure now less frequently performed in many Western surgical practices. IPLA has done well in this group of patients.[74,75] There is, however, some work done in thoracotomy patients that is not complimentary of IPLA.[73,76,77] IPLA is often ineffective in thoracotomy patients because the chest drain, if not clamped for a period after the block, prevents adequate contact time for the local anesthetic. There is little reason to doubt the applicability of IPLA to the aortic surgery patient with the appropriate incision. Like other specialized techniques, the patient with coexisting pulmonary disease may enjoy special benefit from IPLA.[78]

The mechanism of action of IPLA is probably related to global unilateral intercostal nerve blockade.[79] While the intercostal nerves, which lie just deep to the parietal pleura, may be the primary target of the local anesthetic effect, the posterior reflection of the pleura comes close to some other interesting structures. The paravertebral sympathetic chain may be involved in sustaining the pain response via small afferents. A large portion of the sympathetic chain, including the cervical end, may be affected by IPLA.[80,81] In any case, the effect of IPLA on the intercostals is more diffuse and may reach more posteriorly than classical intercostal blocks.

The catheter can be placed at the time of surgery or at any time postoperatively. The intrapleural space is commonly identified by a loss of resistance to injection of fluid. The technique is familiar to anesthesiologists as a variation of the technique for epidural blockade, and there are many permutations. An electronic sensor for locating the pleural space has been described.[82] The disposable kits and catheters made for epidural anesthesia are useful and completely acceptable for intrapleural catheterization. Like epidural catheterization, the technique for IPLA is not perfect and may result in occasional failure and, rarely, in lung puncture. The presence of blood and effusion in the pleural space will render IPLA less effective, probably because of dilution of local anesthetics by effusion fluid or because of an acidotic environment created by the effusion pathology.[68] The occasional pneumothorax resulting from IPLA may be due either to accidental lung puncture or to direct introduction of air at the time of insertion.

IPLA is administered as a bolus every 6–8 hours. The usual volumes are 20–30 ml, and the usual local anesthetic is bupivacaine 0.25–0.50%. The use of 0.5% bupivacaine results in a longer duration of action and in serum levels closer to the toxic threshold.[79,83] The addition of epinephrine in the familiar concentration of 3–10 µg/ml is routine and will substantially lower the serum bupivacaine levels.[68] However, epinephrine may be reduced or omitted if absorption of epinephrine could harm the patient (e.g., in the presence of coronary artery disease or hypertension). The cumulative dosage of bupivacaine for this procedure as well as most continuous local techniques should not exceed 0.3–0.4 mg/kg/hour after an initial bolus, which is not to exceed 2 mg per kg. Lidocaine appears to be less satisfactory than bupivacaine for IPLA use.[84]

If a chest tube is present, IPLA can be administered through it. The complexity of the modern chest tube drainage system may make it more practical to pass a separate catheter for IPLA. A device combining the two catheters has been described.[85] Either way, passing the IPLA catheter can be done with almost total safety at the time of surgery. The disadvantage is that the chest tube must be off suction for some time after each IPLA dose (usually about 20–30 minutes). If the patient cannot tolerate 30 minutes without the chest tube on suction, or if the tube is draining constantly, the patient is not an IPLA candidate.[86]

Pain Management and Organ Failure

Once one has an understanding of the physiology of analgesia and a knowledge of dosages and sched-

ules, most stable patients can be treated with satisfactory results. The remaining question is how analgesic therapy must be modified in the face of major organ failure syndromes that are encountered in aortic surgery patients. Specifically, what can the patient in shock tolerate, and is analgesia really needed? Are our modern opioids affected to any great degree by renal and hepatic failure? In the patient with limited pulmonary reserve, how does one walk the fine line between analgesia that facilitates care and oversedation and respiratory depression?

The patient with organ system failure is not less in need of analgesia than the robust individual. If anything, the stress response associated with pain may be harmful to the very sick patient. As already discussed, the stress response is basically a recruitment of organ reserve not needed under basal conditions. It is the very sick patient who almost by definition does not have reserve to recruit. For example, tachycardia may present a diagnostic problem and may also compromise diastolic ventricular filling and coronary perfusion. Pulmonary hypertension may exacerbate right-sided ventricular failure. Catabolism may be worsened.

The problems with analgesia in the sicker patient are twofold. The simpler aspect to deal with is the altered pharmacokinetics in the face of organ failure.[87–90] This phenomenon should present no difficulties if the basics of drug metabolism are understood, and if therapy is titrated to effect (Table 13-12). The more difficult questions are: How do you titrate therapy if the patient is too ill to communicate need? What, if anything, is administered for analgesia in the face of hypotension and shock? Do you administer opioid even if it appears that pharmacologic support of the circulation will have to be increased as a result? The difficulty of answering the last question sometimes leads to denial of patient analgesic care.

It is probably inappropriate to completely withhold opioid analgesics unless absolutely necessary. Since the sickest patients cannot communicate the need for analgesia, the dosage they receive will represent a guess. Fentanyl is an excellent choice, because it is relatively free of hemodynamic side effects. The most common hemodynamic effect seen with fentanyl in stable patients is bradycardia, which is secondary to decreased sympathetic output from the central nervous system. The critically ill patient in shock usually has tachycardia as a re-

Table 13-12. Some Analgesic Considerations in the Patient with Organ Failure*

Opioid choice: systemic administration

    Meperidine: Toxic metabolite accumulates, especially in renal failure. May also cause hypertension/hypotension/ tachycardia. Avoid completely.

    Morphine: Sedative nontoxic metabolite accumulates in renal failure. Be aware of the possibility and adjust subsequent doses. May cause hypertension/tachycardia.

    Fentanyl or hydromorphone: Excellent choices in organ failure.

    Methadone: May be useful because of long duration of action.

Mode of administration

    If patient is very ill, he or she probably cannot use PCA. Administer by continuous infusion or around-the-clock doses, supplemented by breakthrough doses or nurse-controlled PCA pump.

Route of administration

    Intramuscular administration may be contraindicated because of edema, coagulopathy

    Initiation of regional block may be problematic because of coagulopathy

    If continuous regional catheter is present:

        Use of opioids is no different than in healthier patients

        Caution in use of local anesthetics because of possible sympathectomy

Determination of dose: systemic administration

    If patient cannot communicate, use standard intravenous dosages supplemented when signs of pain are present:

        Morphine, 2–6 mg/hour, boluses of 2–4 mg

        Fentanyl, 25–200 µg/hour, boluses of 50–100 µg

        Hydromorphone, 0.3–1.0 mg/hour, boluses of 0.3–0.5 mg

    Dilemma of tachycardia: common in critical patient, may be related to pain, more often related to toxic state:

        Consider bolus of two to three times hourly infusion dose if heart rate does not decrease, tachycardia probably is not due to pain. May give further opioid doses if systemic and pulmonary hypertension persist.

---

*A few simple modifications are necessary for the analgesic care of the aortic surgery patient who is especially ill with renal disease, liver disease, or multiple organ failure syndrome. In these patients, even more than in their healthier peers, inadequate analgesia is unacceptable because they cannot tolerate the resulting stress response.

sult of the body trying to match increased metabolic rate with an increase in cardiac output. This tachycardia is relentless and is usually not affected by opioid analgesics. Arterial blood pressure may decrease after the administration of opioids. This is addressed by infusing the opioid slowly in small boluses and making the necessary adjustments in hemodynamic support.

In the patient who does not have a history of opioid use and tolerance, and who is too sick to communicate the need for pain relief, fentanyl at a dosage of 0.5–2.0 µg/kg/hour will provide basal analgesia. As these patients are usually mechanically ventilated, higher dosages may be used if needed. The hemodynamic effects of fentanyl can be further minimized if the dosage is increased gradually.

Patients with various organ failure syndromes may demonstrate altered pharmacokinetics. Changes in protein binding, volumes of distribution, and hepatic and renal clearances are common. The protein binding influences free fraction of drug, and when diminished may accentuate drug effect (i.e., render

the drug more potent). The other three factors are the major determinants of elimination half-life of the drug. If the resulting prolongation of the drug effect is not appreciated, accumulation may lead to sedation, respiratory depression, and other side effects. On the other hand, some patients will gradually develop tolerance to opioids, especially when infusion is continued for a number of days. Again, fentanyl has a fairly simple pharmacokinetic profile and is an excellent choice for the critically ill.

Progression or Discontinuation of Advanced Analgesic Techniques

The initial analgesic plan must be altered to accommodate the patient's progress. The question of serious central nervous system infection and its increased incidence with longer indwelling catheter times is also an issue. There are many patients who have had SA and epidural catheters in place for weeks and who have had no problems, but such situations cannot be the guide. The "magic duration," below which infection is rare, is not known. In several institutions the author (M.C.) has practiced at or surveyed, a loose maximum of 4–5 days is observed for epidurals. Regarding SA catheters, the study of Bevacqua et al. implies but does not prove that a period of several days is safe.[40]

It is fairly standard to remove either type of catheter with the onset of a significant fever. This is done out of fear that a bacteremia may seed the catheter. Additionally, there is always the remote possibility that an epidural abscess or meningitis is causing the infection. This possibility is further evaluated according to the clinical findings. In the case of an SA catheter, a specimen of spinal fluid may be aspirated for culture and analysis if there is any question. For both SA and epidural catheters the tip may be cultured. However, the study of Bevacqua et al. demonstrates that this test is nonspecific.[40] A false-positive culture result can be caused by contamination from skin flora during catheter removal. If this is prevented by prepping the skin with an antibacterial solution before removal, one risks a loss of sensitivity.

After catheters are removed or in patients who do not have one, oral analgesic therapy can begin as soon as tolerated. Other than in the elderly and frail, this transition is more likely to be successful if there is initially a component of around-the-clock analgesia, with some additional drug available for rescue doses (for breakthrough pain). If oral therapy is not yet practical, a combination of IVPCA or nurse-administered parenteral therapy is used.

There is no rational reason to have an arbitrary number of days after which IVPCA therapy, or other systemic opioid therapy, is discontinued. As the recovery of these patients progresses, it is far more important to have them pain-free and ambulating than in too much pain to move but free from opioids. The risk of drug habituation in the surgical population is exceptionally low, and most patients taper their use of opioids. It is, however, appropriate to treat anxiety and insomnia with benzodiazepines to avoid the use of opioids for these indications.

The transition to less acute methods of pain relief depends on many factors and is highly facility dependent. Various hospitals must deal with local practice regarding how long epidural catheters may remain in place before infection

becomes a serious risk, how long nasogastric tubes are left in before oral intake is permitted, how long patients remain in the ICU, and what kinds of patient-controlled devices are tolerated on the regular hospital wards.

Nonincisional Pain

Not all postoperative pain is incisional. The sore throat from tracheal intubation and the generalized myalgia from the use of succinylcholine and positioning are treated with acetaminophen, ice, gentle heat, and reassurance. The discomfort of abdominal bloating resulting from the return of bowel function can be worsened if addressed with opioids, which is a fact that patients with opioid PCA should be made aware of. The discomfort is best relieved by increased activity. If the patient is already on a diet, the judicious modulation of its composition to exclude foods that contain natural sugars, such as apple juice, is helpful. Such sugars are readily metabolized by gas-producing intestinal bacteria.

The postthoracotomy patient frequently complains of shoulder pain. This distressing problem is often the primary complaint of patients when visited by the acute pain service. Its etiology is multifactorial. A recent suggestion that it is sympathetically mediated deserves consideration.[91,92]

Adjunctive Analgesic Techniques

A number of adjunctive measures for analgesia should be considered because of their possible benefit and safety. Some of these, such as ketorolac, are documented to reduce opioid requirement, whereas measures such as transcutaneous electrical nerve stimulation deserve consideration because of their almost absolute safety.

Wound instillation of long-acting local anesthetics, a maneuver attractive because there are no contraindications except allergy to the agent, has unfortunately not been shown to be effective, even when practiced repeatedly in the postoperative period.[93]

Nonopioid Analgesics

Acetaminophen is a useful adjunct to opioid analgesics. While acetaminophen has little role as an analgesic in the early postoperative period, it can be helpful after the first 2–3 days when analgesic requirements are more modest. Opioids can contribute to drowsiness and delayed return of bowel function. However, the addition of acetaminophen may reduce the required dosage of opioids and facilitate recovery. The dosage is 10 mg/kg administered orally or rectally every 4–6 hours around the clock.

Ketorolac is an analgesic of the nonsteroidal class. A potent analgesic, ketorolac is capable of reducing the opioid requirement in postoperative patients without contributing to respiratory depression. It is available in a parenteral form approved in the United States for IM, as well as IV, use. Ketorolac is thus the first parenteral nonsteroidal agent released.

In the general surgical population, ketorolac has a profound opioid-sparing effect and is capable of increasing the quality of analgesia in the patient who reports inadequate relief despite apparently adequate dosages of opioids. Ketorolac is especially useful in the patient on opioids who reports pain with movement but not at rest. Its use in the aortic surgery patient would seem to be desirable.

We avoid ketorolac early in the postoperative course of the aortic surgery patient for two reasons. As discussed previously, all nonsteroidal drugs have the potential to exacerbate renal failure by interfering with prostaglandin-mediated renal vasodilatation.[94] In healthy patients, vasodilatation is prostaglandin dependent only in the hypovolemic state. However, in the aortic surgery patient, the nephron may perceive hypovolemia in any state of low renal blood flow, whether cardiogenic, mechanical, or hypovolemic.

The mild impairment of platelet function that can occur with ketorolac is not clearly problematic in the aortic surgery patient. In fact, some antiplatelet effect could be beneficial if medium-size arteries were anastomosed. Nevertheless, postoperative bleeding is a feared complication and the surgeon has a right to demand that any drug that may cause bleeding be avoided. Therefore, at the present time the use of ketorolac is not advised during the early postoperative period in the aortic surgery population. Its use may be an option after the first three postoperative days in the relatively healthy aortic surgery patient who had a stable early recovery.

Nonpharmacologic Adjuncts

The use of transcutaneous electrical nerve stimulation does seem to reduce opioid use in some settings. The electrodes are placed under the dressing at the conclusion of surgery. Therefore, surgical cooperation is required. The stimulator units are reusable and available from most physical therapy departments. If the surgeon's reluctance to try a new procedure can be overcome, the modest cost and inservice training required is the only downside to this therapy.[46]

Conclusion

Given the infinite possible permutations of machines, routes of administration, drugs, dilutions, dosages, lockout intervals, safety checks, and so on, errors are almost inevitable in the absence of specific protocols and dedicated personnel. The application of modern postoperative analgesic technology will be most successful if the personnel of an acute pain service are in charge and available 24 hours a day. Nurse specialists, nurse educators, pharmacists, and anesthesia residents can all function successfully as first-line acute pain providers, but backup by an attending physician expert in acute pain management must be available. The lines of communication between the acute pain service and the ICU personnel must be kept open.

References

1. Pansard JL, Mankikian B, Bertrand M, et al. Effects of thoracic extradural block on diaphragmatic electrical activity and contractility after upper abdominal surgery. Anesthesiology 1993;78:63.
2. Honig MP, Mason RA, Giron F. Wound complications of the retroperitoneal approach to the aorta and iliac vessels. J Vasc Surg 1992;15:28.
3. Yeager MP, Glass DD, Neff RK, Brinck-Johnson T. Epidural anesthesia and analgesia in high-risk surgical patients. Anesthesiology 1987;66:729.
4. Marks RM, Sachar EJ. Undertreatment of medical inpatients with narcotic analgesics. Ann Intern Med 1973;78:173.
5. Donovan M, Dillon P, McGuire L. Incidence and characteristics of pain in a sample of medical-surgical inpatients. Pain 1987;30:69.

6. Woolf CJ, Wall PD. Morphine sensitive and morphine insensitive actions of C-fiber input on the rat spinal cord. Neurosci Lett 1986;64:221.

7. Armitage EN. Postoperative pain-prevention or relief. Br J Anaesth 1989;63:136.

8. Wall PD. The prevention of postoperative pain [editorial]. Pain 1988;33:289.

9. Katz J, Kavanagh BP, Sandler A, et al. Preemptive analgesia. Clinical evidence of neuroplasticity contributing to postoperative pain. Anesthesiology 1992;77:439.

10. Tverskoy M, Cozacov C, Ayache M, et al. Postoperative pain after inguinal herniorrhaphy with different types of anesthesia. Anesth Analg 1990;70:29.

11. Negre I, Gueneron JP, Jamali SJ, et al. Preoperative analgesia with epidural morphine. Anesth Analg 1994;79:298.

12. Wilson RJ, Leith S, Jackson IJ, Hunter D. Pre-emptive analgesia from intravenous administration of opioids. No effect with alfentanil. Anaesthesia 1994;49:591.

13. Quintin L, Bonnet F, Macquin I, et al. Aortic surgery: effect of clonidine on intraoperative cathecholaminergic and circulatory stability. Acta Anaesthesiol Scand 1990;34:132.

14. Davison JK, Cambria RP, Vierra DJ, et al. Epidural cooling for regional spinal cord hypothermia during thoracoabdominal aneurysm repair. J Vasc Surg 1994;20:304.

15. Baron J, Bertrand M, Barre E, et al. Combined epidural and general anesthesia versus general anesthesia for abdominal aortic surgery. Anesthesiology 1991;75:611.

16. Hjortso NC, Neumann P, Frosig F, et al. A controlled study on the effect of epidural analgesia with local anaesthetics and morphine on morbidity after abdominal surgery. Acta Anaesthesiol Scand 1985;29:790.

17. Davies MJ, Silbert BS, Mooney PJ, et al. Combined epidural and general anaesthesia versus general anaesthesia for abdominal aortic surgery: a prospective randomized trial. Anaesth Intensive Care 1993;21:790.

18. de Leon-Casasola OA, Parker BM, Lema MJ, et al. Epidural analgesia versus intravenous patient-controlled analgesia. Reg Anesth 1994;19:307.

19. Dershwitz M, Sherman EP. Acute myocardial infarction symptoms masked by epidural morphine? J Clin Anesth 1991;3:146.

20. Blomberg S, Curelaru I, Emanuelsson H, et al. Thoracic epidural anaesthesia in patients with unstable angina pectoris. Eur Heart J 1989;10:437.

21. Blomberg S, Emanuelsson H, Ricksten SE. Thoracic epidural anesthesia and central hemodynamics in patients with unstable angina pectoris. Anesth Analg 1989;69:558.

22. Blomberg S, Emanuelsson H, Kvist H, et al. Effects of thoracic epidural anesthesia on coronary arteries and arterioles in patients with coronary artery disease. Anesthesiology 1990;73:840.

23. Kataja J. Thoracolumbar epidural anaesthesia and isoflurane to prevent hypertension and tachycardia in patients undergoing abdominal aortic surgery. Eur J Anaesthesiol 1991;8:427.

24. Breslow MJ, Jordan DA, Christopherson R, et al. Epidural morphine decreases postoperative hypertension by attenuating sympathetic nervous system hyperactivity. JAMA 1989;261:3577.

25. Smeets HJ, Kievit J, Dulfer FT, van Kleef JW. Endocrine-metabolic response to abdominal aortic surgery: a randomized trial of general anesthesia versus general plus epidural anesthesia. World J Surg 1993;17:601.

26. Katz S, Reiten P, Kohl R. The use of epidural anesthesia and analgesia in aortic surgery. Am Surg 1992;58:470.

27. Cuschieri RJ, Morran CG, Howie JC, McArdle CS. Postoperative pain and pulmonary complications: comparison of three analgesic regimens. Br J Surg 1985;72:495.

28. Modig J, Borg T, Karlstrom G, et al. Thromboembolism after total hip replacement: role of epidural and general anesthesia. Anesth Analg 1983;62:174.

29. Christopherson R, Beattie C, Frank SM, et al. Perioperative morbidity in patients randomized to epidural or general anesthesia for lower extremity vascular surgery. The Perioperative Ischemia Randomized Anesthesia Trial Study Group. Anesthesiology 1993;79:422.

30. Naylor AR, Ah See AK, Engeset J. Graft occlusion following aortofemoral bypass for peripheral ischaemia. Br J Surg 1989;76:572.

31. Tuman KJ, McCarthy RJ, March RJ, et al. Effects of epidural anesthesia and analgesia on coagulation and outcome after major vascular surgery. Anesth Analg 1991;73:696.

32. Gibbs NM, Crawford GP, Michalopoulos N. The effect of epidural blockade on postoperative hypercoagulability following abdominal aortic bypass surgery. Anaesth Intensive Care 1992;20:478.

33. Gibbs NM, Crawford GP, Michalopoulos N. Postoperative changes in coagulant and anticoagulant factors following abdominal aortic surgery. J Cardiothorac Vasc Anesth 1992;6:680.

34. Rosenfeld BA, Faraday N, Campbell D, et al. Hemostatic effects of stress hormone infusion. Anesthesiology 1994;81:1116.

35. Mason RA, Newton GB, Cassel W, et al. Combined epidural and general anesthesia in aortic surgery. J Cardiovasc Surg (Torino) 1990;31:442.

36. Rao TKL, El-Etr AA. Anticoagulation following placement of epidural and subarachnoid catheters: an evaluation of neurologic sequelae. Anesthesiology 1981;55:618.

37. Reiz S, Balfors E, Sorenson MB, et al. Coronary hemodynamic effects of general anesthesia and surgery: modification by epidural analgesia in patients with ischemic heart disease. Reg Anesth 1982;7:8.

38. Horlocker TT. When to remove a spinal or epidural catheter in an anticoagulated patient. Reg Anesth 1993;18:264.

39. Kang SB, Goudnough DE, Lee YK, et al. Comparison of 26- and 27-gauge needles for spinal anesthesia for ambulatory surgery patients. Anesthesiology 1991;76:734.

40. Bevacqua BK, Slucky AV, Cleary WF. Is postoperative intrathecal catheter use associated with central nervous system infection? Anesthesiology 1994;80:1234.

41. Hanley JA, Lippman-Hand A. If nothing goes wrong, is everything all right? JAMA 1983;249:1743.

42. Parker RK, Holtmann B, White PF. Effects of nighttime opioid infusion with PCA therapy on patient comfort and analgesic requirements after abdominal hysterectomy. Anesthesiology 1992;76:362.

43. Sinatra R, Chung KS, Silverman DG, et al. An evaluation of morphine and oxymorphone administered via PCA or PCA plus basal infusion in post cesarean-delivery patients. Anesthesiology 1989;71:502.

44. Davies FW, White M, Kenny GN. Postoperative analgesia using a computerized infusion of alfentanil following aortic bifurcation graft surgery. Int J Clin Monit Comput 1992;9:207.

45. Sandler AN, Baxter AD, Katz J, et al. A double-blind, placebo-controlled trial of transdermal fentanyl after abdominal hysterectomy. Anesthesiology 1994;81:1169.

46. Calis KA, Kohler DR, Corso DM. Transdermally administered fentanyl for pain management. Clin Pharm 1992;11:22.

47. Gourlay GK, Kowalski SR, Plummer JL, et al. The efficacy of transdermal fentanyl in the treatment of postoperative pain: a double blind comparison of fentanyl and placebo systems. Pain 1990;40:21.

48. Holley FO, Van-Steennis C. Postoperative analgesia with fentanyl: pharmacokinetics and pharmacodynamics of constant-rate IV infusion and transdermal delivery. Br J Anaesth 1988;60:608.

49. Varvel JR, Shafer SL, Hwang SS, et al. Absorption characteristics of transdermally administered fentanyl. Anesthesiology 1989;70:928.

50. Weightman WM. Respiratory arrest during epidural infusion of bupivacaine and fentanyl. Anaesth Intensive Care 1991;19:283.

51. D'Angelo R, Anderson MT, Phillip J, Eisenach JC. Intrathecal sufentanil compared to epidural bupivacaine for labor analgesia. Anesthesiology 1994;80:1209.

52. Hansdottir V, Hedner T, Weostenborghs R, Nordberg G. The CSF and plasma pharmacokinetics of sufentanil after intrathecal administration. Anesthesiology 1991;74:264.

53. Stevens RA, Petty RH, Hill HF, et al. Redistribution of sufentanil to cerebrospinal fluid and systemic circulation after epidural administration in dogs. Anesth Analg 1993;76:323.

54. Gourlay GK, Murphy TM, Plummer JL, et al. Pharmacokinetics of fentanyl in lumbar and cervical CSF following lumbar epidural and intravenous administration. Pain 1989;38:253.

55. Coda BA, Brown MC, Schaffer R, et al. Pharmacology of epidural fentanyl, alfentanil, and sufentanil in volunteers. Anesthesiology 1994;81:1149.

56. Loper KA, Ready LB, Downey M, et al. Epidural and intravenous fentanyl are clinicaly equivalent after knee surgery. Anesth Analg 1990;70:72.

57. Ellis DJ, Millar WL, Reisner LS. A randomized double-blind comparison of epidural versus intravenous fentanyl infusion for analgesia after cesarean section. Anesthesiology 1990;72:981

58. Salomaki TE, Leppaluoto J, Laitinen JO, et al. Epidural versus intravenous fentanyl for reducing hormonal, metabolic and physiologic responses after thoracotomy. Anesthesiology 1993;79:672.

59. Salomaki TE, Laitinen JO, Nuutinen LS. A randomized double-blind comparison of epidural versus intravenous fentanyl infusion for analgesia after thoracotomy. Anesthesiology 1991;75:790.

60. Sandler AN, Stringer D, Panos L, et al. A randomized double-blind comparison of lumbar epidural and intravenous fentanyl infusions for postthoracotomy pain relief. Anesthesiology 1992;77:626.

61. George KA, Chisakuta AM, Gamble JA, Browne GA. Thoracic epidural infusion for postoperative pain relief following abdominal aortic surgery: bupivacaine, fentanyl, or a mixture of both? Anaesthesia 1992;47:388.

62. Wilhelm AJ, Dieleman HG. Epidural fentanyl and sufentanil for intra- and postoperative analgesia. A randomized, double-blind comparison. Pharm World Sci 1994;16:7.

63. Roerig SC, Hoffman RG, Takemori AE, et al. Isobolographic analysis of analgesic interactions between intrathecally and intracerebroventricularly administered fentanyl, morphine, and d-Ala-d-Leu-enkephalin in morphine tolerant and non-tolerant mice. J Pharmacol Exp Ther 1991;257:1091.

64. Slade JM. Epidural bupivacaine for aortic surgery. The effect of dilution on the quality of analgesia. Anaesthesia 1994;49:21.

65. Ready LB, Loper KA, Nessly M, Wild L. Postoperative epidural morphine is safe on surgical wards. Anesthesiology 1991;75:452.

66. Boogaerts JG, Lafont ND, Declercq AG, et al. Epidural administration of liposome-associated bupivacaine for the management of postsurgical pain: a first study. J Clin Anesth 1994;6:315.

67. Bailey PL, Rondeau S, Schafer PG, et al. Dose response pharmacology of intrathecal morphine in human volunteers. Anesthesiology 1993;79:49.

68. Kambam JR, Hammon J, Parris WC, Lupinetti FM. Intrapleural analgesia for post-thoracotomy pain and blood levels of bupivacaine following intrapleural injection. Can J Anaesth 1989;36:106.

69. Thompson GE, Hecher BR. Peripheral Nerve Blocks for Management of Thoracic Surgical Patients. In GP Gravlee, RL Rauck (eds), Pain Management in Cardiothoracic Surgery. Philadelphia: Lippincott and the Society of Cardiovascular Anesthesiologists, 1993.

70. Thompson GE, Moore DC. Celiac Plexus, Intercostal and Minor Peripheral Blockade. In MJ Cousins, PO

Bridenbaugh (eds), Neural Blockade in Clinical Anesthesia and Pain Management (2nd ed). Philadelphia: Lippincott, 1988.

71. Kvalheim L, Reiestad F. Interpleural catheter in the management of postoperative pain. Anesthesiology 1984;61:231.

72. Reiestad F, Stromskag KE. Interpleural catheter in the management of postoperative pain: a preliminary report. Reg Anesth 1986;11:89.

73. McIlvaine WB, Knox RF, Fennesseyt PV, Goldstein M. Continuous infusion of bupivacaine via interpleural catheter for analgesia after thoracotomy in children. Anesthesiology 1988;69:261.

74. Frank ED, McKay W, Rocco A, Gallo JP. Interpleural bupivacaine for postoperative analgesia following cholecystectomy: a randomized prospective study. Reg Anesth 1990;15:26.

75. VadeBoncouer TR, Reigler FX, Gautt RS, Weinberg GL. A randomized double-blinded comparison of the effects of interpleural bupivacaine and saline on morphine requirements and pulmonary function after cholecystectomy. Anesthesiology 1989;71:339.

76. Seltzer JL, Bell SD, Moritz H, Cantillo J. A double-blind comparison of intrapleural bupivacaine and epidural fentanyl for post-thoracotomy pain. Anesthesiology 1989;71:665.

77. Rosenberg PH, Scheinin BMA, Lepantalo MJA, Lindfors O. Continuous intrapleural infusion of bupivacaine for analgesia after thoracotomy. Anesthesiology 1987;67:811.

78. Bruce DL, Gerken V, Lyon GD. Postcholecystectomy pain relief by intrapleural bupivacaine in patients with cystic fibrosis. Anesth Analg 1987;66:1187.

79. Turner D, Williams S, Heavner J. Pleural permeability to local anesthetics: the influence of concentration, pH and local anesthetic combinations. Reg Anesth 1989;14;128.

80. Sihota MK, Holmblad BR. Horner's syndrome after interpleural anesthesia with bupivacaine for postherpetic neuralgia. Acta Anaesthesiol Scand 1988;32:593.

81. Pellegrino DA, Laurito CE, Albrecht RF. Does interpleural local anesthetic administration produce a sympathetic block? Anesthesiology 1990;73(3A):A755.

82. DeAndres J, Gomar C, Calatrava P. Detection of the interpleural space using a new electronic device, the episensor. Reg Anesth 1990;15:28.

83. Stromskag KE, Reiestad F, Holmquist EVO, Ogenstad S. Intrapleural administration of 0.25%, 0.375%, and 0.5% bupivacaine with epinephrine after cholecystectomy. Anesth Analg 1980;67:430.

84. Raffin L, Fletcher D, Sperandio M, et al. Interpleural infusion of 2% lidocaine with 1:200,000 epinephrine for postthoracotomy analgesia. Anesth Analg 1994;79:328.

85. Kizelshteyn G, Gargiulo J, DelGuercio L. Management of post thoracotomy pain through a double-lumen chest tube. Reg Anesth 1990;15:86.

86. Abraham ZA. Interpleural Analgesia. In RS Sinatra, AH Hord, B Ginsberg, L Preble (eds), Acute Pain, Mechanisms and Management. St. Louis: Mosby–Year Book, 1992.

87. Hudson RJ, Thomson IR, Cannon JE, et al. Pharmacokinetics of fentanyl in patients undergoing abdominal aortic surgery. Anesthesiology 1986;64:334.

88. Hudson RJ, Bergstrom RG, Thomson IR, et al. Pharmacokinetics of sufentanil in patients undergoing abdominal aortic surgery. Anesthesiology 1989;70:426.

89. Hudson RJ, Thomson IR, Burgess PM, Rosenbloom M. Alfentanil pharmacokinetics in patients undergoing abdominal aortic surgery. Can J Anaesth 1991;38:61.

90. Hudson RJ. Midazolam pharmacokinetics in patients undergoing abdominal aortic surgery. Anesth Analg 1994;79:219.

91. Burgess FW, Anderson DM, Colonna D, et al. Ipsilateral shoulder pain following thoracic surgery. Anesthesiology 1993;78:365.

92. Garner L, Coats RR. Ipsilateral stellate ganglion block effective for treating shoulder pain after thoracotomy. Anesth Analg 1994;78:1195.

93. Pfeiffer U, Dodson ME, Van-Mourik G, et al. Wound instillation for postoperative pain relief: a comparison between bupivacaine and saline in patients undergoing aortic surgery. Ann Vasc Surg 1991;5:80.

94. Murray MD, Brater DC. Adverse effects of nonsteroidal anti-inflammatory drugs on renal function. Ann Intern Med 1990;112:559.

Index

Note: Page numbers in *italic* indicate figures; page numbers followed by t indicate tables.

Artery of Adamkiewicz
  anatomy of, 7, 81, 186–187, *187*, 240
  aortic cross clamping and, 187–188, 240
  occlusion of, 186
Ascending aorta
  anatomy of, 1, *2*, 39, 135, *136*
  injuries to, 40
  surgical procedures for, 150–153, *151*, *152*
Ascending aortic aneurysm, 12–14, *15*, 43, *136*
  surgical repair, 150–153
    anesthesia management for, 149–150
    arterial pressure monitoring, 65
ASTST. *See* Automated ST-segment trending
      (ASTST)
Atherosclerosis
  abdominal aortic aneurysm associated with, 63,
      137, 229
  aortic, 8, 9, 16, 19, *19*, 45
  aortic arch aneurysm, 159
Atrial natriuretic peptide (ANP), 326
Autologous blood donation, 128, 130, 237–238,
      318
Automated pressure-area analysis (APAA), 79
Automated ST-segment trending (ASTST), 66–67,
      67, 236, *236*, 235t
Automatic border detection, 79–80
Autoprothrombins, 116t

Balloon angioplasty, for aortic coarctation, 211
Barbiturates
  brain protection by during hypothermia, 165
  use in children, 222
  use in thoracic aortic cross clamping, 191
Basal metabolic rate (BMR), 333
Behçet's disease, 11
Benzodiazepines
  postoperative use of, 272, 273
  somatosensory evoked potentials and, 89t
  use in children, 222
Beta-blockers
  postoperative use of, 283
  thoracic aortic aneurysm, treatment with, 148
  use after aortic coarctation surgery, 214–215
  use in aortic coarctation surgery, 216
  use in thoracic aortic cross clamping, 180
Biliary disease, postoperative, 331–332
Bleeding. *See also* Coagulation
  after cardiopulmonary bypass, 123–130, 124t,
      170–172
  controlling, 115, 123t

during thoracic aortic surgery, 194–195
evaluating, 170
gastrointestinal, 331
heparin rebound, 172
Blood clotting. *See* Coagulation
Blood conservation, in aortic surgery, 128–129
Blood donation, autologous, 128, 130, 237–238,
      318
Blood pressure. *See also* Hypertension; Hypoten-
      sion
  monitoring for aortic surgery, 64–65, 65t, 216,
      218
  postoperative hypertension, 280–285
Blood salvage, 128–129, *130*, *131*
Blood supply
  to brain, 3, 5t, 6, *6*
  to spinal cord, 5t, 6, *6*, 7, 80–82, *81*, 186–188,
      187
Blood transfusion, in aortic surgery, 123–130
  in abdominal aortic aneurysectomy, 237–238
  aortic arch surgery, 171
  autologous blood donation, 128, 130, 237–238,
      318
  coagulation factor replacement, 123–125
  complications of, 128–130, 195
  end-organ integrity, 3316–318, 317t
  fresh whole blood, 171
  hemostasis-altering drugs, 125–127
  hyperthermia, 129
  intraoperative blood salvage, 128–129, *130*,
      131
  reactions to, 129
  in thoracic aortic surgery, 194–195
  viral transmission in, 237–238, 238t
  volume therapy, 127–128
Blood transfusions, postoperative, 315–318
Blood urea nitrogen (BUN), preoperative testing
      of, 32
Blood vessels, coagulation and, 113–114
Blood volume, redistribution of during aortic cross
      clamping, 177, *179*
Blood warmers, 315
Body temperature, monitoring of, 63, 100–101,
      103, 149, 238
Bowel ischemia, 327–330
Brachiocephalic artery, anatomy of, 39, *41*, *42*
Brain
  blood supply to, 3, 5t, 6, *6*
  cerebral ischemia, 100, 164, 193, 193t
  evoked potentials, 85

X